2nd edition

preventive medicine and public health

The National Medical Series for Independent Study

2nd edition

preventive medicine and public health

Brett J. Cassens, M.D., M.B.A., F.A.C.P.
Clinical Assistant Professor of Medicine
University of California–San Diego School of Medicine
San Diego, California

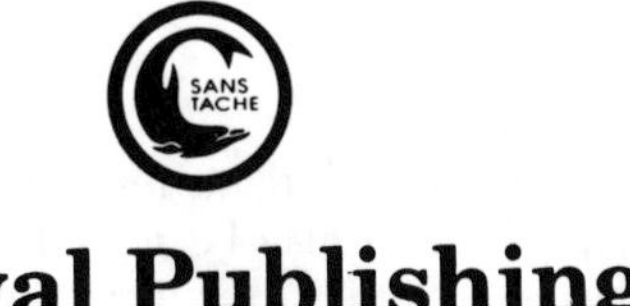

Harwal Publishing

Philadelphia • Baltimore • Hong Kong • London • Munich • Sydney • Tokyo

A Waverly Company

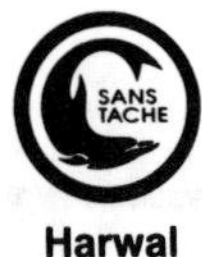

Harwal

Library of Congress Cataloging-in-Publication Data

Preventive medicine and public health / [edited by] Brett J. Cassens.
—2nd ed.
p. cm. — (The National medical series for independent study)
Includes bibliographical references and index.
ISBN 0-683-06262-X
1. Medicine, Preventive—Outlines, syllabi, etc. 2. Public health—Outlines, syllabi, etc. 3. Medicine, Preventive—Examinations, questions, etc. 4. Public health—Examinations, questions, etc. I. Cassens, Brett J. II. Series.
[DNLM: 1. Preventive Medicine—examination questions. 2. Preventive Medicine—outlines. 3. Public Health—examination questions. 4. Public Health—outlines. WA 18 P944]
RA430.5.P75 1992
614'.076—dc20
DNLM/DLC
for Library of Congress 91-24486
CIP

ISBN 0-683-06262-X

10 9 8 7 6 5

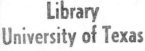

Dedication

To Samuel P. Martin III, M.D., in appreciation of his many acts of kindness and encouragement, and to Donald H. Stille, whose many years of devotion and patience have made this project feasible.

This edition is additionally dedicated to the many public health officers in this country with whom I have had the opportunity to work. In particular, Robert Sharrar, M.D., remains a respected friend and tutor in the area of public health.

Contents

Contributors

Donald J. Balaban, M.D.
Medical Director
Healthcare Management Alternatives, Inc.
Philadelphia, Pennsylvania

Lawrence D. Budnick, M.D., M.P.H.
Clinical Assistant Professor
Department of Environmental and Community Medicine
University of Medicine and Dentistry of New Jersey
Piscataway, New Jersey
Occupational Medicine Advisor
Exxon Biomedical Sciences, Inc.
East Millstone, New Jersey

Anthony J. Buividas, M.B.A.
Chief Operating Officer
Freedom Health Care
Wayne, Pennsylvania

Brett J. Cassens, M.D., M.B.A., F.A.C.P.
Clinical Assistant Professor of Medicine
University of California–San Diego School of Medicine
San Diego, California

Sally Faith Dorfman, M.D., M.S.H.S.A.
Assistant Professor
Cornell University Medical Center
New York, New York
Commissioner of Health, Orange County
Goshen, New York

Christina L. Herring, M.D.
Clinical Associate Professor of Psychiatry and Human Behavior
Jefferson Medical College
Philadelphia, Pennsylvania
Assistant Attending Psychiatrist
Bryn Mawr Hospital
Bryn Mawr, Pennsylvania

Stephen M. Hessl, M.D., M.P.H.
Associate Professor of Medicine
University of Illinois at Chicago College of Medicine
Chairman, Division of Occupational Medicine
Cook County Hospital
Chicago, Illinois

Anne Krantz, M.D., M.P.H.
Attending Physician
Division of Occupational Medicine
Cook County Hospital
Chicago, Illinois

Marie C. McCormick, M.D., Sc.D.
Professor and Chair
Department of Maternal and Child Health
Harvard School of Public Health
Associate Professor of Pediatrics
Joint Program in Neonatology
Harvard Medical School
Boston, Massachusetts

Thomas K. McElhinney, Ph.D.
Professor, Department of Humanities, Social Sciences, and Biometrics
Hahnemann University
Philadelphia, Pennsylvania

Peter Orris, M.D., M.P.H., F.A.C.P., F.A.C.O.E.M.
Associate Professor of Medicine
University of Illinois at Chicago College of Medicine
Attending Physician
Division of Occupational Medicine
Cook County Hospital
Chicago, Illinois

Arnold J. Rosoff, J.D.
Professor of Legal Studies and Health Care Systems
Chair, Department of Legal Studies
The Wharton School
University of Pennsylvania
Senior Fellow
Leonard Davis Institute of Health Economics
University of Pennsylvania
Philadelphia, Pennsylvania

Samuel L. Rotenberg, Ph.D.
Regional Toxicologist
United States Environmental Protection Agency, Region III
Philadelphia, Pennsylvania

Robert G. Sharrar, M.D., M.Sc.
Assistant Health Commissioner for Disease Prevention
Department of Public Health
Philadelphia, Pennsylvania

William C. Steinmann, M.D., M.Sc.
Associate Professor of Medicine
Vice-Chairman, Department of Medicine
Chief of General Medicine
Tulane University School of Medicine
New Orleans, Louisiana

Robert A. Velin, Ph.D.
Assistant Research Psychobiologist
Department of Psychiatry
University of California–San Diego
San Diego, California

Preface

The objective of the second edition of NMS *Preventive Medicine and Public Health* remains that of the first edition: to provide the student with an appreciation of the fundamental importance of epidemiology and preventive medicine. As the United States enters one of the most turbulent and controversial periods for medicine in the country's history, forces of politics and economics likely will prevail. The success or failure of the changes implemented by the politicians and economists, however, will be measured by the epidemiologist and the practitioner of preventive medicine. While it is hoped that any reform of the health care system will provide greater well-being to the many rather than to the select few, only the student of public and community medicine will be properly positioned to evaluate whether such goals are achieved.

To the Reader

Since 1984, the National Medical Series for Independent Study has been helping medical students meet the challenge of education and clinical training. In this climate of burgeoning knowledge and complex clinical issues, a medical career is more demanding than ever. Increasingly, medical training must prepare physicians to seek and synthesize necessary information and to apply that information successfully.

The National Medical Series is designed to provide a logical framework for organizing, learning, reviewing, and applying the conceptual and factual information covered in basic and clinical studies. Each book includes a concise but comprehensive outline of the essential content of a discipline, with up to 500 study questions. The combination of distilled, outlined text and tools for self-evaluation allows easy retrieval and enhanced comprehension of salient information. Each question is accompanied by the correct answer, a paragraph-length explanation, and specific reference to the text where the topic is discussed. Study questions that follow each chapter use current National Board formats to reinforce the chapter content. Study questions appearing at the end of the text in the Comprehensive Exam vary in format depending on the book; the unifying goal of this exam, however, is to challenge the student to synthesize and expand on information presented throughout the book. Wherever possible, Comprehensive Exam questions are presented in the context of a clinical case or scenario intended to simulate real-life application of medical knowledge.

Each book in the National Medical Series is constantly being updated and revised to remain current with the discipline and with subtle changes in educational philosophy. The authors and editors devote considerable time and effort to ensuring that the information required by all medical school curricula is included and presented in the most logical, comprehensible manner. Strict editorial attention to accuracy, organization, and consistency also is maintained. Further shaping of the series occurs in response to biannual discussions held with a panel of medical student advisors drawn from schools throughout the United States. At these meetings, the editorial staff considers the complicated needs of medical students to learn how the National Medical Series can better serve them. In this regard, the staff at Harwal Publishing welcomes all comments and suggestions. Let us hear from you.

1
General Principles of Epidemiology

Robert G. Sharrar

I. DEFINITIONS AND GENERAL INFORMATION

A. Health. According to the Constitution of the World Health Organization (WHO) of 1946, "Health is a state of complete physical, mental and social well-being . . ." (World Health Organization, 1948).

1. Health is not necessarily the absence of disease or infirmity.

2. Many productive and useful members of society have a disease or an infirmity. Franklin D. Roosevelt was a paraplegic throughout most of his adult life.

B. Preventive medicine is the branch of medicine that concentrates on keeping people well. Preventive medicine is an accredited medical specialty and is one of 23 recognized graduate medical education programs with its own American Board of Preventive Medicine.

1. **Goals.** Preventive medicine consists of disease prevention and health promotion.
   a. **Disease prevention** deals with techniques that prevent the occurrence of disease (physical, mental, or emotional) or lead to an early diagnosis where therapy may cure, prevent, or modify the progression of disease.
   b. **Health promotion** deals with techniques that foster physical and emotional well-being and increase the length and quality of life. It deals with the fact that many diseases are not caused by unknown or unpredictable factors, but by personal, modifiable lifestyle habits. Modifying a few lifestyle habits, such as poor diet, infrequent exercise, unprotected sexual intercourse, lack of prenatal care, failure to use seat belts, and the use of tobacco, alcohol, and drugs, could reduce one-third of all cases of acute disability, two-thirds of all cases of chronic disability, and 40%–70% of all premature deaths (Sullivan, 1990).

2. **Preventive medicine activities** can be divided into two broad areas.
   a. **Public health** involves those programs and activities directed at the community level that either benefit everyone (e.g., clean air and water) or benefit those individuals who are not currently under the care of a physician (e.g., categorical sexually transmitted disease clinics and large-scale screening programs).
   b. **Risk factor evaluation** includes programs and activities directed at individuals who are under the care of a physician who **evaluates** them for high-risk factors (e.g., smoking, drug abuse, obesity) that cause disease, **educates** them about good health habits (e.g., the use of seat belts), and **screens** them for appropriate conditions (e.g., hypertension, various cancers). These activities were recently evaluated (U.S. Preventive Services Task Force, 1989).

3. **Levels of prevention**
   a. **Primary prevention** is the prevention of disease or injury. Primary prevention activities can be directed at individuals or at the environment.
      (1) **Health education** efforts are directed at encouraging people to develop good health habits (nutrition, exercise) and to avoid harmful substances (alcohol, tobacco, drug abuse) and harmful circumstances (driving while intoxicated). **Specific protective measures** (e.g., immunizations, condom use) can also prevent diseases from occurring.
      (2) **Environmental modification** can decrease injuries from falls, fires, or automobile accidents. Environmental sanitation is used to provide an adequate sewage system, safe drinking water, clean air, and an environment free of toxic substances.

b. **Secondary prevention** is the early detection and prompt treatment of a disease.
   (1) **Screening programs** are used to detect diseases in the early preclinical stages, when effective therapy may either cure the disease or limit its progression. Examples of effective screening programs include the neonatal detection of phenylketonuria (PKU), the Pap test to detect in situ carcinoma of the cervix, and glaucoma testing.
   (2) **Primary medical care** is the predominant form of secondary prevention. Most health care dollars are spent on, and most health care personnel are employed in, primary care.

c. **Tertiary prevention** is the limitation of disability and the rehabilitation from disease. It emphasizes a person's remaining abilities and attempts to restore the person to as normal a life as possible.

d. **Examples.** All three levels of prevention can be used to control the harmful effects of a single disease process.
   (1) Treating a person with an acute communicable disease such as tuberculosis (secondary prevention) may prevent transmission to another person (primary prevention).
   (2) The control of a chronic disease such as a stroke requires health education to reduce or eliminate risk factors (primary prevention), screening programs for hypertension with early treatment (secondary prevention), and rehabilitation (tertiary prevention) if and when neurologic deficits occur.

4. **Side effects of immunization.** The preventive medicine patient population is basically well. The process that keeps them well may, however, cause them to become sick. Immunizations, which prevent a great deal of illness and death, occasionally have adverse side effects. From 1973 to 1984, there were 138 cases of paralytic polio in the United States. Of these cases, 105 (76%) were related to the use of oral polio vaccine. Nevertheless, the oral polio vaccine has prevented far more disease than it has ever caused.

C. **Public health** is the application of preventive medicine techniques to a population.

1. Public health can be defined as those activities of government agencies or community groups not normally done by the private sector that improve the health status of the community or of individuals in the community.

2. According to a study by the Institute of Medicine (1988) on the status of public health in the United States entitled *The Future of Public Health,* "This nation has lost sight of its public health goals and has allowed the system of public health activities to fall into disarray." Included in the report were recommendations for improving the system.

   a. The report defines the **mission of public health** as "fulfilling society's interest in assuring conditions in which people can be healthy." To accomplish this mission, certain criteria must be met.
      (1) Efforts to prevent disease and promote health must be based on scientific and technical knowledge.
      (2) Public health activities must reflect community values and have a community consensus. They must be established by private organizations, community advocacy groups, and individuals, as well as by public agencies working together.

   b. The report assigns the **responsibility for carrying out this mission** to the governmental public health agencies. The core functions of public health agencies at all levels of government are assessment, policy development, and assurance.
      (1) **Assessment** is the systematic collection and analysis of available data that describe the health status of the community, the needs of the community, and other epidemiologic studies of health problems.
      (2) **Policy development** must be based on the level of scientific and technical knowledge and on the content of public values and popular opinions. Public health officials must educate the public, but the true priorities must be established by the community through the normal democratic political process.
      (3) **Assurance.** Public health agencies must assure their constituents that the agreed-upon goals are being met. These services do not have to be provided by public health agencies; they just have to be guaranteed.

   c. The **breakdown of responsibilities** for carrying out the mission of public health is as follows.
      (1) The **federal government** should make assessments at the national level, establish nationwide health objectives and priorities, and provide necessary technical assistance and funds to assure the agreed-upon services.
      (2) The **state governments** should be the central force in public health in terms of assessing state health needs, establishing state health objectives, and assuring a minimum standard of essential health services.

(3) **Local governments** should assess and monitor local health problems, develop local leadership and policies, and assure high-quality services.

D. ***Healthy People 2000: National Health Promotion and Disease Prevention Objectives*** (Department of Health and Human Services, 1990). In this report, the Department of Health and Human Services has identified 298 specific objectives in 22 separate priority areas. The **three principal goals for the 1990s** are:

1. To increase the span of healthy life for Americans
2. To reduce health disparities among Americans
3. To provide access to preventive services for all Americans

II. EPIDEMIOLOGY is the science that forms the basis for public health action and unites the public health professions.

A. Definitions

1. Derived from three Greek roots (*epi* meaning upon, *demos* meaning people, and *logia* meaning study), the term epidemiology was originally applied to the study of outbreaks of acute infectious diseases and was defined as the science of epidemics.
2. Epidemiology now refers to the study of the distribution and determinants of diseases or conditions in a defined population. Epidemiology is based on two fundamental assumptions.
   - **a.** Diseases do not occur by chance.
   - **b.** Diseases are not distributed randomly in the population; thus, their distribution indicates something about how and why that disease process occurred.
3. Maxcy defined epidemiology as "the field of science dealing with the relationship of the various factors which determine the frequencies and distributions of an infectious process, a disease, or a physiologic state in a human community" (Last, 1986). Three aspects of this definition need emphasis. Epidemiology is a:
   - **a.** Science concerned with the observation, identification, description, experimental investigation, and theoretical explanation of natural phenomena
   - **b.** Study of cause and effect—that is, the relationships among variables that determine an outcome
   - **c.** Study of events in a defined population
4. Frost (1936) states that epidemiology "at any given time is something more than the total of its established facts. It includes their orderly arrangements into chains of inference which extend more or less beyond the bounds of direct observation." This definition emphasizes the fact that epidemiology is primarily a method of reasoning—that is, a way of looking at a complex population with many variables and making sense out of the events that occur within the population. It is applied common sense.

B. Epidemiologists. Since epidemiology is a multidisciplinary subject, epidemiologists have diverse backgrounds, including human and animal medicine, microbiology, statistics, computer programming, administration, toxicology, and entomology.

1. The **goals** of the epidemiologist are to:
   - **a.** Identify factors that cause disease or disease transmission
   - **b.** Prevent the spread of communicable and noncommunicable diseases and conditions
2. An epidemiologist is trained to identify and prevent diseases in a given population, while a clinician is trained to identify and treat disease in an individual.
3. An epidemiologist studies diseases in a population with many variables over which one has no control, while a basic scientist studies diseases in a laboratory, modifying one variable at a time.

C. Types of epidemiologic studies

1. **Descriptive studies** describe the distribution of cases by the variables of person, place, and time in order to study and explain acute outbreaks of disease, to follow secular trends of disease occurrence over time, and to develop hypotheses about disease transmission.

2. **Analytic studies,** such as the retrospective (case-control) studies and the prospective (cohort) studies, identify causal relationships or factors associated with disease. Analytic studies do not prove cause and effect, but they are used to generate hypotheses that can be tested (see Ch 2 II D, E).

3. **Experimental studies,** such as vaccine field trials and clinical studies that evaluate therapy, are carefully designed to prove an association between a factor and disease outcome (see Ch 2 II F).

D. Uses of epidemiology. Study of the distribution and determinants of disease in a defined population helps to:

1. Identify factors that cause disease
2. Identify factors or conditions that can be used or modified to prevent the occurrence or spread of disease
3. Explain how and why diseases and epidemics occur
4. Evaluate the effectiveness of vaccines and different forms of drug therapy
5. Establish a clinical diagnosis of disease
6. Identify the health needs of the community
7. Evaluate the effectiveness of health programs
8. Predict the future health needs of a population

III. INFECTIOUS DISEASE PROCESS.
The following factors are required to produce an infectious disease.

A. Etiologic agent. Agents that can produce infectious disease include the following.

1. **Protozoa** are unicellular parasites of the animal kingdom (e.g., plasmodia, amebae).

2. **Metazoa** are multicellular parasites of the animal kingdom (e.g., tapeworms, blood flukes).

3. **Fungi** are unicellular structures of the plant kingdom. Fungi can exist in either the **yeast phase,** characterized by cells that reproduce asexually by budding, or the **mycelial phase,** characterized by long branching filaments. Most fungi are beneficial to humans. Examples of diseases caused by fungi include ringworm and histoplasmosis.

4. **Bacteria** are unicellular structures that reproduce sexually or asexually, grow on cell-free media, and can exist in an inanimate environment. Some bacteria enter a dormant state and form spores, where they are protected from the environment and remain viable for years.
   a. The **indigenous flora** (i.e., bacteria normally found on the skin and in the mouth, gastrointestinal tract, and vagina) are necessary for life.
   b. **Pathogenic mechanisms.** Bacteria can cause disease in humans by:
      (1) **Invading and multiplying in a portion of the body that is normally sterile,** such as the lungs, urine, and bloodstream
      (2) **Producing a toxin or poison** that can exert its influence at a body site distant from where bacterial replication is occurring. For example, tetanus is caused by a certain type of wound infection, but it presents clinically as a central nervous system (CNS) disorder.
      (3) **Initiating a hypersensitivity response.** An individual with a group A β-hemolytic streptococcal infection may develop rheumatic fever or acute glomerulonephritis. In the process of eliminating the infection, an antibody is produced that also attacks the heart valves or the glomeruli of the kidney. Thus, the heart valve and glomeruli are damaged by antibodies (not the *Streptococcus* organism) that combine with these tissues to form immune complexes.
   c. **Response to treatment.** Bacteria, for the most part, infect the extracellular body space and have different metabolic pathways than humans. Consequently, antimicrobial agents have been developed that selectively kill bacteria without harming the host.

5. **Rickettsiae** are microorganisms that are between bacteria and viruses in terms of size and characteristics. Like bacteria, rickettsiae respond to some antimicrobial agents; like viruses, they are obligate intracellular parasites.

a. In humans, rickettsiae must live intracellularly, where they borrow certain enzymes and coenzymes, which they cannot make, from the cell. Usually, they infect the endothelial cells lining the walls of blood vessels.

b. Most rickettsial species exist in nature in ticks and mites; humans are not necessary for survival of rickettsial species. Rocky Mountain spotted fever is a rickettsial infection.

6. **Viruses** are obligate intracellular parasites that are among the smallest of the biologic agents known to infect humans. Viruses consist of encapsulated genetic material (DNA or RNA).

a. **Pathogenic mechanism.** To infect humans, a virus must first attach to a cell, then squirt its genetic material inside the cell. The genetic material migrates to the nucleus, where it combines with the genetic material of the host cell and takes control. Normal cell functions cease, and the cell begins to exist for the sole purpose of making more viral particles. When sufficient viral particles are made, the cell breaks open, releasing the viral particles, which infect new cells.

b. **Response to treatment.** Viral infections are difficult to treat.

(1) The location of the virus in the cell makes it difficult to develop antiviral agents that selectively kill viruses without harming the host cell.

(2) Viruses destroy cells, which may result in permanent damage. For example, polioviruses and arboviruses destroy certain nerve cells that do not regenerate. However, the lining of the trachea, which can be destroyed by influenza viruses, and the hepatocytes, which can be destroyed by hepatitis viruses, do regenerate.

B. **Reservoir.** A reservoir must exist where the biologic agent can propagate (i.e., live, multiply, and die in the natural state). There are three reservoirs.

1. **Humans.** Certain biologic agents can multiply only in humans, causing either an acute clinical or subclinical problem. **Clinical cases** are not normally a public health problem, since affected individuals stay home from work, school, or other activities and seek medical attention. However, **asymptomatic cases** are problematic, as these individuals may transmit the agent to others without knowing that they are infected. These asymptomatic individuals are called **carriers**. There are four carrier states.

a. **Subclinical cases** are patients who never develop clinical symptoms of disease. For example, most individuals infected with hepatitis A virus (HAV) never develop symptoms.

b. **Incubatory carrier.** Patients incubating a communicable disease may transmit the infection shortly before they become symptomatic, as is the case with chickenpox.

c. **Convalescent carriers.** Patients who have recovered from an acute illness may continue to shed the organism, particularly in cases of enteric infections caused by *Salmonella* or *Shigella*.

d. **Chronic carriers.** Patients may develop chronic infections and transmit the infection for long periods of time, usually over 1 year. *Salmonella typhi,* hepatitis B virus (HBV), and human immunodeficiency virus (HIV) can cause lifelong infections.

2. **Animals.** Diseases that can be transmitted under natural conditions from vertebrate animals to humans are called **zoonoses** (e.g., rabies, tularemia, leptospirosis).

3. **Environment.** Certain biologic agents, such as *Cryptococcus neoformans,* live in the environment.

C. **Portal of exit.** There must be a portal of exit from a reservoir in order for the biologic agent to cause disease elsewhere. There are five portals of exit from a human or animal reservoir.

1. **Respiratory tract.** Organisms in the respiratory tract (e.g., influenza virus, *Mycobacterium tuberculosis*) can be spread by expectoration.

2. **Genitourinary tract.** Organisms can exit the body via urine and secretions of the genital tract. For example, *Leptospirae* are found in the urine of infected animals, and sexually transmitted diseases are transmitted via secretions of the genital tract.

3. **Alimentary tract.** Organisms can exit the body via saliva (e.g., rabies virus) or the lower gastrointestinal route [e.g., HAV, agents of enteric diseases].

4. **Skin.** Organisms in superficial lesions, such as the lesions of impetigo, syphilis, and chickenpox, can be dislodged easily. Other organisms (e.g., plasmodia, HBV) exit the body via the percutaneous route through breaks in the skin, insect bites, and needles.

5. **In utero transmission.** During pregnancy, certain infectious diseases (e.g., rubella, cytomegalovirus infection, syphilis) can be transmitted from the mother across the placenta to the developing fetus, resulting in a wide range of fetal abnormalities.

D. **Transmission.** An organism must be transmitted, either directly or indirectly, from one place to another. Furthermore, an organism may have more than one mode of transmission (see VI A 2 c).

1. **Direct transmission** occurs when the reservoir and the susceptible host are in close proximity, that is, closer than 6 feet.
   a. **Direct contact transmission** occurs from skin-to-skin (person-to-person) contact, as with sexually transmitted diseases (e.g., syphilis, herpes, hepatitis B) or direct contact with a free-living organism in the environment (e.g., sporotrichosis).
   b. **Droplet spread** occurs when infectious aerosols produced by coughing, talking, and sneezing transmit infection to susceptible hosts. These infectious aerosols are large particles that are pulled to the ground by the force of gravity and can only infect a new host within a distance of 6 feet [e.g., mumps, rhinovirus (common cold)].

2. **Indirect transmission** occurs when the reservoir and the susceptible host are separated. This separation can be as small as 6 feet or as large as thousands of miles.
   a. **Vector spread** involves the transmission of an infectious agent in or on an animate thing, such as mosquitoes, fleas, mites, and ticks. Infectious agents may be transmitted through purely mechanical means, such as on the feet or wings of the insect, or it may actually grow and multiply in the vector. For example, the mosquito is not only a means of spreading malaria but also is an important part of the life cycle of the malaria parasite.
   b. **Vehicle spread** involves the transportation of an infectious agent on inanimate objects (fomites) such as toys, school supplies, bedding, or biologic equipment, or in contaminated food, water, milk, or biologic supplies. An epidemiologic investigation of 29 cases of *Salmonella newbrunswick,* a rare serotype, involving 17 states suggested that a commercial product—instant nonfat dry milk—was the vehicle of infection (Collins, et al, 1968).
   c. **Airborne spread** involves droplet nuclei 1–5 μm in size, which are produced by talking, singing, coughing, or sneezing and float on air currents over large distances for varying periods of time. Droplet nuclei may also be created by a variety of atomizing devices, such as a dentist's drill, or laboratory procedures, such as centrifugation. Particles this small can reach the lungs, settle by gravity, and produce disease (e.g., influenza, tuberculosis). The airborne route is obviously the most difficult to block.

E. **Portal of entry.** There must be a portal of entry into a susceptible host. In general, the portal of entry is similar to the portal of exit. For example, if an individual releases an agent by coughing, the susceptible host will inhale it, and if an organism leaves one genitourinary tract, it will enter another genitourinary tract.

F. **Susceptible host.** There must be a susceptible host for disease transmission to occur. Microbiologic agents surround and abound in humans. In general, people stay healthy because of their own host defense mechanisms.

1. **General factors of resistance**
   a. **Intact skin** prevents most organisms from entering the body.
   b. The **cough reflex** eliminates organisms from the lungs.
   c. **Gastric juices** digest food as well as swallowed organisms.
   d. **Diarrhea** eliminates harmful agents from the gastrointestinal tract.
   e. **Normal bacterial flora** prevent pathogenic organisms from growing.

2. **Specific factors of resistance**
   a. **Leukocytes,** with the assistance of serum factors, ingest and destroy bacteria (phagocytosis).
   b. **Serum factors and fibroblasts** encapsulate invading organisms.
   c. **The immune system** consists of cell-mediated immunity and circulating antibodies.
      (1) **Cell-mediated immunity** is responsible for delayed hypersensitivity and the regulation of antibody production. For example, patients with acquired immune deficiency syndrome (AIDS) have abnormalities in the T-cell subpopulations and, consequently, are infected by common organisms that typically do not cause disease in healthy people.
      (2) **Circulating antibodies** are proteins that inactivate specific antigens or organisms and prevent replication in the body. Antibodies are disease-specific (e.g., the measles antibody only protects against measles).

(a) **Active immunity** occurs when the host develops long-lasting antibodies to fight infection. Antibody production results from either natural disease or vaccines. It normally takes several weeks of exposure or immunization before protective antibodies are produced.

(b) **Passive immunity** occurs when antibodies are given to the host. Although of short duration, passive immunization provides immediate protection. Passive antibodies protect the newborn during the first several months of life and can also be used to prevent certain diseases, such as hepatitis A and measles, if immune serum globulin is given shortly after exposure.

IV. EPIDEMIOLOGIC CONCEPTS

A. The epidemiologic triangle states that, in order for a disease process to occur, there must be a unique combination of events: a **harmful agent** that comes into contact with a **susceptible host** in the **proper environment**. A disease or outcome is never caused by one event but rather a chain of events that form a web (epidemiologic web), which, because of its complexity, may be hard to understand. The occurrence of a disease can be blocked by intersecting the triangle at any of its three angles.

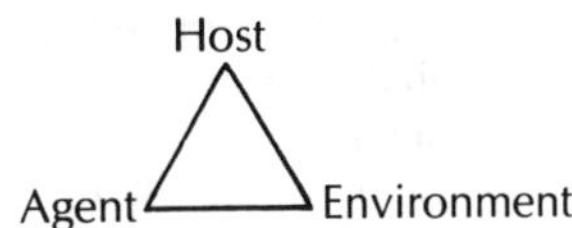

The triangle model is consistent with the infectious disease process outlined in section III, but it also can be applied to chronic noninfectious diseases.

1. **The agents of disease** can be biologic (e.g., microorganisms), chemical (e.g., toxins, poisons), nutritional (e.g., excess food, lack of food, vitamin deficiency), physical forces (e.g., automobiles), or energy (e.g., ionizing radiation).

   a. **Agent factors.** While an agent may be necessary for a disease, exposure to an agent does not always cause clinical symptoms.

      (1) **Inoculum size,** or **dose,** is important. There is a dose-response relationship for most toxic substances. For example, it takes the ingestion of 100,000 *Salmonella* organisms to cause disease as compared to 100 *Shigella* organisms, which represents a 1000-fold difference. Heavy smokers are more likely to get lung cancer than occasional smokers.

      (2) **Particular serotypes,** or **strains,** of a species may be more likely to cause disease than other strains of the same organism [e.g., *Hemophilus influenzae* type B (Hib) is more likely to cause invasive disease than other encapsulated and unencapsulated strains].

      (3) **Host entry.** The agent must be able to enter the host (e.g., being in the same room with someone who is infected with the AIDS virus is not sufficient for transmission to occur).

   b. A disease may be prevented by **eliminating the agent**. The strategy of the WHO to eradicate smallpox worldwide was to eliminate the smallpox virus, which no longer exists in its natural state. Most cases of lung cancer would not occur if the agent (tobacco smoke) were eliminated. Fewer automobile accidents would occur if the host would not drive under the influence of alcohol (agent).

2. **Host factors** that determine the occurrence of a disease include **biologic traits,** with which a host is born, and **social traits,** which a host develops or acquires.

   a. **Biologic traits** include genetic characteristics, race, ethnic origin, sex, and age. Biologic traits cannot be modified. **Age** is one of the most important epidemiologic factors in determining what disease a person gets.

      (1) Young children are more likely to have subclinical infection. An infant infected with the wild poliovirus will have no symptoms, while an older sibling may have paralytic disease.

      (2) Adults are immune to certain diseases because of prior exposure. Meningococcal meningitis is rare after the age of 25 years because of prior exposure to the meningococcal organism.

      (3) Children and adults are exposed to different agents of disease. Children are more likely to be exposed to biologic agents that cause acute communicable diseases, while adults are more likely to be exposed to agents that cause chronic diseases (i.e., drugs, alcohol, tobacco).

b. **Social traits** are acquired as the host goes through life. Marital status, lifestyle, diet, residence, and travel are a few factors that determine disease outcome.
   (1) Modification of dietary habits or use of tobacco or alcohol, as well as changes in employment or area of residence, can prevent disease.
   (2) Vaccines can make a host resistant to certain diseases. For example, individuals immunized against measles by a vaccine will not contract the disease even if they come into contact with the measles virus circulating in the community.

3. **Environmental factors** that determine the occurrence of disease may be physical, biologic, or social.
   a. **Physical factors** include climate (e.g., temperature, moisture), setting (e.g., urban versus rural), and pollution (e.g., water, air).
      (1) Diseases can be prevented by modifying the physical environment. For example, the simple processes of filtering and chlorinating the water supply and separating the water and sewage systems have virtually eliminated typhoid fever in most urban areas in the United States.
      (2) Some injuries could be prevented by the widespread use of smoke detectors, by installing handrails on all stairs, and by modifying traffic patterns.
   b. **Biologic factors** include environmental factors that are necessary to maintain the agent or allow for its transmission. For example, malaria does not occur in Katmandu, Nepal, because the mosquitoes that transmit malaria cannot fly at high altitudes.
   c. **Social factors** include the political, social, and economic bases of society and its institutions. For example, certain diseases and conditions, such as tuberculosis, are more common in the lower socioeconomic strata, where overcrowding may play a role. There is an association between poverty, drug and alcohol abuse, and violence.

B. **Spectrum of disease** describes the varied expression of illness in a population.

1. **Infectious diseases.** In some diseases (e.g., polio), the clinical cases represent only the "tip of the iceberg," while in others (e.g., measles), subclinical cases are thought to be rare. If a group of susceptible people is exposed to a biologic agent, the following outcomes will occur.
   a. A certain proportion will have no clinical or laboratory evidence of infection.
   b. Others will have no clinical evidence of infection but may have laboratory evidence of infection. These individuals will continue normal daily activities but are capable of spreading the disease.
   c. Others will develop mild to severe clinical illness. These individuals will interrupt normal daily activities, seek medical help, and modify their behavior. Therefore, they are less likely to spread the illness.
   d. Some will die from the disease.

2. **Chronic diseases** also present as a spectrum of illnesses. Some individuals who smoke may have no or few symptoms. Others may have a chronic cough, chronic bronchitis, or severe chronic obstructive pulmonary disease (COPD) and die from pulmonary insufficiency.

3. **Clinical presentations.** Many different agents can produce the same clinical disease. For example, the clinical manifestations of pneumonia are fever, cough, and an abnormal chest x-ray; however, these symptoms and findings can be caused by chemicals, parasites, fungi, bacteria, rickettsiae, or viruses. Lung cancers can be caused by tobacco, radon, and various types of chemicals.

C. **Herd immunity** describes the spread of a communicable disease within a group based on the proportions of susceptible and immune individuals in the group. Epidemics or outbreaks of disease occur when the proportion of susceptible individuals is high and disappear as the proportion of immune individuals increases.

1. The proportion of immune individuals within a group that is necessary to prevent an outbreak of disease varies according to the disease and its mode of transmission. In general, diseases spread by the airborne route require a higher proportion of immune individuals to prevent an outbreak than diseases spread by direct contact.

2. Vaccine-preventable diseases (e.g., measles) may occur in immunized individuals because of improper immunization (e.g., immunization at the wrong age), poor storage of vaccine, or unidentifiable host factors. Thus, because of these vaccine failures and because measles is an airborne transmitted disease, measles outbreaks have occurred in populations that were 90% immunized.

3. Because of herd immunity, a disease can be eradicated without achieving 100% immunization levels. For example, smallpox was eradicated by immunizing around a case to prevent further spread and not by achieving 100% immunization levels (see IV E).

D. Disease surveillance refers to the process of determining the frequency with which certain diseases occur in the community by collection, consolidation, analysis, and dissemination of relevant data. The legal bases for disease surveillance are regulations adapted by state boards of health, which derive their authority to issue regulations from acts of the state legislatures.

1. **Objectives** of disease surveillance are to:
   - **a.** Know what diseases are occurring so effective control can be initiated
   - **b.** Evaluate the effectiveness of the control programs
   - **c.** Increase the knowledge of disease processes, either because gaps exist in the available knowledge of many acute and chronic diseases or because shifts from the customary pattern of a particular disease have occurred

2. **Surveillance activities** can be either active or passive.
   - **a. Active surveillance** occurs when the health department calls health care providers to see if they have seen any cases of a particular disease.
   - **b. Passive surveillance** occurs when a health department simply waits for health care providers to report cases.

3. **Sources** of disease surveillance data include:
   - **a.** Individual case reports
   - **b.** Laboratory reports
   - **c.** Emergency room visit records
   - **d.** Hospital discharge summaries
   - **e.** Case investigations revealing additional cases
   - **f.** Death certificates
   - **g.** Surveys

E. Disease eradication requires the total annihilation of the agent so that the epidemiologic triangle will never occur again. Smallpox was eradicated because of unique epidemiologic features of this disease.

1. The agent of smallpox was a virus that only lived in humans and that always caused clinical disease. There were no subclinical cases and no chronic carriers of this virus.

2. A susceptible host could be made immune to this disease by immunization with an effective vaccine.

3. Disease surveillance identified all known cases, and mass immunization campaigns around these cases eliminated the susceptible hosts so that the virus had no reservoir in which to reside. The smallpox virus then became extinct and can no longer cause disease. Therefore, smallpox vaccinations are no longer required.

4. Because of herd immunity, eradication was achieved without 100% immunization levels.

F. Vital statistics refer to the registration or recording of vital events such as births, deaths, fetal deaths, abortions, marriages, and divorces. These vital events must be reported by law, and an analysis of these data provides the best information about the health of a population (see V B). All states use forms that are based on standard certificates developed by the National Center for Health Statistics (NCHS). These standard forms, which were last revised in 1987, enable the NCHS to collect data that are comparable from state to state and can be consolidated at the national level.

1. The **Certificate of Live Birth** (birth certificate) must be certified by the attending physician, licensed midwife, or designated person for unattended births. The birth certificate contains the following information:
   - **a.** Information about the event (i.e., date, time, place of birth)
   - **b.** Demographic data (i.e., age, race, sex) about the newborn and the mother and father of the child
   - **c.** Information about the pregnancy, medical risk factors for the pregnancy, complications of labor or delivery, and congenital anomalies of the newborn

2. The **Certificate of Death** must be certified by a physician, medical examiner, or coroner (Figure 1-1). The death certificate contains the following information:
   a. Information about the event (i.e., date, time, place of death)
   b. Information about the deceased (i.e., names and place of births of parents, date and place of birth, mailing address, actual address, usual occupation, kind of business, any service in United States armed forces, educational level achieved, marital status, and whether or not there is a surviving spouse)
   c. Information about the cause of death; this information is exceedingly important and must be completed accurately by the certifying physician because it is used for much of the public health analyses that are done
      (1) On every death certificate there is an immediate cause of death, an underlying cause of death, and the length of time for each condition. There also is a portion that deals with other significant conditions contributing to death but not resulting in the underlying cause.
         (a) The **immediate cause of death** is the final disease, injury, or complication that resulted in death.
         (b) The **underlying cause of death** is the disease or injury that initiated the chain of events that resulted in death. For statistical purposes, this is the cause of death incorporated into public health statistics.
      (2) The diagnostic terms used on the death certificate must conform to the *International Classification of Diseases, Ninth Revision, Clinical Modification (ICD-9-CM)* [1978]. The *ICD* gives a number for every medical diagnosis or condition. These numbers are also used on discharge summaries, as well as for insurance purposes.

V. TOOLS OF THE TRADE.

To determine factors that cause disease, epidemiologists must be able to describe and compare the occurrence of disease within a population. The characteristics of the populations affected most by disease are used to determine the factors that cause the disease.

A. Quantitative measurements

1. **Ratio** is the expression of the relationship between two items. These items may be either related to or independent of each other. Mathematically, a ratio is expressed as **X:Y,** where X is the count of one item and Y is a count of another. Both counts are taken during the same time interval. For example, in a classroom of 15 boys and 5 girls, the male to female ratio is 15:5, or 3:1.

2. **Proportion** is the expression of the relationship of one part to the whole. The numerator is always included in the denominator, and since the base always equals 100, a proportion is expressed as a percent. Mathematically, a proportion is expressed as

$$\frac{X}{Y} \times K$$

   where X is a count of one item in the population, Y is the total population, and K is the base number. The values of X and Y are determined during the same time interval. For example, in a classroom of 15 boys and 5 girls, the proportion of female students is 5/20, or 25%.

3. **Rate** (see V B for examples) is the expression of the probability of occurrence of a particular event in a defined population during a specified period of time. Mathematically, a rate is expressed as

$$\frac{X}{Y} \times K$$

   where X = the number of events or cases, Y = 5 the total population at risk, and K is a round number, or base, chosen to express the rate as a number greater than one. The values of X and Y are determined during the same time interval.
   a. Since the total population changes during the time interval, the estimated midinterval population is used.
   b. The estimated midinterval population is determined by adding the population at the beginning of the time interval to the population at the end of the time interval and dividing by two.

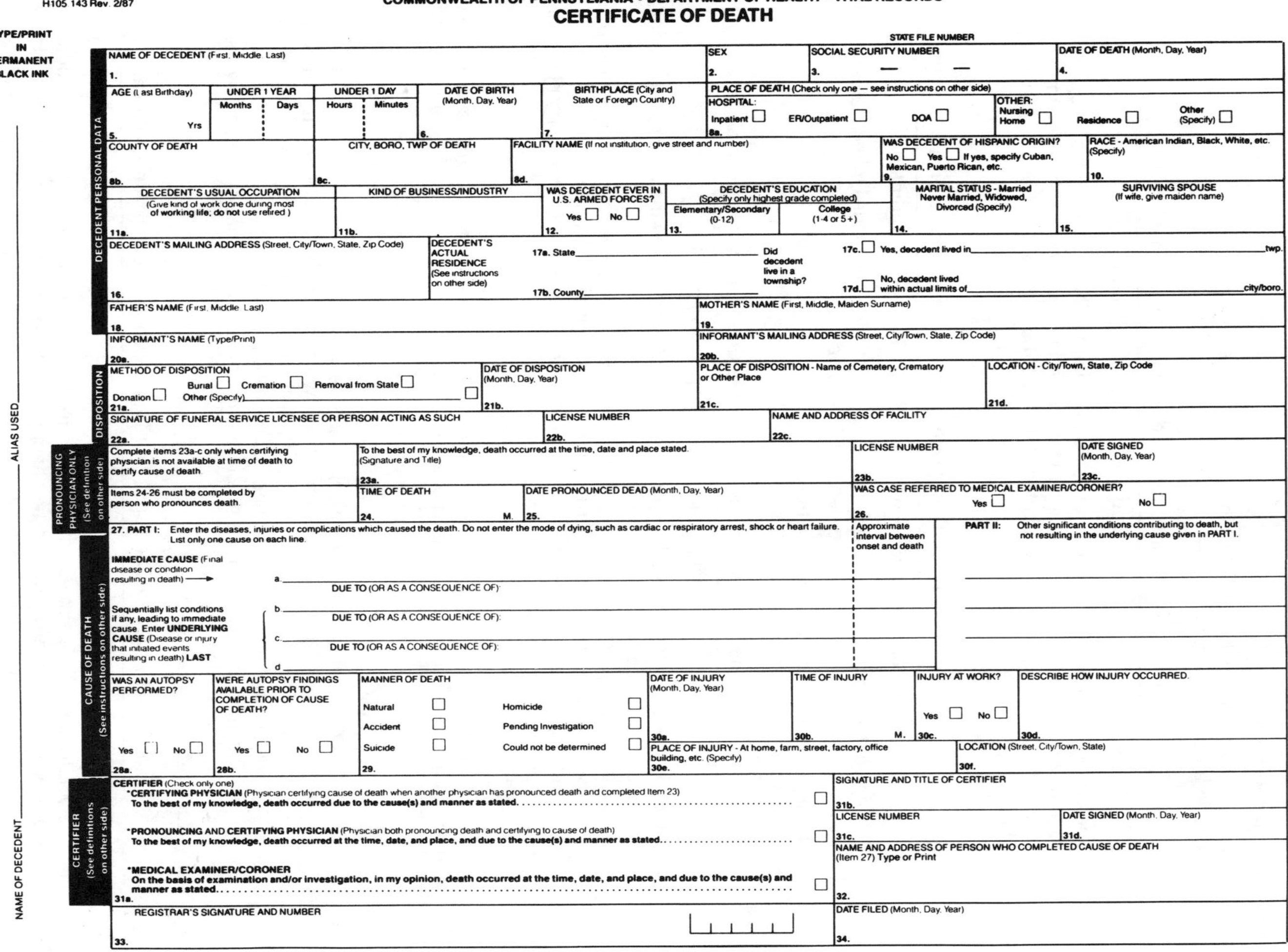

H105 143 Rev. 2/87

TYPE/PRINT IN PERMANENT BLACK INK

COMMONWEALTH OF PENNSYLVANIA • DEPARTMENT OF HEALTH • VITAL RECORDS

CERTIFICATE OF DEATH

STATE FILE NUMBER

DECEDENT PERSONAL DATA

1. NAME OF DECEDENT (First, Middle, Last)
2. SEX
3. SOCIAL SECURITY NUMBER
4. DATE OF DEATH (Month, Day, Year)
5. AGE (Last Birthday) Yrs — UNDER 1 YEAR: Months / Days — UNDER 1 DAY: Hours / Minutes
6. DATE OF BIRTH (Month, Day, Year)
7. BIRTHPLACE (City and State or Foreign Country)
8a. PLACE OF DEATH (Check only one — see instructions on other side) HOSPITAL: Inpatient ☐ ER/Outpatient ☐ DOA ☐ OTHER: Nursing Home ☐ Residence ☐ Other (Specify) ☐
8b. COUNTY OF DEATH
8c. CITY, BORO, TWP OF DEATH
8d. FACILITY NAME (If not institution, give street and number)
9. WAS DECEDENT OF HISPANIC ORIGIN? No ☐ Yes ☐ If yes, specify Cuban, Mexican, Puerto Rican, etc.
10. RACE - American Indian, Black, White, etc. (Specify)
11a. DECEDENT'S USUAL OCCUPATION (Give kind of work done during most of working life; do not use retired.)
11b. KIND OF BUSINESS/INDUSTRY
12. WAS DECEDENT EVER IN U.S. ARMED FORCES? Yes ☐ No ☐
13. DECEDENT'S EDUCATION (Specify only highest grade completed) Elementary/Secondary (0-12) College (1-4 or 5+)
14. MARITAL STATUS - Married, Never Married, Widowed, Divorced (Specify)
15. SURVIVING SPOUSE (If wife, give maiden name)
16. DECEDENT'S MAILING ADDRESS (Street, City/Town, State, Zip Code)

DECEDENT'S ACTUAL RESIDENCE (See instructions on other side)
17a. State
17b. County
Did decedent live in a township?
17c. ☐ Yes, decedent lived in ______ twp.
17d. ☐ No, decedent lived within actual limits of ______ city/boro.

18. FATHER'S NAME (First, Middle, Last)
19. MOTHER'S NAME (First, Middle, Maiden Surname)
20a. INFORMANT'S NAME (Type/Print)
20b. INFORMANT'S MAILING ADDRESS (Street, City/Town, State, Zip Code)

DISPOSITION

21a. METHOD OF DISPOSITION Burial ☐ Cremation ☐ Removal from State ☐ Donation ☐ Other (Specify) ☐
21b. DATE OF DISPOSITION (Month, Day, Year)
21c. PLACE OF DISPOSITION - Name of Cemetery, Crematory or Other Place
21d. LOCATION - City/Town, State, Zip Code
22a. SIGNATURE OF FUNERAL SERVICE LICENSEE OR PERSON ACTING AS SUCH
22b. LICENSE NUMBER
22c. NAME AND ADDRESS OF FACILITY

PRONOUNCING PHYSICIAN ONLY (See definition on other side)

Complete items 23a-c only when certifying physician is not available at time of death to certify cause of death.
23a. To the best of my knowledge, death occurred at the time, date and place stated. (Signature and Title)
23b. LICENSE NUMBER
23c. DATE SIGNED (Month, Day, Year)
Items 24-26 must be completed by person who pronounces death.
24. TIME OF DEATH M.
25. DATE PRONOUNCED DEAD (Month, Day, Year)
26. WAS CASE REFERRED TO MEDICAL EXAMINER/CORONER? Yes ☐ No ☐

CAUSE OF DEATH (See instructions on other side)

27. PART I: Enter the diseases, injuries or complications which caused the death. Do not enter the mode of dying, such as cardiac or respiratory arrest, shock or heart failure. List only one cause on each line.

Approximate interval between onset and death

IMMEDIATE CAUSE (Final disease or condition resulting in death) → a.
DUE TO (OR AS A CONSEQUENCE OF):
Sequentially list conditions if any, leading to immediate cause. Enter UNDERLYING CAUSE (Disease or injury that initiated events resulting in death) LAST b.
DUE TO (OR AS A CONSEQUENCE OF):
c.
DUE TO (OR AS A CONSEQUENCE OF):
d.

PART II: Other significant conditions contributing to death, but not resulting in the underlying cause given in PART I.

28a. WAS AN AUTOPSY PERFORMED? Yes ☐ No ☐
28b. WERE AUTOPSY FINDINGS AVAILABLE PRIOR TO COMPLETION OF CAUSE OF DEATH? Yes ☐ No ☐
29. MANNER OF DEATH Natural ☐ Accident ☐ Suicide ☐ Homicide ☐ Pending Investigation ☐ Could not be determined ☐
30a. DATE OF INJURY (Month, Day, Year)
30b. TIME OF INJURY M.
30c. INJURY AT WORK? Yes ☐ No ☐
30d. DESCRIBE HOW INJURY OCCURRED.
30e. PLACE OF INJURY - At home, farm, street, factory, office building, etc. (Specify)
30f. LOCATION (Street, City/Town, State)

CERTIFIER (See definitions on other side)

31a. CERTIFIER (Check only one)
*CERTIFYING PHYSICIAN (Physician certifying cause of death when another physician has pronounced death and completed Item 23) To the best of my knowledge, death occurred due to the cause(s) and manner as stated. ☐
*PRONOUNCING AND CERTIFYING PHYSICIAN (Physician both pronouncing death and certifying to cause of death) To the best of my knowledge, death occurred at the time, date, and place, and due to the cause(s) and manner as stated. ☐
*MEDICAL EXAMINER/CORONER On the basis of examination and/or investigation, in my opinion, death occurred at the time, date, and place, and due to the cause(s) and manner as stated. ☐
31b. SIGNATURE AND TITLE OF CERTIFIER
31c. LICENSE NUMBER
31d. DATE SIGNED (Month, Day, Year)
32. NAME AND ADDRESS OF PERSON WHO COMPLETED CAUSE OF DEATH (Item 27) Type or Print
33. REGISTRAR'S SIGNATURE AND NUMBER
34. DATE FILED (Month, Day, Year)

ALIAS USED ______
NAME OF DECEDENT ______

Figure 1-1. Certificate of death used by the Commonwealth of Pennsylvania.

4. **Index** (see V B 3 c for an example) is used when the true denominator, or population at risk, cannot be determined. A related denominator is used as a measure of the population at risk. An index is then a **pseudorate**.

B. Specific measurements

1. **Natality rates** measure the rate of birth.
   a. **Crude birth rate** is expressed as

$$\frac{\text{number of live births reported during a given time interval}}{\text{estimated midinterval population}}$$

The crude birth rate is expressed per 1000 population. (Note that the total population is used in the denominator even though many individuals are not at risk of becoming pregnant.) The crude birth rate in the United States in 1988 was 15.9 live births per 1000 population (3,909,510 live births).

   b. **Fertility rate** is expressed as

$$\frac{\text{number of live births reported during a given time interval}}{\text{estimated number of women age 15–44 years at midinterval}}$$

Fertility rate is expressed per 1000 population. The fertility rate in the United States in 1988 was 67.2 live births per 1000 women age 15–44 years.

2. **Morbidity rates** measure the rate of illness.
   a. **Incidence rate** is expressed as

$$\frac{\text{number of new cases of a specific disease during a given time interval}}{\text{estimated midinterval population at risk}}$$

A **high incidence rate** means a high occurrence of disease; a **low incidence rate** means a low occurrence of disease.

   (1) Because incidence rate is a measure of the rate at which healthy people develop disease during a specific time period, it is a statement of probability.
   (2) Since incidence rates are affected by any factor that affects the development of a disease, they can be used to detect etiologic factors.

   b. **Prevalence rate** is expressed as

$$\frac{\text{number of current cases [old (i.e., people who contracted disease before time period began and who still have the disease) and new] of a specified disease during a specified time period}}{\text{estimated midinterval population at risk}}$$

   (1) **Point prevalence** refers to a specific point in time.
   (2) **Period prevalence** refers to a given time interval.
      (a) Since prevalence rate contains all known cases in the numerator, it is used primarily to measure the amount of illness in a community and, thus, can be used to determine the health care needs of that community.
      (b) Prevalence rates are influenced by both the incidence of disease and by the duration of illness.

   c. **Attack rate** is expressed as

$$\frac{\text{number of new cases of a specific disease during a specific time interval}}{\text{total population at risk during the same time interval}}$$

Attack rate normally is expressed as a percentage. It is an incidence rate that is calculated in an epidemic situation using a particular population observed for a limited period of time.

   d. **Secondary attack rate** is expressed as

$$\frac{\text{(number of new cases in a group)} - \text{(index case or cases during a specified time period)}}{\text{(number of susceptible individuals in the group)} - \text{(index case or cases)}}$$

Note that the index case or cases that introduced the disease into the group are removed from both the numerator and denominator. The secondary attack rate measures spread within an epidemiologic unit. **Coindex cases** are two or more cases that, based on the incubation period of the disease, were infected by someone outside the group.

3. **Mortality rates** measure the rate of death.
   a. **Crude death rate** is expressed as

$$\frac{\text{total number of deaths reported during a given interval}}{\text{estimated midinterval population}}$$

   Crude death rate is expressed per 1000 population. (Note that the total population is used even though the risk of death is different for different age-groups.) The crude death rate in the United States in 1988 was 8.8 deaths per 1000 population.

   b. **Cause-specific death rate** is expressed as

$$\frac{\text{number of deaths assigned to a specified cause during a given time interval}}{\text{estimated midinterval population}}$$

   Cause-specific death rate is expressed per 100,000 population. The cause-specific death rate for diseases of the heart in the United States in 1988 was 311.3 deaths per 100,000 population.

   c. **Maternal mortality rate** is expressed as

$$\frac{\text{number of deaths related to pregnancy during a given interval}}{\text{number of live births reported during the same time interval}}$$

   Although the true population at risk should be the number of pregnant women, this is an impossible figure to determine. The number of live births is chosen because it reflects the number of pregnant women; thus, this is a **pseudorate,** or **index**. The maternal mortality rate in the United States in 1988 was 8.4 deaths per 100,000 live births.

   d. **Case-fatality rate** is expressed as

$$\frac{\text{number of deaths assigned to a specific disease}}{\text{number of cases of the disease}}$$

   Case-fatality rate is frequently expressed as a percentage. It predicts the risk of dying if the disease is contracted. Tetanus has a case-fatality rate of 30%–90%, depending on the age of the host, the length of the incubation period, and the type and length of therapy.

   e. **Years of potential life lost (YPLL)** is a quantitative measure of premature mortality (see also Ch 8 III A 3).
      (1) It reflects the **mortality trends of younger age-groups** by taking into account not only the cause of death but also the age at which it occurs.
      (2) The **Centers for Disease Control (CDC) defines YPLL** as the number of years of potential life lost by each death occurring before age 65. There is controversy about these calculations, since the older age-groups are underrepresented by this upper age limit. Some calculations use the remaining life expectancy as the upper age limit.
      (3) The **YPLL for a specific disease is calculated** as follows.
         (a) To determine **the total number of deaths caused by a specific disease in a specific age-group,** the age-specific rate for that specific disease is multiplied by the estimated population of the age-group.
         (b) To determine **the YPLL caused by a specific disease in a specific age-group,** the number of deaths in that age-group is multiplied by the difference between the midpoint of the age range and the designated 65-year endpoint.
         (c) The **total YPLL** is the summation of all of the YPLL for each age-group up to 65 years of age.
      (4) The YPLL can also be calculated for a specific risk factor (e.g., alcohol, tobacco) to determine the number of YPLL caused by that factor.
      (5) When comparing YPLL over time and in different populations, YPLL rates per 1000 population can be calculated. Age-, sex-, and race-adjusted YPLL rates can be calculated to compare premature mortality in different segments of the population.
         (a) In 1982, blacks had an increased risk of premature deaths (99.2 YPLL per 1000 population) as compared to whites (53.6 per 1000). The leading cause of premature mortality was suicide and homicide in blacks and unintentional injuries in whites.

(b) In 1982, males had nearly twice the rate of premature mortality as compared to females (77.6 YPLL per 1000 population as compared to 41.6 per 1000).

(6) The **10 leading causes of death** in the United States are determined by comparing the cause-specific death rates. A different ranking occurs if the leading causes of mortality are ranked by YPLL (Table 1-1).

f. Proportionate mortality ratio (PMR) is expressed as

$$\frac{\text{number of deaths from a given cause in a specified time period}}{\text{total deaths in the same time period}}$$

PMR usually is expressed as a percentage.

(1) The PMR is not a rate and does not measure the probability of dying from a particular cause.

(2) The PMR is primarily used to determine the relative importance of a specific cause of death in relation to all causes of death within a population.

(3) In 1988, the PMR for the top three leading causes of death in the United States was reported as follows:

(a) Heart disease: 35.3%

(b) Malignant neoplasms: 22.4%

(c) Cerebrovascular disease: 6.9%

C. Types of rates. The type of rate calculated depends on the available data and the purpose of the calculation.

1. Crude rates, such as the crude birth and death rates, are summary rates for an entire population.

a. They are simple to calculate because only the number of events and the total population are necessary.

b. They cannot be used to compare events in different populations because the rate depends on the age-sex composition of the total population. For example, a high death rate and a low birth rate would be expected in a community with many senior citizens as compared to a community with many young people.

2. Adjusted rates are summary rates for the total population, but they are fictitious rates. They can be used for international comparison.

a. Statistical techniques are used to calculate summary rates for populations differing in some important characteristics, the most important of which is age. Thus, adjusted rates equalize the differences in the population at risk so that the rates are comparable. However, adjusted rates are difficult to calculate because the demographic composition of the population must be known.

Table 1-1. Rankings of the 10 Leading Causes of Mortality and Years of Potential Life Lost (YPLL) before Age 65, United States, 1987

Ranking	Cause of Death	YPLL (0–65 years)
1	Diseases of the heart	Unintentional injuries
2	Malignant neoplasms	Malignant neoplasms
3	Cerebrovascular diseases	Diseases of the heart
4	Unintentional injuries	Suicide, homicide, and legal intervention
5	Chronic obstructive pulmonary disease and allied conditions	Congenital anomalies
6	Pneumonia and influenza	Human immunodeficiency virus (HIV)
7	Suicide, homicide, and legal intervention	Prematurity
8	Diabetes mellitus	Sudden infant death syndrome (SIDS)
9	Chronic liver disease and cirrhosis	Cerebrovascular disease
10	Nephritis, nephrotic syndrome, and nephrosis	Chronic liver disease and cirrhosis

b. Age-adjusted rates are most frequently used to compare mortality in different populations. Age-adjusted rates are computed either by the direct or indirect method.

(1) The **direct method** calculates the rate that would have been observed if the populations being compared had the same age distribution. It is calculated as follows.

(a) The age-specific rates in the populations being compared must be known.

(b) A standard population from elsewhere must be borrowed (this standard population can be a composite of all populations being compared, the United States population, or a hypothetical population).

(c) The known age-specific rates are multiplied by the chosen standard population in that age-group to determine the number of events that would have occurred (the total number of events divided by the standard population chosen is the adjusted rate).

(2) The **indirect method** calculates the number of events that would have been observed if the two populations being compared had the same age-specific rates. The indirect method is used when the age-specific rates are unknown, as in developing countries, or unstable because of small numbers in the population being studied. It is calculated as follows.

(a) The age composition of the populations being compared and the total number of observed events in each population must be known.

(b) Age-specific rates from a larger population with more stable rates must be borrowed.

(c) The known population in a specified age-group is multiplied by the borrowed age-specific rate to determine the expected number of events that would have occurred in that age-group (the total expected number of events would be the sum of the expected events in each age-group).

(d) The standardized ratio (SR), then, is calculated. The SR is the total observed events in a population divided by the total expected events in that population times 100.

(i) If the SR is over 100, it means that more events are occurring in the population than expected.

(ii) If the SR is less than 100, it means that fewer events are occurring than expected.

(iii) When mortality or morbidity is being compared, the SR is called the standardized mortality or morbidity ratio (SMR).

3. Specific rates are calculated for various segments of the population.

a. These rates are difficult to calculate because more information about the demographic composition of the population must be known than with other rates (i.e., the number of observed events and the number of individuals at risk in each segment of the population).

b. Because these rates are specific for a particular population segment, they can be used to compare events in different populations.

D. Examples of rates. Table 1-2 compares observed death rates in community A and community B.

1. The **crude death rate** can be calculated from Table 1-2 as 10/1000 in both communities. Thus, it might be concluded that the risk of death is equal in both communities. However, crude rates cannot be used to compare rates in different populations.

Table 1-2. Observed Death Rates of Two Communities

	Community A			Community B		
Age-Group	**Number of Deaths**	**Number in Age-Group**	**Age-Specific Death Rate***	**Number of Deaths**	**Number in Age-Group**	**Age-Specific Death Rate***
0–20	10	4000	2.5	40	8000	5.0
21–49	40	9000	4.4	60	10,000	6.0
50–69	100	10,000	10.0	100	6000	16.7
70+	100	2000	50.0	50	1000	50.0
Total	250	25,000	10.0	250	25,000	10.0

*Per 1000 population.

2. **Adjusted rates** also can be calculated from the data in Table 1-2.
   a. **Direct method.** A standard population must be borrowed. In Table 1-3, the composite of the two separate populations (communities A and B) is used.
      (1) The direct age-adjusted death rate of community A is

$$\frac{423.6}{50{,}000} \times 1000 = \frac{8.5}{1000}$$

      (2) The direct age-adjusted death rate of community B is

$$\frac{591.2}{50{,}000} \times 1000 = \frac{11.8}{1000}$$

      (3) Since the direct age-adjusted death rate in community B is higher than that in community A, it can be concluded that the risk of death is higher in community B.
   b. **Indirect method.** Standard age-specific rates from a larger population must be borrowed, as has been done in Table 1-4.
      (1) The standardized mortality ratio (SMR) of community A is

$$\text{SMR} = \frac{\text{observed deaths (Table 1-2}}{\text{expected deaths (Table 1-4)}} \times 100 = \frac{250}{288.2} \times 100 = 86.7$$

      (2) The SMR of community B is

$$\text{SMR} = \frac{250}{204.4} \times 100 = 122.3$$

      (3) Since the SMR in community B is higher than that in community A, it can be concluded that the risk of death is higher in community B.
3. In Table 1-2, the age-specific death rates in all age-groups but the over 70 age-group are higher in community B than in community A. These rates are directly comparable without any need for adjusting.

VI. EPIDEMIOLOGIC VARIABLES.

The characteristics and circumstances of a given population that forms a community are various, and environmental factors are in constant flux. These epidemiologic variables are grouped into the primary categories of time, person, and place. The analysis of the distribution of cases by these variables (descriptive epidemiology) is frequently used to determine how and why diseases occur. Specifically, the epidemiologist looks for a clustering of cases in a segment of the population during a short period of time in a definite geographic space.

A. **Time** refers to the date and, in some instances, the hour of the onset of illness. The occurrence of a disease can be observed over a long period of time (years) to determine secular trends, over a moderate period of time (months) to determine seasonal variation, or over a short period of time (days or weeks) in an epidemic situation.

   1. **Secular trends** reflect changes in the periodicity and the natural history of a disease over many years.

Table 1-3. Adjusted Death Rates for Two Communities Using Standard Population Figures for Comparison

	Community A			**Community B**		
Age-Group	**Age-Specific Death Rate***	**Standard Population**	**Expected Number of Deaths**	**Age-Specific Death Rate***	**Standard Population**	**Expected Number of Deaths**
0–20	2.5	12,000	30.0	5.0	12,000	60.0
21–49	4.4	19,000	83.6	6.0	19,000	114.0
50–69	10.0	16,000	160.0	16.7	16,000	267.2
70+	50.0	3,000	150.0	50.0	3,000	150.0
Total		50,000	423.6		50,000	591.2

*Per 1000 population.

Table 1-4. Adjusted Death Rates for Two Communities Using Borrowed Death Rates for Comparison

	Community A			Community B		
Age-Group	**Number in Age-Group**	**Borrowed Age-Specific Rate***	**Expected Number of Deaths**	**Number in Age-Group**	**Borrowed Age-Specific Rate***	**Expected Number of Deaths**
0–20	4000	3.3	13.2	8000	3.3	26.4
21–49	9000	5.0	45.0	10,000	5.0	50.0
50–69	10,000	13.0	130.0	6000	13.0	78.0
70+	2000	50.0	100.0	1000	50.0	50.0
Total	25,000		288.2	25,000		204.4

*Per 1000 population.

a. Many diseases have a **periodicity** that can be used to predict their future behavior. This periodicity is believed to be related to the proportion of susceptible and immune individuals in the population. For example, because of slight changes (**antigenic drift**) on the surface of the influenza virus, increased influenza activity is seen every few years. Major changes (**antigenic shift**) on the surface of the influenza virus occur at longer intervals and are capable of causing worldwide epidemics (pandemics), which happened in 1947, 1957, and 1968.

b. Changes also occur in the **natural history** of a disease. Figure 1-2 shows the reported cases of viral hepatitis by 4-week periods in the United States from July 1952 to July 1972. [Note that the separate reporting of infectious hepatitis (hepatitis A) and serum hepatitis (hepatitis B) did not occur until 1966.] This graph shows that the 7-year periodicity between 1954 and 1961 was not repeated in 1968. Note also that the baseline has shifted upward and that the seasonal pattern (winter peaks and summer troughs) of the 1950s and 1960s has flattened. These data suggest that there has been a change in the natural history of hepatitis (see VI B 3).

2. Seasonal variations that occur with some diseases may provide information about the reservoir or the mode of transmission. Human susceptibility does not vary significantly throughout the year. Influenza, which is a fall-winter disease in the temperate zone, also occurs in the tropics, which is warm year-round.

a. Legionnaires' disease is more common in the summer months because it is caused by contaminated air-cooling systems. However, since cases occur throughout the year, there must be other sources of infection.

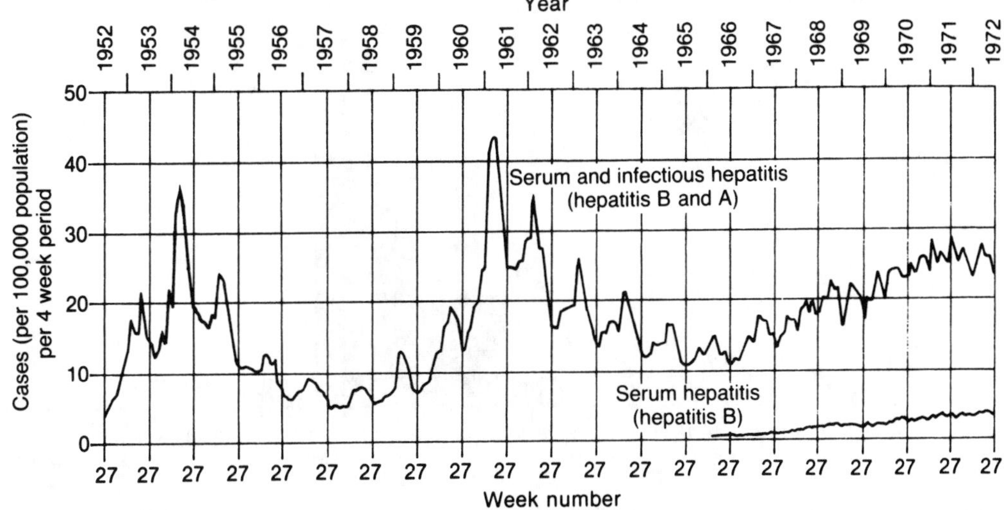

Figure 1-2. Reported cases of viral hepatitis by 4-week periods in the United States between July 1952 and July 1972. (Reprinted from Centers for Disease Control: *Hepatitis Surveillance Report*, no 35. Atlanta, CDC, July 1972, p 5.)

b. **Arthropod-borne viral encephalitis,** which is transmitted by the bite of infective mosquitoes, occurs in temperate regions in the late summer and early fall. Environmental factors, such as temperature and rainfall, influence the size of the vector population.

c. **Tularemia** is a zoonotic disease (see III B 2) that is more common in the summer months in the western states and in the winter months in the eastern states. In western states, tularemia is primarily transmitted by the bite of a tick; in eastern states, it is primarily contracted by skinning rabbits and muskrats during the hunting season, eating insufficiently cooked food, or drinking water contaminated by animals that have died of tularemia.

3. **Epidemic curves** are used to describe the distribution of cases during short periods of time and are helpful in determining the source of infection and the possible mode of transmission. In food-borne outbreaks, the calculation of the incubation period (i.e., the time interval from exposure to onset of clinical disease) can be used to determine the etiologic agent (see VII C 1 e).

a. **Type I epidemic curves** are characterized by a rapid rise and fall of cases so that all cases fall within the range of one incubation period. They are caused by a common source of exposure at one point in time. If the incubation period of the disease is known and if all of the cases occur within one incubation period, the days can be counted backward and the source of infection determined. Figure 1-3 shows the epidemic curve describing an outbreak of infectious hepatitis in Ogemaw County, Michigan. One of the two cases that occurred in early April was responsible for the subsequent 61 cases. The other case was unrelated to this outbreak.

(1) The curve suggests a common-source outbreak since all of the cases fall within a 30-day period, which is consistent with the known incubation period for hepatitis A [i.e., 15–50 days (average 25–30)].

(2) The cases were epidemiologically linked to the index case (onset April 6) who prepared glazed doughnuts and applied icing to pastry.

b. **Type II, or propagated, epidemic curves** are characterized by cases occurring over more than one incubation period of the disease. The shape of the curve suggests either person-to-person transmission or a continuing common-source outbreak. Figure 1-4 shows the epidemic curve describing an outbreak of viral hepatitis A transmitted from person to person.

B. **Person** refers to characteristics that describe the host (see IV A 2). While no two people are exactly alike, many people share certain characteristics that place them in a certain segment of the population. For example, people in a segment of the population because of a particular characteristic (age) may be placed in a different segment of the population with a different characteristic (sex). The occurrence of a disease in certain segments of the population can reveal information about host immunity, host exposure, or source of infection.

1. In the era before measles vaccine, 90% of reported cases occurred in children younger than age 10 years, and 95% occurred by age 15 years. Adults did not get measles because they were immune from childhood exposure.

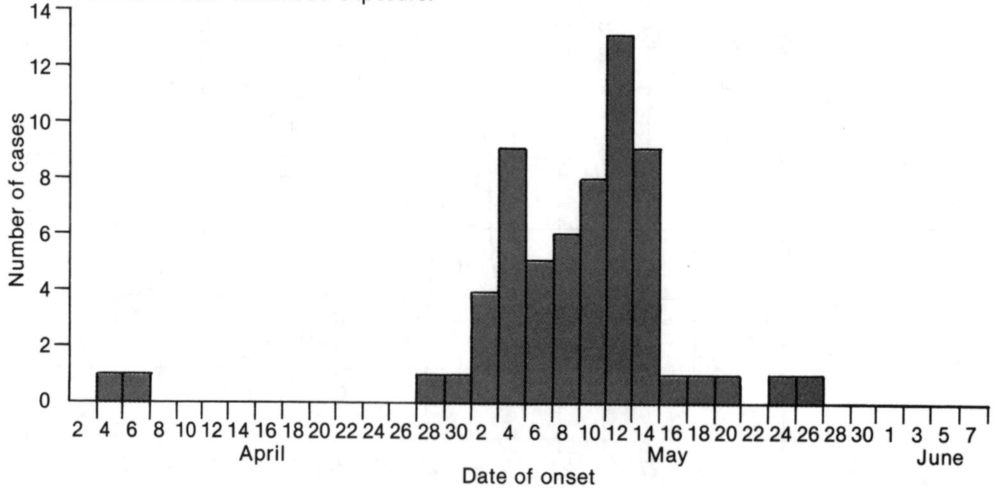

Figure 1-3. Reported cases of infectious hepatitis in Ogemaw County, Michigan, from April to May 1968. (Reprinted from National Communicable Disease Center: *Hepatitis Surveillance Report*, no 29. Atlanta, NCDC, September 1968, p 13.)

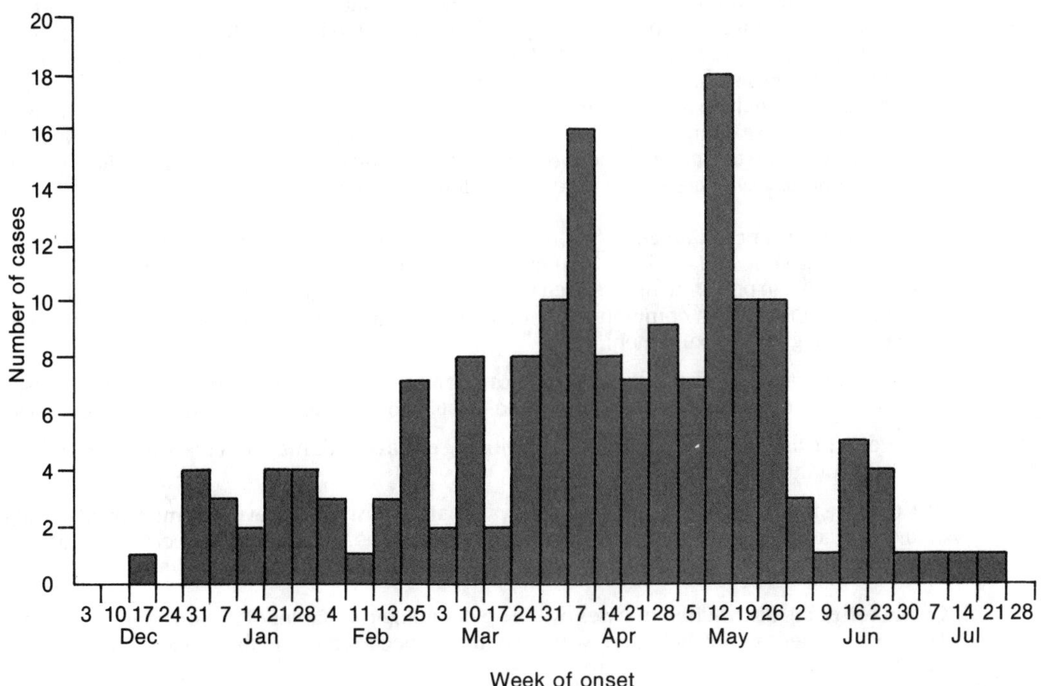

Figure 1-4. Reported cases of viral hepatitis by week of onset in Santa Lucía, Uruguay, from December 1967 to July 15, 1968. (Reprinted from National Communicable Disease Center. *Hepatitis Surveillance Report,* no 29. Atlanta, NCDC, September 1968, p 24.)

2. In the adult population, certain diseases are more common in one sex than the other, primarily because of differences in exposure to biologic agents that cause disease. In the 1960s and 1970s, malaria was more common in men, many of whom acquired the disease during military service in Southeast Asia.

3. During the 1960s and 1970s, the pattern of hepatitis changed. Before 1965, it was primarily hepatitis A that was more common in rural areas in individuals age 5–14 years. Since then, hepatitis has shown a higher urban than rural incidence and a shift to males age 15–29 years. Since many of these men admitted to parenteral drug abuse, this shift is probably due to hepatitis B.

4. In a foodborne outbreak, a particular food can be incriminated by showing that people who ate a particular item (exposed) were more likely to get sick than the group who did not (not exposed).

C. **Place** refers to a specific geographic point or area and to the features, factors, or conditions that exist in or describe the environment **in which the disease occurred**. It is the spot where the agent of disease and the susceptible host come together (see IV A 3). It can be as specific as a place of residence or as broad as an urban area. Place is primarily used to determine the source of infection, but it may be used to determine the mode of transmission.

VII. INVESTIGATION OF AN EPIDEMIC.

Epidemics, like diseases, do not occur by chance; they require that a harmful agent comes into contact with a group of susceptible hosts in the proper environment. The purpose of an investigation of an epidemic is to describe the outbreak and to explain how and why the outbreak took place. There are seven basic steps in conducting an investigation.

A. **Verify the diagnosis** of the disease under investigation.

1. **Laboratory tests** may be used; however, make certain that the results are reliable by having the tests confirmed by another laboratory, repeated, or both.

2. **Clinical criteria** may be used when laboratory results are not available or are unreliable.
   a. Subclinical or mild illnesses will be missed.
   b. Similar, but unrelated illnesses, will be included in the case count.

3. **Epidemiologic criteria** may be added to the clinical and laboratory diagnosis to restrict further the cases under investigation. For example, during the 1976 investigation of legionnaires' disease in Philadelphia, no laboratory test was available to confirm a diagnosis. Consequently, a clinical diagnosis of a febrile respiratory illness was created. Since the clinical definition was so broad as to include a large number of unrelated cases, an epidemiologic component was added to the case definition. To be counted as a case of legionnaires' disease, an individual must have had certain clinical findings; he or she must also have attended the American Legion convention or have entered the hotel where the convention was held.

B. **Establish the existence of an epidemic.** An unusual occurrence of the disease in a defined population must be shown. It could be a common disease in an unusual segment of the population (e.g., pneumonia in persons who attended the 1976 American Legion convention in Philadelphia) or an unusual disease in a common segment of the population (e.g., *Pneumocystis carinii* pneumonia in young homosexual men).

1. **Look for unrecognized or unreported cases** that may be part of the outbreak. Additional cases may be found by surveying physicians, hospitals, laboratories, and friends of known cases.

2. **Determine the population at risk** for developing disease. This may be a classroom, the whole school, or the entire community.

3. **Compare the incidence of disease in the population now with previous time periods,** using the case count as a numerator and the population at risk as a denominator. Because of seasonal variations, compare the incidence with the same time period in previous years.

C. **Characterize the distribution of cases** by the epidemiologic variables of person, place, and time. The key to understanding how and why the outbreak occurred lies in the proper analysis of the distribution of cases.

1. **The variable time** is used to construct an epidemic curve—that is, a graph showing the distribution of cases by date of onset in hours, days, weeks, or months. The shape of the curve may suggest either a common-source outbreak or person-to-person transmission (see VI A 3).
   a. If all cases occur within one incubation period of the disease, it suggests a point source of exposure.
   b. If the cases occur over several incubation periods, it suggests either person-to-person transmission or a continuing common source of exposure.
   c. If the incubation period of the disease is known, the curve could tell the probable time and possible source of infection.
   d. If the time of exposure can be determined, the incubation period of the disease can be determined.
   e. If the time of exposure is known, the incubation period can be used to establish a diagnosis in foodborne outbreaks. Chemical food poisoning due to ingestion of cadmium or copper has incubation periods that can be measured in minutes. Staphylococcal food poisoning has an onset in 2–6 hours, *Bacillus cereus* and *Clostridium perfringens* in 12–18 hours, and *Salmonella* and *Shigella* in 24–72 hours.

2. **The variable place** can be used to detect a source of infection by looking for possible clustering. Cases can be plotted by place of residence, place of work, position in a classroom, or any other geographic coordinates. Since clustering may only reflect population density, maps should be drawn comparing rates in different areas.

3. **The variable person** can be used to examine a population from different angles (segments) to determine the characteristics of the segment contracting the disease compared to the characteristics of the segment without the disease.

D. **Develop an hypothesis** that can adequately explain the distribution of cases observed. In developing an hypothesis, the odd case is extremely helpful. The exceptions frequently provide important information. The hypothesis should explain:

1. The source of infection

2. The mode of transmission

3. Every case (epidemic disease often overlies endemic disease, and some cases may be part of the normal background pattern)

E. Test the hypothesis

1. **Demonstrate differences in attack rates** in people exposed and not exposed to the source of infection. The ill group (cases) must be shown to be more often exposed to the risk factor than the well group (controls).
2. **Apply statistical tests** to data to determine if variations are random or if they are statistically significant (see Ch 3 III B 2 b). A statistically significant result may not be epidemiologically significant.
3. **Collect clinical and environmental specimens** for processing in a laboratory.
4. **Ignore the laboratory data** if they do not support the epidemiologic data.

F. Formulate a conclusion based on all pertinent evidence and the results of the hypothesis testing. A final report describing all aspects of the investigation should be prepared.

G. Institute control measures. Control measures should be instituted as early as possible in the outbreak investigation. Control measures are directed at one of the conditions or events in the infectious disease process (see III). The control measure selected depends on the disease under consideration.

BIBLIOGRAPHY

Centers for Disease Control: Premature mortality in the United States: public health issues in the use of years of potential life lost. *MMWR* 35:(suppl 2S), 1986.

Centers for Disease Control: *Principles of Epidemiology: A Three-day Training Course Prepared by the Training Program, Health Agencies Branch, Epidemiology and Demonstrations Activity.* Atlanta, CDC, 1974.

Centers for Disease Control: Years of potential life lost before age 65 and 85—United States, 1987 and 1988. *MMWR* 39:20–22, 1990.

Collins RN, Treger MD, Goldsky JB, et al: Interstate outbreak of *Salmonella newbrunswick* infection traced to powdered milk. *JAMA* 203:118–124, 1968.

Department of Health and Human Services, Public Health Service: *Healthy People 2000: National Health Promotion and Disease Prevention Objectives—Conference Edition.* Washington, DC, DHHS 1990.

Frost WH: *Snow on Cholera.* Originally published 1936. Reprint, New York, Hafner Publishing Company, 1965.

Institute of Medicine, Committee for the Study of the Future of Public Health: *The Future of Public Health.* Washington, DC, National Academy Press, 1988.

Last JM (ed): *Maxcy-Rosenau Public Health and Preventive Medicine,* 12th edition. Norwalk, CT, Appleton & Lange, 1986.

Lilienfeld AM, Lilienfeld DE: *Foundations of Epidemiology,* 2nd edition. New York, Oxford University Press, 1980.

Manual of the International Statistical Classification of Diseases, Injuries, and Causes of Death, 9th revision. Geneva, World Health Organization, 1978.

Mausner JS, Kramer S: *Epidemiology: An Introductory Text.* Philadelphia, WB Saunders, 1985.

National Center for Health Statistics: *Monthly Vital Statistics Report.* 39:17–18, 1990.

Sullivan LW: Healthy people 2000. *N Engl J Med* 323:1065–1067, 1990.

U.S. Preventive Services Task Force: *Guide to Clinical Preventive Services: An Assessment of the Effectiveness of 169 Interventions.* Baltimore, Williams & Wilkins, 1989.

World Health Organization: *The First Ten Years of the World Health Organization.* Geneva, WHO, 1948.

STUDY QUESTIONS

Directions: Each of the numbered items or incomplete statements in this section is followed by answers or by completions of the statement. Select the **one** lettered answer or completion that is **best** in each case.

Questions 1–3

In a classroom of 25 students (15 males and 10 females), 5 males develop hepatitis A over a 2-week period. During the next 6 weeks, an additional 3 males and 2 females develop the infection.

1. The attack rate of hepatitis A in this classroom is

(A) 25%
(B) 30%
(C) 35%
(D) 40%
(E) 45%

2. The secondary attack rate is

(A) 25%
(B) 30%
(C) 35%
(D) 40%
(E) 45%

3. The source of this outbreak is most likely

(A) common-source outbreak
(B) continuing common-source outbreak
(C) person-to-person transmission
(D) common-source outbreak with secondary person-to-person transmission
(E) continuing common-source outbreak with person-to-person transmission

4. Epidemiologic principles can be applied for all of the following purposes EXCEPT

(A) to evaluate drug therapy
(B) to determine a patient's prognosis
(C) to plan future health needs of the community
(D) to help to establish a diagnosis

5. The most important biologic trait that determines what disease an individual will contract is

(A) sex
(B) genetic predisposition
(C) ethnic origin
(D) age
(E) race

6. The most difficult mode of transmission to prevent is

(A) person-to-person spread
(B) droplet spread
(C) vector spread
(D) vehicle spread
(E) airborne spread

7. The first step in conducting an epidemic investigation is to

(A) determine the case count
(B) calculate the incubation period
(C) determine the population at risk
(D) verify the diagnosis
(E) collect appropriate samples

8. Etiologic agents that cause disease can be detected by using the

(A) incidence rate
(B) prevalence rate
(C) case-fatality rate
(D) adjusted rate
(E) disease index

1-D 4-B 7-D
2-A 5-D 8-A
3-D 6-E

Directions: Each item below contains four suggested answers of which **one or more** is correct. Choose the answer

A if **1, 2, and 3** are correct
B if **1 and 3** are correct
C if **2 and 4** are correct
D if **4** is correct
E if **1, 2, 3, and 4** are correct

9. YPLL has which of the following characteristics?

(1) It is a probability statement
(2) It is a measure of premature mortality
(3) It is used to determine the major causes of death in a population
(4) It can be used to compare premature mortality in different segments of the population

10. True statements about vital statistics include which of the following?

(1) The underlying cause of death is used to calculate vital statistics
(2) Vital statistics are used to determine public health priorities and programs
(3) Vital statistics provide the best information about the health of a population
(4) In documenting vital statistics, the death certificate can be certified by the funeral director

11. To calculate an indirect age-adjustment rate, one must

(1) know the age composition of the population being compared
(2) know the age-specific rates of the population being compared
(3) borrow age-specific rates from a larger population with more stable rates
(4) borrow the age composition of a standard population

12. The prevalence rate of a disease has which of the following characteristics?

(1) It measures all of the current cases of the disease in the community
(2) It depends on the duration of the disease process
(3) It depends on the incidence of the disease
(4) It can be used to determine the health care needs of a community

13. Adjusted rates have which of the following characteristics?

(1) They are easy to calculate
(2) They can be used for international comparisons
(3) They are frequently used in epidemic investigations of acute disease
(4) They are fictitious rates

9-C
10-B
11-B
12-E
13-C

Directions: Each group of items in this section consists of lettered options followed by a set of numbered items. For each item, select the **one** lettered option that is most closely associated with it. Each lettered option may be selected once, more than once, or not at all.

Questions 14–17

For each epidemiologic concept listed below, select the term that most appropriately describes it.

(A) Epidemiologic triangle
(B) Infectious disease spectrum
(C) Herd immunity
(D) Disease surveillance
(E) Disease eradication

14. Group expression of an illness

15. A unique combination of events resulting in disease

16. Explanation of why periodic outbreaks of certain diseases occur

17. Determination of the frequency with which disease occurs

Questions 18–22

For each condition listed below, select the angle or angles in the epidemiologic triangle that could be modified to prevent or decrease the occurrence of disease.

(A) Agent
(B) Agent and environment
(C) Host and environment
(D) Agent and host
(E) Agent, host, and environment

18. Lung cancer

19. Automobile accidents

20. Smallpox

21. Heart disease

22. Homicides

Questions 23–27

For each characteristic listed below, select the rate that is best described by it.

(A) Crude rate
(B) Direct age-adjusted rate
(C) Indirect age-adjusted rate
(D) Incidence rate
(E) Age-specific rate

23. Can be compared in different populations

24. Is used as an attack rate in epidemic investigations

25. Is a summary rate for the entire population

26. Is expressed as a standardized ratio

27. Borrows a standard population

Questions 28–32

For each disease listed below, select the factor in the infectious disease process that should be blocked to prevent disease.

(A) Agent
(B) Reservoir
(C) Transmission
(D) Portal of entry
(E) Susceptible host

28. Meningococcal meningitis

29. Polio

30. Sexually transmitted diseases

31. Tuberculosis

32. *Salmonella* infection

14-B 15-A 16-C 17-D 18-B 19-E 20-A 21-D 22-E 23-E 24-D 25-A 26-C 27-B 28-A 29-E 30-D 31-B 32-C

ANSWERS AND EXPLANATIONS

1–3. The answers are: 1-D *[V B 2 c]*, **2-A** *[V B 2 d]*, **3-D** *[VI A 3 a, b; VII C 1 a, b]*.
The attack rate of hepatitis A in this classroom is 40%. The attack rate is the number of cases divided by the population at risk, that is, 10 cases divided by 25 students, or 40%. Note that the sex-specific attack rate differs: 8/15 = 53% for males as compared to 2/10 = 20% for females.

The secondary attack rate is 25%. To calculate the secondary attack rate, subtract the initial case(s) from both the numerator and the denominator. Since the first five cases developed during a 2-week period, they must have been infected by the same external source. The secondary attack rate, therefore, is (10 − 5)/(25 − 5) = 5/20 = 25%. Note that the secondary attack rate for males (3/10 = 30%) is similar to the secondary attack rate for females (2/10 = 20%).

This epidemic curve suggests a common-source outbreak (five initial cases) with secondary person-to-person transmission (five cases) over one incubation period of 6 weeks. It could have been a continuing common-source outbreak, but this is unlikely because the initial cases were all in males, and the secondary cases were equally divided in both sexes.

4. The answer is B *[II D 1–8]*.
Epidemiologic principles are used to evaluate drug therapy, to plan future health needs of the community, and to help establish a diagnosis. Epidemiology is the study of the distribution and determinants of diseases or conditions in a defined population and, as such, cannot determine the prognosis of a disease process in a particular patient. Since the social and occupational characteristics determine what diseases an individual will be exposed to, these factors can be used to establish a diagnosis. Clinical trials use epidemiologic principles to evaluate the effectiveness of new drugs. Because epidemiology can be used to predict future occurrence of disease, it can also predict future health care needs of a community.

5. The answer is D *[IV A 2 a]*.
The most important biologic trait that determines what disease an individual will contract is age. Host factors that determine the occurrence of a disease include biologic traits (i.e., genetic characteristics, race, ethnic origin, sex, age) with which a host is born and social traits (i.e., lifestyle, diet, employment, residence, marital status), which a host acquires or develops. Age is the most important biologic factor because it is directly related to the ability of the body to respond to disease, acquired immunity, and exposure. For example, susceptible children are more likely to have subclinical disease than susceptible adults, and adults who have acquired immunity over time because of prior exposure are more likely to have no disease. In addition, adults in the workplace are exposed to different agents than children in school.

6. The answer is E *[III D 2 c]*.
The most difficult mode of transmission to prevent is airborne spread. An organism must be transmitted, either directly or indirectly, from one place to another. Direct transmission includes person-to-person spread by skin contact and droplet spread produced by coughing, sneezing, talking, or singing within close proximity of a susceptible host. Indirect transmission occurs when the reservoir and the susceptible host are separated; this type of transmission involves vector spread, vehicle spread, and airborne spread. Diseases disseminated by the airborne route are the most difficult to prevent and, thus, are able to infect large numbers of individuals in a relatively short period of time. For example, a new strain of influenza virus can spread throughout the world in a relatively short period of time.

7. The answer is D *[VII A]*.
The first step in conducting an epidemic investigation is to verify the diagnosis of the disease under investigation. The establishment of a clinical, laboratory, or epidemiologic case definition is necessary to determine an accurate case count so that the existence of an epidemic can be established. Once the existence of an epidemic has been established, the full investigation can then begin.

8. The answer is A *[V B 2 a]*.
Etiologic agents that cause disease can be detected by using the incidence rate. An incidence rate is defined as the number of new cases of a specific disease during a specified time period divided by the estimated midinterval population at risk. Because incidence rate is a measure of the rate at which healthy people develop disease during a specified time period, it is a statement of probability, and, as such, it can be used to determine factors that cause disease. A prevalence rate contains all current cases (old and new) in the numerator and is, therefore, determined by both the incidence and duration of disease and cannot be used to determine etiologic factors. Case-fatality rate only reveals what happens once the disease

occurs. Adjusted rates are fictitious rates and are used only to compare overall rates in different populations. Indexes are used when the true population at risk cannot be determined.

9. The answer is C (2, 4) *[V B 3 e].*
Years of potential life lost (YPLL) takes into consideration the age and cause of death and, hence, is a quantitative measure of premature mortality. Premature mortality can be compared in different segments of the population by calculating YPLL per 1000 population. Since YPLL takes into consideration only deaths in individuals under a specified age, it is not a probability statement, and it is not used to determine the major causes of mortality.

10. The answer is B (1, 3) *[IV F 1–2].*
Vital statistics provide the best information about the health of the population. The underlying cause of death is used to calculate public health statistics such as vital statistics. The underlying cause of death is the disease or injury that initiated the chain of events that resulted in death, and it is used to determine the major causes of mortality in the population. Death certificates must be certified by a physician, medical examiner, or coroner. Public health priorities are not determined by data analysis but by political considerations.

11. The answer is B (1, 3) *[V C 2 b (2) (a), (b)].*
To calculate an indirect age-adjustment rate, the age composition of the populations being compared must be known, and age-specific rates from a larger population with more stable rates must be borrowed. An indirect age-adjustment rate is a summary rate for the entire population. It is used to compare two populations and is used when the age-specific rates are unknown (as in developing countries) or when the age-specific rates of a population are unstable because of small numbers.

12. The answer is E (all) *[V B 2 b (1), (2)].*
The prevalence rate is the number of current cases (old and new) of a specified disease during a specified time period divided by the estimated midinterval population at risk. Since the prevalence rate includes all cases in the community, it is determined by both the incidence and the duration of the disease process. It can also be used to determine the health needs of the community, because it measures the total illness within the community.

13. The answer is C (2, 4) *[V C 2].*
Adjusted rates can be used for international comparisons, and they are fictitious; that is, by using a standard population or standard age-specific rates, adjusted rates equalize the differences in the population at risk so that the rates are comparable. Adjusted rates are difficult to calculate because the demographic composition of the population must be known. They are frequently used to compare birth and death rates in different populations and for international comparisons, because they take into consideration the age composition of the different populations. Adjusted rates are seldom used for epidemic investigations of acute diseases.

14–17. The answers are: 14-B, 15-A, 16-C, 17-D *[IV A–E].*
The infectious disease spectrum describes a group expression of illness in response to exposure to a particular biologic agent. Group expression ranges from no clinical evidence of disease to death from the disease.

The epidemiologic triangle describes the unique combination of events that results in disease. A harmful agent must come in contact with a susceptible host in the proper environment. The disease process can be prevented by eliminating the agent likely to cause disease, by immunizing susceptible hosts, or by modifying the physical environment.

Periodic outbreaks of disease occur when the proportion of susceptible individuals is high; these outbreaks subside as the proportion of immune individuals increases (herd immunity). Herd immunity explains why epidemics occur in a cyclic or periodic fashion. Outbreaks occur when the population contains a lot of susceptible individuals and disappear when most of the population is immune from either natural exposure or immunizations.

Disease surveillance refers to the process of determining the frequency with which certain diseases occur in the community. A good surveillance program consists of the collection, consolidation, analysis, and dissemination of relevant data.

18–22. The answers are: 18-B, 19-E, 20-A, 21-D, 22-E *[IV A 1–3].*
The agent and environment angles of the epidemiologic triangle could be modified to prevent or decrease the occurrence of lung cancer. Lung cancer can be prevented by eliminating the agents that cause

lung cancer. Most cases of lung cancer (90%–95%) are caused by smoking tobacco. A smaller percentage may be caused by environmental pollutants. Cigarette smoking is the major cause of preventable deaths in the United States. Approximately 320,000 deaths (16% of the total deaths) in 1984 were due to smoking.

The agent, host, and environment angles could be modified to prevent or decrease the occurrence of automobile accidents. The host can be taught to be a better driver. Agents that contribute to accidents, such as alcohol, can be eliminated. Environmental factors (stop signs, traffic lights) also can be modified to prevent injuries.

Smallpox was eliminated from the world by eliminating the agent that causes smallpox. There is no need to modify the host or the environment.

Heart disease is caused primarily by host factors and by agent factors. Host factors, such as genetics, cannot be modified. However, the host can improve his or her prognosis by exercise, diet, and the avoidance of tobacco (agents) that cause heart disease.

Homicides are a difficult public health problem that involve the agent, host, and environment. Environmental factors, such as crowding, and host factors, such as poverty and unemployment, are not easy to change. Control of the agent (i.e., guns and knives) may or may not solve this problem. Homicides are a major cause of death among minority groups.

23–27. The answers are: 23-E *[V C 3]*, **24-D** *[V B 2 a, c]*, **25-A** *[V C 1]*, **26-C** *[V C 2 b (2)]*, **27-B** *[V C 2 b (1)]*.
Rates are precise terms with precise definitions in terms of what constitutes the numerator and the denominator when they are expressed mathematically. They were developed to quantify or describe certain events in a population.

Age-specific rates are calculated for various segments of the population. Although they are difficult to calculate because more information about the demographic composition of the community must be known than with other rates, they can be used to compare events in similar age-groups in different populations.

Attack rates are a form of incidence rates—that is, the number of new cases of a specified disease during a specific time interval divided by the total population at risk during the same time interval. They are used in epidemic investigations using a particular population observed for a limited period of time.

Crude rates are summary rates for an entire population. They are easy to calculate because only the number of events and the total population are needed. They cannot, however, be used to compare events in different populations because the rate is dependent on the age-sex composition of the total population.

The indirect age-adjusted rate is expressed as a standardized ratio. It calculates the number of events that would have been observed if the two populations being compared had the same age-specific rates, which in this case are unknown. The age composition of the populations being compared and the total number of observed events in each population must be known, but age-specific rates from a larger population with stable rates must be borrowed. The total observed events is divided by the total expected events in that population multiplied by 100 and is expressed as a standardized ratio.

The direct age-adjusted rate calculates the rate that would have been observed if the populations being compared had the same age distribution; the age-specific rates in the populations being compared must be known, but the standard population from elsewhere must be borrowed.

28–32. The answers are: 28-A, 29-E, 30-D, 31-B, 32-C *[III A–F]*.
The agent should be blocked to prevent meningococcal meningitis. Chemoprophylaxis with either rifampin or sulfonamide is used to eliminate pharyngeal carriage of *Neisseria meningitidis* from household contacts of a known case of meningococcal meningitis and thus prevent secondary spread. The hope is that the family will be recolonized by a less pathogenic strain of the meningococcus, which would stimulate a natural immunity.

The susceptible host should be blocked to prevent polio. Polio vaccine is used to immunize a susceptible host against the wild poliovirus. Once immunity has been established in the host, exposure to the wild virus will not cause disease.

Most sexually transmitted diseases can be prevented by using a condom, which blocks the portal of entry into a susceptible host. Note that the condom does not block the agent's portal of exit from its reservoir.

New cases of tuberculosis can be prevented by eliminating the reservoir of infection. The reservoir of infection consists of individuals who have been infected with the tubercle bacillus, including patients with sputum-positive pulmonary tuberculosis, who can infect other people, and individuals with only a positive tuberculin skin test, in whom a dormant infection can be reactivated, causing disease. Chemotherapy can prevent spread from a patient with pulmonary tuberculosis, and chemoprophylaxis with isoniazid can prevent reactivation.

The mode of transmission should be blocked to prevent *Salmonella* infection. *Salmonella* infections are spread by poor personal hygiene or by a common vehicle such as contaminated food. *Salmonella* infections are controlled by emphasizing good hand-washing techniques and by not allowing infected individuals to work in an occupation that prepares or serves food for public consumption. *Salmonella* organisms are commonly found in chickens and turkeys purchased at market. Proper cooking of this common vehicle can prevent further transmission. The spread of all enteric diseases is prevented by having a safe water supply and an adequate sewage system.

2
Study Designs and Research Approaches

Brett J. Cassens
William C. Steinmann

I. GENERAL PRINCIPLES OF CLINICAL RESEARCH

A. Types of studies. Clinical studies usually are one of two major types.

1. **Observational studies** use existing phenomena in an attempt to understand aspects of health or illness. In these studies, the investigator controls neither the population nor the factors to which the population is exposed.
2. **Experimental studies** test the effect of some intervention on a certain aspect of health or illness. In these studies, the investigator controls both the population and the factors to which the population is exposed.

B. Purpose. The basic aim of clinical research is to advance knowledge of human health and illness. By nature, these studies require the participation of humans or, at least, a scrutiny of medical histories. Specific goals of medical studies may be to:

1. **Assess the health status or clinical characteristics** of a well-defined population or group of subjects. Examples of information that could be sought include:
   - **a.** The annual rate for suicide in teenagers
   - **b.** The immunization status of children in the community
   - **c.** The incidence of rabies in the state
2. **Probe the natural history of disease.** Examples of information that could be sought include:
   - **a.** The clinical course of retinopathy in diabetics over a 10-year follow-up period
   - **b.** The prognosis of patients with a solitary calcified pulmonary nodule
3. **Examine clinical decision-making processes.** Examples of information that could be sought include:
   - **a.** The best sequence of tests for screening and diagnosis of a patient with a solitary pulmonary nodule
   - **b.** The best screening test for glaucoma in the general population by general practitioners
   - **c.** The likelihood of colorectal cancer in patients with bright red blood per rectum
4. **Determine and assess treatment outcomes.** Examples of information that could be sought include:
   - **a.** Tumor response of laryngeal cancer in patients who receive radiation treatment
   - **b.** Benefit of medical treatment versus coronary artery bypass surgery for angina pectoris
5. **Identify and assess risk factors.** Examples of information that could be sought include:
   - **a.** The incidence of lung cancer in smokers compared to nonsmokers
   - **b.** The likelihood of rheumatoid arthritis in the offspring of affected patients
   - **c.** The likelihood of colorectal cancer in patients with colonic polyps

C. Study design principles

1. **Study characteristics** that are determined by the clinical information sought include:
   - **a.** The specific **type of study design** that will be employed
   - **b.** The **manner in which the study will be conducted,** including the criteria used for subject selection and treatment and the way in which data are collected and analyzed

2. **Strengths and limitations** of a clinical study are defined by the study methodology, which, in turn, affects the validity and generalizability of the results and possible conclusions.
   a. Each study design has well-defined and well-recognized strengths or weaknesses.
   b. The methods employed within any study design for the selection and treatment of subjects, data collection, and analysis can vary greatly, thereby strengthening or weakening the study design.

3. **Major methodologic considerations** are important in the conduct of a study, particularly issues of subject selection, data collection, and statistical analysis.
   a. **Subject selection**
      (1) It is important to consider whether or not the clinical subjects represent the target population (e.g., the general population).
      (2) How the subjects are selected also is important.
         (a) For example, if selected at random, it is important to determine whether all eligible subjects had an equal chance to be included in the study, who was excluded, and how those who were excluded may differ from those who participated.
         (b) If subjects were not selected at random, were the selection criteria objective enough to eliminate systematic error?
      (3) Was there a group (controls) with which to compare results?
   b. **Data collection**
      (1) **Prospective data collection** involves the collection of data after the study objectives are defined and the study design has been completed.
      (2) **Retrospective data collection** involves collection of data from sources that existed before the study objectives and design were defined. The data usually have been collected in the course of medical care or other statistical studies and are reviewed. For example, the data can be abstracted from medical charts to assess quality of care.
      (3) **Methods of data collection**
         (a) Data can be collected **directly** by examination of patients or **indirectly** by review and abstraction from hospital case records.
         (b) Treatments can be standardized to eliminate the possible influence of systematic error (**bias**).
         (c) Observations of outcomes or results can be standardized to prevent bias.
         (d) Treatments or other interventions can be allocated randomly—that is, patients have an equal chance of falling into any of the treatment groups.
         (e) Observers and subjects can be "masked," or "blinded," to ensure that observations are made and treatments are administered in an unbiased manner.
         (f) There may or may not be a control group with which to compare results.
   c. **Statistical analysis**
      (1) The **number of subjects should be sufficient** to generate enough statistical power to determine a true difference that may have existed between the comparison groups. Otherwise, a **type II (β) error** occurs, which is the failure to detect a true difference when it exists because the sample size is too small (see Ch 3 III B 4 b).
      (2) The **appropriate statistical tests or methods should be employed** based on characteristics of the data collected, including whether or not the distribution of the variables is normal (gaussian) and whether it is continuous or discrete.
      (3) The likelihood that differences found between two or more groups were due to chance (i.e., that no real difference existed) should be determined. Detection of a difference in the absence of a real difference is called **type I (α) error** (see Ch 3 III B 4 a).

4. **Other considerations** in assessing study methodologies include:
   a. The **limitations** of the study—all studies have limitations; the key is to determine whether those limitations affect the validity of the study design and the generalizability of results (e.g., can they be generalized for comparison to individual practices?)
   b. The **resources** that were available for the study
   c. The **ethical constraints** that were imposed by the study design
   d. The **population** that reasonably could have been expected to participate in the study
   e. The **costs and risks** that had to be considered in the design of the study

D. Principles used in assessing study data

1. **Efficacy** describes the true treatment or intervention effect under ideal conditions.

2. **Effectiveness** describes the true treatment or intervention effect under clinical conditions or in "routine" practice.

3. **Reliability** describes the reproducibility of test results.
4. **Validity** describes the accuracy and reliability of a test (i.e., the extent to which the test measures what it is supposed to measure).
5. **Causality** denotes direct effect. It requires that criteria, such as biologic plausibility, reproducibility, consistency, and temporal association, be met. Rarely can cause and effect be defined by a single clinical study.
6. **Bias** is a systematic error that is unintentionally made.
7. **Sensitivity** of a test describes the population of true abnormals or test-positives correctly identified (see Ch 3 IV E 1).
8. **Specificity** of a test describes the population of true normals or test-negatives correctly identified (see Ch 3 IV E 2).

II. SPECIFIC STUDY DESIGNS

A. Case report

1. **Description.** A case report is a brief, objective report of a clinical characteristic or outcome from a single clinical subject or event.
2. **Study questions.** A case report can address almost any clinical question or issue, including screening test results or treatment outcomes, or natural history findings. It commonly is used to report unusual or unexpected events, such as adverse drug reactions, or previously unrecognized diseases or disease characteristics.
3. **Examples**
   - **a.** A report of advanced proliferative diabetic retinopathy in a patient with no other clinical evidence of diabetes is an appropriate subject for a case report.
   - **b.** The initial report of phocomelia in a newborn of a woman on thalidomide is an example of how a single case report triggered further important investigations.
4. **Methodology**
   - **a.** A single noteworthy event first must be identified.
   - **b.** Data collection generally is retrospective, with a review and a descriptive summary of subjects or events.
   - **c.** No statistical analysis or comparison group is included in the design.
   - **d.** Although few conclusions can be drawn based on evidence from a single event or observation, case reports provide:
     - **(1)** A first report of unexpected findings
     - **(2)** Hypotheses for testing
     - **(3)** Definitions of issues for further study
5. **Strengths and limitations.** A case report often is the first evidence of an unexpected or unusual event, but the results rarely are generalizable.

B. Case series report

1. **Description.** A case series report is an objective report of a clinical characteristic or outcome from a group of clinical subjects.
2. **Study questions.** A case series report can address almost any clinical issue, including screening test results or treatment outcomes and natural history findings. However, it is most commonly used to describe clinical characteristics, such as signs and symptoms of disease or disease outcomes (e.g., the natural history of a series of patients with a specific disease).
3. **Examples**
   - **a.** A study of intraocular pressure control in 100 consecutive patients with primary open-angle glaucoma who were treated with laser trabeculoplasty and followed for 1 year is an appropriate subject for a case series report.
   - **b.** A well-known case series report is one that identified several children with birth defects who were born to mothers who had taken thalidomide.
4. **Methodology**
   - **a.** Subjects must be identified with regard to the clinical events or characteristics in question.

b. Data collection may be retrospective or prospective, but **a comparison or control group usually is not included**.
c. Descriptive statistics are calculated to define the proportion of subjects with the characteristics under study. Results often are compared incorrectly with the results from other populations or studies of similar subjects.
d. Conclusions generally are limited because there is no comparison group within the study.

5. **Strengths and limitations**
   a. Because the selection of study subjects often is unrepresentative or otherwise biased, the generalizability of the results usually is limited. The population from which the subjects were drawn as well as the selection criteria for subjects rarely are defined, which further limits generalizability.
   b. The lack of a control or comparison group also limits the generalizability of results.
   c. Conclusions often are incorrectly considered to be generalizable and valid based on the large number of study subjects.
   d. Study results are strengthened when a consecutive series of subjects (i.e., all eligible subjects) are included over a specified period of time.

C. Incidence and prevalence studies

1. **Description.** Incidence and prevalence studies actually are a type of case series report in which the entire study population is well defined and then uniformly surveyed regarding the parameters in question.

2. **Study questions.** Incidence and prevalence studies usually concern the occurrence of disease, but they also address the rate of other events (e.g., adverse side effects of drugs, death rate for a certain disease).
   a. **Incidence** is the occurrence of an event or characteristic over a period of time (e.g., the rate of staphylococcal food poisoning following lunch in a particular restaurant). Incidence is used to:
      (1) Describe the rate of disease occurrence over time (the time interval must be specified)
      (2) Assess patient survival, that is, the incidence of death over time or at a specific time after follow-up (e.g., the 5-year survival rate for breast cancer)
      (3) Compare the risk of disease between two or more populations
   b. **Prevalence** is the presence of an event or characteristic at a single point in time (e.g., the rate of previously undiagnosed glaucoma in a population of elderly individuals screened for ophthalmic disorders). Prevalence is used to:
      (1) Describe the burden of disease, especially undiagnosed disease
      (2) Define the rate of clinical characteristics in subjects with a specified disease (e.g., weight loss in patients presenting with terminal disorders)

3. **Examples**
   a. **Incidence.** The rate at which colon carcinoma develops in an elderly population over 1 year is an appropriate subject for an incidence study.
   b. **Prevalence.** The rate of unrecognized heart murmur in children presenting for their first preschool physical is an appropriate subject for a prevalence study.

4. **Methodology**
   a. A target population, which will be followed over a period of time for an incidence study or will be surveyed at a single point in time for a prevalence study must be identified.
   b. Events or characteristics must be measured and recorded by periodic reassessment over time for the incidence study and at a particular time for the prevalence study.
   c. A rate—the occurrence of the measured target event divided by the entire population —must be calculated.
   d. No statistical analytic component is included, although rates within populations or subpopulations can be compared.

5. **Strengths and limitations.** True rates are determined, which can serve as comparison measures between populations. However, these rates may provide poor estimates of infrequent or rare events. They may be affected adversely by sampling, which may be unrepresentative. True rates usually require description of population characteristics, such as age, race, and sex, to be meaningful.

D. Case-control study

1. **Description.** A case-control study is an **observational study** in which diseased and nondiseased (or affected and nonaffected) subjects are identified after the fact and then compared regarding specific characteristics to determine possible association or risk for the disease in question.

2. **Study questions**
   - **a.** Most often, case-control studies address issues relating to risk factors for disease by comparing the effect of a particular factor in diseased populations to that in nondiseased populations (e.g., comparison of the rate of cigarette smoking in lung cancer patients to that in persons without lung cancer).
   - **b.** Case-control studies also are used in clinical decision analysis to assess the differences in test positivity between diseased and nondiseased populations (e.g., to determine the likelihood that patients with urinary tract infection have more than 10 white cells in unspun urine samples before treatment, compared to those without infection).

3. **Examples**
   - **a.** A comparison of prior estrogen use in uterine cancer patients to that in age-matched controls without cancer to assess possible risk for uterine cancer is an appropriate subject for a case-control study.
   - **b.** The case-control study comparing thalidomide ingestion in mothers of children with phocomelia to ingestion in mothers with normal children clearly demonstrated that thalidomide ingestions were more common in mothers with affected children than in mothers with children who did not have phocomelia.

4. **Methodology**
   - **a.** Diseased and nondiseased populations must be identified, usually retrospectively.
   - **b.** The prevalence of characteristics under study—as well as other attributes that may be related to the presence of the disease or to the characteristics under study—must be determined.
   - **c.** Statistical comparison can be made between study groups of the characteristics under investigation to determine the likelihood that differences in these characteristics between diseased and nondiseased groups are real and not due to chance (α error).
   - **d.** Conclusions are useful for the generation of hypotheses and for initial evidence of putative risk associations. Results cannot be used to define causality.

5. **Strengths and limitations**
   - **a.** A case-control study is relatively easy and inexpensive to conduct, since neither prospective nor long-term follow-up is required.
   - **b.** There is a potential for bias in the selection of subjects, since a case-control study is not population-based.
   - **c.** Bias in data collection also may occur, since the presence or absence of disease usually is known to the subject and may be known to the study observer (making the study **unmasked**). Bias may also influence the recall of previous exposure by the subject if possible associations are known to the subject, such as the association between cigarette smoking and lung cancer.
   - **d.** The incidence rate of disease in a population can be neither determined nor compared between populations to assess possible risk (**relative risk**). However, the **odds ratio,** which provides an estimate of the relative risk of characteristics between diseased and nondiseased populations, can be calculated.

E. Cohort study

1. **Description.** A cohort study is an **observational study** in which exposed and nonexposed populations are identified and followed prospectively over time to determine the rate of a specific clinical disease or event.

2. **Study questions**
   - **a.** Most often, cohort studies address issues relating to risk factors for disease by comparing populations exposed to a factor under study to populations that are not exposed (e.g., an observation of smokers and nonsmokers over time to provide comparison rates for lung cancer).

b. Cohort studies also are used in clinical decision analysis to address the predictive value of test positivity or negativity (e.g., to determine the proportion of patients with positive sedimentation rates at screening who have a diagnosis of cancer on a subsequent definitive workup).

3. Examples

a. Follow-up in a population of adults who were exposed or not exposed as children to radiation of the neck to assess risk for thyroid cancer is an appropriate subject for a cohort study.

b. The cohort study of physicians comparing the incidence of lung cancer in smokers to that in nonsmokers was a landmark study in defining the association of cigarette smoking and lung cancer.

4. Methodology

a. A population of exposed and nonexposed (or test-positive and test-negative) individuals must be identified and followed prospectively.

b. Exposure to the risk factors under study and other potentially associated variables must be quantitated initially and over time.

c. The incidence of the target event, such as cancer, over time must be measured.

d. The incidence rate of an event for both exposed and nonexposed populations must be calculated. This calculation then can be compared to determine the relative risk and incidence in exposed and nonexposed individuals.

(1) Statistical comparison of the rates of disease occurrence or outcome parameters between the exposed and nonexposed groups allows one to assess the likelihood that the observed differences are real and not due to chance (α error).

(2) In addition, the **attributable risk** can be determined, which is the difference in the incidence of the event or disease between exposed and nonexposed populations. While relative risk is commonly used to assess possible etiology, attributable risk is used to measure the burden of disease in a population.

5. Strengths and limitations

a. Although costly and time-consuming due to the need for a large number of subjects and the prolonged follow-up, a cohort study allows for determination of a population-based rate of the disease or event under question and the relative risk.

b. Potential bias in recall and observations is lessened, since exposure can be determined prior to the onset of the disease or event.

c. As with a case-control study, causality cannot be determined by results from this type of study, since bias may result from unrecognized **confounding variables**. For example, alcoholism might be considered a risk factor for coronary artery disease (CAD), if it were true (but not recognized) that alcoholics are unusually heavy users of tobacco, a known risk factor for CAD.

F. Clinical trial

1. Description. A clinical trial is an **experimental study** design used to assess differences between two or more groups receiving different interventions or treatments.

2. Study questions

a. A clinical trial usually is used to compare outcomes between different treatments (e.g., antibiotic treatments for a specific disease or chemotherapy for a specific cancer).

b. It can also be used in clinical decision analysis to compare outcomes (e.g., to compare the differences in mortality from cancer among populations receiving different screening interventions).

3. Examples

a. A comparison of chemotherapy to chemotherapy plus radiation for laryngeal carcinoma is an appropriate topic for a clinical trial.

b. A recent randomized controlled clinical trial for breast cancer showed that radical mastectomy was, in some cases, no more effective than lumpectomy.

4. Methodology

a. A population with a clinical characteristic requiring intervention must be identified.

b. Subjects must be allocated, preferably randomly, to each of the treatment interventions. Treatments are administered in an identical or controlled manner to ensure uniformity of nontreatment covariants, which may affect outcomes.

c. Treatment outcomes and other results (e.g., side effects, costs, benefits) must be measured. Preferably, observations should be made while observers and patients are masked to the type of interventions (i.e., **double-blind**).
d. Rates of measured outcomes for the different treatment groups can be compared statistically.
e. The strongest evidence of differences in clinical outcome due to treatment effect is provided by the results of the statistical comparison.

5. **Strengths and limitations**
   a. A clinical trial allows for control of other clinical variables, which can also affect outcomes under investigation. Randomization minimizes the potential adverse effect from systemic error (**bias**).
   b. However, unmasking either the observer or subject often leads to biased observations and may invalidate the results.
   c. An insufficient number of subjects may lead to failure to detect true differences that may exist (**β error**).

III. META-ANALYSIS

META-ANALYSIS is a relatively new form of research that was uncommon in the literature in the early 1980s but is increasingly being used. Readers of medical literature are obliged to evaluate the quality of these reviews as carefully as they would evaluate original trials.

A. Description. Meta-analysis seeks to combine the results of several clinical studies on the same subject to derive a definitive conclusion from the varied, and sometimes contradictory, results. The term meta-analysis was coined by Glass (1976).

1. Similar to a review article, a meta-analysis begins with a literature review identifying studies of a similar research question.
2. Unlike a review article, however, meta-analysis attempts to analyze statistically the aggregate results to derive a single integrated conclusion.

B. Study questions. Meta-analysis may be used to:

1. Decide on the best clinical approach to a problem based on several related studies
2. Scrutinize studies to explain why research results differ
3. Identify new directions for research

C. Examples. Subjects for meta-analysis abound. Recent examples include:

1. Fibrinolytic therapy for acute myocardial infarction
2. Postoperative irradiation in breast cancer treatment
3. Steroid treatment of acute hepatitis and of chronic obstructive pulmonary disease

D. Methodology

1. **Formulation of a meta-analysis** includes qualitative and quantitative techniques.
   a. **Qualitative aspects** include:
      (1) Developing the research question to be analyzed
      (2) Comprehensively reviewing the literature for relevant clinical studies
      (3) Selecting an outcome variable common to the studies
      (4) Evaluating the studies to identify similarities or to explain differences among them
   b. **Quantitative aspects** of meta-analysis employ a variety of statistical tools. Goodman (1991) cautions, however, that the application of these quantitative methods alone does not guarantee a valid meta-analysis unless a careful qualitative evaluation precedes the quantitative work. Quantitative analysis must include:
      (1) A statistical test of homogeneity (i.e., are the studies similar enough to be legitimately compared?); heterogeneous results cannot be combined for a meta-analysis
      (2) A means of pooling appropriate data and statistically analyzing these combined data to derive a "definitive result"

2. **Meta meta-analysis** evaluates the quality of meta-analysis. Halvorsen (1986) has established criteria for such a critique.
   a. **Methods of search.** How did the researchers identify the relevant studies (i.e., was a computerized search or a review of citations of other review articles used)? How complete was the search?
   b. **Eligibility criteria.** How did the meta-analysts decide which pieces of research to include in their evaluations?
   c. **Number of studies.** How many research studies were selected for analysis?
   d. **Outcome variable.** Which variables were selected from each article to be included in the statistical analysis? Each original article may provide several outcome variables, not all of which may be included in the other articles or be of particular interest to the meta-analysis.
   e. **Study design.** What were the specific type or types of studies used in the analysis, and how many of each type were used? Study designs may include retrospective, prospective, open, or blinded, to name a few.
   f. **Results used in combining studies.** Were the data from all studies pooled to arrive at the conclusions, or were the actual results of each study analyzed?
   g. **Test of homogeneity** [see III D 1 b (1)]
   h. **Statistical methods.** To enable the reader to verify the results of the analysis, the researchers should indicate the specific statistical methods and the specific computer program used for the analysis.

E. Weakness of meta-analysis may result when:

1. The qualitative critique of the studies is overshadowed by the single meta-analytic result
2. The pooled results are not germane to a specific patient's situation; variations in individual cases must be accounted for when applying generalized conclusions

IV. ETHICS OF CLINICAL STUDIES

A. Definition. Ethics of clinical studies concern the balance of risks and benefits an individual experiences as a human subject (see Chapter 15). In contemporary society, it is assumed that individuals volunteer freely as research subjects. History shows many examples of coercion however.

1. Under National Socialism, non-Aryan Germans were unwilling subjects (victims) of medical research often designed to "purify" the races. Injection of coloring into the eyes of living subjects to give them the desired blue-grey appearance is one such example.
2. In the United States, prison inmates and military personnel have been assigned to research studies either involuntarily or without full knowledge of the potential risks.
3. More commonly today, unethical practitioners offer untried treatments to terminally ill patients. While still under development, therapies are provided often at substantial cost to desperate individuals blinded to potential risks.

B. Protection of human subjects

1. **Institution Review Boards (IRBs),** or **Human Subjects Committees,** are federally mandated councils. Institutions in which humans are subject to clinical studies must elect these committees to oversee research carried out in the institution.
   a. **Personnel.** IRBs are composed of medical personnel, attorneys, and lay representatives.
   b. **Purpose.** The IRB reviews research proposals for both scientific merit and ethical concerns. IRB approval requires an appropriate consent form, which is provided to all subjects for their signature prior to entry in a study.
2. **Experimental consent forms** may vary in length and detail among different IRBs. Certain elements are uniform in all consent forms.
   a. All consent forms present a brief summary of the **purpose and nature of the experiment.**
   b. **Likely risks and benefits** of the experimental procedure are listed. Particular emphasis is given to potential dangers.
   c. A **guarantee to guard the privacy** of medical results is provided.
   d. The **voluntary nature of participation** is detailed, and the subject is informed of her right to withdraw from the study at any time.

Experimental Subject's Bill of Rights

The faculty and staff of the University of California, San Diego, wish you to know:

Any person who is requested to consent to participate as a subject in a research study involving a medical experiment, or who is requested to consent on behalf of another, has the right to:

1. Be informed of the nature and purpose of the experiment
2. Be given an explanation of the procedures to be followed in the medical experiment, and any drug or device to be used
3. Be given a description of any attendant discomforts and risks reasonably to be expected from the experiment
4. Be given an explanation of any benefits to the subject reasonably to be expected from the experiment, if applicable
5. Be given a disclosure of any appropriate alternative procedures, drugs, or devices that might be advantageous to the subject, and their relative risks and benefits
6. Be informed of the avenues of medical treatment, if any, available to the subject after the experiment if complications should arise
7. Be given an opportunity to ask any questions concerning the experiment or the procedures involved
8. Be instructed that consent to participate in the medical experiment may be withdrawn at any time, and the subject may discontinue participation in the medical experiment without prejudice
9. Be given a copy of a signed and dated written consent form when one is required
10. Be given the opportunity to decide to consent or not to consent to a medical experiment without the intervention of any element of force, fraud, deceit, duress, coercion, or undue influence on the subject's decision

If you have questions regarding a research study, the researcher or his/her assistant will be glad to answer them. You may seek information from the Human Subjects Committee—established for the protection of volunteers in research projects.

Figure 2-1. Example of experimental subject's Bill of Rights. [Reprinted from Human Subjects Committee: *Experimental Subject's Bill of Rights.* University of California, San Diego (based on California State Assembly Bill 1752, 1978).]

e. Potential study participants are assured that they **may withdraw without prejudice** to future medical care. That is, if they decline to participate or enter a study and later drop out, they will still be eligible to receive medical care as they would have before.

f. All study subjects have the **right to question the investigator** directly about the study.

g. **Experimental subject's Bill of Rights.** To assure that research subjects are aware of their rights as subjects, all researchers must provide study participants with a list of the items required to be included in the study consent form. Such lists are called experimental subject's Bill of Rights and include items discussed in IV B 2 a–f. Figure 2-1 shows a sample Bill of Rights.

BIBLIOGRAPHY

Bailer JC III, Mosteller F (eds): *Medical Uses of Statistics.* Waltham, MA, NEJM Books, 1986.

Glass GV: Primary, secondary and meta-analysis of research. *Educ Res* 5:3–8, 1976.

Goodman, SN: Have you ever meta-analysis you didn't like? *Ann Intern Med* 114:244–246, 1991.

Halvorsen KT: Combining results from independent investigations: meta-analysis in medical research. In: *Medical Uses of Statistics.* Edited by Bailer JC, Mosteller F. Waltham, MA, NEJM Books, 1986, pp 392–416.

Hulley, SB, Cummings SR (eds): *Designing Clinical Research.* Baltimore, Williams & Wilkins, 1988.

Sachs HS, et al: Meta-analysis of randomized controlled trials. *N Engl J Med* 316:450–455, 1987.

STUDY QUESTIONS

Directions: Each of the numbered items or incomplete statements in this section is followed by answers or by completions of the statement. Select the **one** lettered answer or completion that is **best** in each case.

1. Bias is unlikely to invalidate cohort studies used to assess risk of exposure because

(A) data collection is prospective
(B) large numbers of subjects usually are included
(C) exposure usually is determined prior to disease occurrence
(D) actual relative risk can be determined

2. A case series report is useful for addressing all of the following clinical issues EXCEPT

(A) the natural history of a specific disease
(B) the clinical characteristics of a disease
(C) the outcomes from two different treatments
(D) unusual or unexpected findings resulting from a new treatment

Directions: Each item below contains four suggested answers of which **one or more** is correct. Choose the answer

A if **1, 2, and 3** are correct
B if **1 and 3** are correct
C if **2 and 4** are correct
D if **4** is correct
E if **1, 2, 3, and 4** are correct

3. Clinical study designs that routinely incorporate the use of a control or comparison group include

(1) clinical trials
(2) case-control studies
(3) cohort studies
(4) case series reports

4. Results from clinical trials may be invalidated by

(1) an inadequate number of subjects
(2) biased observations
(3) unmasked observations
(4) an unrepresentative sample

5. Before an individual can participate in a clinical study, which of the following requirements must be met?

(1) The individual must demonstrate a detailed understanding of the study
(2) The IRB must approve the scientific basis of the study
(3) The individual must be offered reasonable compensation for participation
(4) Substantial risks of the study must be explained to the individual subject

---

1-C
2-C
3-A
4-E
5-C

Directions: The group of items in this section consists of lettered options followed by a set of numbered items. For each item, select the **one** lettered option that is most closely associated with it. Each lettered option may be selected once, more than once, or not at all.

Questions 6–10

For each case history described below, select the study design it most appropriately illustrates.

(A) Case series report
(B) Case-control study
(C) Clinical trial
(D) Cohort study
(E) Case report

6. A total of 300 newly diagnosed patients with laryngeal cancer are allocated to treatment with either surgical excision alone or surgical excision plus radiation treatment.

7. A 39-year-old man who presents with a mild sore throat, fever, malaise, and headache is treated with penicillin for presumed streptococcal infection. He returns after a week with hypotension, fever, rash, and abdominal pain. He responds favorably to chloramphenicol, after a diagnosis of Rocky Mountain spotted fever is made.

8. A total of 3500 patients with thyroid cancer are identified and surveyed by patient interviews regarding past exposure to radiation.

9. A total of 10,000 Vietnam veterans, half of whom are known by combat records to have been in areas where Agent Orange was used and half of whom are known to have been in areas where no Agent Orange was used, are asked to give a history of cancer since discharge.

10. Patients admitted for carcinoma of the stomach are age- and sex-matched with fellow patients without a diagnosis of cancer and surveyed as to smoking history to assess the possible association of smoking and gastric cancer.

6-C
7-E
8-A
9-D
10-B

ANSWERS AND EXPLANATIONS

1. The answer is C *[II E 5].*
Bias is unlikely to invalidate cohort studies used to assess relative risk of exposure since exposure is usually determined prospectively (i.e., after the study has begun) and prior to the onset of disease. Hence, subjects are unaware of their disease status as are those who are recording the exposure. Although a large number of subjects may be needed, size alone would not invalidate the results if the investigators ensured that the sample size was adequate to provide the statistical power to determine a true difference in exposure—if a difference truly exists—and, thus, avoid a β error problem. Although prospective data collection will help prevent bias in observations, knowledge of possible associations, if present, could invalidate cohort design.

2. The answer is C *[II B 1–4].*
A case series report is not useful for addressing the outcomes from two different treatments. A case series report is an objective report of a clinical characteristic or outcome from a group of clinical subjects. A case series report can address almost any clinical issue, but it is particularly useful for describing the natural history of disease or treatment outcomes. The major limitation of case series reports is that no control group is included for comparison. Hence, the results or observations may not be valid or generalizable to other populations, since the population studied may be highly selected as may the treatment or other evaluations. It is not acceptable or logical to compare the results of one case series with those of other studies, since there is no way to ensure that the subjects, interventions, or treatments were equal.

3. The answer is A (1, 2, 3) *[II B, D–F].*
Clinical study designs that routinely incorporate the use of a control or comparison group include clinical trials, case-control studies, and cohort studies. Clinical trials, which are most commonly used to compare treatments, routinely use controls who receive a placebo, no active drug, or alternative treatments for comparison of efficacy. In case-control studies, nondiseased subjects (controls) serve as comparison for those with disease. In cohort studies, the comparison is between those who were exposed and those who were not exposed to the possible etiologic agents. Case series reports, which typically do not use a control group, often compare results with the results of other studies; however, these comparisons should never be used for statistical analyses.

4. The answer is E (all) *[II F 5].*
Results from clinical trials may be invalidated by an inadequate number of subjects, biased observations, unmasked observations, or an unrepresentative sample. A clinical trial is an experimental design used to assess differences between two or more groups receiving different interventions or treatments. The design is such that at least one control group is included for comparison of the planned interventions. A population with a clinical characteristic requiring intervention must be identified. Preferably, observations should be made while observers and patients are masked to the type of interventions being made to avoid biased observations. This is called a double-blind study, as compared to a single-blind study when only the subject or the observer is masked to the intervention. An insufficient number of subjects may lead to failure to detect true differences that may exist (β error). It should also be noted that statistically significant results can occur due to chance (α error) even in the most rigorous study design, such as a well-designed clinical trial where treatments are randomized and subjects and observers are masked. An unrepresentative sample of subjects may, by chance, be enrolled in the study. For example, in a trial of antibiotic treatment of pneumonia, a greater number of patients in the experimental medication group might die because of heart attack. Whether the new drug caused heart attack or whether the group taking the experimental treatment was unrepresentative because of a high prevalence of coronary artery disease might be unknown at the time the study results are analyzed.

5. The answer is C (2, 4) *[IV B].*
Before an individual can participate as an experimental subject, the Institution Review Board (IRB) must approve the scientific basis of the study, and substantial risks must be explained to the potential subject. Subjects are expected to have a general knowledge of the nature and purpose of the study but a more detailed, explicit understanding of the risks and benefits. IRB responsibility includes both the scientific and ethical merits of an experiment. Aside from reimbursement for costs incurred as a research participant, subjects often are not compensated. A central concern, among others, is the possible financial coercion a stipend could represent. Potential financial gain could unduly influence a poor person's "option" to decline participation. Conversely, lack of affordable transportation or child-care could prevent poor people from entering studies.

6–10. The answers are: 6-C *[II F 1–4]*, **7-E** *[II A 1–4]*, **8-A** *[II B 1–4]*, **9-D** *[II E 1–4]*, **10-B** *[II D 1–4]*. The laryngeal cancer patients are part of a clinical trial, since subjects receive one treatment or the other with the intent to compare outcomes between the two treatment groups. This study is strengthened if patients are allocated randomly to the treatment groups to minimize possible selection bias. Obviously, it would be difficult to mask patients and observers to treatment regimens to prevent biased observations. Case reports and case series reports do not include comparison groups; cohort and case-control studies, which use controls, are used to assess risk association.

The 39-year-old man represents a case report, which is a description of a single interesting case. It is an important report that serves to alert other physicians of the possibility of misdiagnosing a potentially fatal disease if untreated. No control or comparison subjects are included.

The thyroid cancer patients represent a case series report, because there is no active group for comparison of exposure with those who have the disease. The report processes information on a unique population as to their experience with previous radiation exposure. In a case-control study, the assessment of risk would also be retrospective. In addition, a population of those without disease would be included, from whom a history of past exposure would be obtained for comparison with estimates of relative risk.

The Vietnam veterans represent a cohort study, which relies on classification of subjects as to exposure to Agent Orange and then looks forward in time to assess the incidence of cancer. This type of study, where historic data are used to define previous exposure, is sometimes called a **historic cohort design**. True incidence rates can be determined for this disease in this population in contrast to case-control studies. In case-control studies, those with disease would first be identified, then past exposure would be assessed for possible risk associations. Unlike case series reports, controls are available for comparison.

The patients admitted for stomach carcinoma are part of a case-control study, since the study uses both diseased and nondiseased populations for comparisons of previous exposure to cigarette smoking. Cancer incidence rates among exposed or nonexposed individuals obviously could be determined. There is great potential for bias in recall of exposure by individuals with cancer, given the current knowledge of association of lung cancer and cigarette smoking. Case series do not include control groups for comparison nor can they be used for possible assessment of risk association.

3 Statistics

Lawrence D. Budnick

I. BASIC CONCEPTS

A. Statistics

1. **Definition.** Statistics is a scientific field that deals with the collection, classification, description, analysis, interpretation, and presentation of data.
   a. **Descriptive statistics** concerns the summary measures of data for a sample of a population.
   b. **Analytic statistics** concerns the use of data from a sample of a population to make inferences about the population.
   c. **Vital statistics** is the ongoing collection by government agencies of data relating to events such as births, deaths, marriages, divorces, and health- and disease-related conditions deemed reportable by local health authorities.

2. **Uses.** For the practicing physician, statistics has at least three important functions.
   a. Statistics is a scientific method that uses theory and probability to aid in the evaluation and interpretation of measurements and data obtained by other methods.
   b. Statistics provides a powerful reinforcement for other determinants of scientific causality.
   c. Statistical reasoning, albeit unintentional or subconscious, is involved in all scientific clinical judgments, especially with preventive medicine and clinical medicine becoming increasingly quantitative.

B. Data

1. **Definition.** Data are the basic building blocks of statistics and refer to the individual values presented, measured, or observed.

2. **Characteristics**
   a. **Population versus sample.** Data can be derived from a total population or a sample.
      (1) A **population** is the universe of units or values being studied. It can consist of individuals, objects, events, observations, or any other grouping.
      (2) A **sample** is a selected part of a population. The following are some of the more common types of samples.
         (a) In a **simple random sample,** each member of the population has an equal possibility of being chosen for the sample, with chance alone responsible for the selection of any member. The sample can be chosen by using a table of random numbers. Each individual in the population is numbered, and a list of random numbers is drawn from the table, with the sample size needed determining how many numbers to draw. This list of numbers represents the individuals chosen for the simple random sample.
         (b) In a **systematically selected sample,** a random starting point at the beginning of an ordered population is chosen, and then the remainder of the sample is chosen according to a predetermined selection schedule. For example, 100 students are ranked by age. Beginning with the fourth student, every tenth student is chosen (the students numbered 4, 14, 24, and so on).
         (c) In a **stratified selected sample,** the population is divided into sampling units that contain individuals, and a random sample of individuals **proportionate** to the size of the sampling unit is chosen from each sampling unit. For example, in a city, a proportion of residents who live in randomly selected blocks are chosen. The number of residents included depends on the size of the block.

(d) In a **cluster selected sample,** the population is divided into sampling units, or groups, and a random sample of groups is chosen. A complete count of the individuals in the chosen groups is undertaken. The sample is made up of groups, not individuals. For example, in a city, all of the residents who live in randomly selected blocks are chosen.

(e) In a **nonrandomly selected, or convenience, sample,** members of the population are chosen for the sample based on known factors. For example, of the 100 students ranked by age, the first 10 are chosen.

b. Ungrouped versus grouped

(1) **Ungrouped data** are presented or observed individually. An example of ungrouped data is the following list of weights (in pounds) for six men: 140, 150, 150, 150, 160, and 160.

(2) **Grouped data** are presented in groups consisting of identical data by frequency. An example of grouped data is the following list of weights for the six men noted above: 140 lb (one man), 150 lb (three men), and 160 lb (two men).

c. Quantitative versus qualitative

(1) **Quantitative data** are numerical, or based on numbers. An example of quantitative data is height measured in inches.

(2) **Qualitative data** are nonnumerical, or based on a categorical scale. An example of qualitative data is height measured in terms of short, medium, and tall.

d. Discrete versus continuous

(1) **Discrete data** are data for which distinct categories and a limited number of possible values exist. An example of discrete data is the number of children in a family, that is, two or three children, but not 2.5 children. All qualitative data are discrete.

(2) **Continuous data** are data for which there is an unlimited number of possible values. An example of continuous data is an individual's weight, which may actually be 159.232874 . . . lb but is reported as 159 lb.

e. The quality of measured data is defined in terms of the data's accuracy, validity, precision, and reliability.

(1) **Accuracy** refers to the extent that the measurement measures the true value of what is under study.

(2) **Validity** refers to the extent that the measurement measures what it is supposed to measure.

(3) **Precision** refers to the extent that the measurement is detailed.

(4) **Reliability** refers to the extent that the measurement is stable and dependable.

C. Distributions

1. Definition. A distribution is the complete summary of frequencies or proportions of a characteristic for a series of data from a sample or population.

2. Types of distributions

a. Binomial distribution is a distribution of possible outcomes from a series of data characterized by two mutually exclusive categories (see III D 2).

b. Uniform distribution, also called **rectangular distribution,** is a distribution in which all events occur with equal frequency.

c. Skewed distribution is a distribution that is asymmetric.

(1) A skewed distribution with a tail among the **lower values** being characterized is skewed to the left, or **negatively skewed**.

(2) A skewed distribution with a tail among the **higher values** being characterized is skewed to the right, or **positively skewed**.

d. Normal distribution, also called **gaussian** distribution, is a continuous, symmetric, bell-shaped distribution and can be defined by a number of measures (see III E).

e. Log-normal distribution is a skewed distribution when graphed using an arithmetic scale but a normal distribution when graphed using a logarithmic scale.

f. Poisson distribution is used to describe the occurrence of rare events in a large population.

II. DESCRIPTIVE STATISTICS

A. Measures of central tendency are characteristics that describe the middle or most commonly occurring values in a series; they are used as summary measures for the series. The series can consist of a sample of observations or a total population, and the values can be grouped or ungrouped. In this discussion, ungrouped data are presented and analyzed.

1. Arithmetic mean

a. Definition. The arithmetic mean, or simply, the mean, is the sum of all values in a series divided by the actual number of values in the series.

b. Applications and characteristics

(1) The arithmetic mean is useful when performing **analytic manipulations**.

(2) The arithmetic mean is sensitive to an extreme value in the series.

c. Calculation. The arithmetic mean ($\bar{x}$) is determined as

$$\bar{x} = \frac{\Sigma x_i}{n}$$

where Σ = "the sum of"; x_i = each of the values in the series; and n = the number of values in the series. In describing a total population, the mean is symbolized by $\bar{\mu}$ and the number of the population by N.

d. Example. The ages (in years) of seven children seen in an emergency room after a house fire are: 1, 1, 1, 2, 4, 6, and 6. Since the sum of the ages (Σx_i) is 21 years and the number of children (n) is 7, the arithmetic mean ($\bar{x}$) of the ages is 21 years divided by 7, or 3 years.

2. Median

a. Definition

(1) The median is the value that divides the series into two equal groups so that half of the values are greater than and half are less than the median.

(2) The median is the middle of the **quartiles** (the values that divide the series into quarters) and the middle of the **percentiles** (the values that divide the series into defined percentages).

b. Applications and characteristics

(1) The median is not sensitive to one or more extreme values in a series; therefore, in a series with an extreme value, the median is a more representative measure of central tendency than the arithmetic mean.

(2) The median is used in **cumulative frequency graphs** (see II C 7) and in **survival analysis** (see III M).

c. Calculation

(1) **In a series with an odd number of values,** the values in the series are arranged from lowest to highest, and the value that divides the series in half is the median.

(2) **In a series with an even number of values,** the two values that divide the series in half are determined, and the arithmetic mean of these two values is the median.

(3) An alternative method for calculating the median is to determine the 50% value on a cumulative frequency curve.

d. Example. Among the seven children discussed in II A 1 d, three are younger than and three are older than 2 years. The median age of the children, therefore, is 2 years.

3. Mode

a. Definition. The mode is the most commonly occurring value in a series of values. A series may have no mode (i.e., no value occurs more than once) or it may have several modes (i.e., several values equally occur at a higher frequency than the other values in the series).

b. Applications and characteristics

(1) The mode is useful in **practical epidemiological work,** such as determining the peak of disease occurrence in the investigation of a disease outbreak.

(2) The mode is the most difficult measure of central tendency to manipulate mathematically; no analytic concepts are based on the mode.

c. Calculation. The mode is calculated by determining which value or values occur most in a series.

d. Example. Among the seven children discussed in II A 1 d, the most common age is 1 year. Therefore, the mode of the ages is 1 year.

4. Geometric mean

a. Definition. The geometric mean is the **nth root** of the product of the values in a series of **n values**.

b. Applications and characteristics

(1) The geometric mean is more useful and representative than the arithmetic mean when describing a series of reciprocal or fractional values, such as for a series of serum antibody titers or a series with a skewed distribution.

(2) The geometric mean can be used only for positive values.

(3) It is more difficult to calculate than the arithmetic mean.

c. **Calculation.** The geometric mean is most easily determined by calculating first the logarithms of the values, then the arithmetic mean of the logarithms, and finally the antilogarithm of the calculated arithmetic mean. Any logarithm base can be used. The geometric mean (GM) is determined as

$$GM = \sqrt[n]{(x_1)(x_2)\ldots(x_n)} \quad \text{or} \qquad (1)$$

$$GM = \text{antilog } 1/n\ [\Sigma(\log x_i)] \qquad (2)$$

The geometric mean is easier to calculate using equation (2).

d. **Example.** Five individuals are tested for serum antibody to influenza A/Lilliput and are found to have reciprocal serum titers of 10, 100, 100, 10,000, and 1,000,000 (i.e., the serum titers are 1:10, 1:100, 1:100, 1:10,000, and 1:1,000,000, respectively).

(1) Using a base of 10, the **logarithms of the reciprocal titers** are: 1, 2, 2, 4, and 6, respectively. (Note that with $10^1 = 10$, $10^2 = 100$, $10^3 = 1000$, the logarithms to the base of 10 are 1, 2, 3, respectively.)

(2) Because the sum of the logarithms is 15 and there are five values, the arithmetic mean of the logarithms is calculated as 15 divided by 5, or 3.

(3) Finally, the **geometric mean** is calculated as the antilogarithm of 3 (to the base of 10), or 1000 (recall that $10^3 = 1000$). Therefore, the geometric mean reciprocal serum titer for the five individuals tested is 1000. (Incidentally, the geometric mean serum titer is 1:1000.)

B. **Measures of dispersion** are characteristics that are used to describe the spread, variation, and scatter of a series of values. The series can consist of a sample of observations or a total population, and the values can be grouped or ungrouped.

1. **Range**

a. **Definition.** The range is the difference between the highest and lowest values in a series.

b. **Applications and characteristics**

(1) The range is used to measure data spread.

(2) The range provides no information concerning the scatter within the series.

c. **Calculation.** The range is calculated by subtracting the lowest value in the series from the highest value.

d. **Example.** Five individuals arrested for driving automobiles under the influence of alcohol are age 17, 18, 18, 21, and 26 years. The range of ages is 26 years minus 17 years, or 9 years.

2. **Variance**

a. **Definition.** The variance is the sum of the squared deviations from the mean divided by the number of values in the series minus 1.

b. **Applications and characteristics**

(1) The principal use of the variance is in calculating the standard deviation.

(2) The variance is mathematically unwieldy.

c. **Calculation.** The variance (V; also symbolized by s^2) is determined as

$$V = \frac{\Sigma(\bar{x}-x_i)^2}{n-1}, \quad \text{or} \qquad (3)$$

$$V = \frac{\Sigma x_i^2}{n-1} - \frac{(\Sigma x_i)^2}{n(n-1)} \qquad (4)$$

where Σx_i^2 = the sum of the squares of all x_i; and $(\Sigma x_i)^2$ = the square of the sum of all x_i. Usually, the variance is easier to calculate using equation (4). In describing a total population, the variance is symbolized by σ^2.

d. **Example.** The age variance for the five drunk drivers, whose mean age is 20 years, can be calculated in two ways using the data in Table 3-1.

(1) The variance can be calculated by using equation (3).

(a) The sum of the squares of the deviations, which is 54, is divided by the number of values minus 1, which, in this example, is 5 minus 1, or 4.

(b) The variance, therefore, equals 13.5. In this example, the unit of the variance is years^2.

(2) Alternatively, the variance can be calculated by using equation (4).

(a) The squares of the ages of the five individuals are summed (Σx_i^2) and then divided by the number of values minus 1, which, in this example, is 2054 divided by 4, or 513.5.

Table 3-1. Calculating the Age Variance for Five Individuals

Case Number	Age (years)	Mean Age (years)	Deviation from the Mean	Deviation from the Mean Squared	Age Squared
1	17	20	−3	9	289
2	18	20	−2	4	324
3	18	20	−2	4	324
4	21	20	+1	1	441
5	26	20	+6	36	676
Total	100	. . .	0	54	2054

(b) The squared sum of all the ages is then calculated, which is 100^2, or 10,000.
(c) The squared sum is divided by both the number of values and the number of values minus 1, which, in this example, is 10,000 divided by 20, or 500.
(d) The variance is calculated by subtracting 500 from 513.5, which equals 13.5—the same as calculated using the first formula.

3. Standard deviation

a. Definition. The standard deviation is the positive square root of the variance.

b. Applications and characteristics

(1) The standard deviation is the most useful measure of dispersion. In certain circumstances, quantitative probability statements that characterize a series, a sample of observations, or a total population can be derived from the standard deviation of the series, sample, or population (see III E 3).
(2) When the standard deviation of any sample is small, the sample mean is close to each individual value.
(3) When the standard deviation of a random sample is small, the sample mean is likely to be close to the mean of all the data in the population.
(4) The standard deviation decreases when the sample size increases.

c. Calculation. The standard deviation (SD; also symbolized by s) is determined as

$$SD = +\sqrt{V}$$

In describing a population, the standard deviation is symbolized by σ, and V is variance, as above.

d. Example. The variance of the ages of the five drunk drivers is 13.5 years^2. The standard deviation of the ages, which is the positive square root of the variance, is 3.7 years.

4. Coefficient of variation

a. Definition. The coefficient of variation is the ratio of the standard deviation of a series to the arithmetic mean of the series. The coefficient of variation is unitless and is expressed as a percentage.

b. Applications and characteristics

(1) The coefficient of variation is used to compare the relative variation, or spread, of the distributions of different series, samples, or populations or of the distributions of different characteristics of a single series.
(2) The coefficient of variation can be used only for characteristics that are based on a scale with a true zero value.

c. Calculation. The coefficient of variation (CV) is calculated as

$$CV\ (\%) = \frac{SD}{\bar{x}} \times 100$$

d. Example

(1) In a typical medical school, the mean weight of 100 fourth-year medical students is 140 lb, with a standard deviation of 28 lb. The coefficient of variation for weight is 28 lb divided by 140 lb, or 20%.
(2) The mean height for these students is 66 in, with a standard deviation of 6 in. The coefficient of variation for height is 6 in divided by 66 in, or 9%.
(3) Based on the coefficients of variation, therefore, the relative spread of weight among the students is greater than that of height.

C. Graphic or pictorial presentations of data are useful in simplifying the presentation and enhancing the comprehension of data. All graphs, figures, and other pictures should have clearly stated and informative titles, and all axes and keys should be clearly labeled, including the appropriate units of measurement. Visual aids can take many forms; some basic methods of presenting data are described below.

1. Pie chart

a. Description. A pie chart is a pictorial representation of the proportional divisions of a sample or population, with the divisions represented as parts of a whole circle.

b. Example. Figure 3-1 is an example of a pie chart.

2. Venn diagram

a. Description. A Venn diagram shows the degrees of overlap and exclusivity for two or more characteristics or factors within a sample or population (in which case each characteristic is represented by a whole circle) or for a characteristic or factor among two or more samples or populations (in which case each sample or population is represented by a whole circle). The sizes of the circles (or other symbols) need not be equal and may represent the relative size for each factor or population.

b. Example. Figure 3-2 is an example of a Venn diagram.

3. Bar diagram

a. Description. A bar diagram is a tool for comparing categories of mutually exclusive discrete data. The different categories are indicated on one axis, the frequency of data in each category is indicated on the other axis, and the categories are compared by the lengths of the bars. Because the data categories are discrete, the bars can be arranged in any order with spaces between them.

b. Example. Figure 3-3 is an example of a bar chart.

4. Histogram

a. Description. A histogram is a special form of bar diagram that represents categories of continuous and ordered data. The bars are adjacent to each other on the x-axis (**abscissa**), and there is no intervening space. The frequency of data in each category is depicted on the y-axis (**ordinate**), and the width of the bar represents the interval of each category.

b. Example. Figure 3-4 is an example of a histogram.

5. Epidemic curve

a. Description. An epidemic curve is a histogram that depicts the time course of an illness, disease, abnormality, or condition in a defined population and in a specified location and time period. The time intervals are indicated on the x-axis, and the number of cases during each time interval are indicated on the y-axis. An epidemic curve can help an investigator determine such outbreak characteristics as the peak of disease occurrence (mode), a possible incubation or latency period, and the type of disease propagation (see Ch 1 VI A 3).

b. Example. Figure 3-5 is an example of an epidemic curve.

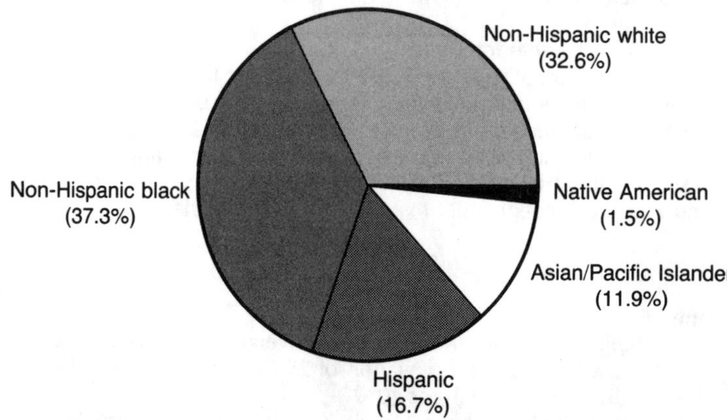

Figure 3-1. Pie chart showing the distribution of cases of tuberculosis by race and ethnicity in the United States in 1989. Because the non-Hispanic black cases are most common, they make up the largest piece of the "pie." [Reprinted from Centers for Disease Control: Summary of notifiable diseases, United States, 1989. *MMWR* 38(54):45, 1989.]

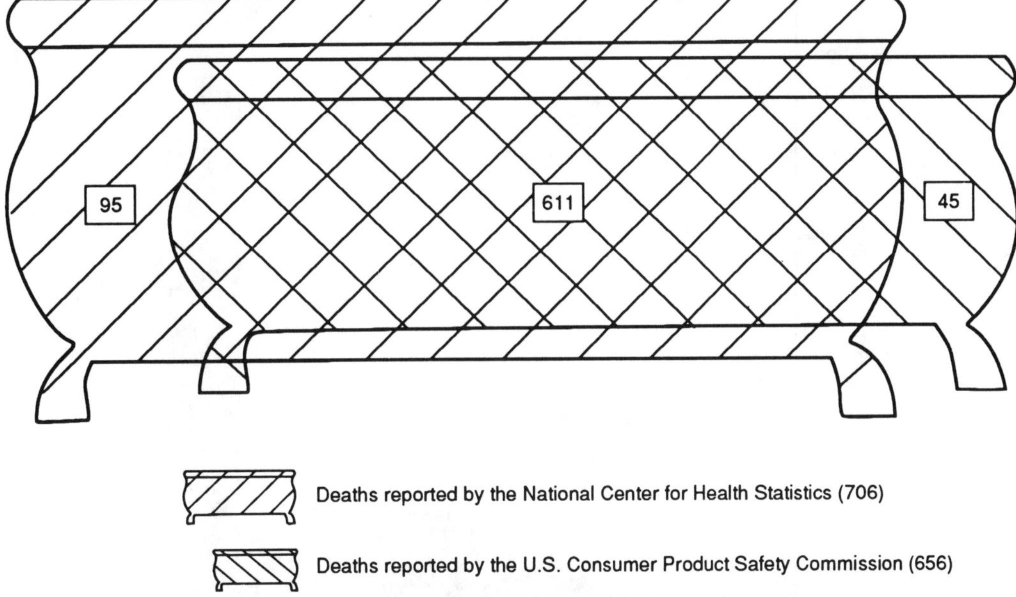

Figure 3-2. Venn diagram showing the number of bathtub-related drownings by reporting source in the United States from 1979 to 1981. While each source reported some deaths that the other did not, most deaths (611 out of 751) were reported through both surveillance systems.

6. **Frequency polygon**
   a. **Description.** A frequency polygon is a representation of the distribution of categories of continuous and ordered data and, in this respect, is similar to a histogram. The x-axis depicts the categories of data, and the y-axis depicts the frequency of data in each category. In a frequency polygon, however, the frequency is plotted against the midpoint of each category, and a line is drawn through each of these plotted points. The frequency polygon can be more useful than the histogram because several frequency distributions can be plotted easily on one graph.
   b. **Example.** Figure 3-6 is an example of a frequency polygon.

7. **Cumulative frequency graph**
   a. **Description.** A cumulative frequency graph also is a representation of the distribution of continuous and ordered data. In this case, however, the frequency of data in each category represents the sum of the data from that category and from the preceding categories. The

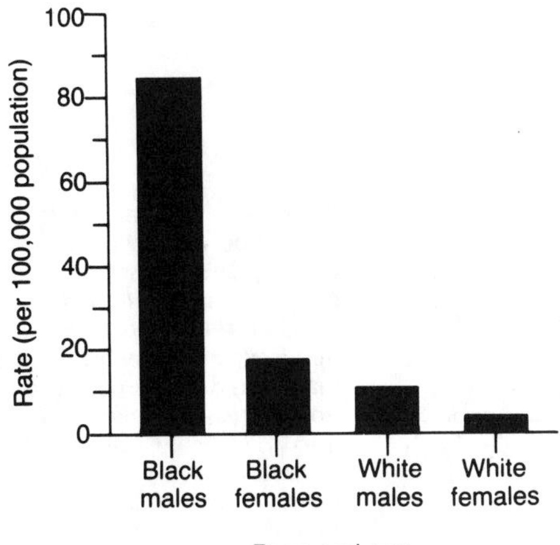

Figure 3-3. Bar chart showing the homicide rate (per 100,000 population) for persons age 15–24 years by race and sex in the United States in 1987. Homicide rates in black males were more than 4, 7, and 21 times greater than homicide rates in black females, white males, and white females, respectively. (Reprinted from Centers for Disease Control: Homicide among young black males —United States, 1978–1987. *MMWR* 39:869–873, 1990.)

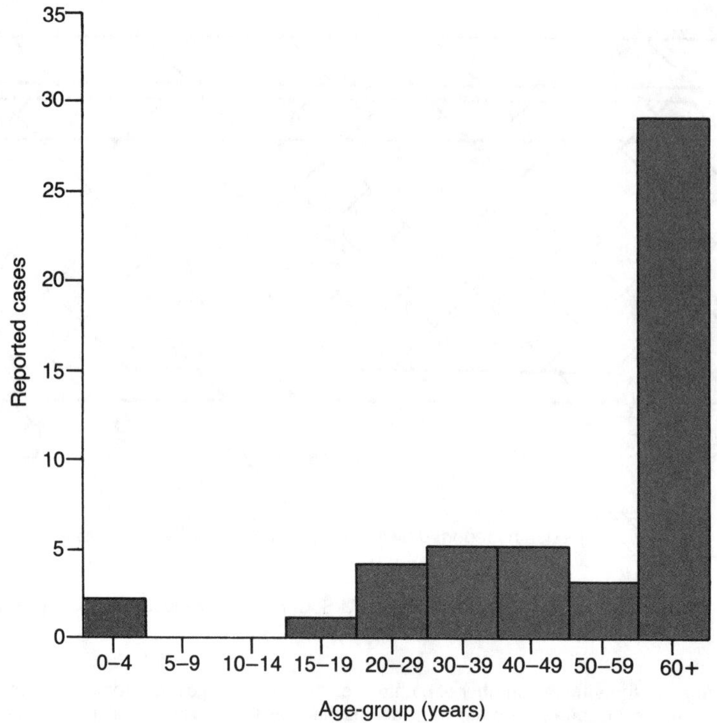

Figure 3-4. Histogram showing the number of reported cases of tetanus by age-group in the United States in 1989. The greatest number of reported cases occurred among persons age 60 years and older. [Reprinted from Centers for Disease Control: Summary of notifiable diseases, United States, 1989. *MMWR* 38(54):41, 1990.]

x-axis depicts the categories of data, and the y-axis is the cumulative frequency of data, sometimes given as a percentage ranging from 0% to 100%. The cumulative frequency graph is useful in calculating distributions by percentile, including the median, which is the category of data that occurs at the cumulative frequency of 50%.

b. Example. Figure 3-7 is an example of a cumulative frequency graph.

8. Box plot

a. Description. A box plot is a representation of the quartiles [25%, 50% (median), and 75%]

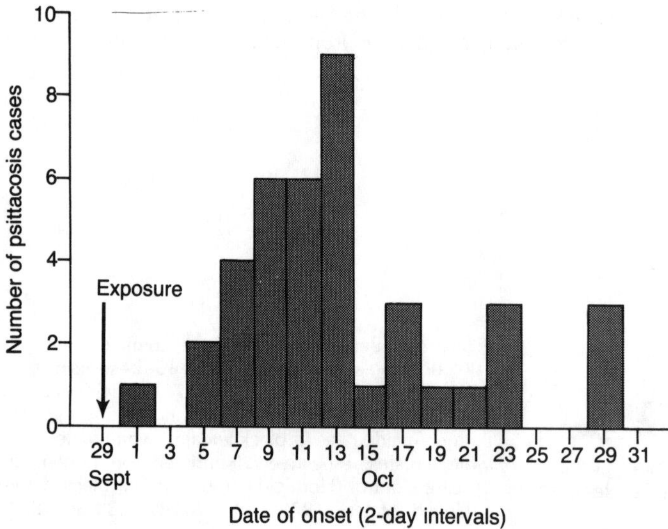

Figure 3-5. Epidemic curve showing the number of confirmed psittacosis cases by date of onset in a turkey processing plant in North Carolina in October 1989. The investigation of this occupational outbreak suggested that it was due to exposure to viscera from diseased turkeys. (Reprinted from Centers for Disease Control: Psittacosis at a turkey processing plant—North Carolina, 1989. *MMWR* 39:460–469, 1990.)

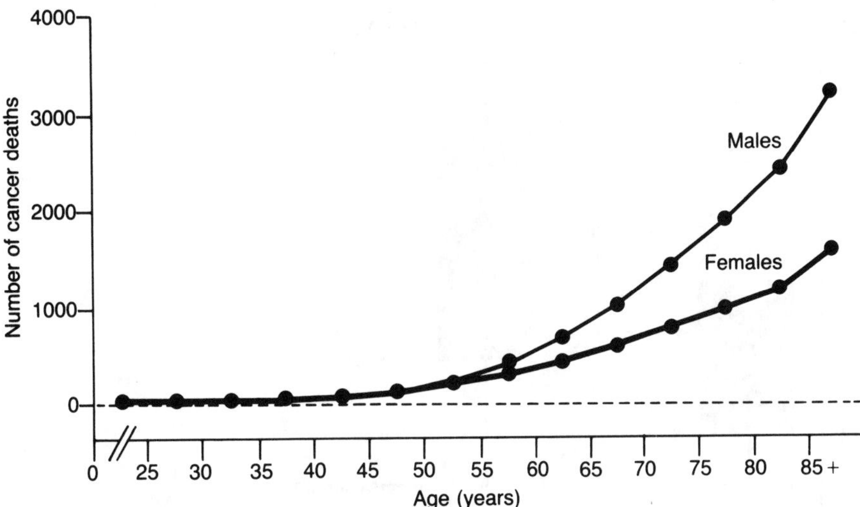

Figure 3-6. Frequency polygon showing cancer mortality by age-group and sex in Canada in 1988. Males had a greater mortality than females, and mortality increased for both sexes with increasing age. (Reprinted from National Cancer Institute of Canada: *Canadian Cancer Statistics 1990*. Toronto, Canada, 1990, p 35.)

and the range of a continuous and ordered data set. The y-axis can be arithmetic or logarithmic. Box plots can be used to compare the different distributions of data values.

b. Example. Figure 3-8 depicts the weights of 50 patients from hospital A and 60 patients from hospital B (the values in the box plot for patients from both hospitals are labeled).

(1) The median weight of patients in hospital B is 60 kg and the interquartile range (from 25% to 75%) is 22.5 kg, which is the difference between 47.5 kg and 70 kg. The range of weights of all the patients in hospital B is 45 kg (the difference between 35 kg and 80 kg).

(2) The patients in hospital A tend to weigh less and to have a narrower distribution of weights (the median weight is 50 kg, the interquartile range is 15 kg, and the total range is 30 kg).

9. Spot map

a. Description. A spot map, also called a **geographic coordinate chart,** is a map of an area with the location of each case of an illness, disease, abnormality, or condition identified by a spot or other symbol on the map. A spot map often is used in an outbreak setting and can help an investigator determine the distribution of cases and characterize an outbreak if the population at risk is distributed evenly over the area.

b. Example. Figure 3-9 is an example of a spot map.

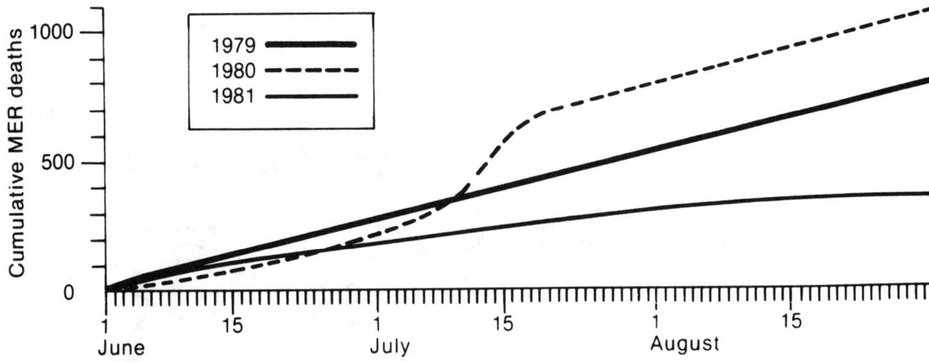

Figure 3-7. Cumulative frequency graph showing the cumulative medical examiner-reported (*MER*) deaths in St. Louis from June through August for the years 1979, 1980, and 1981. Note the increased slope of the curve in mid-July 1980, during which there was a severe heat wave. [Reprinted from Centers for Disease Control: *Surveillance Summaries*, 32 (suppl 1). Atlanta, CDC, February 1983, p 455.]

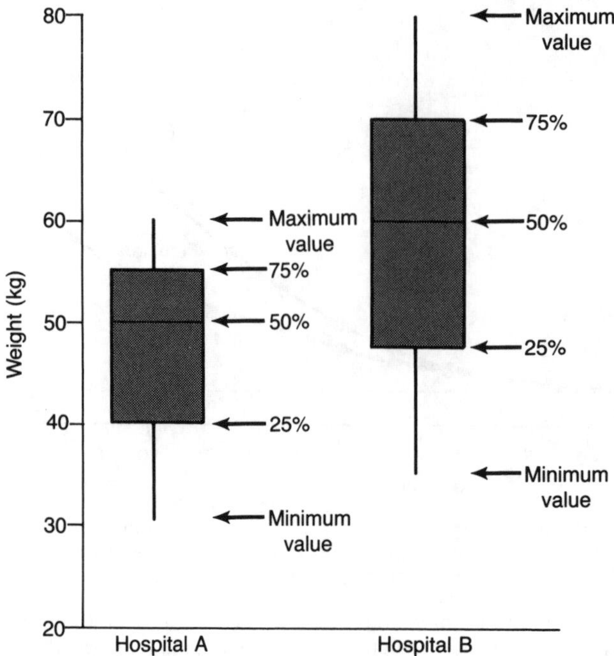

Figure 3-8. Box plots showing the distribution of weights of patients from hospital A and hospital B.

III. ANALYTIC STATISTICS

A. Probability

1. **Definition.** The probability of a specified event is the fraction, or proportion, of all possible events of a specified type in a sequence of almost unlimited random trials under similar conditions. The probability of an event is the likelihood the event will occur; it can never be greater than 1 (100%) or less than 0 (0%).

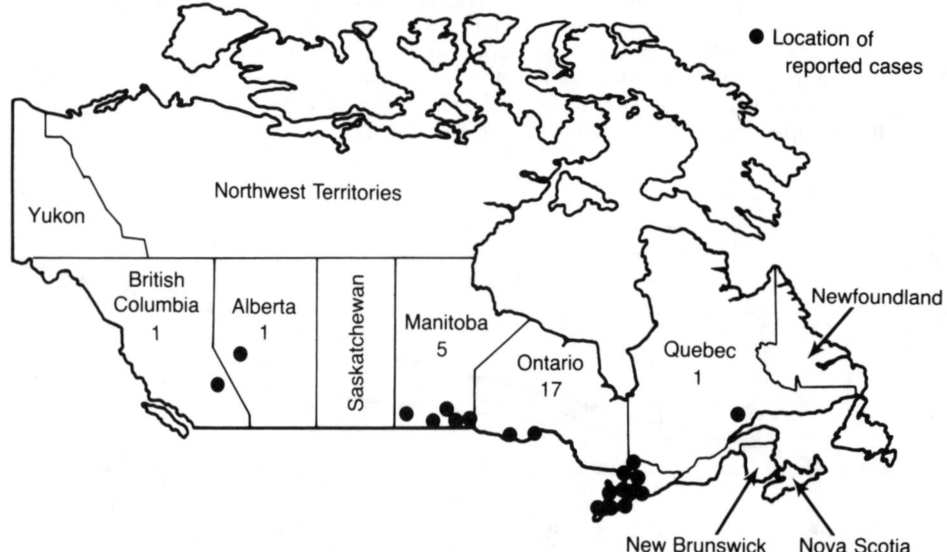

Figure 3-9. Spot map showing the distribution of indigenous Lyme disease cases by province in Canada from 1977 to 1989. Most cases occurred near the southern border with the United States. (Reprinted from Centers for Disease Control: Lyme disease—Canada. *MMWR* 38:677–678, 1989.)

2. Applications and characteristics

- **a.** The probability values in a population are distributed in a definable manner that can be used to analyze the population.
- **b.** Probability values that do not follow a distribution can be analyzed using nonparametric methods (see III K).

3. Types. Some commonly used probability distributions include:

- **a.** Binomial distribution (see III D)
- **b.** Normal distribution (see III E)
- **c.** The t distribution (see III F)
- **d.** Chi-square distribution (see III H)

4. Calculation. The probability of an event is determined as

$$P(A) = A/N$$

where P(A) = the probability of event A occurring; A = the number of times that event A actually occurs; and N = the total number of events during which event A can occur.

5. Example. A medical student performs venipunctures on 1000 patients and is successful on 800 in the first attempt. Assuming that all other factors are equal (i.e., random selection of patients), the probability that the next venipuncture will be successful on the first attempt is 80%.

6. Rules

a. Additive rule

(1) Definition. The additive rule applies when considering the probability of one of at least two mutually exclusive events occurring, which is calculated by adding together the probability value of each event.

(2) Calculation. The probability of only one of two mutually exclusive events is determined as

$$P(A \text{ or } B) = P(A) + P(B)$$

where P(A or B) = the probability of event A or event B occurring.

(3) Example. About 6.3% of all medical students are black, and 5.5% are Hispanic. The probability that a medical student will be either black or Hispanic is 6.3% plus 5.5%, or 11.8%.

b. Multiplicative rule

(1) Definition. The multiplicative rule applies when considering the probability of at least two independent events occurring together, which is calculated by multiplying the probability values for the events.

(2) Calculation. The probability of two independent events occurring together is determined as

$$P(A \text{ and } B) = P(A) \times P(B)$$

where P(A and B) = the probability of both event A and event B occurring.

(3) Example. About 6.3% of all medical students are black and 36.1% of all students are women. Assuming race and sex are independent selection factors, the percentage of students who are black women should be about 6.3% multiplied by 36.1%, or 2.3%.

B. Null hypothesis

1. Definition. The null hypothesis, symbolized as H_0, is the hypothesis that the samples or populations being compared in an experiment, study, or test are similar. Any difference discerned is ascribed to chance and not to any other measurable factor.

2. Applications and characteristics

a. The null hypothesis is initially accepted and considered true for all analytic comparisons. The hypothesis to be tested (the **alternative hypothesis**) must be stated before the study is designed, so the null hypothesis can be tested using statistical techniques.

b. The null hypothesis is used to define **significant difference**. Significant difference, also called **statistical significance,** is the conclusion that a difference between the samples, populations, or both is due to factors other than chance. In other words, a significant difference occurs if the null hypothesis is disproved.

(1) When the null hypothesis is rejected, at least one alternative hypothesis is accepted; that is, factors other than chance account for the difference.

(2) **When no significant difference can be shown** between two populations, they may still be different; that is, accepting the null hypothesis does not necessarily mean the populations are identical.

(3) The **level of confidence** for rejecting the null hypothesis is arbitrary. One conventional cutoff for defining a significant difference is **5%;** that is, if the probability that the difference is due to chance is 5% or less, then the null hypothesis is rejected, and an alternative hypothesis is accepted. This level of confidence refers to the type I error (see III B 4 a).

(4) Statistical testing using probability values evaluates only the null hypothesis and does not evaluate the accuracy of the proposed alternative hypothesis.

(5) The probability value provides no information about the extent that two variables are associated or differ. Statistically significant differences may not be clinically important, and clinically important differences may not be statistically significant.

(6) Probability values are associated with sample size. If the study is large, negligible differences may be associated with highly significant probability values, and if the study is small, strong associations may have insignificant probability values.

c. **Testing.** The null hypothesis can be tested using either one-tailed or two-tailed analytic tests.

(1) **One-tailed tests**

(a) A one-tailed test checks only one of the tails (the upper or lower tail) of the bell-shaped normal distribution curve (see III E 1 a).

(b) A one-tailed test is used to test a null hypothesis for which the alternative hypothesis is assumed to be directional—a situation for which the one-tailed test is more powerful than the two-tailed test.

(c) **Example.** In comparing the rates of cancer between a population exposed to a known carcinogen and a control population, a one-tailed analytic test can be used because the only alternative hypothesis of interest is that the exposure was harmful. It is assumed that the exposure was not beneficial.

(2) **Two-tailed tests**

(a) A two-tailed test checks both the upper and lower tails of the normal distribution curve.

(b) A two-tailed test is used to test a null hypothesis for which no assumptions are made concerning the alternative hypotheses.

(c) Two-tailed tests are especially useful when generating alternative hypotheses and, as such, are used more often than one-tailed tests.

(d) **Example.** In comparing the rates of death between two neighboring communities, a two-tailed analytic test is used to look for significant differences because no assumptions are made about the alternate hypotheses.

3. **Calculation.** The null hypothesis (H_0) and the alternative hypothesis (H_A) are determined as

$$H_0\colon P_1 - P_0 = 0, \text{ or } P_1 = P_0$$
$$H_A\colon P_1 - P_0 \neq 0, \text{ or } P_1 \neq P_0$$

where P_1 = the probability of the characteristic in the observed or studied sample or population; and P_0 = the probability of the characteristic in the hypothetical or control sample or population.

4. **Sampling errors** are errors due to chance and concern incorrect rejection or acceptance of a null hypothesis. The two types of sampling error are **type I** and **type II.**

a. **Type I error**

(1) **Definition.** A type I error, also called an **error of the first kind** or an **α error,** is the rejection of a null hypothesis that is actually true (Table 3-2). If the null hypothesis is false in a study, there can be no type I error. The probability of a type I error is equal to α.

(2) **Applications and characteristics**

(a) Statistical testing is based predominantly on the α error. Many studies testing a null hypothesis arbitrarily use an α error of 0.05 (5%) as the cutoff for rejecting the null hypothesis.

(b) Sample size determinations depend on the type I error and the type II error (see III B 4 b) as well as other parameters, such as the prevalence of the problem under study, the standard deviation, the amount of difference to be detected, and the relative number of experimental-to-control subjects.

Table 3-2. Sampling Errors

	Decision	
Null Hypothesis	**Accept**	**Reject**
True	Correct conclusion	Type I (α) error
False	Type II (β) error	Correct conclusion

(c) In studies designed to generate hypotheses, other values of the α error may need to be considered.

(d) Multiple comparisons and repeated testing for significance increase the likelihood of a type I error.

(i) When the null hypothesis is true, and n independent statistical tests are performed, the probability that at least one test will appear statistically significant ($p \leq 0.05$) is $1.0 - (0.95)^n$.

(ii) In studies that test multiple hypotheses, more stringent (i.e., lower) values for the α error or multivariate computerized methods can be used, but this assigns equal value to all alternative hypotheses. Alternatively, multiple comparisons of measures may best be done using significance tests to eliminate unnecessary alternative hypotheses and then using confidence intervals (see III G 2) to evaluate the remaining alternative hypotheses.

(3) Example

(a) In a study of hemoglobin levels of students in different high schools, the α error is defined as 5%. The mean hemoglobin level in one school is 14 g/dl and in another is 13 g/dl. The probability that this is due to chance is determined to be 15%, which is greater than the acceptable α error. The difference is not considered significant, and the null hypothesis is not rejected.

(b) However, if the study were repeated 100 times, the mean hemoglobin levels may appear significantly different statistically for five (5% of 100) of the trials, although there actually is no true difference between the populations. For these five trials, the null hypothesis has been incorrectly rejected, and a type I error has been made.

(c) If five tests are done, the probability that at least one significance test will appear "significant" by chance alone, even though the null hypothesis is true, is $1.0 - (0.95)^5 = 0.23$. If ten tests are done, then there is a $1.0 - (0.95)^{10} = 0.40$ probability of a type I error.

b. Type II error

(1) Definition. A type II error, also called an **error of the second kind** or a **β error,** is the acceptance of a null hypothesis as true when it actually is false (see Table 3-2). If the null hypothesis is true in a study, there can be no type II error. The type II error is inversely related to the type I error. The probability of a type II error is equal to **β.**

(2) Applications and characteristics

(a) The type II error is used to determine the **power of a study,** which equals **1 minus β**. The power of a study is the probability that the study would reject a null hypothesis as false when it actually is false (i.e., that the study would detect a difference of specified size that actually exists).

(b) As the difference between a false null hypothesis and a true alternative hypothesis increases, the probability of accepting the null hypothesis (the β error) decreases, and the power of the study increases.

(c) As the sample size increases, the power of the study increases.

(d) Power is most important when designing a study, in which the β error generally is at least double the α error. A power of 80% often is considered acceptable.

(3) Example. In the study of high school students, the β error is defined as 20%. Therefore, the power of the study is 80%. If there is a difference between the hemoglobin levels of the students, the probability of the study detecting the difference is 80% and of not detecting the difference is 20%.

C. Contingency table and degrees of freedom

1. Contingency table

a. Definition. A contingency table depicts the cross-classification of data according to two characteristics, each of which can be divided into two or more discrete and mutually exclusive categories.

(1) A contingency table in which there are more than two categories for either or both characteristics is called an **r × c table,** where r = the number of horizontal rows and c = the number of vertical columns.

(2) A contingency table in which the characteristics are divided into only two categories is called a **2 × 2,** or **fourfold, table.**

b. Application. The contingency table is a simple method for displaying data and is useful when performing chi-square and other tests (e.g., Fisher's exact test, Student's t tests, nonparametric tests).

c. Structure. The structure of a contingency table is depicted in Table 3-3, in which the value in each cell is represented by a, b, c, or d; the marginal values, which are subtotals, are represented by a + b, a + c, b + c, and c + d; and the grand total, which equals a + b + c + d, is represented by N.

d. Example. Table 3-4C is an example of a fourfold contingency table in which the sex and eye color of 50 schoolchildren are tabulated.

2. Degrees of freedom

a. Definition

(1) The degrees of freedom is the number of variables in a series or distribution that can be freely assigned values when the sum of the values is fixed.

(2) In a contingency table, the degrees of freedom is the number of cells available in the table that can be freely assigned values, assuming set and established marginal values. Once these cells have been assigned values, the values of all the remaining cells in the table are automatically determined.

b. Application. In a number of probability distributions, such as the **t distribution** and the **chi-square distribution,** the probability values vary with the number of degrees of freedom of the sample.

c. Calculation

(1) When the distribution has either a single row (r) or a single column (c), the number of degrees of freedom (df) is determined as

$$df = c - 1, \text{ if } r = 1, \text{ or}$$
$$df = r - 1, \text{ if } c = 1$$

(2) When the table has at least two rows and two columns, the number of degrees of freedom is determined as

$$df = (r - 1)(c - 1)$$

d. Example. In a fourfold table in which the sex and eye color of 50 schoolchildren are tabulated, the marginal values are 20, 30, 15, and 35, and the total is 50 (see Table 3-4A).

(1) It is determined that five boys have blue eyes, and all the children have either blue or brown eyes (see Table 3-4B). Therefore, the number of boys with brown eyes must be 15, the number of girls with blue eyes must be 10, and the number of girls with brown eyes must be 20 (see Table 3-4C). Because it is necessary to determine the value in only one cell to determine the value of all the cells, this table has 1 degree of freedom.

(2) Alternatively, the number of degrees of freedom could be determined from the equation. Since there are two rows and two columns, the number of degrees of freedom is calculated as

$$(2 - 1)(2 - 1) = 1$$

D. Binomial distribution

1. Definition. A binomial distribution of data is the distribution that results when there are only two mutually exclusive and, therefore, discrete outcomes in a series of independent trials of an event.

Table 3-3. The Structure of a Contingency Table

	Characteristic A		
Characteristic B	**Category A-1**	**Category A-2**	**Total**
Category B-1	a	b	a + b
Category B-2	c	d	c + d
Total	a + c	b + d	N

Table 3-4. The Distribution of Eye Color by Sex for 50 Schoolchildren

Eye Color	Sex: Male	Sex: Female	Total
	A. Marginal Values and Total Are Known		
Blue	a	b	15
Brown	c	d	35
Total	20	30	50
	B. Value in One Cell Is Known		
Blue	5	b	15
Brown	c	d	35
Total	20	30	50
	C. Values in All Cells Are Known		
Blue	5	10	15
Brown	15	20	35
Total	20	30	50

2. **Application.** A binomial distribution is used when a problem relates to the probability of two mutually exclusive outcomes in a known number of trials. The probability of each of the two outcomes is the same in each of the trials, but the result of each trial is independent from the results of the other trials. Standard deviations can be derived from the binomial distribution and confidence limits can be established (see III G 2).

3. **Calculation.** The probability in a binomial distribution is determined as

$$f(x) = \frac{n!}{x!\,(n-x)!}\, p^x q^{n-x}$$

where f(x) = the probability of obtaining x values in n trials; p = the probability of one of two possible outcomes (e.g., a success) in a single trial; q = the probability of the other possible outcome (e.g., a failure) in a single trial; n = the size of each independent trial; x = the number of successes in one trial of size n; n − x = the number of failures in the same trial; and ! = the factorial sign. (The factorial sign, which is also read as "prime," indicates the product of the preceding whole number and all smaller whole numbers to 1. For example, 4! = 4 × 3 × 2 × 1. Both 1! and 0! are defined as being equal to 1.)

4. **Example.** When a woman is pregnant, the probability of having a girl is about 50% (p = 0.50), and the probability of having a boy is about 50% (q = 0.50). If a parent has seven children (n = 7), the probability that two will be girls (x = 2) and five will be boys (n − x = 5) is calculated as

$$\begin{aligned} f(2) &= \frac{7!}{2!5!}\,(0.50^2)\,(0.50^5) \\ &= \frac{5040}{240}\,(0.25)\,(0.03) \\ &= (21)\,(0.25)\,(0.03) \\ &= 0.16, \text{ or } 16\% \end{aligned}$$

A useful shortcut when calculating with factorials is to cancel like terms before multiplying out the factorial expression. In the calculation above, 7!/[(2!)(5!)] can be simplified because 7!, or (7)(6)(5)(4)(3)(2)(1), is equal to (7)(6)(5!). The 5! term, therefore, can be canceled from both the numerator and denominator, which reduces 7!/[(2!)(5!)] to (7)(6)/2.

E. Normal distribution

1. **Definition.** The normal distribution, also called the **gaussian distribution,** is a theoretical, continuous, symmetrical, unimodal distribution of infinite range.

a. **Curve.** The normal distribution curve is **bell-shaped,** with lower and upper tails, and is determined by the mean and the standard deviation of the population.
b. The mean, median, and mode of a normally distributed population are equal.

2. **Applications**
   a. The normal distribution can be used to characterize many populations and samples, especially large ones.
   b. The normal distribution and normal approximations are the bases of a number of analytic tests, such as chi-square tests.

3. The **critical ratio,** or **z score,** is the number of standard deviations that a value in a normally distributed population lies away from the mean.
   a. Increasing the critical ratio corresponds to decreasing the probability for accepting the null hypothesis.
   b. The proportion of the population (or the probability of finding a member of the population) within each critical ratio, within ± each critical ratio, and outside ± each critical ratio are listed in Table 3-5.
   c. In a normally distributed population, about 68.3% of the population lies within 1 critical ratio (i.e., within the mean ± 1 standard deviation), about 95.4% lies within 2 critical ratios of the mean, and about 99.7% lies within 3 critical ratios of the mean (Figure 3-10).
   d. In large samples, the critical ratio is used to calculate confidence intervals around the sample mean.

4. **Calculation.** The critical ratio (z) is determined as

$$z = \frac{x - \bar{\mu}}{\sigma}$$

where x = the value being tested; $\bar{\mu}$ = the population mean; and σ = the population standard deviation.

5. **Example.** One thousand randomly selected men have a mean weight of 160 lb, with a standard deviation of 10 lb. The population is normally distributed with respect to weight.
   a. About 680 (68%) of the men have weights of 160 ± 1(10) lb (mean ± 1 standard deviation), or weights ranging from 150 to 170 lb; about 950 (95%) have weights of 160 ± 2(10) lb (mean ± 2 standard deviations), or weights ranging from 140 to 180 lb; and about 997 (99.7%) have weights of 160 ± 3(10) lb (mean ± 3 standard deviations), or weights ranging from 130 to 190 lb.
   b. Similarly, about 340 (34%) of the men weigh between 160 and 170 lb (mean to mean + 1 standard deviation); about 136 (13.6%) of the men weigh between 140 and 150 lb (mean − 2 standard deviations to mean − 1 standard deviation); and about 23 (2.3%) of the men weigh greater than 180 lb (mean + 2 standard deviations).

F. **Student's t tests**—based on the **t distribution,** which reflects greater variation due to chance than the normal distribution—are used to analyze small samples. The t distribution is a continuous, symmetrical, unimodal distribution of infinite range, which is bell-shaped, similar to the shape of the normal distribution, but more spread out. As the sample size increases, the t distribution closely resembles the normal distribution. At infinite degrees of freedom, the t and normal distributions are identical, and the t values equal the critical ratio values.

Table 3-5. Table of Critical Ratio (abbreviated)

	Probability that Value Lies		
Critical Ratio	**Within the Critical Ratio**	**Within ± the Critical Ratio**	**Outside ± the Critical Ratio**
1.0	.341	.683	.317
1.645	.450	.900	.100
1.96	.475	.950	.050
2.0	.477	.954	.046
2.576	.495	.990	.010
3.0	.499	.997	.003

Reprinted from Centers for Disease Control: *Analytic Statistics: Statistical Methods—Testing for Significance.* Washington, DC, US Department of Health and Human Services, Public Health Service, May 1981.

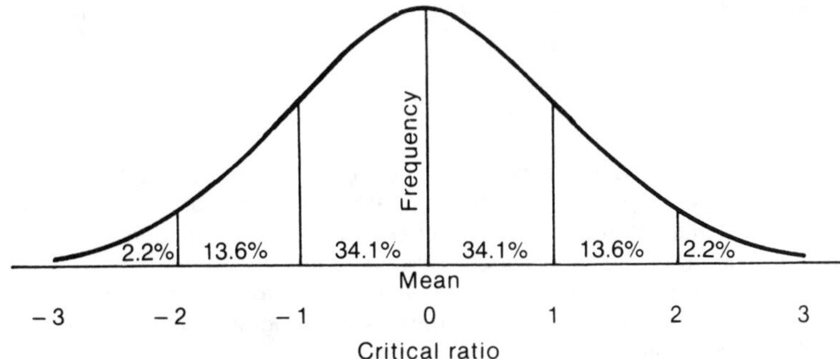

Figure 3-10. The standardized normal distribution (i.e., the *curve*), shown with the percentage of values included between critical ratios from the mean.

1. **Student's t test for a single small sample**
   a. **Definition.** Student's t test for a single small sample compares a single sample with a population.
   b. **Applications and characteristics**
      (1) **Appropriate sample size.** Student's t tests are used to evaluate the null hypothesis for continuous variables for sample sizes less than 30.
      (2) Student's t tests are used in analyses for which a sample standard deviation is substituted as an estimate for an unknown population standard deviation.
      (3) Either the proportions or the actual counts of the variables can be employed in Student's t tests.
      (4) **The t table.** Probability values are derived from the t value and the number of degrees of freedom by using the t table. (Table 3-6 is an abbreviated t table.) For each degree of freedom, a row of increasing t values corresponds to a row of decreasing probabilities for accepting the null hypothesis.
      (5) The **probability statements** derived from Student's t tests are dependent on the sample size in two ways.
         (a) The sample size is related to the value of the t. As the sample size decreases, the t value decreases, and the probability that the difference noted is ascribed to chance increases; that is, there is an increased probability for accepting the null hypothesis.
         (b) The sample size is directly related to the number of degrees of freedom. As the number of degrees of freedom decreases, for a constant t value, the probability that the difference noted is ascribed to chance increases.
         (c) Even though the t distribution is more appropriate than the normal distribution for analyzing small samples, statistically significant differences observed in small samples may be overestimates of true differences.
      (6) **Confidence intervals.** In small samples, especially sample sizes less than 30, the t distribution is used to calculate confidence intervals around the sample mean (see III G 2).

Table 3-6. The t Table (abbreviated)

	Probability		
Degrees of Freedom (df)	**.10**	**.05**	**.01**
1	6.31	12.71	63.66
2	2.92	4.30	9.93
8	1.86	2.31	3.36
9	1.83	2.26	3.25
10	1.81	2.23	3.17
∞	1.64	1.96	2.58

Reprinted from Centers for Disease Control: *Analytic Statistics: Statistical Methods—Testing for Significance.* Washington, DC, US Department of Health and Human Services, Public Health Service, May, 1981.

c. **Calculation.** The t value for comparing a sample mean with a population mean is determined as

$$t(df) = \frac{\bar{x} - \bar{\mu}}{SD/\sqrt{n}}$$

where t (df) = the t value at the degrees of freedom; df = the number of degrees of freedom, which equals n − 1; $\bar{x}$ = the sample mean; $\bar{\mu}$ = the population mean; SD = the sample standard deviation; and n = the number in the sample. The denominator of the equation is the standard error of the sample mean (see III G 1).

d. **Example.** The mean serum sodium concentration for nine patients is 150 mg/dl, with a standard deviation of 6 mg/dl. The mean serum sodium concentration for all individuals in the community is 140 mg/dl.
   (1) The t value—calculated from the equation with $\bar{x}$ = 150, $\bar{\mu}$ = 140, SD = 6, and n = 9—is equal to 5.
   (2) The probability is determined from the t table (see Table 3-6). For (9 − 1), or 8, degrees of freedom and a t value of 5, the probability is less than 0.01 that the observed difference between the sample and population means is due to chance.
   (3) If an arbitrary cutoff of 0.05 is accepted for statistical significance, then the difference between the sample mean and the population mean is significantly greater than the difference expected due to chance alone. The null hypothesis is rejected.

2. **Student's t test for independent samples**
   a. **Definition.** Student's t test for independent samples compares the means of two small samples.
   b. **Applications and characteristics.** The uses and restrictions of Student's t test for independent samples are similar to those for other Student's t tests, except that both sample sizes are less than 30. Student's t test is inappropriate to use if more than two means are compared, unless adjustments for multiple comparisons are made.
   c. **Calculation.** The t value for comparing the means from two independent samples is determined as

$$t(df) = \frac{|\bar{x} - \bar{y}|}{SD_p \sqrt{\frac{1}{n_x} + \frac{1}{n_y}}}$$

with

$$SD_p = \sqrt{\frac{\Sigma(\bar{x} - x_i)^2 + \Sigma(\bar{y} - y_i)^2}{(n_x - 1) + (n_y - 1)}}$$

where t(df) = the t value at the degrees of freedom; df = the number of degrees of freedom, which equals $n_x + n_y - 2$; $\bar{x}$ = the mean from sample x; $\bar{y}$ = the mean from sample y; n_x = the number in sample x; n_y = the number in sample y; SD_p = the pooled standard deviation from both samples x and y; and | | = "absolute value of," or the difference between the values expressed with a positive sign. The denominator of Student's t test is the standard error of the difference between the means.

   d. **Example.** Serum sodium concentration is measured in two groups of patients. The serum sodium levels (in mg/dl) in one group of six patients are: 142, 147, 148, 149, 153, and 155, with a mean of 149 mg/dl; the serum sodium levels in another group of five patients are: 138, 139, 142, 143, and 144, with a mean of 141.2 mg/dl. To determine the probability that the 8 mg/dl difference between the means is due to chance, the t value is determined according to the above equations. In this example: $\bar{x}$ = 149; $\bar{y}$ = 141.2; n_x = 6; n_y = 5; and SD_p = 3.35. The t value at 9 degrees of freedom is equal to 8, and the associated probability that the difference is due to chance, according to Table 3-6, is less than 0.01. The null hypothesis is rejected and the difference is probably not due to chance.

3. **Student's t test for paired samples**
   a. **Definition.** Student's t test for paired samples compares the means of two small paired samples.
   b. **Applications.** The uses and restrictions of Student's t test for paired samples are similar to those for other Student's t tests, except that this test is restricted to samples with matched pairs of less than 30 each.

c. Calculation. The t value for comparing the means from two paired samples is determined as

$$t(df) = \frac{\bar{d}}{SD_p / \sqrt{n}}$$

with

$$SD_p = \sqrt{\frac{\Sigma (d_i - \bar{d})^2}{n-1}}, \quad \text{or} \tag{5}$$

$$SD_p = \sqrt{\frac{\Sigma d_i^2 - (\Sigma d_i)^2/n}{n-1}} \tag{6}$$

where t(df) = the t value at the degrees of freedom; df = the number of degrees of freedom, which equals n − 1; d_i = the difference between each pair; $\bar{d}$ = the mean difference; and n = the number of pairs.

(1) The denominator of Student's t test is the standard error of the difference between the means.
(2) The pooled standard deviation is easier to calculate with equation (6).
(3) The t value is used to determine the probability that the difference between the means of the pairs is due to chance at the calculated degrees of freedom (see Table 3-6).

d. Example. Eleven medical students are given separate tests on the subjects of internal medicine and general surgery. The two scores for each student represent a matched pair and are listed in Table 3-7. To determine the probability that the difference between each paired sample is due to chance (i.e., the null hypothesis is true), the t value is determined according to equations (5) and (6).

(1) The difference between each paired sample is calculated.
(2) The arithmetic mean of the differences is calculated and is 302 divided by 11, or 27.5.
(3) The squares of the differences are calculated, and the sum of the squares is 21,294.
(4) The square of the sum of the differences (91,204) divided by the number of pairs (11) equals 8291, which is subtracted from the sum of the squares (21,294). The resulting difference (13,003) is divided by the number of degrees of freedom (10), which yields the variance (1300).
(5) The standard deviation (36.1), which is the square root of the variance, is divided by the square root of the number of samples (3.3) to yield the standard error (10.9).
(6) The t value equals the mean difference between the samples (27.5) divided by the standard error (10.9) and equals 2.5.
(7) For 10 degrees of freedom, according to Table 3-6, a t value of 2.23 is associated with a probability of 0.05 that the difference between the means of two samples is due to chance. In this example, the t value indicates a probability between 0.05 and 0.01.
(8) With a 0.05 cutoff for rejecting the null hypothesis, the internal medicine and general surgery test scores are significantly different for these students. The null hypothesis is rejected; a factor other than chance appears responsible for the difference in the scores.

Table 3-7. The Association between Internal Medicine and General Surgery Test Scores for 11 Medical Students

Medical Student Number	Internal Medicine Score	General Surgery Score	Difference between Scores	Square of Difference
1	75	90	−15	225
2	85	10	+75	5625
3	93	20	+73	5329
4	55	55	0	0
5	79	60	+19	361
6	86	30	+56	3136
7	90	70	+20	400
8	76	85	−9	81
9	89	25	+64	4096
10	54	75	−21	441
11	92	52	+40	1600
Total	874	572	+302	21,294

G. The standard error and confidence limits

1. Standard error of the mean

a. Definition

(1) The standard error of a measure is based on a sample of a population and is the estimate of the standard deviation of the measure for the population.

(2) The standard error of the mean, one of the most commonly used types of standard error, is a measure of the accuracy of the sample mean as an estimate of the population mean. In comparison, the standard deviation is a measure of the variability of the observations.

(a) When studying a population, many different samples can be chosen, and the values of the mean of a characteristic for each of the samples may be different. Often, the means of the samples follow a normal distribution, even if the original population was not normally distributed. The distribution of the means of the samples has a standard deviation around the population mean, and the standard error of the mean from one sample is an estimate of this standard deviation.

(b) The standard error of the mean is based on the standard deviation of the sample and the sample size. As the sample size increases, the sample better reflects the total population, the sample mean more closely estimates the population mean, and the standard error of the mean from that sample decreases.

b. Applications

(1) The standard error of the mean is used to construct confidence limits around a sample mean.

(2) Standard errors are used in Student's t test.

(3) The standard error is a measure of sampling fluctuation.

c. Calculation. The standard error of the mean (SEM) is determined as

$$\text{SEM} = \frac{\text{SD}}{\sqrt{n}}$$

where n = the number of observations in the sample.

d. Example. The mean weight of 100 randomly selected medical students is 140 lb, with a standard deviation of 28 lb. The standard error of the mean of the weights equals 28 lb divided by the square root of 100, which is 2.8 lb. Therefore, 2.8 lb is the estimate of the standard deviation of the population from which the sample was taken.

2. Confidence limits of a mean

a. Definition

(1) Confidence limits

(a) The upper and lower confidence limits define the range of probability, that is, the **confidence interval,** for a measure of the population based on a measure of a sample and the measure's standard error.

(b) Confidence intervals are expressed in terms of probability based on the α error.

(c) A $(1 - \alpha)$ confidence interval indicates that there is a $(1 - \alpha)$ probability that the population mean lies within the upper and lower confidence limits and an α probability that it lies outside these limits.

(2) The confidence limits of a mean define the confidence interval for the population mean based on a sample mean.

(a) For large samples, confidence limits are based on the critical ratio for the associated probability. For a 95% confidence interval, the estimated sampling error is multiplied by 1.96; the chances are 95% (19 out of 20) that the interval includes the average result of all possible samples of the same size.

(b) For small samples (less than 30), confidence limits are based on the t value for the number of degrees of freedom and the associated probability.

b. Applications and characteristics

(1) Confidence limits of a mean are used to estimate a population mean based on a sample from the population. The confidence interval is the margin of error of the point estimate.

(2) A repeated random sample from the population will yield another point estimate similar to, but not necessarily the same as, the first sample. The 95% confidence interval probably will cluster in the same area.

(3) The most commonly used confidence limits are 95% confidence limits, which indicate that there is a 95% probability that the population mean lies within the upper and lower confidence limits and a 5% probability that it lies outside these limits ($\alpha = 0.05$).

(4) Other commonly used confidence intervals are 90% confidence limits ($\alpha = 0.10$) and

99% confidence limits ($\alpha = 0.01$). All differ in width but cover the same relative position around the point estimate and would yield similar interpretations.

(5) Confidence intervals can be used in analyzing the binomial and Poisson distributions, survival curves, and rates.

(6) Data with confidence intervals provide a quantitative estimate of the measure of effect and give an indication of the likely magnitude of the true value, information that is not available when comparing data on the basis of simple statistical significance ($p \leq 0.05$), which is a qualitative (dichotomous) judgment.

(7) The wider the confidence interval, the less accurate and reliable the point estimate (i.e., there is more uncertainty).

(8) For a given sample size, the confidence intervals of proportions or percentages near 50% are wider than those near either extreme (0% or 100%).

(9) The larger the sample number, the more likely that the computed mean is closer to the true value, and the range of the confidence interval decreases.

(10) Confidence intervals are useful when comparing the results of different studies and in evaluating data to determine if there is a trend toward difference, even if the difference is not significant at $\alpha = 0.05$.

(11) The trend in peer-reviewed medical literature in the 1990s is to report analyses based on confidence intervals, with probability values having a less important role.

c. Calculation

(1) For large samples, the confidence limits of a mean are determined as

$$(1 - \alpha) \text{ confidence limits} = \bar{x} \pm z_\alpha \text{ SEM, or} \tag{7}$$

$$P(\bar{x} - z_\alpha \text{ SEM} \leq \bar{\mu} \leq \bar{x} + z_\alpha \text{ SEM}) = 1 - \alpha \tag{8}$$

(2) And for small samples, the confidence limits of a mean are determined as

$$(1 - \alpha) \text{ confidence limits} = \bar{x} \pm t_{df,\alpha} \text{ SEM, or} \tag{9}$$

$$P(\bar{x} - t_{df,\alpha} \text{ SEM} \leq \bar{\mu} \leq \bar{x} + t_{df,\alpha} \text{ SEM}) = 1 - \alpha \tag{10}$$

where $\bar{x} - z_\alpha$ SEM or $\bar{x} - t_{df,\alpha}$ SEM = the lower confidence limit; $\bar{x} + z_\alpha$ SEM or $\bar{x} + t_{df,\alpha}$ SEM = the upper confidence limit; P = the probability that the population mean ($\bar{\mu}$) lies within the confidence limits; α = the type I error; n = the sample size; z_α = the critical ratio (see III E 3); and $t_{df,\alpha}$ = the t score at (n − 1) degrees of freedom. When a smaller α error is accepted, the confidence interval is wider, and the probability that the population mean lies within the confidence limits is greater.

d. Example. Using again the 100 medical students whose mean weight is 140 lb, with a standard error of 2.8 lb, the following can be calculated.

(1) For 95% confidence limits, $\alpha = 0.05$ and $z = 1.96$ (sometimes approximated by 2).

(a) The 95% lower confidence limit is 140 − (1.96 × 2.8) = 134.5 lb.

(b) The 95% upper confidence limit is 140 + (1.96 × 2.8) = 145.5 lb.

(c) Therefore, there is a 95% probability that the mean weight of the population of medical students from which the sample is drawn is between 134.5 lb and 145.5 lb, inclusive.

(2) For 99% confidence limits, $\alpha = 0.01$ and $z = 2.576$.

(a) The 99% lower confidence limit is 140 − (2.576 × 2.8) = 132.8 lb.

(b) The 99% upper confidence limit is 140 + (2.576 × 2.8) = 147.2 lb.

(c) The 99% confidence interval is between 132.8 lb and 147.2 lb, inclusive.

(3) If the sample size were 20, the calculations would be the same, except that the t values for 19 degrees of freedom (2.09 for 95% confidence limits and 2.86 for 99% confidence limits) would be substituted for the critical ratio values.

H. Chi-square tests

1. The r × c chi-square test

a. Definition

(1) The r × c chi-square test determines the extent that a single observed series of proportions differs from a theoretical, or expected, distribution of proportions or the extent that two or more series, proportions, or frequencies differ from one another, based on the **chi-square distribution**.

(2) The chi-square distribution is a continuous asymmetric probability distribution based on a normal approximation of the binomial distribution. The chi-square distribution at 1 degree of freedom is identical to the distribution of the squares of the critical ratio.

b. Applications and characteristics

(1) The r × c chi-square test is used to determine the extent that an observed distribution differs from a theoretical or expected distribution or that two or more distributions differ from each other.

(2) The categories of data used in chi-square tests must be mutually exclusive and discrete.

(3) Only actual counts of the variables can be employed in chi-square tests.

(4) The r × c chi-square test depends on both the observed and expected values in the cells. The test can be used only if the theoretical or expected value of each variable is equal to or greater than 5. Observed values can be less than 5.

(5) Chi-square tests do not take into account whether the categories of data are ordered.

(6) **Chi-square table.** Probability values are derived from the chi-square value and the number of degrees of freedom by using a chi-square table. For each degree of freedom, a row of increasing chi-square values corresponds to a row of decreasing probabilities for accepting the null hypothesis. (Table 3-8 is an abbreviated chi-square table.)

c. Goodness of fit test is one type of r × c chi-square test, which is used for a contingency table with only one row or one column. The value of the chi-square is determined as for other r × c contingency tables, but the number of degrees of freedom is calculated differently (see III C 2 c).

d. The **Mantel-Haenszel technique** is a summary chi-square test that provides a weighted average or an adjusted summary odds ratio for data that have been stratified to control for confounding or intervening factors.

e. Yates correction factor

(1) Because the chi-square is based on a normal approximation of the binomial distribution, a correction for continuity, called Yates correction factor, often is included in the chi-square test equation.

(2) A chi-square symbol with the correction (c) subscript indicates that the chi-square value was calculated with the correction for continuity. Unless otherwise stated, a chi-square symbol without the correction subscript indicates that the chi-square value was calculated without the correction.

(3) The Yates correction factor is used for small samples.

(4) The Yates correction factor decreases the chi-square value and makes the probability estimate greater than it would have been without the correction.

(5) The Yates correction factor tends to decrease the likelihood of a type I error (i.e., the null hypothesis is less often rejected).

f. Calculation. The chi-square value is determined as

$$\chi^2_c(\mathrm{df}) = \frac{(|O_i - E_i| - 1/2)^2}{E_i}$$

where $\chi^2_c(\mathrm{df})$ = the chi-square value that reflects the correction for continuity at the calculated degrees of freedom; O_i = the observed frequency, or count, for each variable or cell; E_i = the theoretical or expected frequency or count for each variable or cell; and the ½ in the numerator is the Yates correction factor.

g. Example. Over a 4-year period, 95 individuals are electrocuted in bathtubs. The deaths are distributed by season as shown in Table 3-9. The probability that the seasonal distribution differs from what would be expected if there were no seasonal distribution (the null hypothesis) is calculated as follows.

(1) The expected number of deaths in each season is calculated as 24.

Table 3-8. Chi-square Table (abbreviated)

	Probability		
Degrees of Freedom (df)	**.10**	**.05**	**.01**
1	2.71	3.84	6.64
2	4.61	5.99	9.21
3	6.25	7.82	11.35

Reprinted from Centers for Disease Control: *Analytic Statistics: Statistical Methods—Testing for Significance.* Washington, DC, US Department of Health and Human Services, Public Health Service, May 1981.

Table 3-9. Calculating the Chi-square Value for Bathtub-Related Electrocutions by Season

Season	**Observed Frequency (O_i)**	**Expected Frequency (E_i)**	**$O_i - E_i$**	**$(\lvert O_i - E_i\rvert - 0.5)^2$**	**$\frac{(\lvert O_i - E_i\rvert - 0.5)^2}{E_i}$**
Winter	33	24	+9	72.25	3.01
Spring	30	24	+6	30.25	1.26
Summer	14	24	−10	90.25	3.76
Fall	19	24	−5	20.25	0.84
Total	96	96	0	. . .	8.87

(2) The number of deaths that deviated from the expected number is calculated ($O_i - E_i$), the Yates correction factor is subtracted, and the resultant value is squared.

(3) Each of the squared deviates is divided by the respective expected number of deaths for that season.

(4) The sum of these values is the value of the chi-square (8.87).

(5) The number of degrees of freedom is 3.

(6) The probability is determined from a chi-square table (see Table 3-8). For 3 degrees of freedom and a chi-square value of 8.87, the probability is between 0.05 and 0.01 that the seasonal distribution observed is due to chance.

(7) If an arbitrary cutoff of 0.05 is accepted for statistical significance (i.e., to reject the null hypothesis), then the seasonal distribution is significantly different from the distribution expected due to chance alone. The null hypothesis is rejected.

2. The 2 × 2 chi-square test

a. Definition. The 2 × 2 chi-square test, a type of r × c chi-square test, is specific for fourfold, or 2 × 2, contingency tables. The 2 × 2 chi-square always has 1 degree of freedom.

b. Applications. The uses and restrictions of the 2 × 2 chi-square test are the same as for the r × c chi-square test, except that it is restricted to fourfold table data analysis.

c. Calculation. The 2 × 2 chi-square value is determined using the same general chi-square equation as the r × c chi-square value. It is also determined more simply as

$$\chi^2_c = \frac{N(|ad - bc| - N/2)^2}{(a+b)(c+d)(a+c)(b+d)}$$

The symbols are the same as for the fourfold contingency table (see III C 1 and Table 3-3). N/2 is the Yates correction factor.

d. Example. The chi-square value for the distribution of eye color and sex among 50 children discussed in III C 1 d and listed in Table 3-4C can be calculated in two ways.

(1) The chi-square can be calculated by first determining the expected number in each cell. The expected number of boys with blue eyes is (20 × 15)/50 = 6. The expected number in each of the other cells is calculated similarly or is determined from the expected fourfold contingency table, which has the same marginal values as the observed fourfold table. The expected number of girls with blue eyes is 9, of boys with brown eyes is 14, and of girls with brown eyes is 21.

(2) Since the observed and expected values for all four cells are known, the corrected chi-square value is calculated using the r × c chi-square test equation and equals 0.10.

(3) Alternatively, the corrected chi-square value can be calculated using the 2 × 2 chi-square equation, which yields

$$\begin{aligned}\chi^2_c &= \frac{50\,[|(5)(20) - (10)(15)| - 50/2]^2}{(15)(35)(20)(30)} \\ &= \frac{50(25)^2}{315{,}000} \\ &= 0.10\end{aligned}$$

(4) The two methods yield approximately equal results.

(5) The probability is determined from the chi-square table (see Table 3-8). For 1 degree of freedom and a chi-square value of less than 2.7, the probability is greater than 10% that the distribution of eye color and sex among the 50 children is due to chance.

3. The McNemar test

a. Definition. The McNemar test, a type of 2 × 2 chi-square test, is specific for comparisons of variables from matched pairs and uses information only from discordant pairs.

b. Applications and characteristics

(1) Except that the variables being compared are from matched pairs and are not independent, the uses and restrictions of the McNemar test are the same as those for the 2 × 2 chi-square test.

(2) The null hypothesis tested is that the expected frequencies for the discordant pairs are equal.

(3) The McNemar test is more appropriate for testing matched pairs than the simple chi-square test, because it tends to decrease the likelihood of a type I error (i.e., the null hypothesis is less often incorrectly rejected).

(4) In a McNemar test, there is 1 degree of freedom because, with the marginal values constant, one of the values in the discordant pair automatically determines the other value.

c. Calculation. The chi-square value for matched-pair analysis using the McNemar test is determined as

$$\chi^2_c = \frac{(|f - g| - 1)^2}{f + g}$$

where f and g are the values of the discordant pair in the matched pair fourfold contingency table (Table 3-10).

d. Example. In a study to determine risk factors for acquired immune deficiency syndrome (AIDS), 200 AIDS patients are matched with 200 controls (individuals without AIDS). Table 3-11 lists the results of the investigation concerning the prior use of inhalant stimulants. In 18 pairs, the patients had used inhalant stimulants and the controls had not; in 9 pairs, the controls and not the patients had used inhalant stimulants. In the remaining pairs, both the patients and controls had the same history, with 32 pairs having used inhalant stimulants and 141 pairs having not used them. Using the McNemar test, the probability that the difference between the patients and controls with respect to the use of inhalant stimulants is due to chance is determined as follows.

(1) The chi-square value is calculated as $(|9 - 18| - 1)^2/(9 + 18)$, which equals $8^2/27$, or 2.4.

(2) The probability is determined from the chi-square table (see Table 3-8). For 1 degree of freedom and a chi-square value of less than 2.7, the probability is greater than 10% that the difference in the use of inhalant stimulants by patients and controls is due to chance.

I. Fisher's exact test

1. Definition. Fisher's exact test determines the probability due to chance of an association between the two characteristics being analyzed in a fourfold table that does not rely on the chi-square distribution.

2. Applications and characteristics

a. Fisher's exact test is used to determine the probability that an observed distribution is due to chance for a fourfold table in which any of the expected values is less than 5.

b. To determine the probability that an observed distribution (fourfold table) is due to chance, the exact probabilities are calculated for the observed distribution and for more extreme distributions, and the calculated probability values are added together using the additive rule (see III A 6 a).

Table 3-10. Fourfold Table for Matched-Pair Analysis

	Sample A		
Sample B	**Positive**	**Negative**	**Total**
Positive	e	f	e + f
Negative	g	h	g + h
Total	e + g	f + h	N

Table 3-11. Prior Use of Inhalant Stimulants among 200 Patients with Acquired Immune Deficiency Syndrome (AIDS) and 200 Matched Controls

	AIDS Patients		
Controls	**Used Stimulants**	**Did Not Use Stimulants**	**Total**
Used stimulants	32	9	41
Did not use stimulants	18	141	159
Total	50	150	200

c. The Fisher's exact test calculated probability value is always larger than the true probability value for the distribution. Therefore, Fisher's exact test is a conservative test.
d. Fisher's exact test can be used in either one-tailed or two-tailed applications.

3. **Calculation.** Probability using Fisher's exact test is determined as

$$P = \frac{(a+b)!\,(c+d)!\,(a+c)!\,(b+d)!}{N!\,a!\,b!\,c!\,d!}$$

where P = the exact probability that the association between the two characteristics is due to chance in the distribution being tested; and the other symbols are as noted for the fourfold contingency table (see III C 1 and Table 3-3).

4. **Example.** Of 30 individuals at a meeting, 13 became ill with gastrointestinal symptoms within 24 hours. The only foods consumed at the meeting were soda and milk. Everyone had either soda or milk, but no one had both. The distribution of individuals by presence of illness and type of drink consumed is depicted in Table 3-12A.
   a. In this example, Fisher's exact test and not a chi-square test is used to test the association between illness and type of drink consumed, because the smallest expected value—determined by multiplying the smallest columnar total (10) by the smallest row total (13) and dividing by the grand total (30)—is 4.3, which is less than 5.
   b. The exact probability that the observed distribution is due to chance is (13!17!20!10!)/(30!11!2!9!8!), which equals 0.06311.

Table 3-12. Distribution of 30 Individuals by Gastrointestinal Illness and Beverage Consumed

	Beverage Consumed		
Illness	**Milk**	**Soda**	**Total**
	A. Observed Distribution		
Yes	11	2	13
No	9	8	17
Total	20	10	30
	B. More Extreme Distribution		
Yes	12	1	13
No	8	9	17
Total	20	10	30
	C. Most Extreme Distribution		
Yes	13	0	13
No	7	10	17
Total	20	10	30

c. The exact probability of each of the more extreme distributions is calculated by the smallest cell value from the observed fourfold table diminished by 1, with the other cells adjusted accordingly, until the smallest value in a cell is zero.
   (1) The exact probability of the more extreme distribution in Table 3-12B is (13!17!20!10!)/(30!12!1!8!9!), which equals 0.01052. (Note that, because the margins remain the same and only the cells change, the numerator used for each of the extreme distributions is the same as the numerator for the observed distribution.)
   (2) The exact probability of the most extreme distribution in Table 3-12C is (13!17!20!10!)/30!13!0!7!10!), which equals 0.00065.

d. The total probability of seeing the observed distribution or one even more extreme is the sum of the probabilities for each distribution: 0.06311 + 0.01052 + 0.00065 = 0.07428.

e. With an arbitrary cutoff of 0.05 for statistical significance, the difference between the illness attack rates for those who drank soda and milk is not significant, and the null hypothesis is not rejected. [Although the difference is not statistically significant, other factors may incriminate the milk as the causative agent of illness (see Ch 1 VII).]

J. Correlation

1. **Definition.** Correlation is a measure of mutual correspondence between two variables and is denoted by the coefficient of correlation.

2. **Applications and characteristics**
   a. The **simple correlation coefficient,** also called the **Pearson's product-moment correlation coefficient,** is used to indicate the extent that two variables change with one another in a linear fashion.
   b. The correlation coefficient can range from −1 to +1 and is unitless (Figure 3-11).
      (1) When the correlation coefficient approaches −1, a change in one variable is more highly, or strongly, associated with an inverse linear change (i.e., a change in the opposite direction) in the other variable (see Figure 3-11A).
      (2) When the correlation coefficient equals zero, there is no association between the changes of the two variables (see Figure 3-11B).
      (3) When the correlation coefficient approaches +1, a change in one variable is more highly, or strongly, associated with a direct linear change in the other variable (see Figure 3-11C).
   c. A correlation coefficient can be calculated validly only when both variables are subject to random sampling [see I B 2 a (2)], and each is chosen independently.
   d. Although useful as one of the determinants of scientific causality, correlation by itself is not equivalent to causation. For example, two correlated variables may be associated with another factor that causes them to appear correlated with each other.
   e. A correlation may appear strong but be insignificant because of a small sample size.

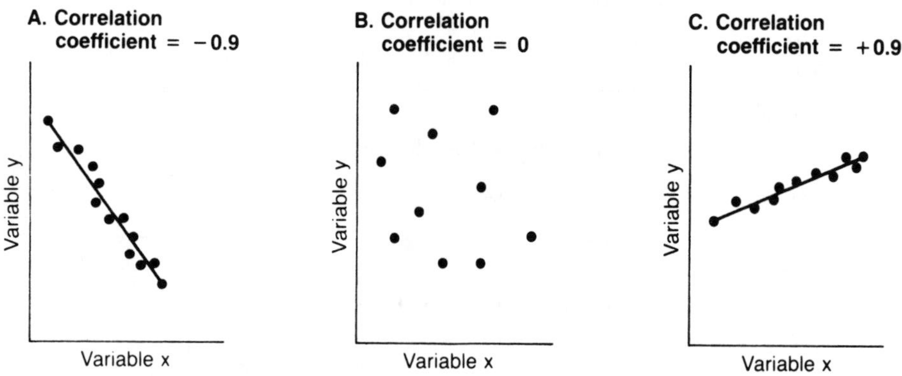

Figure 3-11. Correlation—the mutual correspondence between two variables—is measured by the correlation coefficient.

3. **Calculation.** The correlation coefficient (r) is determined as

$$r = \frac{CoV_{x,y}}{\sqrt{V_x V_y}} = \frac{CoV_{x,y}}{(SD_x)(SD_y)}, \quad \text{or} \qquad (11)$$

$$r = \frac{\Sigma(x_i - \bar{x})(y_i - \bar{y})}{\sqrt{\Sigma(x_i - \bar{x})^2 \, \Sigma(y_i - \bar{y})^2}}, \quad \text{or} \qquad (12)$$

$$r = \frac{\Sigma x_i y_i - (\Sigma x_i)(\Sigma y_i)/n}{\sqrt{[\Sigma x_i^2 - (\Sigma x_i)^2/n]\,[\Sigma y_i^2 - (\Sigma y_i)^2/n]}} \qquad (13)$$

where $CoV_{x,y}$ = the sample covariance between variables x and y; V_x = the variance of the x variable; V_y = the variance of the y variable; and n = the number of paired observations. The correlation coefficient is easier to calculate using equation (13).

4. **Example.** Using equation (13), the following steps are taken to determine the correlation coefficient between age and the number of prior arrests for five drunk drivers (Table 3-13).
   a. The product of the age and the number of prior arrests for each individual is calculated: $(\Sigma x_i y_i) = 155$.
   b. The product of the sum of the ages and the sum of the prior arrests for each individual is calculated and then divided by the number of paired observations: $[(\Sigma x_i)(\Sigma y_i)/n] = (100 \times 7)/5 = 140$.
   c. The numerator is calculated by subtracting 140 from 155, which equals 15.
   d. The denominator is the square root of the respective sums of the squares of the deviations from each of the means.
      (1) For age, the sum of the squares of the deviations equals 54 (see II B 2 d for an example of calculation).
      (2) For prior arrests, the sum of the squares of the deviations from the mean is similarly calculated: $15 - 7^2/5 = 5.2$.
      (3) The product of the two sums of the squares of the deviations from the respective means is: $(54 \times 5.2) = 280.8$, the square root of which is 16.76. This is the denominator.
   e. The correlation coefficient is equal to the numerator (15) divided by the denominator (16.76) and in this example is +0.9. The age and the number of prior arrests for each individual are highly correlated. (Note, however, that the age does not cause the number of arrests nor does the number of prior arrests cause the age.)

K. Nonparametric tests

1. **Definition.** Nonparametric, or **distribution-free,** methods of statistical analysis are tests that evaluate the null hypothesis or determine confidence limits for samples and populations regardless of the underlying population distribution. Although the observations need to come from a continuous scale of measurement, the distribution need not be a defined one (e.g., a normal, chi-square, or t distribution).

2. **Applications and characteristics**
   a. Nonparametric tests require fewer assumptions about the distribution of the samples or populations under study than do parametric tests such as chi-square tests and Student's t tests.

Table 3-13 Calculating the Correlation Coefficient between Age and Number of Prior Arrests for Five Individuals

Case Number	Age (years)	Age Squared	Number of Prior Arrests	Number of Arrests Squared	Age × Number of Arrests
1	17	289	1	1	17
2	18	324	0	0	0
3	18	324	1	1	18
4	21	441	2	4	42
5	26	676	3	9	78
Total	100	2054	7	15	155

b. Nonparametric tests can be used to analyze samples or populations that do not follow a normal distribution or an approximation of the normal distribution and for which parametric methods are inappropriate.
c. Nonparametric tests can be used to analyze samples or populations for which parameters such as mean or standard deviation are unavailable or undeterminable.
d. Nonparametric tests can be used when the observations are described in terms of rank or in a hierarchy.
e. Although nonparametric tests are designed for use in populations regardless of the underlying distribution, they can be used instead of parametric tests to analyze populations that follow normal or approximately normal distributions.

3. **Example.** The internal medicine and general surgery test scores of the 11 medical students that were analyzed by Student's t test for paired samples can be reanalyzed by a nonparametric test. The scores are listed in Table 3-14. The association between the students' scores for the two tests can also be determined using the Wilcoxon signed rank test for pairs, which is a nonparametric alternative to Student's t test for paired samples.
   a. The difference between the internal medicine and general surgery scores is calculated for each student.
   b. The absolute value for each of the calculated differences is determined.
   c. The absolute values are ranked by magnitude from 1 to 10. Differences of zero are discounted and not included in the ranking.
   d. Each rank is assigned the sign of the calculated difference for that pair.
   e. The like-signed ranks are added together. The sum of the positive ranks equals +47; the sum of the negative ranks equals −8. The smaller signed rank sum, which in this example is 8, is used to determine the probability that the two scores are associated.
   f. A table of probability values for the Wilcoxon test for paired samples shows that, for 10 pairs, a smaller rank sum of 8 is associated with a two-tailed probability of 0.05. Therefore, for these students, the internal medicine and general surgery test scores are significantly different if the cutoff for rejecting the null hypothesis is 0.05.
   g. The conclusions reached using the parametric and nonparametric tests are the same.

L. Regression analysis

1. **Definition.** Regression analysis is the mathematical modeling to describe the effect that one or more independent variables have on a dependent, or outcome, variable.

2. **Types**
   a. **Linear regression** describes the effect that one independent variable has on a dependent variable.
   b. **Multiple regression** describes the effect that two or more independent variables have on a dependent variable.
   c. **Nonlinear regression** involves more complicated mathematical forms, including logarithmic functions, in the regression analysis.

Table 3-14. Calculations Needed to Test the Association between Internal Medicine and General Surgery Test Scores for 11 Students Using the Wilcoxon Test

Medical Student Number	Internal Medicine Score	General Surgery Score	Difference between Scores	Absolute Value of Difference	Rank of Absolute Value	Assigned Rank
1	75	90	−15	15	2	−2
2	85	10	+75	75	10	+10
3	93	20	+73	73	9	+9
4	55	55	0	0	...	...
5	79	60	+19	19	3	+3
6	86	30	+56	56	7	+7
7	90	70	+20	20	4	+4
8	76	85	−9	9	1	−1
9	89	25	+64	64	8	+8
10	54	75	−21	21	5	−5
11	92	52	+40	40	6	+6

3. **Applications and characteristics**
   a. The regression model is valid only in the observed range of the dependent variable. **Extrapolations are risky.** When applying linear regression, the actual relationship may not be linear.
   b. The **regression line** is an approximation of the relationship between the independent and dependent variables. The equation of the regression line is the **regression equation**.
   c. The **regression coefficient** is the average change in the dependent variable for each unit of the independent variable. In the regression equation, the slope is the regression coefficient.
   d. The dependent variable also is affected by random variation.

4. **Calculation**
   a. The linear regression equation is determined as

$$y = a + bx$$

   where a = the y-axis intercept (the y value when x = 0); b = the regression coefficient; x = the independent variable; and y = the dependent variable.
   b. In a multiple regression model, each dependent variable has its own regression coefficient and is determined as

$$y = a + b_1x_1 + b_2x_2 + b_ix_i$$

   where b_i = the regression coefficient for each dependent variable, x_i.
   c. The linear regression line determined from a series of data points is based on the **method of least squares,** in which the sum of the squared deviations of the data points from the line is minimal.

5. **Example.** The diastolic blood pressures of 25 adult men randomly chosen from 100 men age 30–50 years are plotted against their ages. The regression line is determined as

$$y = 40 + 1.5x$$

   where y = diastolic blood pressure (in mm Hg); and x = age in years. The regression coefficient is 1.5; each increase in age of 1 year results in an average increase in blood pressure of 1.5 mm Hg between the ages of 30 and 50 years. The predicted diastolic blood pressure of a 30-year-old man in this population is: 40 + (1.5 × 30) = 85 mm Hg; the predicted diastolic pressure of a 50-year-old man is 115 mm Hg. It would be erroneous to use this equation to try to determine the blood pressure of a 5-year-old girl or of any other person not part of the sampled population.

M. **Survival analysis**

1. **Definition.** Survival, or **life table, analysis** is a technique used to measure a defined outcome in a population or sample whose members are followed over a variable time period.

2. **Types**
   a. The **demographic,** or **population,** life table is based on the application of national or other reported age-specific mortality data to a theoretical population.
   b. The **cohort,** or **clinical,** life table is based on data obtained from an observed or studied sample.

3. **Applications and characteristics**
   a. In a clinical life table, each subject has a known initial point and a well-defined endpoint of observation with a dichotomous outcome (e.g., alive or dead).
   b. Subjects are entered independently and observed at different time periods and for varying lengths of time. Some subjects may be lost to follow-up, but they should be included in the analysis for the time period they were observed.
   c. The contribution of each subject is weighted by the time under observation, for example, as measured in **person-years** (one subject observed for 4 years contributes a total of 4 person-years, as do four subjects observed for 1 year each).
   d. The **Kaplan-Meier** method of analysis of a clinical cohort provides nonparametric estimates of cumulative incidence for defined outcomes based on incomplete observations.
   e. In a population life table, needed data include all of the following:
      (1) The time at the beginning of the interval
      (2) The length of the time interval (e.g., the age interval)
      (3) The number who are under observation at the beginning of the time interval

(4) The probability of dying during the interval
(5) The number who migrate or are lost to follow-up

4. **Examples**
   a. Figure 3-12 depicts a Kaplan-Meier survival curve of the cumulative incidence of bladder cancer in 2000 adult residents by number of years living in an industrial town between 1950 and 1990. At 30 years, the cumulative incidence of bladder cancer among men is 1.25% and among women is 0.5%. In this town, a work-related exposure to a bladder carcinogen may account for the greater incidence among men. The survival curve for men terminates when fewer than 10 subjects are under observation for the time period.
   b. Table 3-15 depicts an abridged life table for all persons in the United States in 1987. The proportion of persons in the 35–40 year age-group who died during the time interval is 0.0093, or 900 persons of the 96,273 alive at the beginning of the interval from a hypothetical birth cohort of 100,000. The stationary population refers to the total number of persons alive in the time interval indicated when 100,000 persons are born per year.

IV. SCREENING

A. Basic concepts

1. **Definition.** Screening is the initial examination of an individual to detect disease not yet under medical care. Screening may be concerned with a single disease or with many diseases (called **multiphasic screening**).
2. **Purpose.** Screening separates apparently healthy individuals into groups with either a high or low probability of developing the disease for which the screening test is being used.
3. **Types of diseases.** Screening may be concerned with many different types of diseases, including:
   a. Acute communicable diseases (e.g., rubella)
   b. Chronic communicable diseases (e.g., tuberculosis)
   c. Acute noncommunicable diseases (e.g., lead toxicity)
   d. Chronic noncommunicable diseases (e.g., glaucoma)

B. Testing of patients

1. **Case finding**
   a. **Definition.** Case finding is the examination of an individual for a disease unrelated to the health problem for which medical care was sought.
   b. **Subjects.** Case finding is performed on patients who have sought medical care for a health problem.

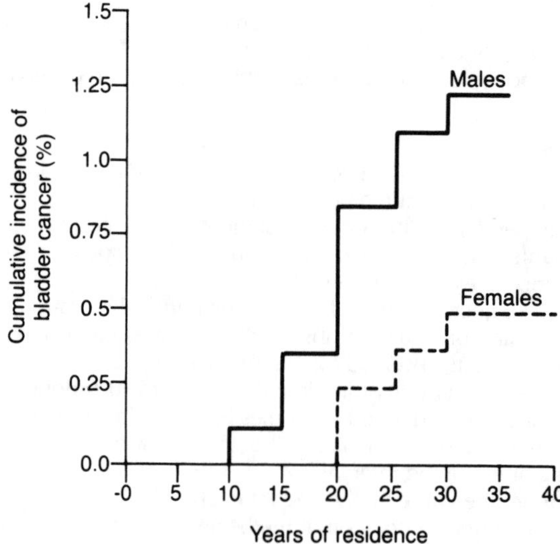

Figure 3-12. A Kaplan-Meier survival curve of the cumulative incidence of bladder cancer in 2000 adult residents of an industrial town between 1950 and 1990.

STUDY QUESTIONS

Directions: Each of the numbered items or incomplete statements in this section is followed by answers or by completions of the statement. Select the **one** lettered answer or completion that is **best** in each case.

1. The critical ratio, or z score, is applicable to which type of distribution?

(A) t
(B) Normal
(C) Chi-square
(D) Binomial
(E) Skewed

2. Confidence limits are calculated using

(A) the median and the range
(B) the median and its standard error
(C) the mean and the range
(D) the mean and its standard error

3. A normal distribution curve is determined by the

(A) mean and sample size
(B) mean and standard deviation
(C) range and sample size
(D) range and standard deviation
(E) mean and range

4. Measures of dispersion include all of the following EXCEPT

(A) mode
(B) range
(C) variance
(D) standard deviation
(E) coefficient of variation

5. An analysis of the race of patients who visit an emergency room reveals that 40% are white, 35% are black, 20% are Native American, and 15% are Asian. These data would best be depicted graphically with a

(A) Venn diagram
(B) cumulative frequency graph
(C) normal curve
(D) histogram
(E) pie chart

6. In a 3×4 contingency table, the number of degrees of freedom equals

(A) 1
(B) 5
(C) 6
(D) 7
(E) 12

7. Two variables, x and y, are studied for a population, and the simple correlation coefficient (r) is equal to $+0.80$. The correlation coefficient indicates that

(A) x and y have the same unit of measure
(B) x and y are causally related
(C) there is an inverse linear relationship between x and y
(D) x and y are strongly associated

8. True statements concerning type I error include all of the following EXCEPT

(A) it is the rejection of a null hypothesis that is actually true
(B) it is often assigned a value of 0.05 in studies
(C) it is also called the α error
(D) it is used to determine sample size
(E) it is equal to 1 minus the β error

9. Characteristics of the subjects in a clinical life table include all of the following EXCEPT that each subject

(A) has a known initial point
(B) is observed for a standard time period
(C) has a dichotomous clinical outcome
(D) lost to follow-up is included in the analysis
(E) is entered in the analysis independently

1-B	4-A	7-D
2-D	5-E	8-E
3-B	6-C	9-B

10. True statements concerning Student's t test and the t distribution include all of the following EXCEPT

(A) Student's t test is appropriate for sample sizes of fewer than 30
(B) as the sample size increases, the t value approaches the value of the critical ratio
(C) the t distribution reflects less variation due to chance than does the normal distribution
(D) the probability value derived from a t value depends on the number of degrees of freedom
(E) proportions can be used in calculating the t value

11. True statements concerning chi-square tests and chi-square values include all of the following EXCEPT

(A) the categories of data used must be mutually exclusive
(B) chi-square values are useful in calculating confidence intervals
(C) chi-square tests do not take into account the ordering of data categories
(D) the probability value derived from a chi-square value depends on the number of degrees of freedom
(E) proportions cannot be used in calculating the chi-square value

12. All of the following statements about screening tests are true EXCEPT

(A) they are used as a basis for therapy
(B) they are performed on apparently healthy individuals
(C) they are measured by sensitivity and specificity
(D) they are applicable to large numbers of individuals
(E) they are performed for diseases amenable to therapy prior to the onset of symptoms

Directions: Each item below contains four suggested answers of which **one or more** is correct. Choose the answer

A if **1, 2, and 3** are correct
B if **1 and 3** are correct
C if **2 and 4** are correct
D if **4** is correct
E if **1, 2, 3, and 4** are correct

13. Measures of central tendency include the

(1) median
(2) range
(3) mode
(4) variance

14. The standard error of the mean of a sample is

(1) an estimate of the standard deviation of the population
(2) based on a normal distribution
(3) used to determine confidence limits
(4) increased as the sample size increases

10-C
11-B
12-A
13-B
14-A

SUMMARY OF DIRECTIONS

A	B	C	D	E
1,2,3 only	1,3 only	2,4 only	4 only	All are correct

15. The sensitivity of a screening test is

(1) the test's ability to identify correctly those persons who truly have the disease
(2) equal to 1 minus the specificity of a test
(3) independent of disease prevalence in the population under study
(4) calculated by dividing the number of persons with the disease who screen positive by the total number of persons who screen positive

16. A confidence interval has which of the following characteristics?

(1) It is based on a critical ratio when the sample is large
(2) It gives an indication of the likely magnitude of the true value
(3) It gives an indication of the certainty of the point estimate
(4) It becomes narrower as the sample size increases

17. True statements concerning the chi-square test include which of the following?

(1) It requires that the expected value in each cell be at least 5
(2) It requires that the observed value in each cell be at least 5
(3) It depends on both the observed and expected values in each cell
(4) It depends on the arithmetic mean of the series under study

18. True statements concerning Fisher's exact test include which of the following?

(1) It is used instead of the chi-square test if the observed value in any cell of the fourfold table is less than 5
(2) It is used instead of the chi-square test if the expected value in any cell of the fourfold table is less than 5
(3) It requires that the probability value determined be adjusted according to the number of degrees of freedom
(4) It requires calculating probability values for the fourfold table under study and for tables that are more extreme

19. Nonparametric tests can be used to compare two populations when

(1) each population is unimodal
(2) both populations have equal numbers
(3) each population is independent
(4) each population is distributed normally

20. In one city, five white children and seven black children are bitten by rats. The white children are age 3, 3, 4, 5, and 6 years; the black children are age 1, 2, 2, 3, 4, 4, and 5 years. Based on this information, it can be determined that

(1) the median age for the black children is less than that for the white children
(2) the mean age for the black children is more than that for the white children
(3) there are two modal ages for the black children and one for the white children
(4) the range of ages for the black children equals that for the white children

15-B
16-E
17-B
18-C
19-E
20-B

SUMMARY OF DIRECTIONS

A	B	C	D	E
1,2,3 only	1,3 only	2,4 only	4 only	All are correct

21. A chi-square test is used during an outbreak of gastroenteritis to test the association between eating chicken salad and becoming ill. The proportion of individuals who ate chicken salad who were ill is statistically significantly greater than the proportion of individuals who did not eat chicken salad and who were ill ($p = 0.02$). Correct interpretations of these data include which of the following?

(1) Two percent of those who ate the chicken salad became ill
(2) The null hypothesis is rejected
(3) The probability for becoming ill after eating the chicken salad was 98%
(4) There is a 2% probability that the difference noted is due to chance

22. A surgery intern has conducted a study of sleeping habits among her 10 colleagues and has developed the following regression equation: $y = 6 + 0.1x$, where x is the number of hours working on one shift, and y is the number of hours sleeping the night after that shift. Each work shift analyzed was between 8 and 24 hours long. True statements about this model include which of the following?

(1) The model is valid only for work shifts between 8 and 24 hours long
(2) The independent variable is also affected by random variation
(3) The regression coefficient is 0.1
(4) This is an example of logarithmic regression

Directions: Each group of items in this section consists of lettered options followed by a set of numbered items. For each item, select the **one** lettered option that is most closely associated with it. Each lettered option may be selected once, more than once, or not at all.

Questions 23–26

The linear regression equation is determined as follows: $y = a + bx$. Match each description below with the appropriate equation characteristic.

(A) a
(B) b
(C) x
(D) y

23. Dependent variable
24. Independent variable
25. Regression coefficient
26. The y-axis intercept

21-C 24-C
22-B 25-B
23-D 26-A

Questions 27–30

A fourth-year medical student has completed five elective rotations, which are weighted equally. The student is graded in each rotation on a scale of 1 to 10 as follows:

Skiing surgery	2
Cross-cultural pharmacology	3
Literary medicine	6
Introductory bartering	7
Clinical kinetics	7

For each descriptive statistic listed below, select the numerical value that is most appropriate.

(A) 3
(B) 4
(C) 5
(D) 6
(E) 7

27. Median

28. Mode

29. Mean

30. Range

27-D
28-E
29-C
30-C

ANSWERS AND EXPLANATIONS

1. The answer is B *[III E 3].*
The critical ratio, or z score, is the number of standard deviations that a value in a normally distributed population lies away from the mean. The critical ratio is used in testing the null hypothesis and in calculating confidence limits in large samples and populations.

2. The answer is D *[III G 2].*
Confidence limits are based on the arithmetic mean and the standard error of the mean. The upper and lower 95% confidence limits are equal to the mean plus and minus, respectively, two times the standard error of the mean. Neither the range nor the median is useful in calculating confidence limits or other probability statements.

3. The answer is B *[III E 1, 3].*
The shape of the normal distribution curve is determined by the mean and the standard deviation. In a normal distribution, 68% of the population lies within 1 standard deviation of the mean and 95% within 2 standard deviations. A normal curve cannot be described by the range or the sample size.

4. The answer is A *[II B].*
Measures of dispersion include the range, variance, standard deviation, and coefficient of variation, which are summary measures for a sample or population that describe the scatter of the series. Measures of central tendency include the mode (which describes the most frequently occurring value), the median (which is the middle value), and the mean, or average.

5. The answer is E *[II C 1].*
Given the choice of a Venn diagram, cumulative frequency graph, normal curve, histogram, or pie chart, a pie chart is the most appropriate figure to represent a population by the proportional distribution of a discrete characteristic, which, in this example, is race. A bar chart would also be appropriate. A Venn diagram is used to show two or more characteristics within a population or one characteristic within two or more populations. A cumulative frequency graph is used for continuous data. A normal curve is a symmetrical curve of continuous and ordered data. A histogram is a special form of bar chart used for continuous and ordered data.

6. The answer is C *[III C 2].*
In a contingency table with 3 rows and 4 columns, the number of degrees of freedom is equal to the product of the number of rows minus 1 and the number of columns minus 1, which is 2×3, or 6. The number of degrees of freedom is the number of variables in a distribution that can be assigned values freely when the sum of the values is fixed.

7. The answer is D *[III J 2].*
The correlation coefficient indicates that x and y are strongly associated. The correlation coefficient is used to indicate the extent that two variables change with one another in a linear manner. The two variables can have the same or different units of measure. Correlation coefficients range from -1 to $+1$ and are unitless. A -1 value indicates a strong inverse linear association (an increase in one variable is associated with a decrease in the other), while $+1$ indicates a strong direct linear association. Causality cannot be determined from the correlation coefficient, because the two variables may be associated through a third variable rather than directly.

8. The answer is E *[III B 4].*
Type I error is not equal to 1 minus the β error. The β error is the acceptance as true of a false null hypothesis, and the formula 1 minus the β error is used to calculate the power of a study. The type I error, or α error, is the rejection of a null hypothesis that is actually true. Type I error is used to determine sample size and to test the null hypothesis, which is often rejected at the arbitrary cutoff of 5% probability due to chance.

9. The answer is B *[III M 3].*
Subjects in a clinical life table have a known initial point and a dichotomous clinical outcome and are entered in the analysis independently. Subjects lost to follow-up are included in the analysis. Each subject is not observed for a standard period of time. A clinical life table, or survival curve, is based on data obtained from an observed or studied sample. The subjects may enter the study at different time periods and be followed for different lengths of time. The clinical outcome must always be defined in dichotomous terms (e.g., dead or alive) for categorization. The contribution of each subject is measured in person-years.

10. The answer is C *[III F 1].*
The t distribution does not reflect less variation due to chance than does the normal distribution. Student's t tests analyze small samples based on the t distribution, which allows for greater variation due to chance than does the normal distribution. As the sample size increases, the sample more closely approximates the population, and the t value approaches the value of the critical ratio. The probability value derived from a t value depends on the number of degrees of freedom, which in turn is based on the sample size. Either actual counts or proportions can be used in calculating the t value.

11. The answer is B *[III H 1].*
Chi-square values are not used in calculating confidence intervals. The chi-square test determines the extent to which an observed distribution differs from a theoretical, or expected, distribution, regardless of the order of the categories of data. The probability value derived from a chi-square value depends on the number of degrees of freedom, which in turn is based on the sample size. The chi-square value is calculated on actual counts, not proportions.

12. The answer is A *[IV A, E 1, 2].*
Screening is not used as a basis for therapy. Screening is the initial examination of an individual to detect disease not yet being treated. Screening tests are applicable to large numbers of individuals and are best if highly sensitive and specific. The ability of the screening test to identify correctly those individuals who truly have the disease is the sensitivity, and its ability to identify correctly those who truly do not have the disease is the specificity. Diagnosis testing is done to determine the cause of a patient's disease and treatment testing to monitor the effectiveness of and the patient's response to therapy. Individuals for whom a screening test is positive should be given follow-up evaluation.

13. The answer is B (1, 3) *[II A].*
Measures of central tendency include the median, mode, and mean, which are summary measures for a sample or population that describe the middle values or the values occurring most often. Measures of dispersion include the range, variance, standard deviation, and coefficient of variation, which are summary measures for a sample or population that describe the scatter of the series.

14. The answer is A (1, 2, 3) *[III G 1 a, b].*
The standard error of the mean is an estimate of the standard deviation of the population based on the standard deviation of a sample. The standard error of the mean is based on the fact that the means of the samples follow a normal distribution, even if the samples do not. The standard error of the mean is used to determine confidence limits. The standard error of the mean is equal to the standard deviation of the sample divided by the square root of the sample size; therefore, the standard error of the mean decreases as the sample size increases.

15. The answer is B (1, 3) *[IV E 1].*
The sensitivity of a screening test is the test's ability to identify correctly those persons who truly have the disease. It is independent of disease prevalence in the population under study. Screening test parameters are measures of the clinical usefulness of a test when compared with a definitive diagnostic test. Sensitivity is calculated by dividing the number of persons with the disease who screen positive by the total number of persons with the disease. The positive predictive value is a test's ability to identify those persons who truly have the disease from among all those persons whose screening tests are positive.

16. The answer is E (all) *[III G 2 a (2), b (1), (6), (9)].*
A confidence interval is based on a critical ratio when the sample size is large, it gives an indication of the likely magnitude of the true value, it gives an indication of the certainty of the point estimate, and it becomes narrower as the sample size increases. A confidence interval is the probable range for a population measure around a point estimate from a sample. For large populations, the critical ratio is used, and, for small samples, a t value is used. When the confidence interval is wider, the point estimate is likely to be less accurate and reliable. As the sample size increases, it approaches the population size; therefore, the confidence interval decreases in size.

17. The answer is B (1, 3) *[III H 1].*
The chi-square test determines the extent that an observed distribution differs from a theoretical, or expected, distribution. Although the expected value in each cell must be at least 5 for the test to be valid, observed values can be less than 5. The chi-square value is independent of the arithmetic mean.

18. The answer is C (2, 4) *[III I].*
Fisher's exact test is used instead of the chi-square test if the expected value in any cell of the fourfold table is less than 5, regardless of the observed value. It requires calculating probability values for the fourfold table under study and for tables that are more extreme. Fisher's exact test determines the exact probability due to chance of an association between two variables that are being analyzed in a fourfold table. The test yields the exact probability for the observed distribution and for more extreme distributions. No adjustment is necessary for varying degrees of freedom. (There is always only 1 degree of freedom in a fourfold table).

19. The answer is E (all) *[III K 1–2].*
Nonparametric tests can be used to compare two populations when each population is unimodal, independent, and distributed normally, and when both populations have equal numbers. Nonparametric tests are analytic tests of the null hypothesis for samples and populations regardless of their size or the underlying distribution. The populations being compared may be dependent or independent.

20. The answer is B (1, 3) *[II A 1–3, B 1].*
The median age for the black children is less than that for the white children. There are two modal ages for the black children and one for the white children. The median is the value in a series that divides the series into two equal parts. The median age for the black children (3 years) is less than that for the white children (4 years). The mode is the value that occurs most frequently in a series. Among the black children there are two modal ages—2 and 4 years—whereas among the white children the modal age is 3 years. The mean is the sum of all values in a series divided by the number of values. The mean age for the black children (3 years) is less than the mean age for the white children (4.2 years). The range of ages, or the difference between the highest and lowest ages, is higher among the black children (4 years) than it is among the white children (3 years).

21. The answer is C (2, 4) *[III B 2 b (1), (3), (4)].*
The probability is 2% that the distribution of illness in those who ate chicken salad compared with those who did not is due to chance. Because the report states that the difference is statistically significant, the null hypothesis (i.e., that the difference is due to chance) can be rejected, and alternative hypotheses (e.g., the chicken salad was contaminated) must be considered. The proportion of individuals who were ill cannot be deduced from the given probability value.

22. The answer is B (1, 3) *[III L].*
The model is valid only for work shifts between 8 and 24 hours long, and the regression coefficient is 0.1. Regression analysis is the mathematical modeling used to describe the effect that one or more independent variables have on a dependent variable. A regression equation is valid only in the observed range of the dependent variable and only for the population under study. The dependent variable (the number of hours sleeping), not the independent variable (the number of hours working), is also subject to random variation. The regression coefficient is the average change in the dependent variable for each unit in the independent variable. In this model, there is a linear and nonlogarithmic relationship between the independent and dependent variables.

23–26. The answers are: 23-D, 24-C, 25-B, 26-A *[III L].*
A regression equation is the mathematical model to describe the effect that one or more independent variables have on a dependent variable. In the equation $y = a + bx$, the dependent variable (y) is determined by the independent variable (x). The average change in the dependent variable for each unit in the independent variable is the regression coefficient (b) or slope of the equation. The y-axis intercept (a) is the value of the dependent variable when the independent variable is equal to zero.

27–30. The answers are: 27-D, 28-E, 29-C, 30-C *[II A 1–3, B 1].*
The median is the value that divides a series of values into two equal parts. Because the number of test scores greater than 6 equals the number of scores less than 6, the median test score equals 6. The mode is the value that occurs most frequently in a series. In this distribution, the mode is 7. The mean is the sum of all the values in a series (25) divided by the number of values (5) and, therefore, in this example, is 5. The range is the spread between the highest and lowest values in a series, which is determined by subtracting the lowest value (2) from the highest value (7). In this example, then, the range is 5.

4
Epidemiology and Prevention of Selected Acute Illnesses

Robert G. Sharrar

I. INTRODUCTION. This chapter focuses on acute communicable diseases of public health importance, emphasizing the various recommendations for controlling the spread of these diseases. Each section presents important epidemiologic features of the disease, the infectious disease process, and current recommendations for control.

II. GENERAL METHODS OF CONTROL AND PREVENTION

A. Agent. There are three methods of control.

1. **Eliminating the disease-causing agent**
   a. **Chemotherapeutic or chemoprophylactic agents** kill biologic agents internally so they cannot infect others.
   b. **Disinfectants** kill organisms outside the body. Blood spills are cleaned with detergent and water and the area disinfected with a 1:10 dilution of household bleach, which inactivates hepatitis B virus (HBV) and human immunodeficiency virus (HIV), the virus that causes acquired immune deficiency syndrome (AIDS).
   c. **Chlorination** of the water supply prevents the spread of many microorganisms.
   d. **Heat** is used to pasteurize milk, to destroy certain bacteria that are part of the food chain (e.g., *Salmonella*), and to inactivate botulinal toxin in contaminated food. Heat also is used to sterilize certain equipment.

2. **Preventing the organism from multiplying to the level at which it can cause disease**
   a. **Proper temperatures for storing and serving food** should be used so the small number of organisms that frequently contaminate food are not able to multiply to a sufficient number **(inoculum)** to cause disease.
   b. **Chlorinating air-cooling towers** can prevent *Legionella pneumophila* (the agent responsible for legionnaires' disease) from reaching a sufficient inoculum to cause disease.

3. **Eliminating the reservoir so that the agent has no natural place to multiply.** Certain agents (e.g., measles, smallpox) die out when there are no susceptible hosts in which to live. The virus that causes smallpox has been eradicated from the general population in this way.

B. Reservoir

1. **Human**
   a. **Isolation or quarantine.** The object is to isolate the agent that causes disease not the patient.
      (1) **Total physical isolation** rarely is indicated. It is used in special circumstances (e.g., hospitalized patients) and for certain diseases that are highly contagious, usually by the airborne route. A case of pneumonic plague would require total isolation.
      (2) **Limited physical isolation** is used to restrict certain actions of the patients. Individuals with certain infections [e.g., due to *Salmonella, Shigella,* or acute hepatitis A virus (HAV)] are not allowed to work in occupations that prepare or serve food for public consumption.
   b. **Chemotherapeutic agents** can eliminate the organism from symptomatic or asymptomatic (carrier) individuals. For example, rifampin is used to eliminate the pharyngeal carriage of *Neisseria meningitidis* and *Hemophilus influenzae,* and proper antituberculosis therapy can eliminate *Mycobacterium tuberculosis* from infected patients.

c. **Active immunization** can prevent the carrier state. Dentists who receive HBV vaccine will not become infected with HBV or become chronic carriers of the hepatitis B surface antigen (HBsAg).

2. **Animals**

a. **Wild animals. Rabies infection** is known to be endemic in certain wild animals, such as skunks, raccoons, bats, and foxes. Thus, contact (especially bites) by potentially rabid animals should be avoided. These wild animals should not be helped in emergency situations, because the injured animals may be rabid. They should not be fed or approached by individuals inexperienced in handling them.

b. **Pets.** Only certain animals are appropriate as household pets, and they should be properly immunized and seen regularly by a veterinarian. Raccoons and skunks should not be kept as pets, since some of these animals become rabid. Pet dogs should be examined periodically for the presence of ticks.

3. **Environment**

a. **Natural environment.** Certain environmental factors can serve as a breeding ground for agents or vectors of disease.

(1) **Bird droppings.** *Histoplasma capsulatum* can grow in certain bird droppings. Areas containing bird droppings should be decontaminated with a formaldehyde solution before they are cleaned.

(2) **Mosquitoes.** Stagnant water can serve as a breeding ground for mosquitoes. Many communities have vector control programs that prevent the breeding of mosquitoes.

b. **Man-made environment.** Cooling towers and air-conditioning units have served as breeding grounds for *L. pneumophilia.*

C. **Portal of exit.** Since microorganisms exit the human and animal reservoirs in normal body functions (e.g., breathing, defecating), the portal of exit cannot be blocked. Percutaneous exit can be prevented by avoiding needle sticks and insect bites. When the environment is the reservoir, any change, such as construction activity, may cause dissemination of organisms.

D. Mode of transmission

1. **Direct transmission,** which is the transfer of organisms directly from one person to another, can be blocked by simple processes.

a. **Hand washing** is the most important procedure for preventing the spread of most infections (e.g., enteric diseases such as shigellosis).

(1) The **microbial flora of the skin** consists of **resident microorganisms,** which are not virulent, and **transient microorganisms,** which are acquired from colonized or infected people or from the individual's own gastrointestinal tract. These transient microorganisms may be pathogens capable of causing serious systemic disease.

(2) **Good hand-washing technique** consists of a vigorous rubbing together of all surfaces of lathered hands for at least 10 seconds, followed by thorough rinsing under a stream of water. Plain soap can be used in routine situations, but antimicrobial hand-washing products should be used in a health care setting when handling newborns or touching immunocompromised patients.

(3) **When hand washing is necessary.** Hands should be washed before preparing food for consumption by someone else, after defecating or urinating, and after handling items that may be contaminated. In a health care environment, most routine, brief patient-care contacts do not require hand washing. However, hand washing is required in the following settings:

(a) Before performing invasive procedures
(b) Before touching susceptible or immunocompromised patients or open wounds
(c) Between contact with patients in high-risk areas
(d) After removing gloves
(e) After touching body fluids, secretions, or excretions
(f) After touching potentially contaminated environmental items

b. **Protective apparel** is used primarily in a health care setting to protect the health care worker from microorganisms transmitted in blood or body fluids that might contain blood.

(1) **Universal Blood and Body Fluid Precautions** are recommended in the care of all patients, since it is impossible to tell who is infected with what on the basis of a medical history or physical examination.

(a) These precautions apply to:

(i) Blood and other body fluids containing visible blood

(ii) Semen and vaginal secretions, even though they have not been implicated in occupational transmission in a health care setting

(iii) Certain tissues and fluids, such as cerebrospinal fluid (CSF), and synovial, pleural, peritoneal, pericardial, and amniotic fluids

(b) These precautions do not apply to saliva, feces, nasal secretions, sputum, sweat, tears, urine, and vomitus, unless they contain visible blood.

(2) Protective apparel may include gloves, gowns, masks, protective eyewear, and in some instances, boots and hats. Protective garments should be worn only once and then discarded in appropriate receptacles.

(a) Gloves are used to prevent the transfer of organisms from the patient to the staff and vice versa and to prevent personnel from becoming transiently colonized by pathogenic organisms. Gloves should be worn for touching blood and body fluids, mucous membrane surfaces or broken skin of all patients; for handling items or surfaces soiled with blood or body fluids; and for performing venipuncture and other vascular access procedures. Gloves should be changed after contact with each patient.

(b) Gowns should be worn when individuals will be exposed to blood, body fluids that might contain blood, or infective secretions or excretions. Sterile gowns should be worn when changing dressings on extensive wounds or burns.

(c) Masks are used primarily to prevent airborne transmitted diseases; however, they also protect against those diseases spread by direct contact or by transfer between mucous membrane surfaces, by preventing personnel from touching the mucous membranes of their eyes, nose, and mouth until after they have washed their hands and removed their masks. Masks should be worn during procedures that are likely to generate droplets of blood or other body fluids to prevent exposure of mucous membranes of the mouth, nose, and eyes. High-efficiency disposable masks, which cover the nose and the mouth, are more effective than cotton gauze or paper tissue masks. Masks become ineffective after they become moist.

(d) Protective eyewear should be used by dentists and all health care workers who are exposed to aerosols of saliva and blood.

c. Patient education

(1) Condom use can prevent the transfer of most sexually transmitted diseases (STDs), including herpes simplex virus (HSV) infection, chlamydial infection, syphilis, gonorrhea, and AIDS.

(2) Organisms that spread by **large airborne droplets** can be blocked by patients covering their mouths when coughing or sneezing and by using disposable tissues.

2. Indirect transmission

a. Avoiding bites from arthropod vectors. Diseases transmitted by arthropod vectors (e.g., mosquitoes, mites, ticks) can be prevented by avoiding bites from these insects. Lyme disease and Rocky Mountain spotted fever can be prevented with the following precautions:

(1) Door and window screens can prevent insects from entering.

(2) Protective clothing, such as long pants and long-sleeved shirts, should be worn when exposure is expected.

(3) Insect repellents should be used on exposed skin surfaces, preferably repellents containing over 30% active ingredient of *N,N*-diethyl-*m*-toluamide (deet).

(4) Ticks should be removed from the body immediately, with tweezers if possible, using a gentle, steady motion to avoid leaving mouth parts in the skin. The tick that causes Rocky Mountain spotted fever must be attached to the body for several hours to allow transmission of the rickettsial organism.

b. Avoiding diseases spread by common vehicle can be accomplished by eliminating the vehicle or by preventing significant contamination.

(1) Disposable patient-care equipment should be used when possible and properly discarded. Articles contaminated with infectious material should be discarded or bagged and labeled before being sent for decontamination and reprocessing.

(2) Blood should be screened for serologic markers of biologic agents that cause disease. Those units that are positive should not be used for transfusion purposes. Table 4-1 lists the tests used by the American Red Cross to screen every unit of blood for specific diseases.

Table 4-1. Blood-Screening Tests for Specific Diseases

Disease	Screening Test
Syphilis	Rapid plasma reagin (RPR)
Hepatitis B virus (HBV)	Hepatitis B surface antigen (HBsAg)
AIDS/HIV	HIV antibodies
Hepatitis C (HCV)	HCV antibody (anti-HCV)
Hepatitis non-A, non-B	Hepatitis B core antibody (anti-HBVc) and alanine aminotransferase as markers or surrogate markers
Human T cell lymphotropic virus types I/II (HTLV-I/II)	HTLV-I/HTLV-II antibodies
Cytomegalovirus (CMV)*	CMV antibodies

*Only blood given to immunocompromised patients and premature infants is screened for CMV. CMV infection can be severe in these patients.

(3) **Proper canning, preparation, serving, and storage of food** can prevent contamination of food or prevent a small bacterial inoculum from multiplying to the point at which it can cause disease.

(a) **Canning** requires a processing temperature of 250° F (120° C) or higher (steam under pressure) to destroy the spores of *Clostridium botulinum*.

(b) **Poultry,** which is frequently contaminated with *Salmonella,* must be heated to an internal (core) temperature of 165° F (75° C).

(c) **Steam serving tables** should maintain a minimum temperature of 140° F (60° C).

(d) **Refrigeration.** Food should be refrigerated at temperatures below 45° F (8° C). Many foods require lower temperatures.

(e) ***Staphylococcus* enterotoxin.** Food contaminated with *Staphylococcus* enterotoxin must be discarded, since the enterotoxin cannot be inactivated by heat.

c. **Diseases spread by the airborne route** are much more difficult to control. The droplet nuclei remain suspended in the air and can be widely dispersed by air currents. Ultraviolet lights and isolation of patients in well-ventilated rooms have been used.

E. Portal of entry. Since most microorganisms enter the host through normal body functions (e.g., breathing, eating), the portal of entry is difficult to block. **Percutaneous entry** can be prevented by using sterile needles, by avoiding insect bites, and by covering open cuts or sores.

F. Susceptible host

1. **Good health habits** such as rest, exercise, and a balanced diet may protect a person from certain communicable diseases. While no one has proven that good health habits are effective, no one has proven that they are not.
   a. Studies have shown that **excessive alcohol intake** interferes with serum bactericidal properties and white cell function.
   b. **Tobacco smoke** interferes with the ciliary motion in the lining of the respiratory tract and leads to anatomic changes, which can result in chronic bronchitis and recurrent episodes of bacterial and viral pneumonias.
2. **Prevention of skin breakdown** (e.g., avoiding dryness, preventing decubitus ulcers) is important since skin is an effective barrier against all biologic agents.
3. **Natural immunity** is acquired immunity. All children are born with some antibody protection, which they acquire from their mothers. This **passive immunity** lasts about 6 months. When the maternal protection disappears, the infant must develop her own immunity. This **naturally acquired immunity** occurs when the child is exposed to biologic agents as she begins the socialization process. This may begin when the child is exposed to other children in school or day-care centers. Unfortunately, socialization brings exposure, and exposure brings disease. However, children handle many diseases better than adults.
4. **Artificially acquired immunity** occurs when individuals are immunized with **vaccines**. It is artificial since it is caused by a man-made vaccine. It is acquired since the individual makes his own antibodies. Vaccines do not provide immediate protection since it may take 2 weeks

for antibody production to occur. Vaccines make susceptible hosts resistant to circulating organisms. They have been used to eradicate smallpox from the globe and to eliminate measles and polio from most parts of the United States. As the proportion of immune (immunized plus previously infected) individuals increases, the amount of wild virus in the population decreases and the amount of clinical disease decreases, since there are fewer susceptible people exposed to the biologic agent.

5. **Chemoprophylaxis** can protect temporarily a susceptible host during periods of intense exposure. Chloroquine phosphate or mefloquine hydrocloride is used to prevent malaria in individuals traveling in malarious areas. Isoniazid (INH) is used to protect household or close contacts of patients with pulmonary tuberculosis until their tuberculin skin test can be determined accurately (3 months after exposure) and until the index case is no longer communicable.

III. IMMUNOBIOLOGIC AGENTS

A. Types of agents

1. **Vaccine** is a suspension of attenuated live or killed microorganisms (bacteria or viruses), or fractions thereof, administered to induce immunity, thereby preventing an infectious disease. Commonly used vaccines include:
   a. **Live attenuated viral vaccines,** such as measles, mumps, rubella, polio, and yellow fever vaccines
   b. **Killed or fractionated viral vaccines,** such as influenza, hepatitis B, polio, and rabies vaccines
   c. **Killed or fractionated bacterial vaccines,** such as *H. influenzae* type B (Hib) vaccine, meningococcal or pneumococcal polysaccharide vaccines, and cholera vaccines

2. **Toxoid** is a modified bacterial toxin that has been rendered nontoxic but that retains the ability to stimulate the formation of antitoxin. Commonly used toxoids include diphtheria and tetanus toxoids.

3. **Immune globulin (IG)** is a sterile solution of human antibodies prepared by cold ethanol fractionation of large pools of blood plasma. It is primarily used for passive immunization against measles and HAV and for routine maintenance of certain immunodeficient individuals.

4. **Specific IG** is a special sterile solution of human antibodies prepared from donor pools preselected for a high antibody titer content against a specific disease. Commercially available preparations include:
   a. Hepatitis B immune globulin (HBIG)
   b. Rabies immune globulin (RIG)
   c. Tetanus immune globulin (TIG)
   d. Varicella zoster immune globulin (VZIG)

5. **Antitoxin** is a solution of antibodies derived from the serum of animals immunized with specific antigens. Antitoxins are used to provide passive immunity as treatment for certain bacterial infections or poisonous snakebites. Examples of antitoxins include:
   a. Botulism antitoxin
   b. Diphtheria antitoxin
   c. Crotalus antitoxin against the venum of rattlesnakes

B. Disease prevention.
Immunobiologic agents were created to prevent the following types of diseases.

1. **Common diseases** cause a great deal of illness. In the era before vaccines, almost every child experienced measles, mumps, and rubella.

2. **Serious diseases,** which can include common diseases, have significant sequelae.
   a. **Measles,** which can cause pneumonia, encephalitis, mental retardation, and death
   b. **Rubella,** which can cause congenital birth defects
   c. **Polio,** which can cause paralysis and death

3. **Untreatable or difficult to treat diseases.** Examples include:
   a. **Viral infections** (e.g., rabies, HBV)

b. **Toxogenic infections** (e.g., diphtheria, tetanus), which still have a high case-fatality rate (even with penicillin therapy, pneumococcal pneumonia is fatal in 5% of hospitalized cases)

C. **Recommendations for use of immunobiologic agents.** Since no vaccine is completely safe or completely effective and since scientific data concerning all possible circumstances are incomplete, the decision to administer an immunobiologic agent must lie with the clinician who has some understanding of these vaccines and who knows the patient. The balance between benefits (prevention of a disease) and risks (side effects of the vaccine), which may be significant, must be considered in each instance.

1. **Sources of vaccine information**
   a. **Recommendations of the Advisory Committee on Immunization Practices (ACIP)** are issued by the U.S. Public Health Service (USPHS), Centers for Disease Control (CDC) and periodically are updated in the *Morbidity and Mortality Weekly Report (MMWR).*
   b. ***Report of the Committee on Infectious Diseases of the American Academy of Pediatrics* (AAP)** is commonly referred to as the "red book" (AAP, 1988) and is periodically updated in *Pediatrics.*
   c. **Package inserts** also are published in the *Physician's Desk Reference (PDR).*
   d. ***Technical Bulletin of the American College of Obstetricians and Gynecologists*** contains information about immunizing pregnant women.
   e. ***Health Information for International Travel*** is published annually by the CDC as a guide to requirements and recommendations for specific immunizations and health practices for travel to various countries.
   f. **Advisory memoranda** are published periodically by the CDC and advise international travelers about specific outbreaks of communicable diseases abroad.
   g. ***Guide for Adult Immunization*** is published by the American College of Physicians. In addition to discussing various vaccines, it includes immunization recommendations for special groups (e.g., family member exposures, occupational groups, lifestyles), for immunocompromised adults (e.g., individuals who are HIV positive, alcoholics, patients with diabetes mellitus or renal failure), for accidental or unavoidable exposures (e.g., animal bites, specific infections), and for international travel.

2. **General guidelines for administration.** The package insert should be consulted for information about the manufacturing, nature, and content of an immunobiologic agent as well as information about contraindications, side effects, and storage of the agent.
   a. **The ACIP recommended immunization schedule** for adults is shown in Table 4-2 (see Tables 7-1 and 7-2 for immunization schedules for normal infants and children).
   b. **Split doses or intradermal administration** should be avoided unless specifically recommended.
   c. **Multiple doses or periodic reinforcements** are necessary for full protection by some vaccines.
      (1) It is not necessary to restart or add extra doses to an interrupted series of an immunobiologic agent. The immunization schedule can be continued as if it had not been interrupted.
      (2) Doses given at less than recommended intervals should not be counted as part of the primary series (e.g., two polio immunizations given a week apart should be counted as one polio immunization).

Table 4-2. Recommended Immunization Schedules for Normal Adults*

Indications	Vaccine
> 18 years	Td every 10 years (see III D 1)
Born after 1956	Measles (see IV A 3)
Women in reproductive years	Rubella (see III D 3 c)
High-risk adults	Hepatitis B (see VI B 3 d) Pneumococcal (see III D 7) Influenza (see IV B 3 b)

Td = tetanus and diphtheria.

*From Advisory Committee on Immunization Practices (ACIP)

d. Simultaneous administration of several immunobiologic agents. Most widely used vaccine antigens can be given safely and effectively simultaneously.

(1) **Inactivated vaccines** can be administered simultaneously at separate sites.

(2) **Live attenuated viral vaccines** can be given on the same day; otherwise, they should be given at least 1 month apart.

(3) **Inactivated and live attenuated vaccines** may be administered at the same time. However, cholera and yellow fever vaccines should be separated by at least 3 weeks.

e. Administration of IG and vaccines

(1) **Inactivated vaccines** have a large antigenic load, do not require multiplication in the body, and can be given anytime after IG. When administered simultaneously, they should be given at different sites.

(2) **Live attenuated viral vaccines** have a small antigenic load, require multiplication in the body, and cannot be given with IG.

(a) A live vaccine should not be given for at least 6 weeks and preferably 3 months after the administration of IG.

(b) If IG has to be given less than 14 days after administration of a live vaccine, the vaccine should be repeated 3 months after the IG.

(c) IG does not interfere with oral polio or yellow fever immunizations.

f. Reactions to vaccine components

(1) **Egg hypersensitivity.** Some vaccines (e.g., yellow fever, measles, mumps, influenza) are grown in embryonated chicken eggs.

(a) If an individual can eat eggs without adverse effects, then he can be immunized with measles, mumps, yellow fever, or influenza vaccines.

(b) Any vaccine grown on embryonated eggs should not be given to anyone with a known anaphylactic hypersensitivity to eggs.

(2) **Preservative hypersensitivity.** Some vaccines contain preservatives, such as **thimerosal** (a mercurial), or trace amounts of an antibiotic **(neomycin)**. They should not be given to individuals who have had anaphylactic reactions to these agents.

(3) **Penicillin allergy.** No currently recommended vaccine contains penicillin or its derivatives. Therefore, a history of penicillin allergy is not a contraindication to immunization.

(4) **Immunocompromised individuals** should not be given a live attenuated viral vaccine. Since recipients of oral poliovirus vaccine (OPV) excrete the vaccine strain in their stool, OPV should not be given to individuals who live in households with immunocompromised hosts.

(5) **Individuals with severe febrile illnesses** (an oral temperature greater than 100° F) should not be immunized until they have recovered, primarily to avoid blaming a vaccine for a manifestation of the underlying illness.

(6) **Adverse events following immunizations** may or may not be related to the vaccine. All temporally associated events severe enough to require medical attention should be reported to local or state health officials, to the vaccine manufacturer, and to the Food and Drug Administration (FDA).

g. Vaccination during pregnancy

(1) Although no studies show teratogenic effects, live attenuated viral vaccines should not be given to pregnant women or to those likely to become pregnant within 3 months of receiving the vaccine.

(2) Pregnant women at substantial risk of exposure may receive a live viral vaccine. When possible, it should be given during the second or third trimester.

(3) There is no evidence that inactivated vaccines or IG poses any risk to the fetus. In fact, women incompletely immunized against tetanus should complete their primary series during the last two trimesters of pregnancy.

(4) **Children of pregnant women** should receive age-appropriate immunizations. There is no evidence that children given measles-mumps-rubella (MMR) vaccine can transmit these diseases.

h. Misconceptions concerning contraindications to vaccination. The following conditions are *not* reasons for delaying or discontinuing routine immunizations:

(1) Soreness, redness, or swelling at the injection site or a temperature of less than 105° F (40.5° C) in reaction to a previous dose of diphtheria and tetanus toxoids and pertussis (DTP) vaccine; more severe reactions to DTP [see III D 1 c (4) (a)] are contraindications to future DTP immunizations

(2) Mild acute illness with low-grade fever or mild diarrheal illness in an otherwise well child
(3) Current antimicrobial therapy or the convalescent phase of illnesses
(4) Prematurity; immunizations should be given on the basis of chronologic age, and the vaccine dose should not be reduced
(5) Pregnancy of mother or other household contact
(6) Recent exposure to a communicable disease
(7) Breast-feeding
(8) A history of nonspecific allergies or relatives with allergies
(9) Family history of convulsions in persons considered for pertussis or measles vaccination
(10) Family history of sudden infant death syndrome in children considered for DTP vaccination
(11) Family history of an adverse event, unrelated to immunosuppression, following vaccination

D. Vaccines available for routine immunization

1. **Diphtheria and tetanus toxoids and pertussis (DTP) vaccine.** DTP and diphtheria and tetanus toxoids (DT) vaccines are used for children under 7 years of age. Tetanus and diphtheria toxoids (Td) vaccine is used for individuals 7 years of age or older. Single antigen preparations also are available. Diphtheria and tetanus toxoids are prepared by formaldehyde treatment of the respective toxins. Pertussis vaccine is a suspension of inactivated *Bordetella pertussis.*

a. Diphtheria

(1) **Incidence.** Diphtheria is a rare disease in the United States with less than five reported cases each year. Cases primarily occur in inadequately immunized persons.
(2) **Presence of bacteria.** Immunization does not eliminate *Corynebacterium diphtheriae* in the nasopharynx or on the skin.
(3) **Serosurveys.** Results of serosurveys suggest that many adults are not protected against diphtheria.
(4) **Conferred immunity.** Diphtheria infection may not confer immunity since some strains that cause disease are nontoxicogenic. Active immunization should be initiated at the time of recovery.

b. Tetanus

(1) **Incidence.** Fewer than 100 cases of tetanus have been reported per year for the past 10 years. Approximately two-thirds of the patients are over 50 years old.
(2) **Morbidity and mortality.** There were 101 reported cases in 1987–1988.
   (a) Twenty-five percent of the reported cases had no identified acute injury. The most frequently reported injuries were puncture wounds (29%), lacerations (18%), and abrasions (13%).
   (b) Of the 61 patients whose circumstances of injury were known, 33% were injured indoors, 41% during farming or gardening activities, and 26% in outdoor settings.
   (c) Fifty-eight percent of tetanus patients with acute injuries did not seek medical care for their injuries; of those who did, 81% did not receive prophylaxis as recommended by ACIP guidelines.
   (d) The case-fatality ratio was 21% for 1987–1988.
(3) **Presence of bacteria.** The spores of *Clostridium tetani* are ubiquitous.
(4) **Serosurveys** show that over 50% of individuals over 60 years old have inadequate levels of antitoxin.
(5) **Conferred immunity.** Clinical tetanus does not confer immunity. Active immunization should be instituted at the time of recovery.
(6) **Prevention.** For tetanus prophylaxis in wound management, the physician must:
   (a) Determine if the patient has completed a primary series (two doses)—individuals who have had military service since 1941 have received at least one dose; uncertain immunizations should not be counted
   (b) Administer Td or DT to anyone who has not completed the primary series or if more than 10 years have passed since the last dose
   (c) Give Td or DT for certain wounds (e.g., wounds contaminated with dirt, feces, soil, or saliva; puncture wounds; avulsions; wounds resulting from missiles, crushing, burns, or frostbite) if more than 5 years have passed since the last dose
   (d) Use TIG in individuals who have not had a primary series and who have wounds that call for Td or DT [see III D 1 b (6) (c)].

c. Pertussis

(1) Incidence. There were 8682 reported cases of pertussis during 1986–1988. However, it is estimated that only 5%–10% of cases get reported.

(2) Morbidity and mortality

(a) Although 46% of the reported cases were in children under 1 year of age, they accounted for 80% of the hospitalizations.

(b) Of the 26 patients who died, 14 were less than 6 months of age, giving this group a case-fatality rate of 0.5%.

(c) Two-thirds of the pertussis cases in children age 7 months to 4 years could have been prevented with age-appropriate immunizations.

(3) Communicability. Pertussis is highly communicable, with secondary family attack rates of over 90% in unimmunized household contacts.

(4) Contraindications

(a) Serious reactions (and frequency of occurrence per dose of vaccine administered), which can occur following DTP immunizations, represent an absolute contraindication for further immunizations with a vaccine containing pertussis. These reactions are:

(i) Persistent, inconsolable crying lasting 3 hours or more (1/100 doses) or an unusual, high-pitched cry occurring within 48 hours (1/900 doses)

(ii) Fever of 105° F (40.5° C) or greater (orally) within 24 hours (1/330 doses)

(iii) Collapse or shock-like state (hypotonic-hyporesponsive episode) within 48 hours (1/1750 doses)

(iv) Convulsions with or without fever occurring within 3 days (1/1750 doses); children who have convulsions within 4–7 days should be evaluated carefully before receiving additional DTP immunizations

(v) Acute encephalopathy within 7 days, including severe alterations in consciousness with generalized or focal neurologic signs (1/110,000 doses)

(vi) Permanent neurologic deficit occurring within 7 days (1/310,000 doses)

(b) Children or infants with an evolving neurologic disorder should not receive pertussis vaccine. These disorders include:

(i) Uncontrolled epilepsy

(ii) Infantile spasms

(iii) Progressive encephalopathy

(5) Children with stable conditions (e.g., cerebral palsy, developmental delay, controlled seizures, corrected neurologic disorders) may be immunized with a pertussis vaccine.

2. Oral, attenuated poliovirus vaccine (OPV) [containing poliovirus types 1, 2, and 3] and inactivated poliovirus vaccine (IPV)

a. Incidence. Poliomyelitis is rare in the United States today. Fewer than 12 cases of paralytic polio are reported each year. Most of these are in vaccinates or their contacts. In 1954, more than 18,000 cases of paralytic disease were reported.

b. Presence of virus. Wild polioviruses have diminished markedly. Inapparent infection with wild strains early in life no longer play a significant role in establishing immunity. Universal immunization of all infants and children with OPV is a necessity.

c. Prevention with OPV

(1) The primary series of OPV consists of three doses. A supplementary dose is recommended upon entry into school (4–6 years of age).

(2) Breast-feeding does not interfere with successful OPV immunizations.

(3) OPV has been associated with paralytic disease in vaccine recipients and their close contacts. There were 138 cases of paralytic polio from 1973–1984; 105 (76%) were vaccine-associated.

(a) Thirty-five of these cases occurred in recipients of OPV, 50 in contacts to OPV-vaccinated individuals, 14 in immunodeficient individuals, and 6 in individuals who had no history of receiving OPV or contact with recent OPV recipients.

(b) Seventy-nine percent of these vaccine cases occurred with the first dose of OPV.

(c) The risk of paralytic polio from the first dose of OPV is approximately one case per 520,000 doses as compared to one case per 12.3 million for subsequent doses.

(d) The overall risk of vaccine-associated paralytic disease in immunologically normal contacts of OPV recipients is approximately one case per 5.5 million doses of OPV distributed.

(4) OPV should not be given to immunodeficient patients or to household contacts of immunodeficient patients.

d. Prevention with IPV

(1) An enhanced potency IPV with greater antigenic content was distributed commercially in 1988. It is produced in human diploid cells.

(2) The primary series of enhanced-potency IPV consists of three doses. The need for additional doses is unknown.

(3) IPV is used to immunize susceptible adults and immunodeficient patients.

(4) IPV is used to immunize children who cannot be isolated from immunodeficient household contacts.

e. Prevention in adults. Routine immunization of adults (18 years old or older) residing in the United States is not recommended. However, adults who are at risk for exposure to wild poliovirus should be immunized, including:

(1) Travelers to areas where poliomyelitis is epidemic or endemic

(2) Members of communities or specific population groups with disease caused by wild polioviruses

(3) Laboratory workers handling specimens that may contain polioviruses

(4) Health care workers in close contact with patients who may be excreting polioviruses

3. Live attenuated measles-mumps-rubella virus (MMR) vaccine. Measles-rubella, mumps-rubella, and single antigen vaccines also are available. All three vaccines should be given as MMR.

a. Measles (see IV A)

b. Mumps

(1) **Incidence.** There has been a 98% decrease in reported mumps cases since the vaccine was licensed. Approximately 5000 cases were reported in 1990. However, there has been a shift to older age-groups, with more than one-third of the cases occurring in individuals over the age of 15. Part of this is due to the recent outbreaks in high schools, on college campuses, and in occupational settings.

(2) **Complications. Meningoencephalitis, deafness,** and **orchitis** are complications of mumps disease. Meningeal signs occur in up to 15% of cases and orchitis in 20%–30% of postpubertal males. Sterility is rare. Encephalitis occurs in 5 per 1000 reported cases and deafness in up to 5 per 100,000 reported cases.

(3) **Morbidity.** Although mumps vaccine became commercially available in 1967, it was not recommended for routine use until 1977. Since the peak age-specific incidence for mumps in the prevaccine era was in children age 5–9 years, most persons born before 1957 are likely to have been infected between 1957 and 1977 and probably are immune.

(4) **Immunization recommendations.** Mumps vaccine is recommended for anyone who is unsure of their mumps disease history. Clinical vaccine efficacies have ranged from 75%–90%.

c. Rubella

(1) **Incidence.** Since the vaccine was licensed in 1969, there has been a marked decline in reported rubella cases and in cases of congenital rubella syndrome (CRS). In 1990, there were only 1093 reported cases of rubella and 10 reported cases of CRS.

(2) **Complications.** The major reason for developing rubella vaccine was to prevent the abortions, miscarriages, stillbirths, and fetal anomalies that result from rubella infection in early pregnancy, especially in the first trimester. CRS can cause mental retardation, blindness, deafness, and cardiac defects. From 25%–80% of infants born to women with rubella in the first trimester will be affected.

(3) **Immunization recommendations**

(a) Because of a theoretical risk to the fetus, rubella vaccine should not be given to pregnant women, and women should not become pregnant for 3 months after vaccination. However, the risk of teratogenicity from rubella vaccine is quite small, and rubella immunization during pregnancy is not a reason to recommend interruption of the pregnancy.

(b) Rubella immunization of a woman who has no history of vaccination is justifiable without serologic testing.

4. Hib conjugate vaccine (diphtheria toxoid conjugate) [see VIII A 3 a]

5. Influenza vaccine (see IV B 3 b)

6. **Hepatitis vaccine** (see VI B 3 d)

7. **Pneumococcal polysaccharide vaccine** contains purified capsular materials of 23 types of *Streptococcus pneumoniae* that are responsible for 88% of recent bacteremia pneumococcal diseases in the United States.
   a. **Incidence.** Pneumococcal pneumonia accounts for 10%–25% of all pneumonias and an estimated 40,000 deaths annually in the United States. In some high-risk patients, mortality has been reported to be greater than 40% for bacteremic disease and 55% for meningitis, despite appropriate antimicrobial therapy.
   b. **Immunization recommendations.** This vaccine can be given to everyone. However, vaccination is particularly recommended for:
      (1) **Adults** who are
         (a) **Elderly** (age 65 or older)
         (b) **Chronically ill** due to cardiovascular or pulmonary disease, diabetes mellitus, alcoholism, cirrhosis, or CSF leaks
         (c) **Immunocompromised** due to splenic dysfunction or anatomic asplenia, Hodgkin's disease, AIDS, lymphoma, multiple myeloma, chronic renal failure, nephrotic syndrome, or some other immunosuppressive condition
      (2) **Children age 2 years or older** who are
         (a) **Chronically ill** due to anatomic or functional asplenia, nephrotic syndrome, or CSF leaks
         (b) **HIV infected** or immunosuppressed
   c. **Reimmunization.** Individuals who received the earlier pneumococcal polysaccharide vaccine containing 14 types of *S. pneumoniae* should not be reimmunized with the newer vaccine. However, revaccination should be considered in high-risk adults who were immunized 6 or more years previously and for those who have a rapid decline in antibody.

E. **Immunization schedules** (see Table 4-2 and Tables 7-1 and 7-2). Every patient-physician encounter requires an evaluation of a patient's immunization status. No one in the 20th century should ever develop a vaccine-preventable illness because of lack of immunization.

1. **Documentation.** Administered immunizations should be well documented on the medical record and on the patient's permanent, personal, comprehensive immunization record. The record should contain the type of vaccine administered, the lot number, and the manufacturer, as well as the month, day, and year of administration. The patient should be instructed to keep this record in a safe place so that it is accessible when needed.

2. **Individuals who are traveling abroad** and need additional immunizations should consult their local or state health departments for current recommendations.

IV. MEASLES AND INFLUENZA

A. Measles (rubeola)

1. **Epidemiologic features**
   a. **Prevaccine era (before 1963)**
      (1) **Incidence.** Measles was a common disease of childhood. From 1950 to 1962, over 500,000 cases were reported annually. However, since virtually all children acquired measles, the true number of cases probably exceeded 4 million cases per year, that is, the entire birth cohort.
      (2) **Outbreaks.** Community-wide outbreaks were common and tended to occur every couple of years. Large families often had several children ill at the same time. Outbreaks were most likely to occur in the late winter or early spring.
      (3) **Age distribution**
         (a) Ninety percent of reported cases occurred in individuals less that 10 years of age.
         (b) An estimated 95% of Americans had measles by 15 years of age.
         (c) Over 50% of the cases occurred in children 5–9 years of age.
   b. **Postvaccine era**
      (1) **Incidence.** Measles is now an uncommon disease of childhood. However, there were 27,672 reported cases in 1990. This is the largest number of reported cases since 1977.
         (a) In 1990, 48.1% of the cases were under 5 years of age, and 22.5% were over 20 years of age.

(b) Information on race and ethnicity was available for 11,083 cases. Of these, 56% were non-Hispanic white, 22% were non-Hispanic black, 19% were Hispanic, and 3% were other racial or ethnic groups.
(c) Only 18.4% of the reported cases were appropriately immunized with measles vaccine on or after their first birthday.

(2) **Outbreaks.** In recent years, two types of outbreaks have occurred in the United States.
(a) There have been outbreaks in **unvaccinated preschool-age children in inner city areas,** including those under 15 months of age. Approximately 90% of these children were unimmunized, and 26% of these cases occurred in children under 16 months of age in whom vaccination was not indicated.
(b) There have also been outbreaks in **vaccinated school-age children** with immunization levels of greater than 98%. Some of these outbreaks have occurred on college campuses, where some students were immunized at age 12–14 months or where documentation of immunization was lacking.

c. Morbidity and mortality

(1) **Encephalitis,** with resulting brain damage and mental retardation, occurs in approximately 1 of 2000 reported cases.
(2) **Death** from respiratory or neurologic complications occurs in 1 in 2000 reported cases. There were 89 measles-associated deaths in 1990 for a death-to-case ratio of 3.2 deaths per 1000 cases. Fifty-five percent of the deaths occurred among children less than 5 years of age, and 30.3% of deaths occurred among adults 20 years of age or older.

2. Infectious disease process

a. Agent. The agent is a paramyxovirus, an RNA virus.

b. Reservoir. Humans with clinical disease are the reservoir for measles.

(1) **Subclinical cases** do not occur, or they are extremely rare. There is no carrier state.
(2) **Communicability.** The patient is communicable from just before the prodromal period to about 4 days after the onset of rash. The peak period of communicability is during the prodromal period.

c. Portal of exit is via respiratory secretions.

d. Mode of transmission is primarily by contact with airborne infectious droplets.

e. Portal of entry is via the respiratory tract. Entry via the conjunctiva also has been postulated.

f. Susceptible host

(1) Everyone is susceptible. The onset of disease can occur 6–18 days after exposure.
(2) Clinical disease confers lifelong immunity.
(3) Immunity is acquired by immunization with a live attenuated measles vaccine.
(4) Clinical disease is more severe in malnourished individuals.

3. Control and prevention strategies

a. Measles vaccine development

(1) From 1963 to 1967, a killed measles vaccine was available. Approximately 1.8 million doses were distributed, and an estimated 600,000–900,000 individuals received this vaccine. However, this vaccine was discontinued because it was not effective and was associated with atypical measles, which occurred after exposure to natural measles.
(2) From 1963 to 1974, a live attenuated measles vaccine (Edmonston B strain) was available. Approximately 19 million doses were distributed. Since this vaccine caused a rectal temperature of 103° F (39.5° C) in 30%–60% of recipients, a dose of IG was administered with it.
(3) In 1965 and 1968, further attenuated strains (Schwartz and Moraten) of measles vaccine were marketed. The Moraten vaccine currently is used in the United States.

b. Prior recommendations for vaccine usage

(1) In 1963, the recommendations were to administer the vaccine at age 9 months when maternal antibodies were presumably absent. IG was administered with this vaccine.
(2) In 1965, the age for administering measles vaccine was raised to 12 months, because maternal antibodies were shown to persist to 11 months.
(3) In 1976, the age for administering measles vaccine was raised to 15 months because of better seroconversion.
(4) In 1989, a two-dose MMR immunization schedule was recommended because of outbreaks occurring in older school-age children and young adults who had received a single previous immunization.

c. Immunization recommendations

(1) Individuals born before 1957 usually have immunity from measles as a result of infection with the natural disease and do not need to be immunized.

(2) The ACIP and the AAP now recommend a two-dose MMR immunization schedule.

(a) The first dose should be given at 15 months of age in most areas of the United States but may be given at age 12 months in areas with recurrent measles transmission.

(b) The ACIP recommends that the second dose be given at entry into school (age 4–6 years), while the AAP recommends that it be given just before puberty (age 10–12 years).

(3) Since measles can be a severe disease in HIV-infected patients, and since the administration of MMR vaccine to these patients has not been associated with severe or unusual adverse effects, MMR vaccine should be used to immunize both symptomatic and asymptomatic HIV-infected individuals.

d. Several **national programs** have been initiated by the USPHS to eliminate indigenous measles in the United States.

(1) The strategy consists of:

(a) Achieving and maintaining high immunization levels in the population

(b) Detecting the presence of measles through effective surveillance

(c) Preventing the further spread of measles through aggressive outbreak control

(2) The strategy has been moderately successful at decreasing the number of reported cases, but it has failed to eliminate measles, because it has not been possible to achieve or maintain high immunization levels in all segments of the population.

e. Results of control strategies. Figure 4-1 shows the reported measles cases in the United States from 1960 to 1990.

(1) From 1981 to 1990, the number of reported cases has ranged from 1500 (1983) to 27,672 (1990) cases per year. This represents a decrease of over 95% as compared to the era before vaccine.

(2) In 1990, almost 36% of the reported cases occurred in the preschool-age population. Immunization of preschoolers at the proper age has always been difficult, especially in the lower socioeconomic segments of the urban population.

(3) The current measles vaccine has an efficacy of around 95%. Therefore, some cases of measles will occur in properly immunized persons.

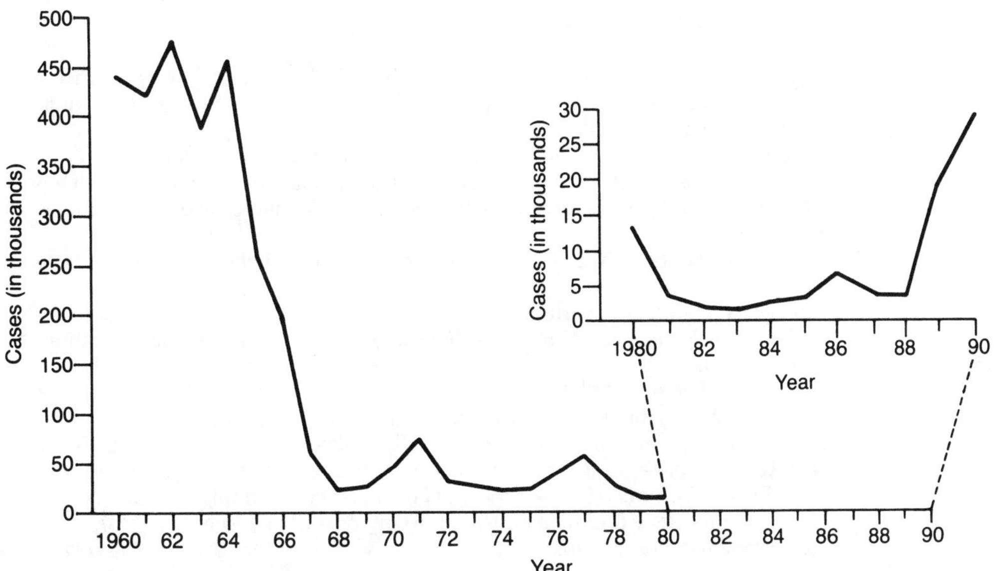

Figure 4-1. Measles (rubeola) cases reported in the United States, by year—1960–1990. The insert shows detail of cases reported from 1980–1990. Data for 1990 are provisional. (Reprinted from Centers for Disease Control: Measles—United States, 1990. *MMWR* 40:369–372, 1991.)

(4) The two-dose MMR immunization schedule should protect against primary vaccine failure (i.e., the failure to seroconvert with the initial vaccine dose) and secondary vaccine failure (i.e., waning immunity) and, therefore, prevent measles outbreaks in older children and young adults.

B. Influenza

1. **Epidemiologic features.** Influenza occurs as sporadic cases, localized outbreaks, epidemics, and pandemics.

a. **Outbreaks**

(1) Influenza outbreaks have a **characteristic pattern**. The virus normally seeds the population with isolated sporadic cases. The actual epidemic begins abruptly, spreads quickly so that peak activity occurs in 2–3 weeks, and is over in 5–6 weeks, depending on the size of the community. The **amount of influenza activity in a community** is measured by:

(a) Increased absenteeism in schools and industries

(b) Increased visits to emergency rooms for upper respiratory illness symptoms

(c) Increased hospitalizations for pneumonia

(d) Increased pneumonia-influenza mortality; this excess mortality normally occurs 2 or more weeks after the epidemic has peaked, and it is considered an index of the severity of the outbreak

(2) During an outbreak, several different strains of influenza virus may circulate at the same time, although one strain is normally predominant. It is difficult to isolate an influenza virus between epidemic periods.

b. **Epidemics**

(1) **Nationwide epidemics** occur every 2–3 years; **worldwide epidemics** occur at longer intervals and normally are preceded by a major change in the antigenic structure.

(2) **Seasonal tendency.** In temperate zones, epidemics occur in the winter months, but in the tropics, they can occur at any time.

(3) **Attack rates** during epidemics range from 10%–50%. Although the highest clinical attack rates are in the school-age population, the highest case-fatality rates are in the older or more debilitated segments of the population.

(4) **Morbidity and mortality.** In interpandemic years, widespread influenza activity and excess mortality normally occurs in January through March. In pandemic years, widespread influenza activity and excess mortality normally occurs between October and December.

2. **Infectious disease process**

a. **Agent**

(1) **Types.** Influenza is an RNA virus. There are three distinct types of influenza viruses—A, B, and C. Types A and B cause widespread epidemics; type C causes local outbreaks of mild disease.

(2) **Antigens.** The surface of the virus has two main antigenic structures:

(a) **Hemagglutinin (H) spike,** which is the site for attachment of the virus to host cell

(b) **Neuraminidase (N) spike,** which may play a role in releasing virus particles from the cell

(3) **Antigenic variation.** The H and N antigens undergo antigenic variation. This is particularly true for type A.

(a) **Types of antigenic variation**

(i) **Antigenic drift** refers to minor changes that continuously occur within a subtype.

(ii) **Antigenic shift** refers to major changes that occur periodically. The new virus has very little or no serologic relationship with previous strains of influenza virus. Pandemic years are normally preceded by a major antigenic shift.

(b) **Recent strains.** In this century, five new H and two N antigens have appeared (Table 4-3). Since 1977, a variety of H_1N_1 and H_3N_2 strains have been circulating simultaneously (the subscripts refer to the type of H and N antigens).

(c) **Nomenclature.** Because of the antigenic variations that occur, influenza isolates have a special nomenclature. The strain designation consists of the virus type, geographic origin, laboratory reference number, and year of occurrence. The antigen description follows in parentheses and describes the antigenic character of the hemagglutinin and the neuraminidase.

Table 4-3. Antigenic Variation of the Influenza Virus

Year	Subtype Designation	No. Years in Circulation
1918	$H_{sw1}N_1$	11
1929	H_0N_1	17
1946	H_1N_1	11
1957	H_2N_2	11
1968	H_3N_2	9
1977	H_1N_1, H_3N_2	...

b. Reservoir. Humans are the reservoir for the strains that cause disease in humans. Animal strains of influenza viruses do exist, but they rarely infect humans.

c. Portal of exit is via the respiratory tract. The period of communicability begins at the onset of clinical disease and persists for about 5 days.

d. Mode of transmission is by the airborne route. Infected individuals cough out large numbers of virus particle aerosols, less than 5 μm in size. The explosive nature of most epidemics suggests that a single infected person can infect a large number of individuals in a relatively short period of time.

e. Portal of entry is via the respiratory tract.

f. Susceptible host

(1) Everyone is susceptible to a new strain of influenza virus.

(2) Since antigenic types of H and N tend to recirculate periodically, and since some immunity develops from prior exposure, the highest incidence rates are in school-age children.

(3) Influenza infection in a young healthy individual is a nuisance but seldom serious.

(4) Infection in the elderly or in those debilitated by chronic cardiac, pulmonary, renal, or metabolic diseases may cause death.

3. Control strategies. Because of the unique characteristics of the virus, influenza is uncontrollable. Pneumonia and influenza are the only communicable diseases that are among the top ten causes of death worldwide.

a. The **World Health Organization (WHO)** has established a worldwide network, consisting of two international centers (London and Atlanta) and nearly 100 collaborating laboratories in over 70 countries, which collects and disseminates laboratory and epidemiologic information on influenza. The main purpose of this network is to monitor the strains of influenza viruses in circulation and to detect any significant antigenic changes that may precede a pandemic. The information also is used to update the formulation of influenza vaccines.

b. Control programs have been directed at high-risk individuals and consist of immunizations with an inactivated influenza vaccine or chemoprophylaxis with amantadine.

(1) Immunization. The PHS recommends that immunizations be offered to:

(a) Adults and children with chronic cardiovascular or pulmonary disorders that require regular medical evaluation

(b) Residents of nursing homes and other care facilities

(c) Adults over 65 years of age

(d) Adults and children with other chronic disorders requiring regular medical follow-up or long-term aspirin therapy, which places the patient at increased risk for developing Reye's syndrome after an influenza infection

(e) Medical personnel who can transmit an influenza infection to their high-risk patients

(f) Persons with HIV infection or immunosuppression

(g) Employees of nursing homes and chronic care facilities who have contact with patients and residents

(h) Providers of home care to, or household members of, high-risk individuals

(2) Composition of vaccine. The antigenic components of the vaccine are based on the types of influenza viruses that were circulating in the community in the previous year. Consequently, the vaccine is almost always at least a year behind. The strains that were used in the 1991–1992 vaccine were A/Taiwan/1/86-like (H_1N_1), A/Beijing/353/89-like (H_3N_2), and B/Panama/45/90-like.

(3) **Chemoprophylaxis**
   (a) **Amantadine** interferes with the uncoating step in the virus replication process and reduces viral shedding.
   (b) It is only effective against type A and must be taken throughout the influenza season.

V. SEXUALLY TRANSMITTED DISEASES (STDs)

A. General characteristics of STDs

1. **Terminology.** The term STD, which describes the mode of transmission rather that the site of infection, came into common use during the 1970s as the medical community became aware of the large number of infections spread from person to person during sexual contact. Since these diseases were found to be not restricted to the genital tract and since many of them were found to be of a systemic nature, the term STD has gradually replaced the term venereal disease.

2. **Diagnostic laboratory tests.** The development of better and more rapid diagnostic laboratory tests has helped to define the problem and its many ramifications. STDs comprise more than 50 different disease entities, including 25 different syndromes, and are caused by more than 20 different organisms. The list includes HAV, HAB, cytomegalovirus (CMV), enteric infections, and ectoparasites, to name only a few.

3. **Incidence.** There has been a marked increase in the total number of cases and in the incidence of STDs.
   a. Approximately 12 million cases of STDs occur each year, including:
      (1) 4 million cases of chlamydial infection
      (2) 3 million cases of trichomoniasis
      (3) 1.4 million cases of gonorrhea
      (4) 1.2 million cases of urethritis (nongonococcal and nonchlamydial)
      (5) 1 million cases of mucopurulent cervicitis (nonchlamydial)
      (6) 1 million cases of human papillomavirus (HPV)
      (7) 200,000–500,000 cases of genital herpes
      (8) 300,000 cases of HBV
      (9) 130,000 cases of syphilis
   b. Approximately 3 million teenagers are affected with STDs annually.
   c. Approximately 63% of all cases occur in individuals under 25 years of age.

4. **Epidemiologic factors.** Not all individuals in the sexually active age-group are at risk for STDs, either because they are not sexually active or because they are in mutually monogamous relationships. The population at risk for STDs is determined by behavioral factors.
   a. **Behavioral risk factors** for STDs include:
      (1) The exchange of sex for drugs
      (2) Casual date or pickup sex—in 1988, 6% of men and 1.2% of women age 18 and over had sex with at least one casual date or pickup within the preceding 12 months
      (3) Multiple sex partners—in 1988, 4.6% of 18- to 29-year-old and 2.9% of 30- to 40-year-old never-married men reported 10 or more sex partners over the preceding 12 months
   b. **Trends in sexual behavior.** In 1988, 60% of men and 50% of women age 15–19 were sexually active.
      (1) Sexually active adults are either remaining single or postponing marriage. In 1980, 28% of 25-year-old women and 43% of 25-year-old men were single compared to 10% and less than 20%, respectively, in 1970.
      (2) Contraceptive practices in the United States have changed. Women now use oral contraceptives to prevent pregnancy. This may have caused a corresponding increase in sexual activity and a decrease in the use of condoms and other barrier contraceptive methods, which are thought to be somewhat protective against STDs. The AIDS epidemic has caused some women to modify their sexual behavior patterns to have less intercourse and fewer partners. However, only 17% of women age 15–19 used condoms in 1988.

5. **Complications.** The extent of human suffering caused by STDs has been recognized by health officials and clinicians. Women and newborn children have the most significant complications of these diseases.

a. **Pelvic inflammatory disease (PID)** is, perhaps, the most severe complication in women.
   (1) PID occurs in 10%–20% of women infected with *Neisseria gonorrhoeae.* It also can be caused by other organisms, such as *Chlamydia* and *Mycoplasma.*
   (2) Approximately 4% of women become infertile following a single episode of PID, 33% after the second episode, and 60% after the third episode.
   (3) Over 750,000 cases of PID are diagnosed and treated each year. Over 180,000 women 15–44 years of age were hospitalized with PID in 1988, and almost 29,200 had hysterectomies.

b. **Infertility.** Officials estimate that 100,000–150,000 women become sterile each year because of pelvic infection due to STDs. Eight percent of all married couples were infertile in 1988; PID was the cause in a significant number of these couples.

c. **Ectopic pregnancies** in the United States have nearly quadrupled since 1970, with almost 88,000 cases in 1987.
   (1) Studies have shown that 6% of pregnancies occurring in women with a previous history of PID were ectopic.
   (2) Women with a history of PID are 10 times more likely to experience an ectopic pregnancy than those without such a history.

d. **Cancer.** At least four viruses (HSV, HPV, HBV, CMV) have been associated with cancers that include the following:
   (1) Cervical intraepithelial neoplasia (HSV and HPV)
   (2) Carcinoma of the cervix (HSV)
   (3) Vulvar carcinoma (HSV)
   (4) Penile carcinoma (HPV and HSV)
   (5) Anal carcinoma (HPV)
   (6) Hepatocellular carcinoma (HBV)
   (7) Kaposi's sarcoma (CMV)

e. **Teratogenicity.** The impact on the fetus and newborn can be devastating. Syphilis and infections caused by HSV, CMV, and *Chlamydia* all result in significant morbidity and mortality, including miscarriages, stillbirths, neonatal deaths, mental retardation, neonatal conjunctivitis, and pneumonia.

6. **Financial costs.** The tremendous economic costs of STDs to society have been recognized by health officials. The total cost of STDs is estimated to exceed $5 billion annually. The total cost (direct and indirect) of PID and its complications of infertility and ectopic pregnancies exceeded $2.6 billion in 1985.

7. **Primary prevention of STDs.** It is important to prevent the acquisition of certain STDs because they are untreatable (e.g., herpes, AIDS) or difficult to treat (e.g., HPV) or because they cause a destructive process in the subclinical state (e.g., latent and congenital syphilis).

a. **Modification of sexual activity** decreases the likelihood of exposure to or contact with infectious agents. For maximal safety, a person should:
   (1) Engage in a mutually monogamous relationship
   (2) Limit the number of sexual partners
   (3) Inspect and question new partners
   (4) Avoid sexual practices involving anal or fecal contact

b. **Barrier methods of contraception** (i.e., condoms, diaphragms, spermicides) provide protection against STDs.
   (1) **Condoms** must be used properly at all times. Advantages include:
      (a) Protection for both partners
      (b) Prevention of the transfer of infected body secretions from one person to another
      (c) Prevention of mucosal surfaces from coming into contact with infected lesions
   (2) **Diaphragms** cover the cervix and, therefore, block an important portal of entry for many infectious agents. When used with a spermicide, they may decrease a woman's risk of acquiring an STD. However, there is no evidence that a diaphragm protects a man from acquiring an STD.

c. **Vaccines.** The only STD that can be prevented with a vaccine is HBV. However, this vaccine is expensive, requires three injections, and does not work well in immunosuppressed individuals.

d. **Prophylactic antibiotics** should not be taken before or after exposure because of the following.
   (1) No single antibiotic covers all potential STDs.
   (2) Allergic reactions may occur.
   (3) They may lead to the emergence of resistant organisms.

e. **Ineffective methods.** There is no evidence that postcoital urination, washing, or douching prevents the acquisition of an STD.

B. Syphilis

1. Epidemiologic features

a. **Rank.** Syphilis ranks as the third most prevalent reportable communicable disease in the United States. Other diseases (e.g., chickenpox) and other STDs (e.g., infections caused by *Chlamydia,* HSV, and HPV; trichomoniasis) occur more frequently but are not reportable to health departments. In 1989, there were approximately 115,000 reported cases of syphilis (all stages), including 46,000 primary and secondary cases.
b. **Geographic distribution.** In 1989, 61% of reported cases occurred in 35 counties nationwide, which include large urban areas.
c. In 1989, the **highest case rates** for primary and secondary syphilis were in men aged 30–34 years and women aged 20–24 years.
d. The **increase in early syphilis** over the last several years has occurred in low-income, inner-city, heterosexual minority populations. Syphilis rates in 1989 were 52 times higher in blacks and 10 times higher in Hispanics than in whites. This increase has been linked to the exchange of sex for drugs.
e. **Congenital syphilis** is most likely to occur in the newborn infants of young, unmarried women who have not received proper prenatal care.
f. **Untreated syphilis infection** can cause blindness, psychosis, or cardiovascular disease.

2. Infectious disease process

a. **Agent.** *Treponema pallidum* is a spirochete that causes syphilis; it is indistinguishable from the spirochetes that cause pinta or yaws.
   (1) *T. pallidum* is 6–15 μm long and 0.15 μm wide.
   (2) It can only be seen with darkfield microscopy, which shows a rotary motion with flexion and back-and-forth motion.
   (3) It is extremely fragile and can be destroyed by soap, antiseptics, and drying.
   (4) It is sensitive to penicillin and several other antimicrobial agents.
b. **Reservoir** of infection is humans who are most likely to transmit the agent during the first year of the disease, when cutaneous lesions are present (primary and secondary stages). Communicability may persist for several years. Untreated women may infect their fetuses for many years; however, this risk declines and may no longer be present after 8 years.
c. **Portal of exit** is:
   (1) **Percutaneously** through cutaneous lesions (e.g., chancre, mucous patch, condyloma latum, lesions of secondary syphilis)
   (2) **Transplacental** from mother to child
   (3) **By a sanguineous nasal discharge** (snuffling, which contains spirochetes (may be the earliest sign of congenital syphilis)
d. **Mode of transmission**
   (1) **Direct contact** with infectious exudates from moist mucosal or cutaneous lesions is the most common mode of transmission.
      (a) The **risk** of getting syphilis from a sexual partner with early syphilis is estimated to be around 30% (range of 10%–60%).
      (b) The **prevalence** of syphilis among contacts with prolonged and repeated exposure (marital partners) may approach 90%.
   (2) **Transplacental transmission** has been documented as early as the 9th week of pregnancy.
   (3) **Transmission by blood transfusions** no longer occurs because the spirochete is killed by a 24–48-hour refrigeration process before red blood cells are transfused.
   (4) **Transmission by accidental needle sticks** is highly unlikely.
e. **Portal of entry** is believed to be through tiny abrasions produced during sexual intercourse. Although the organisms cannot enter through intact skin, they can probably penetrate unbroken mucous membranes. However, they can enter directly into the bloodstream by the transplacental route.
f. **Susceptible host**
   (1) Everyone is susceptible.
   (2) There is no natural or acquired immunity.
   (3) Reinfection is common. No vaccine is available.

3. **Diagnosis**
   a. The antibody response that is invoked can be used for diagnostic purposes.
      (1) **A fourfold rise in the rapid plasma reagin (RPR) test**—a nontreponemal titer test—can be used to diagnose a recent infection that requires treatment.
      (2) The **fluorescent treponemal antibody absorption (FTA-ABS) test** remains positive for life and, therefore, cannot be used to diagnose repeat infections.
   b. Simultaneous HIV infection may alter the clinical presentation, serologic response, or response to therapy. Follow-up serologies are recommended at 1, 2, 3, 6, 9, and 12 months on HIV-infected patients.

4. **Control strategies**
   a. **Routine screening** with serologic tests for syphilis should be done on:
      (1) All individuals with multiple sexual partners
      (2) Any individual with another STD
      (3) Any pregnant women as a means of preventing congenital syphilis; women who have positive serologies should be rescreened during the third trimester or at the time of delivery
   b. **Routine premarital testing and testing of all hospitalized patients** is probably not a cost-effective way of controlling syphilis.
   c. **Case investigation and contact tracing** by experienced investigators have been shown to interrupt the transmission of syphilis. All identified sexual contacts during the communicable stage must be located and treated epidemiologically. For primary, secondary, and early latent syphilis, the periods of concern are 3 months, 6 months, and 1 year, respectively.
   d. **A control program** conducted by federal, state, and local health officials has been in effect since the early 1940s. The success of this program can be documented.
      (1) The number of reported cases of all stages of syphilis has decreased by 89%.
      (2) Reported cases of congenital syphilis have declined by 98%, and infant deaths directly related to syphilis have decreased by 99%. However, over the past several years, the number of cases of congenital syphilis has increased dramatically.
      (3) First admissions to mental hospitals with the diagnosis of syphilis psychosis (general paresis) have declined by 98%.

C. **Gonorrhea**

1. **Epidemiologic features**
   a. **Rank.** Gonorrhea ranks as the number one reportable communicable disease in the United States.
   b. The **number of reported cases** tripled between fiscal year 1965 (325,000 cases) and fiscal year 1976 (over 1 million cases). The number of reported cases has declined for the past 5 years (Figure 4-2). This may be a reporting artifact, since the other STDs seem to be on the rise. There are an estimated 1–1.5 million cases that are not reported.
   c. The **highest case rates** are in individuals age 15–24 years. The incidence rate in large cities (over 200,000 population) is twice the rate of smaller cities and rural areas.
   d. **Reinfection rate.** In certain veneral diseases clinics, 40% of infected patients return within 12 months, and 20% of these reinfections return within 6 weeks.
   e. **Penicillin-resistant strain.** Penicillinase-producing *N. gonorrhoeae* was first detected in the United States in 1976 when 98 cases were reported from 17 states. Most of these cases could be traced to military personnel or civilians who acquired the disease in the Far East and transmitted it to their sexual partners in the United States. By 1982, penicillinase-producing *N. gonorrhoeae* had been documented in every state.
   f. The **National Gonococcal Isolate Surveillance Project** was established in 1987 to monitor trends in antimicrobial resistance.
      (1) Resistance in the gonococcus can be mediated by either plasmids or chromosomal mutations.
      (2) Of the gonococcal isolates tested in 1989, 17% were resistant to tetracycline and 12% to penicillin. Seventy-four percent of the strains showed no resistance to the commonly used antibiotics. Although there have been sporadic cases resistant to spectinomycin, there has been no clinical resistance to ceftriaxone.

2. **Infectious disease process**
   a. **Agent**
      (1) *N. gonorrhoeae,* the cause of gonorrhea, is a gram-negative diplococcus. There are many different strains that can be distinguished on the basis of:
         (a) Nutritional requirements (auxotyping)

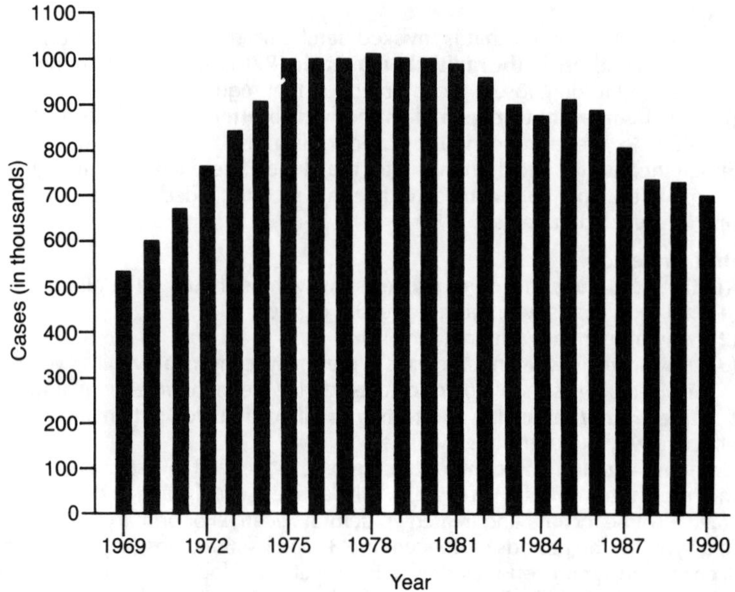

Figure 4-2. Gonorrhea cases reported in the United States, by year—1969–1990. [Reprinted from Centers for Disease Control: Guidelines for prevention of transmission of human immunodeficiency virus and hepatitis B virus to health-care and public-safety workers. *MMWR* 38(S-6), 1989.]

(b) Antibiotic sensitivity patterns

(c) Antigenic diversity

(d) Plasmid analysis

(2) Different strains circulate in different segments of the population and have different clinical characteristics.

(a) One strain, which is more sensitive to penicillin and tetracycline and which is more common in whites than blacks, is more likely to cause asymptomatic urethral infection in men and also accounts for most of the cases of disseminated gonococcal infection.

(b) Another strain, which is more resistant to antibiotics and fecal lipids, is more common in homosexual men.

(c) Strains resistant to penicillin, tetracycline, and spectinomycin have been isolated. Penicillin resistance can be caused by a **plasmid** (β-lactamase positive-penicillinase-producing *N. gonorrhoeae*), or it can be **chromosomally mediated** (**β-lactamase-negative**).

b. Reservoir of infection is humans who may be symptomatic or asymptomatic. (Asymptomatic carriage may persist for many months.) The exact proportion of asymptomatic infections probably varies from area to area.

(1) About 5% of men with urethral infections are asymptomatic.

(2) About 10% of homosexual men with rectal infections are asymptomatic.

(3) Asymptomatic infections in women range from 25%–80%.

(4) Over 90% of pharyngeal infections are asymptomatic.

c. Portal of exit. The organism, which can only infect columnar and transitional epithelium, is already on the body surface of infected individuals and can be easily dislodged.

d. Mode of transmission

(1) Most cases are transmitted through **sexual activity** when mucous membrane surfaces come into contact with infected exudates.

(a) The risk of a male acquiring the gonococcus from a single exposure to an infected female is estimated to be around 18%–25%. Multiple exposures increase the risk.

(b) The risk of a female acquiring the gonococcus from an infected male is unknown, but it is believed to be high (maybe 75% or higher).

(c) Transmission of the organism from pharyngeal carriage to other sites is uncommon.

(2) **Nonvenereal transmission** may occur between an infected mother and her newborn.
(3) **Transmission by fomites or by nonsexual personal contact** over the age of 1 year probably occurs infrequently or not at all.

e. **Portal of entry** is via the mucous membrane surfaces of the body lined by nonsquamous epithelium.

f. **Susceptible host**
(1) Everyone is susceptible.
(2) There is no natural or acquired immunity, and no vaccine is available.
(3) Reinfection is common.
(4) Prepubertal women with columnar or transitional vaginal epithelium may develop a vulvovaginitis, while adult women with squamous epithelium will not.
(5) Women using intrauterine contraceptive devices have a high risk for developing salpingitis.
(6) Complement-deficient individuals are more likely to develop bacteremia.

3. **Control strategies**

a. **Diagnosis.** Appropriate and multiple cultures should be performed on individuals being evaluated in STD clinics.
(1) A positive culture is indicated by the growth of bacterial colonies of *N. gonorrhoeae.*
(2) Women should have endocervical and rectal cultures.
(3) Homosexual men should have urethral and rectal cultures.
(4) Individuals who have oral sex should have pharyngeal cultures.

b. **Therapy and follow-up**
(1) Every individual with a positive gonococcal culture should be properly treated with an approved antimicrobial regimen. Because of widespread drug resistance to penicillin and tetracycline, ceftriaxone is the recommended therapy. All identified sexual contacts of a known case of gonorrhea should receive similar treatment even before their culture results are known.
(2) All gonococcal isolates should be tested for β-lactamase production.
(3) A test of cure should be done on all patients, especially women who may be asymptomatic, 4–7 days after completion of therapy. These isolates should be tested further for antibiotic sensitivity.
(4) **Patients with penicillinase-producing *N. gonorrhoeae.*** Health officials are concerned about this strain of gonorrhea because the cost of treating it is more than ten times the cost of treating a penicillin-sensitive organism.

c. **Screening.** Because of the high number of asymptomatic gonorrhea infections in women, screening gonorrhea cultures are recommended for sexually active women in high-incidence areas. Screening occurs in health department clinics, hospitals, emergency rooms, family planning clinics, student health centers, correction centers, and in certain obstetrics and gynecology clinics. In fiscal year 1989:
(1) A total of 5.1 million culture specimens were obtained from women as part of a nationwide screening program.
(2) Of these, 188,200 (3.7%) were positive for gonorrhea, and 152,100 (81%) of these women were located and treated.
(3) About 61% of total gonorrhea cases were identified through screening.

d. **Interviewing and contact tracing.** Although it is not possible to interview or do contact tracing on all infected individuals, it should be done on the following groups.
(1) **Women with PID.** Studies have shown that 50% of the male contacts of women with PID have gonorrhea, and since multiple episodes of PID lead to sterility, reinfection must be prevented.
(2) **Individuals with recurrent gonorrheal infections** should be interviewed so that their partners can be treated to prevent reinfection.

e. **Prophylaxis in newborns.** Every state has regulations requiring the prophylactic instillation of a 1% silver nitrate solution or an erythromycin (0.5%) or tetracycline (1.0%) ophthalmic ointment in the eyes of newborn infants to prevent gonococcal conjunctivitis. This should be done as soon as possible after birth and never later than 1 hour after birth. Single-use tubes or ampules are preferable to multiple-use tubes.

f. The **national program to control gonorrhea,** which was implemented in 1972, has been moderately successful.
(1) Between 1965 and 1975, the morbidity rate increased at an annual rate of 12%.

(2) Between 1976 and 1983, the number of reported cases of gonorrhea leveled, and the rates actually declined.
(3) This decline has continued into fiscal year 1990 (see Figure 4-2). These data are remarkable considering that the larger number of people entering the sexually active cohort should have driven the case count even higher.

D. Acquired immune deficiency syndrome (AIDS)

1. **Definition.** AIDS is the end stage of a chronic infection caused by HIV. The **surveillance definition** requires the patient to have a definite specific opportunistic infection, or a specific cancer with no underlying cause of immunodeficiency, or specific conditions (e.g., recurrent bacterial infections, encephalopathy, wasting syndrome) and a positive HIV antibody test.

2. **Epidemiologic features.** AIDS is a new disease that began to appear in the United States in the late 1970s but was not recognized until the summer of 1981.
   a. The **number of reported cases** continues to rise. As of May 1991, there were 179,136 reported cases, with 176,047 cases in adults and adolescents and 3089 cases in children less than 13 years of age.
      (1) It took over 6 years for the first 50,000 cases to be reported; there were 43,339 cases reported in 1990.
      (2) It is estimated that, by the end of 1991, AIDS will be the second leading cause of death among men 25–44 years of age and one of the five leading causes of death among women 15–44 years in the United States.
      (3) WHO estimates that there are 8–10 million adults and 1 million children infected with HIV worldwide.
   b. **Occurrence.** AIDS has occurred primarily in young men of all racial and ethnic groups.
      (1) Eighty-eight percent of cases have occurred in individuals age 20–49 years.
      (2) Eighty-nine percent of cases have occurred in men and eleven percent in women.
      (3) Nationally, 54% of patients have been white, 29% have been black, 16% have been Hispanic, and 1% is of unknown or other ethnic origin.
   c. **Adult and adolescent cases** have been reported in certain high-risk groups.
      (1) Homosexual and bisexual men account for 59% of cases. The risk is increased for homosexual men who:
         (a) Have had multiple sexual partners
         (b) Have had anonymous contacts
         (c) Practice certain sexual acts, such as receptive anal intercourse
      (2) Male homosexual and bisexual intravenous (IV) drug abusers account for 7% of cases.
      (3) IV drug abusers account for 22% of the total cases and for over 64% of the cases in the heterosexual population.
      (4) Patients with hemophilia or other coagulation disorders account for 1% of cases. These people contracted AIDS through infected plasma products (clotting factor concentrates) used to treat their coagulation disorders.
      (5) Heterosexual contacts of patients with AIDS or contacts of individuals in high-risk groups account for 6% of cases.
         (a) About 25% of these cases occur in individuals from foreign countries where heterosexual transmission is a major mode of transmission.
         (b) About 75% of these cases occur in the United States from heterosexual transmission.
            (i) Approximately 60% of these cases are women whose sexual partners are either IV drug abusers or bisexual men.
            (ii) About 40% of these cases are men whose sexual partners are IV drug abusers.
      (6) Individuals transfused with infected blood products account for about 2% of cases.
      (7) Five patients, all of whom had invasive procedures, became infected with HIV while receiving care from a dentist with AIDS. This is the only documented instance of HIV transmission from an infected health care worker to patients. The exact mode of transmission and the reasons for transmission to multiple patients in a single practice are not known.
      (8) Individuals without a known cause account for 4% of reported adult cases. These can be further subdivided.
         (a) Seventy-one percent of these cases are still under epidemiologic investigation and may be reclassified as additional information is obtained.

(b) Twenty-two percent of these cases either died before adequate information could be obtained, were lost to follow-up, or refused to answer questions.

(c) Seven-percent of these cases cannot be explained. Many of these individuals have serologic evidence of other STDs (e.g., syphilis, HBV infection), suggesting that they probably contracted the disease from sexual activity.

d. Pediatric patients account for 1.7% of cases. This group divides into:

(1) Children born to parents who belong to a high-risk group (84%)

(2) Children who have had blood transfusions (14%), of whom 58% are hemophiliacs

(3) Children in an unknown category (2%); that is, there are insufficient data on both parents to classify them

e. Household spread. There have been no documented instances of household spread of HIV from one adult to another or from one child to another through normal casual (nonsexual) contact. The only household contacts found to be infected were sexual partners, infants born to infected mothers, and household members with other known risk factors.

f. Health care workers. AIDS cases have occurred in health care workers.

(1) Ninety-five percent of those infected acquired the disease via standard nonoccupational exposure.

(2) Health care workers are less likely to get the disease from IV drug abuse and are more likely to get the disease from homosexual/bisexual activity.

(3) Some cases have been reported in health care workers

(a) Without documented exposure or documented seroconversion

(b) With documented exposure but without documented seroconversion

(c) With documented exposure and documented seroconversion

(4) The risk of becoming infected with HIV following a needle-stick is about 0.4%. The risk of becoming infected from a mucocutaneous exposure is less than 0.4%.

g. AIDS in the United States

(1) AIDS has been documented in all 50 states, the District of Columbia, and the three United States territories. (It has been documented in at least 149 countries worldwide.) Sixty-two percent of all reported cases have occurred in five states—New York, California, Florida, New Jersey, and Texas—states that have large populations in high-risk groups. They also are the areas in which the disease has existed for the longest period of time.

(2) Table 4-4 shows the changing epidemiologic characteristics of AIDS as it continues to spread in the population.

(a) Because of massive educational efforts and the impact of AIDS cases in the homosexual community, homosexual men have modified their sexual behavior, and HIV transmission has decreased in this group.

(b) HIV transmission continues unabated among IV drug abusers, especially in black and Hispanic communities, and from sexual transmission in the heterosexual population.

Table 4-4. Comparisons by Category of Reported Cases of Acquired Immune Deficiency Syndrome (AIDS) in the United States

	Year	
Category	**1981**	**1990**
Total number of cases	189	43,339
Type of exposure		
Male homosexual and bisexual activity	77%	55%
Intravenous drug abuse	7%	23%
Homosexual/bisexual male intravenous drug use	11%	5%
Other	5%	17%
Sex		
Male	97%	88%
Female	3%	12%
Geography		
New York and California, combined	76%	33%
Remainder of United States	24%	67%

(c) A higher proportion of cases are now occurring throughout the United States.

3. Infectious disease process

a. Agent

(1) **HIV** is an RNA retrovirus that requires an enzyme, **reverse transcriptase,** to multiply. Reverse transcriptase, which is made by the RNA virus, permits viral replication by forming DNA from viral RNA. Humans do not have reverse transcriptase.

(2) The **antigenic structure** of the surface of the virus undergoes continuous change. This change occurs inside the patient so that antigenically different viruses can be isolated at different times.

(3) The virus attacks and destroys the $CD4^+$ (helper) lymphocyte. It can also live in certain nerve cells.

(4) HIV is fragile outside the body and can be inactivated by a number of disinfectants (e.g.,1:10 dilution of household bleach, gluteraldehyde, hydrogen peroxide, isopropyl alcohol, ethyl alcohol). Under laboratory conditions and using high concentrations of HIV, the virus can live for several days in a wet or dry state outside the body. However, these concentrations are not achieved in normal body fluids, so this fact does not appear to be of any epidemiologic significance.

b. Reservoir of infection is humans in both the symptomatic and asymptomatic state. Based on seroprevalence data in high-risk groups and on estimates of the number of people in these groups, the PHS estimates that 1–2 million Americans have been infected with this virus.

(1) Most of these HIV-infected individuals are asymptomatic; that is, they look and feel normal and do not know that they are infected. Consequently, they can transmit this disease to others unknowingly.

(2) Most, if not all, HIV antibody–positive patients have circulating infectious HIV particles in their plasma and in their peripheral blood mononuclear cells.

(3) Patients with advanced disease have higher plasma titers of HIV.

(4) Most of the cell-associated virus in the blood is in the $CD4^+$ lymphocytes.

(5) **Azidothymidine (AZT)** has been shown to lower plasma titers of HIV, but it has little or no effect on cell-associated virus levels.

c. Portal of exit. The portals of exit for this virus are the percutaneous route (blood), the genital tract (semen and vaginal secretions), and the transplacental route. The virus also has been isolated in saliva, tears, breast milk, and urine.

d. Modes of transmission

(1) **Documented modes of transmission**

(a) **Sexual transmission** includes both male homosexual transmission and heterosexual (man-to-woman and woman-to-man) transmission. Rectal and vaginal intercourse carry the highest risks of transmission. Sexual transmission is enhanced when a genital lesion (ulcer) is present.

(b) **Percutaneous exposure** to contaminated blood includes sharing needles in IV drug abuse or receiving contaminated blood or blood products. Blood donors are not at risk.

(c) **Transmission from mother-to-child** can occur either in utero, at the time of delivery, or shortly thereafter. There have been a couple of cases transmitted from mother to child through breast milk.

(2) **Unlikely modes of transmission.** Since there has been no documented spread to household contacts through casual (nonsexual) exposure and since there has been no significant spread to health care workers or to individuals not in the well-defined risk groups, it can be argued that this disease cannot be transmitted by:

(a) **Airborne route.** AIDS cannot be contracted by being in the same room with an AIDS patient.

(b) **Casual contact.** It appears that AIDS cannot be transmitted by saliva or tears.

(c) **Foodborne route.** AIDS cannot be contracted by eating food prepared by an individual infected with the AIDS virus.

(d) **Vectors.** AIDS cannot be transmitted by mosquito or other insect bites.

e. Portal of entry. The virus enters the body through breaks in the skin or mucosal surfaces.

f. Susceptible host

(1) Everyone is susceptible to AIDS.

(2) No cofactors have been identified as being necessary for this disease.

(3) There is no scientific evidence that exercise, rest, or good nutrition can prevent the progression of AIDS.
(4) A study of homosexual men in San Francisco suggests that approximately 54% develop AIDS within 10 years of seroconversion and that ultimately up to 99% may develop AIDS.

4. **Control strategies.** Although there is no current treatment for HIV infection and no vaccine for preventing HIV infection, this disease can be controlled. Some control measures have already been implemented, and educational programs for behavior modification have been developed.
   a. **Blood screening.** Control measures that make the blood supply safe have already been implemented.
      (1) Individuals who should not donate blood include:
         (a) Any man who has had sexual contact with another man since 1977
         (b) Present or past IV drug abusers
         (c) Individuals from countries where AIDS is common (Central Africa and Haiti) even when not associated with any known risk factors
         (d) Sexual partners of the above groups
         (e) Any individual who has had sex with a prostitute or with one of the above-named groups in the past 6 months [consideration is being given to raise the time interval to 12 months because of the longer incubation period of hepatitis C (HCV)]
      (2) Every unit of blood that is collected is screened for antibodies against the AIDS virus, and the positive units are discarded. The current positivity rate is about 1–2 per 10,000 screened units.
      (3) The manufacturing process for factor VII concentrate now includes heat treatment, which inactivates HIV.
   b. **Educational programs** for behavior modification in homosexual men, heterosexual men and women, and IV drug abusers have been developed in some parts of the country.
   c. **Safe sex recommendations** (see also V A 7). (Many homosexual men have adopted these recommendations as indicated by the declining incidence of rectal and pharyngeal gonorrhea.) Safe sex recommendations include:
      (1) Limiting the number of sexual partners
      (2) Avoiding the transfer of body fluids from one partner to the other (i.e., avoiding unprotected vaginal or rectal intercourse) by using condoms
      (3) Limiting activities to hugging and touching, which will not transmit HIV
   d. **IV drug abusers** are strongly advised not to use drugs, but if they persist, they are advised to refrain from sharing equipment and to clean their equipment with bleach solution.
   e. **Other control strategies** include the treatment of other STDs and drug detoxification programs. It is important to emphasize that, since AIDS is a new disease, new strategies might be necessary for control; society may be compelled to impose controls that have not been imposed previously.

E. Chlamydial infection

1. **Epidemiologic features**
   a. Although health officials do not keep statistics on the number of cases that occur, *Chlamydia* is believed to be the most common sexually transmitted bacterial pathogen in the United States today. An estimated 4 million cases occur each year.
   b. Infection is more common in urban areas with low socioeconomic groups, particularly those individuals under 20 years of age with multiple partners.
   c. **Prevalence rates**
      (1) Adult heterosexual men: 2%–31%
      (2) Homosexual men: 5%–10%
      (3) Heterosexual women: 3%–27%

2. **Infectious disease process**
   a. **Agent.** *Chlamydia trachomatis,* the causative agent, is a bacteria with the following characteristics.
      (1) It grows only intracellularly.
      (2) It contains both DNA and RNA.
      (3) It divides by binary fission.
      (4) It has cell walls similar to gram-negative bacteria.

b. **Reservoir** of infection is humans in both the clinical and asymptomatic states. Most women with cervical infections, most homosexual men with rectal infections, and as many as 30% of heterosexual men with urethral infections have few or no symptoms.
c. **Portal of exit.** The organism mainly infects the squamocolumnar-columnar epithelial cells lining mucosal surfaces. These cells are destroyed as a result of the infection and are discarded with the inflammatory debris.
d. **Mode of transmission**
   (1) Most cases are transmitted through sexual activity when a mucosal surface comes into contact with infected exudates.
   (2) An infant can acquire a chlamydial infection coming through the birth canal.
e. **Portal of entry** is the mucosal surfaces of the body.
f. **Susceptible host**
   (1) There is no natural or acquired immunity.
   (2) Approximately 45% of gonorrhea cases have coexisting chlamydial infections.
   (3) *Chlamydia* causes:
      (a) Approximately 50% of all cases of nongonococcal urethritis and acute epididymitis in men
      (b) Mucopurulent cervicitis and approximately 40% of cases of PID
      (c) Inclusion conjunctivitis and afebrile interstitial pneumonia in infants born to infected mothers

3. **Control strategies**
   a. **Diagnosis.** Chlamydial infections now can be diagnosed by culture or by two different antigen tests.
      (1) Culture is the preferred method, but it takes several days and is costly.
      (2) Direct smear fluorescent antibody test can be done quickly, but it takes trained personnel and high-quality equipment. Only a limited number of tests can be done because it is a labor-intensive process.
      (3) Enzyme-linked immunoabsorbent assay (ELISA) can be used to test large numbers of specimens, but it takes about 4 hours to complete.
   b. **Empirical treatment**
      (1) Certain individuals should receive empirical treatment for chlamydial infection, including:
         (a) Those with certain clinical conditions caused by *Chlamydia* (e.g., nongonococcal urethritis, acute epididymitis, mucopurulent cervicitis, PID)
         (b) Those with gonococcal infections
         (c) Sexual partners of the above-mentioned groups
      (2) **Test of cure.** Since *Chlamydia* organisms are very sensitive to tetracycline and erythromycin, test of cure cultures are not necessary.
   c. **Screening.** Certain populations that should be screened for chlamydial infection include:
      (1) Individuals attending an STD clinic who would not otherwise receive therapy for chlamydial infection
      (2) Health care facilities that may have a high prevalence of infections, such as adolescent and family planning clinics
      (3) Young, urban individuals of low socioeconomic status who have multiple sexual partners and who would not otherwise receive therapy for chlamydial infection
      (4) Certain groups of pregnant women, including:
         (a) Adolescents (< 20 years of age)
         (b) Unmarried women
         (c) Married women who may be at high risk because of multiple sexual partners or a history of another STD.
   d. **Prophylaxis in newborns.** Chlamydial ophthalmia can be prevented by instilling either erythromycin (0.5%) ophthalmic ointment or tetracycline (1%) ointment into the eyes of all neonates (see V C 3 e).

VI. VIRAL HEPATITIS

A. Hepatitis A virus (HAV)

1. **Epidemiologic features.** Infection with HAV **(infectious hepatitis)** has a worldwide occurrence.
   a. **Seroprevalence.** High seroprevalence rates occur in very early life in developing countries

where sanitation is inadequate and at a later age (i.e., school-age children, adults) in developed countries. In the United States, most cases occur in older children and young adults.

b. Epidemics have occurred in institutions, day-care centers, in families who have children attending day-care centers, rural areas where sanitation may be poor, and overcrowded areas.

c. Incidence. About 30,000 cases are reported in the United States each year. The actual number of cases is probably several times the reported number.

d. Identifiable risk factors. Although most of the cases have no recognized risk factors for infection, HAV infection is more likely to occur in individuals who have close contact with:

(1) Individuals with HAV infection
(2) Homosexual men
(3) Foreign countries with inadequate sanitation systems
(4) Children who attend day-care centers

2. Infectious disease process

a. Agent

(1) HAV is a small (25–29 nm), nonenveloped, RNA-containing virus (picornavirus).
(2) Only one antigenic class has been identified.
(3) The virus remains stable at 4° F (−20° C) for long periods of time and at 140° F (60° C) for at least 39 minutes. In some outbreaks, the virus appears to have survived brief steaming or cooking or refrigeration for 48 hours.
(4) HAV has been found in blood and stools but not in urine and other body fluids.

b. Reservoir

(1) Humans are the primary reservoir, although nonhuman primates have been infected.
(2) There are no chronic carriers. There is a brief period of viremia that precedes the onset of hepatic disease.
(3) HAV appears to be maintained in nature by serial transmission during the incubation period.
(4) The patient is infectious from about 2 weeks before the onset of clinical disease to about 1 week after. The greatest period of infectivity is before the onset of jaundice.

c. Portal of exit

(1) HAV multiplies in the hepatocytes and reaches the intestinal tract by way of the bile duct.
(2) It is then excreted in large quantities (10^8 particles/g) via the stool. Peak virus excretion occurs during the last half of the incubation period rather than during acute illness.
(3) The amount of virus shed in the stool appears to be unrelated to the severity of clinical illness.
(4) Percutaneous transmission from needle sticks during the brief periods of viremia is possible, but documented instances of percutaneous transmission or transfusion-related infections are very rare.

d. Mode of transmission is primarily person-to-person via the fecal-oral route or by common vehicle via contaminated food or water.

(1) Transmission is facilitated by:
  (a) Poor personal hygiene
  (b) Poor sanitation
  (c) Intimate (intrahousehold or sexual) contact
(2) Sharing utensils (e.g., drinking out of the same cup) or cigarettes or kissing does not transmit the infection.
(3) Foodborne outbreaks are almost always caused by:
  (a) Foods that are not cooked thoroughly or are consumed raw
  (b) Foods contaminated by human hands after cooking
  (c) Ingesting raw shellfish (e.g., clams, oysters) harvested from sewage-contaminated waters

e. Portal of entry almost always is by ingesting the virus.

f. Susceptible host

(1) Infection is related to age and socioeconomic status. Approximately 20% of Americans are infected by age 20 and 50% by age 50. Incidence appears to be declining. In developing countries, over 90% of individuals have antibodies by adulthood.
(2) The **incubation period** is 15–50 days with an average of 28–30 days.
(3) **Severity of clinical disease** is related to age. Young children are more likely to have subclinical infections, whereas adults are more likely to have overt disease. Less than 20% of children in day-care centers are believed to develop clinical disease, while over 80% of infected adults probably become symptomatic.

(4) The **case-fatality rate** among reported cases is about 0.6%
(5) Infection confers lifelong immunity.

3. **Control strategies** for HAV infection include good personal hygiene, removal of known hepatitis patients from occupations that prepare or serve food for public consumption, and the postexposure prophylactic administration of IG.
   a. **Strict isolation of the patient is not necessary** if the following precautions and hygienic practices are instituted (see also Ch 14 VIII B 4 a).
      (1) All patients and household contacts should wash their hands with soap and water before eating and after using the toilet.
      (2) Toothbrushes, washcloths, and towels should not be shared.
      (3) Eating utensils should be washed carefully with soap and water.
      (4) Bathroom facilities may be shared by all household members.
   b. **Prophylaxis.** IG should be given in the standard single intramuscular dose (0.02 ml/kg body weight) as soon as possible after exposure but not later than 2 weeks. Serologic confirmation of HAV in an index case is recommended, but not necessary, before treatment of contacts. IG may either prevent infection altogether, or it may modify the severity of the disease. IG is recommended for the following groups.
      (1) **Intimate contacts.** All household and sexual contacts of persons with HAV should receive IG.
      (2) **Children and employees in day-care centers**
         (a) In day-care centers with children in diapers, IG should be given to all children and staff if one case of HAV occurs in either a child or in an employee or if cases occur in two or more of the children's households. If cases occur in three or more families, IG should also be administered to household members of the children's families.
         (b) In day-care centers without diapered children, IG should only be given to classroom contacts of an index case.
      (3) **Food handlers** who work in a restaurant or cafeteria where another food handler has been diagnosed as having HAV should receive IG. Although IG is not usually recommended for patrons, it may be given to patrons when:
         (a) The infected person handled food that was not cooked before it was eaten
         (b) The hygienic practices of the infected food handler were deficient or the food handler had diarrhea
         (c) Patrons can be identified and treated within 2 weeks of exposure
      (4) **Travelers to tropical areas or developing countries** should receive IG. This is especially true for tourists who travel to out-of-the-way places where they may be exposed to infected persons or contaminated food and water. The actual dose of IG depends on body weight and length of stay.
         (a) A single dose of IG (0.02 ml/kg body weight) is recommended if travel is for less than 3 months.
         (b) For prolonged travel or residence in developing countries, 0.06 ml/kg body weight should be given every 5 months.
         (c) For persons who require repeated IG prophylaxis because of extensive travel, screening for total anti-HAV before travel is useful to eliminate those who are immune and do not need IG.
      (5) **Individuals at risk.** IG is recommended for controlling outbreaks after an epidemiologic investigation has identified individuals at risk.
   c. **IG is not recommended for:**
      (1) Casual contacts at work or school
      (2) Classmates of elementary or secondary schools after a single case
      (3) Hospital personnel caring for a patient
      (4) Individuals exposed to a common source (e.g., food) of HAV infection when cases begin to occur after the 2-week period at which point IG is ineffective

B. Hepatitis B virus (HBV)

1. **Epidemiologic features.** Infection with HBV **(serum hepatitis)** has a **worldwide occurrence,** with the highest incidence in China and Southeast Asia, most parts of Africa, most Pacific islands, parts of the Middle East, and in the Amazon Basin where infection occurs in early infancy and childhood. In the United States, most cases occur in young adults between 15 and 30 years of age in urban areas.

a. **Incidence.** There are approximately 300,000 new HBV infections in the United States each year. Approximately 75,000 become symptomatic with jaundice, 10,000 require hospitalization, and 250 die of fulminant hepatitis.
b. **Seroprevalence.** A seroprevalence study of HBV infection in the United States [Second National Health and Nutrition Examination Survey (NHANES II) conducted from 1976 to 1980] showed that 3.2% of white participants and 13.7% of black participants had serologic markers of HBV infection.
c. **Lifetime risk** of developing HBV infection in the general population in the United States is 3%–14% but may be as high as 85%–100% in certain groups.
d. **Carriers.** There are between 750,000 and 1,000,000 carriers in the United States.
e. **Long-term sequelae** of HBV infection include:
   (1) Chronic active hepatitis, which occurs in approximately 25% of carriers
   (2) HBV-related cirrhosis, which causes about 4000 deaths each year
   (3) Primary hepatocellular carcinoma, which is 12–300 times more common in HBV carriers and accounts for approximately 800 deaths each year

2. **Infectious disease process**
   a. **Agent**
      (1) **Structure and antigenic composition.** HBV is a 42-nm, double-shelled DNA virus (hepadnavirus). At one time, it was called the Dane particle. HBV contains the following antigenic components:
         (a) **Hepatitis B surface antigen (HBsAg),** found on the surface of the virus, is produced in excess amount and can be found circulating in blood as 22-nm spherical and tubular particles. There are four distinct subtypes (i.e., *adr, adw, adyw, adyr*), which vary geographically and, thus, are useful in epidemiologic studies. HBsAg appears 30–60 days after exposure and persists for variable periods of time.
         (b) **Hepatitis B core antigen (HBcAg),** is the internal core of the virus.
         (c) **Hepatitis B e antigen (HBeAg)** is associated with HBV replication and high infectivity. It parallels the presence of DNA polymerase, which is associated with complete virons.
      (2) **Stability.** The virus is apparently quite stable and can survive for hours and days outside the body.
      (3) **Serologic response to HBV infection**
         (a) Antibody to HBsAg (anti-HBs) indicates past infection, immune response to HBV vaccine, or passive antibody from hepatitis B immune globulin (HBIG).
            (i) The development of anti-HBs eliminates HBsAg and prevents the development of the carrier state.
            (ii) Anti-HBs also is associated with long-term immunity. Infection with one subtype confers protection against infections with other subtypes.
         (b) Antibody to HBcAg (anti-HBc) indicates past infection with HBV.
         (c) IgM class antibody to HBcAg (IgM anti-HBc) indicates recent HBV infection and may persist for 4–6 months.
         (d) Antibody to HBeAg (anti-HBe) suggests a low titer of HBV and a low degree of infectivity.
   b. **Reservoir.** Humans are the only known reservoir.
      (1) **Carriers** of HBV, who maintain the virus in nature, are individuals who are HBsAg positive two or more times within a period of at least 6 months or who are HBsAg positive and IgM anti-HBc negative when a single serum specimen is tested. Certain groups (patients on hemodialysis, clients in institutions for the mentally retarded) are more likely to become chronic carriers; thus, other factors, (e.g.,immunocompetence) are also important (Table 4-5 shows the prevalence of HBV markers in various population groups). The likelihood of developing the carrier state also depends on the age at which infection occurs.
         (a) Only 6%–10% of infected adults become chronic carriers of HBsAg.
         (b) Between 25% and 50% of children infected before 5 years of age become carriers.
         (c) Approximately 90% of infants infected in the perinatal period become carriers.
      (2) HBV has been **found in almost all body secretions and excretions,** including blood, serum, semen, vaginal fluid, saliva, breast milk, urine, and feces. The highest concentration of HBV is in blood and serous fluid. A lower concentration is found in other body fluids (e.g., saliva, semen).

Table 4-5. Prevalence of Hepatitis B (HBV) Serologic Markers in Various Population Groups

	Serologic Markers	
Population Group	**HBsAg (%)**	**Any Marker (%)**
High risk		
Immigrants and refugees from areas of high HBV endemicity	13	70–85
Alaskan natives/Pacific Islanders	5–15	40–70
Clients in institutions for the developmentally disabled	10–20	35–80
Users of illicit parenteral drugs	7	60–80
Sexually active homosexual men	6	35–80
Household contacts of HBV carriers	3–6	30–60
Patients of hemodialysis units	3–10	20–80
Intermediate risk		
Health care workers who have frequent blood contact	1–2	15–30
Prisoners (male)	1–8	10–80
Staff of institutions for the developmentally disabled	1	10–25
Heterosexuals with multiple partners	0.5	5–20
Low risk		
Health-care workers with no or infrequent blood contact	0.3	3–10
General population		
Blacks	0.9	14
Whites	0.2	3

Reprinted from Advisory Committee on Immunization Practices: Recommendations for protection against viral hepatitis. *MMWR* 39(RR-2):9, 1990.

c. Portal of exit

(1) HBV can leave the body via cuts, wounds, weeping lesions, or needle sticks, or it can exit via body fluids (semen, vaginal fluid, saliva).

(2) Individuals who are HBeAg positive are more likely to shed higher numbers of organisms.

d. Mode of transmission is primarily by direct person-to-person contact via infected body fluids or by common vehicle, such as a contaminated needle. Approximately 28% of cases acquire the disease from IV drug abuse, 22% from heterosexual contact with infected persons or multiple partners, and 8% from homosexual activity. In addition, 30% of cases deny any of the recognized risk factors for infection.

(1) HBV transmission occurs by infective blood or body fluids introduced at birth, through sexual contact, or by contaminated needles. Transmission is more likely to occur:

(a) In overcrowded populations with lack of sanitation and poor personal hygiene

(b) In settings of continuous close personal contact (e.g., in households or among children in institutions for the developmentally disabled), presumably via inapparent or unnoticed contact of infective secretions with skin lesions or mucosal surfaces; epidemiologic studies have shown especially high transmission rates in families who adopt antigen-positive children

(c) In sexual partners of infected adults

(d) In IV drug abusers who share contaminated needles

(e) In infants born to HBsAg-positive mothers, especially those mothers who are also HBeAg positive; only a minority of the infants born to these mothers are infected at birth; however, some become infected at the time of birth, and others become infected during the first year of life

(2) HBV transmission does not occur:

(a) By the fecal-oral route

(b) By foodborne or waterborne transmission

(c) By arthropod (mosquito) transmission

e. Portal of entry of HBV occurs through breaks in the skin (percutaneous) or through permucosal exposure to infective body fluids.

f. Susceptible host

(1) All ages are susceptible, but clinical expression of disease occurs in only 20% of children infected and in 25%–50% of adults infected.

(2) The **incubation period** is 45–160 days with an average of approximately 120 days.
(3) The **case-fatality rate** for reported cases is 1.4%.

3. Control strategies

a. **Good personal hygiene.** The same factors described for HAV infection [see VI A 3 a (1)–(4)] apply to HBV infection; in addition, razors also should not be shared.

b. **Avoiding contact with blood.** Gloves and gowns should be worn when handling or being exposed to blood or body fluids containing blood. All blood spills should be cleaned with soap and water and disinfected with a 1:10 dilution of household bleach.

c. **HBIG** contains anti-HBs and has a titer of higher than 1:100,000 by radioimmunoassay. HBIG is used for postexposure prophylaxis. IG should not be used in postexposure prophylaxis for HBV.

d. **Vaccines.** Plasma-derived HBV vaccine became available in June 1982, and genetically engineered recombinant HBV vaccines became available in July 1986. All vaccines are composed of 17–25 nm spherical surface antigen particles. Plasma-derived vaccine is no longer being produced in the United States.

(1) **Dosage.** Three intramuscular injections at 0, 1, and 6 months, respectively, in the deltoid muscle have been shown to produce antibodies in over 90% of healthy adults. Field trials have shown an 80%–95% efficacy in preventing infection among susceptible individuals. The vaccine costs about $120 for the three doses. Larger vaccine doses or an increased number of doses may be necessary to provide protective antibody in a high proportion of hemodialysis patients and other immunocompromised persons.

(2) **Contraindications** to the use of HBV vaccine are minimal and consist primarily of allergic reactions to vaccine components.

(a) Pregnancy or lactation is not a contraindication.
(b) Administration of the vaccine to HBsAg carriers or to previously infected individuals has neither therapeutic nor adverse consequences.
(c) Passively acquired antibody from either HBIG or IG will not interfere with active immunization.

(3) **Side effects.** The most common side effect has been soreness at the injection site. Guillain-Barré syndrome has occurred following the first vaccine dose of the plasma-derived vaccine, but it was of borderline significance and occurred at a rate of 0.5 per 100,000 vaccines.

(4) **Testing for immunity after vaccination** is not routinely recommended. When necessary, testing should be done between 1 and 6 months after completion of the vaccine series. Revaccination of people who did not respond to the primary series can produce an adequate antibody response in 25%–50% of nonresponders. Postvaccination testing is required for:

(a) Persons whose subsequent management depends on knowing their immune status (i.e., persons at occupational risk, dialysis patients, staff)
(b) Persons for whom a suboptimal response may be anticipated (e.g., those who have received vaccine in the buttock, those ≥ 50 years of age, those with known HIV infection)

(5) **Long-term protection by HBV vaccine.** Although antibody levels decline and become undetectable in 30%–50% of cases within 7 years, protection against clinical (or viremic) HBV infection persists. Resultant infections almost always are innocuous and do not cause detectable viremia, liver inflammation, or clinical illness.

(6) **Recommendations for booster doses**

(a) Booster doses are not recommended for adults and children with normal immune status.
(b) Booster doses may be indicated for hemodialysis patients and for people who experience percutaneous or needle exposure to HBsAg-positive blood.

e. **Pre-exposure immunization.** Although most cases of acute HBV now occur in homosexual men, parenteral drug abusers, and persons acquiring the disease through heterosexual exposure, 85% of the distributed vaccine has been used to immunize persons at occupational risk of developing HBV infection. Occupational exposure accounts for only 4% of the cases that occur. Susceptible individuals at risk for acquiring HBV infection include:

(1) Individuals with **occupational risk,** especially health care and public safety workers who are exposed to blood or blood products or potential accidental needle sticks; vaccination of health care workers should be completed while they are still in school.

(2) Clients and staff of institutions for the developmentally disabled or of residential settings with known HBV carriers and the staff and clients of nonresidential day-care programs attended by known HBV carriers

(3) Hemodialysis patients

(4) Homosexual men, as soon as their homosexual activity begins

(5) Users of illicit injectable drugs

(6) Patients with clotting disorders who receive clotting factor concentrates

(7) Household and sexual contacts of HBV carriers

(8) Families adopting or providing foster care for HBsAg-positive children

(9) Children in classrooms or child-care centers containing HBV carriers who behave aggressively or have special medical problems that increase the risk of exposure to their blood

(10) Populations with high endemicity of HBV infection (e.g., Alaskan Natives, Pacific Islanders, refugees from HBV-endemic areas); in these groups, universal HBV vaccination of children younger than 7 years is recommended because of the high rate of interfamilial spread of HBV infection

(11) Inmates of long-term correctional facilities

(12) Heterosexually active individuals with multiple sexual partners

(13) International travelers who plan to visit areas with high levels of endemic HBV, particularly if they plan to:

(a) Have contact with blood

(b) Have sexual contact with residents

(c) Reside in these areas for more than 6 months

f. Postexposure prophylaxis is indicated in the following situations.

(1) Perinatal exposure is one of the most efficient modes of HBV transmission. Infants born to HBsAg- and HBeAg-positive mothers have a 70%–90% chance of becoming infected and a 90% chance of becoming chronic HBV carriers. More than 25% of these carriers will die from primary hepatocellular carcinoma or cirrhosis of the liver.

(a) All pregnant women should be tested for HBsAg during an early prenatal visit or at the time of delivery.

(b) Infants born to HBsAg-positive mothers should receive HBIG and HBV vaccine as soon as possible after delivery, preferably in the delivery room. Children who receive HBIG at birth should receive their routine immunizations at 2 months of age. The HBV vaccine should be repeated at 1 and 6 months. This regimen has been shown to prevent the HBV carrier state in 85%–90% of infants.

(c) Household members and sexual partners of HBV carriers (identified) should be evaluated and, if susceptible, should receive HBV vaccine.

(2) Percutaneous or permucosal (ocular or mucous membrane) exposure to HBsAg-positive blood has been shown to transmit HBV infection. The risk of developing an HBV infection following a needle-stick injury with a needle contaminated with HBsAg blood is about 6%–30%. This risk can be decreased by 75% with two injections of HBIG: one immediately after exposure and one a month later. Since this type of exposure usually occurs in health care workers, the incident can be used to encourage immunization.

(a) The **decision to administer prophylaxis** in the case of percutaneous or permucosal exposure depends on several factors:

(i) Whether the source of the blood is available

(ii) The HBsAg status of the source

(iii) The HBV vaccination and vaccine-response status of the exposed person

(b) Table 4-6 summarizes the **recommendation for prophylaxis** for percutaneous or permucosal exposure to blood according to the vaccination status and vaccine response of the exposed person and to the HBsAg status of the source of exposure. Attempts should be made to determine the HBsAg status of the source patient whenever possible. All immunized or incompletely immunized patients should complete the HBV vaccine series.

(3) Sexual partners of persons with acute HBV infection or of HBsAg-positive individuals should receive HBIG (0.06 ml/kg body weight), provided that it can be given within 14 days of the last exposure. HBIG has been shown to be 75% effective in preventing such infections.

Table 4-6. Recommendations for Hepatitis B Prophylaxis Following Percutaneous or Permucosal Exposure

	Treatment When Source Is Found To Be:		
Exposed Individual	**HBsAg Positive**	**HBsAg Negative**	**Not Tested or Unknown**
Unvaccinated	HBIG x 1* and initiate HBV vaccine†	Initiate HBV vaccine†	Initiate HBV vaccine†
Previously vaccinated			
Known responder	Test exposed for anti-HBs: If adequate, no treatment; if inadequate, HBV vaccine booster dose	No treatment	No treatment
Known nonresponder	Two doses HBIG 1 month apart; HBIG x 1 plus one dose HBV vaccine	No treatment	If known high-risk source, may treat as if source were HBsAg positive
Response unknown	Test exposed for anti-HBs: If adequate, no treatment; if inadequate,‡ HBIG x 1 plus HBV vaccine booster dose	No treatment	Test exposed for anti-HBs: If adequate, no treatment; if inadequate,‡ HBV vaccine booster dose

Adapted from Advisory Committee on Immunization Practices: Recommendations for protection against viral hepatitis. *MMWR* 39(RR-2):20, 1990.

HBsAg = hepatitis B surface antigen; HBIG = hepatitis B immune globulin; HBV = hepatitis B virus; anti-HBs = antibody to hepatitis B surface antigen.

*HBIG dose; 0.06 ml/kg body weight intramuscularly administered as soon as possible after exposure; effectiveness beyond 7 days postexposure is unclear.

†HBV vaccine dose; dose depends on age or type of vaccine.

‡Adequate anti-HBs can be ≥ 10 milli-international units per milliliter (mIU/ml), approximately equivalent to 10 sample ratio units (SRU) by radio immunoassay, or positive by enzyme immunoassay.

(a) Testing sexual partners for HBV susceptibility is recommended if it does not delay treatment beyond 14 days after the last exposure. Testing for anti-HBc is the most efficient prescreening test to use in this population.

(b) The HBV vaccine series should be initiated if the susceptible individual is a member of a high-risk group (i.e., homosexuals, heterosexuals with multiple sexual contacts) or if the steady sexual contact is or becomes an HBsAg carrier.

(c) If the exposed individual is not from a high-risk group in whom immunization is routinely recommended and if the index individual had acute HBV infection, HBV vaccine is unnecessary. A second dose of HBIG should be given 3 months later if sexual contact is continuous and if the index patient is still HBsAg positive. Ninety percent of adults with acute HBV infection become HBsAg negative within 15 weeks of diagnosis.

(d) Nonsexual household contacts of patients with acute HBV infection do not need postexposure prophylaxis. However, household contacts of chronic HBsAg carriers need to be immunized with HBV vaccine.

(4) Infants under 12 months of age who have close contact with a primary care provider with an acute HBV infection should obtain prophylaxis with HBIG (0.5 ml) and be immunized with HBV vaccine.

C. Non-A, non-B hepatitis. There are at least two types of viral hepatitis caused by at least two different agents.

1. **Parenterally transmitted (PT) non-A, non-B hepatitis** is similar to HBV infection and may be caused by several different agents, since multiple episodes of infection have been observed among the same individuals. A portion of the genome of a virus thought to be responsible for PT non-A, non-B hepatitis has been cloned. The proposed name of this virus is **hepatitis C virus (HCV).**

a. **High-risk groups** include transfusion recipients, parenteral drug users, dialysis patients, and possibly health care workers and household and sexual contacts. It is the most common cause of post-transfusion hepatitis in the United States.
b. The **carrier state** may exist in 1%–3% of the population.
c. Approximately 50% of infected individuals later develop **chronic hepatitis.**
d. **Control methods** consist of:
   (1) Screening all blood for antibodies to a part (epitope) of the HCV (anti-HCV)
   (2) Administering IG (0.06 ml/kg body weight) to people with percutaneous exposure to blood from a patient with PT non-A, non-B hepatitis

2. **Enterically transmitted (ET) non-A, non-B hepatitis** is similar to HAV infection and has caused epidemic or sporadic disease in parts of Asia, North and West Africa, and Mexico. It has not been recognized as an endemic disease in the United States or Western Europe.
   a. A 27–30 nm virus-like particle has been identified in stool samples, but no serologic tests have been developed.
   b. **Young to middle-aged adults** are most often affected, with an unusually high mortality rate among pregnant women.
   c. **Waterborne epidemics** have occurred as well as person-to-person transmission via the fecal-oral route.
   d. The **incubation period** is approximately 40 days.
   e. The **chronic carrier state** does not exist and complete recovery occurs.
   f. United States–manufactured IG does not provide protection.
   g. **Control methods** consist of avoiding potentially contaminated food or water.

3. There are other unidentified viruses that cause non-A, non-B hepatitis.

D. Hepatitis D virus (HDV)

1. **Infectious disease process**
   a. **Agent**
      (1) The **delta agent** of the HDV (delta hepatitis) is a defective virus, 35–37 nm in size, consisting of RNA genetic materials with an internal protein antigen (delta antigen) surrounded by a coat of HBsAg.
      (2) Since the delta agent requires the presence of HBV for synthesis, **coinfection** must take place for the clinical expression of the disease. Infection of an HBV carrier leads to a chronic delta infection and chronic active hepatitis. In the United States, 25%–50% of fulminant HBV cases have a concurrent delta agent infection.
   b. **Mode of transmission** is similar to HBV.

2. **Control strategies** consist of preventing the HBV infections and of preventing the HBV carrier state. Superinfection of HBsAg carriers cannot be prevented with any known biologic agent.

VII. TUBERCULOSIS

A. Epidemiologic features. Worldwide disease has caused significant morbidity and mortality. Tuberculosis will continue to be a problem in the United States as long as it remains a worldwide problem.

1. **Testing.** Infection with the tubercle bacilli is determined by a positive skin test to an intradermal injection of 5 international units (IU) of the international standard of purified protein derivative (**Mantoux test**).
   a. The reaction becomes positive about 2–10 weeks after infection and remains positive throughout life. It is a measure of tuberculous infection not tuberculous disease.
   b. Cutaneous anergy may occur in individuals with advanced tuberculous disease or in immunosuppressed individuals.
   c. In individuals over age 35 years, a booster phenomenon exists. When tuberculin skin tests are applied 1 week apart, the second test may show a marked increase in size of the reaction. The size of the induration in the second test should be the baseline reading for that patient.
   d. **Interpretation of Mantoux test**
      (1) A reaction of **≥ 5 mm induration** is considered positive in the following individuals.
         (a) Persons with HIV infection or with risk factors for HIV infection who have an unknown HIV antibody status

(b) Close recent contacts of an infectious tuberculosis case
(c) Persons with a chest radiograph consistent with old healed tuberculosis

(2) A reaction of ≥ **10 mm induration** is considered positive in persons who have risk factors for tuberculosis.

(a) Foreign-born individuals from high-prevalence countries in Asia, Africa, and Latin America
(b) IV drug abusers who are HIV antibody negative
(c) Medically underserved low-income populations, including high-risk racial or ethnic minority populations
(d) Residents of long-term care facilities
(e) Persons with medical conditions that have been reported to increase the risk of tuberculosis (e.g., silicosis, gastrectomy, jejunoileal bypass, being 10% or more below ideal body weight, chronic renal failure, diabetes mellitus, high-dose corticosteroids and other immunosuppressive therapy, some hematologic disorders such as leukemia and lymphomas, and other malignancies)

(3) A reaction of ≥ **15 mm induration** is considered positive in all other individuals.

2. **Tuberculous disease** (i.e., clinical symptoms) can occur from a primary infection, but most adult cases occur from reactivation of a latent infection—that is, one that was acquired many years previously (the original infection could have been asymptomatic or so mild as to be unrecognized as tuberculosis).

3. **Incidence.** In 1989, 23,495 cases of tuberculosis were reported. About 90% of these cases occurred from reactivation of a latent infection, and only 10% represented new infections.

4. **Prevalence** of tuberculosis infection as determined by positive tuberculin skin tests increases with increasing age. Most individuals born in the United States today remain tuberculin-negative. However, high tuberculin positivity rates occur in certain segments of the population, such as the elderly, nonwhites, and in individuals with low socioeconomic status. Tuberculosis infection is also common in immigrants from Asia, Latin America, and the Caribbean. It is estimated that perhaps 50% of the people in developing countries are infected with the tubercle bacilli.

5. **Case rates** for tuberculosis parallel the prevalence rates of tuberculosis infection. Cases are more likely to occur in older individuals (> 45 years of age) than in younger age-groups, in nonwhites (more than five times higher in nonwhite older age-groups) than in whites, and in men than in women. The racial differences may be related to socioeconomic factors, or there may be genetic differences in susceptibility. Tuberculosis morbidity is not evenly distributed in the United States.

   a. The highest case rates are along the southeastern seaboard, through the Appalachian mountain region, along the United States border with Mexico, and in scattered areas of the northwest containing many native Americans.
   b. The case rate per 100,000 population in 1989 ranged from 0.0 (Wyoming) to 66.4 (Newark, NJ) with an overall United States rate of 9.5. The higher case rates were in cities of more than 250,000 population and increased as the population increased.
   c. Tuberculosis is not only an urban problem, since 60% of the cases in 1989 occurred in communities of less than 250,000 population.

B. Infectious disease process

1. **Agent.** The causative agent is *M. tuberculosis* var. *hominis*.
   a. Drug-resistant organisms often initially cause illness in certain population groups, such as Asians and Hispanics.
   b. Drug resistance can also develop while individuals are on therapy, either because they have not taken their medications properly or because therapy was inappropriate.
   c. Tubercle bacilli can be destroyed by direct sunlight, ultraviolet light, heat, and some disinfectants, such as phenol or tricresol solution.
   d. Organisms can remain viable in dried sputum for long periods of time. Droplet nuclei may remain infectious for 8–10 days. However, when exposed to sunlight, the organisms die more quickly.

2. **Reservoir** of infection is humans.

3. **Portal of exit** is via the respiratory tract. The organism exits the body in respiratory secretions by coughing, sneezing, talking, singing, or other respiratory action. Patients with cavitary pulmonary lesions and large numbers of organisms in their sputa are highly infectious. Extrapulmonary tuberculosis is noncommunicable.

4. **Mode of transmission** is by inhalation of droplet nuclei, the airborne route. These droplet nuclei can remain suspended in the air, float to all parts of a room, and infect people in other rooms via ventilating systems. However, transmission is not easily achieved; it normally requires prolonged exposure to an infectious case.

5. **Portal of entry** is via the respiratory tract. Most primary lesions in the lungs are found in the periphery, suggesting that the site of implantation is the alveoli.

6. **Susceptible host.** Once infection has occurred, the outcome depends on several factors.
   a. **Age at the time of infection** is important. Infants and adolescents are more likely to experience severe disease.
   b. **The risk of developing clinical disease** is greatest (about 5%) within the year following infection (i.e., conversion of skin test from negative to positive). However, the risk of developing acute disease never disappears as long as living tubercle bacilli are present in the host.
   c. **Reactivation of a latent infection** is more likely to occur in the elderly, in patients with diabetes or silicosis, and in immunosuppressed individuals.
   d. **Clinical disease in patients with AIDS or HIV infection** is normally extensive and presents with atypical manifestations. Extrapulmonary forms, such as lymphatic and disseminated (miliary) disease are more common, and pulmonary disease with mediastinal or hilar lymphadenopathy occurs in any lobe and without cavitation.

C. **Control strategies.** Morbidity and mortality from tuberculosis has been declining since the beginning of the 20th century. Although improvements in diet, housing, and living conditions have contributed significantly to this decline, the advent of effective chemotherapy in the late 1940s and early 1950s has accelerated this decline. The objectives of a tuberculosis control program are to eliminate morbidity and mortality in infected individuals and to interrupt transmission of the tubercle bacilli in the community. Control programs can be divided into two components—surveillance and containment.

1. **Surveillance** refers to the process of identifying infected patients.
   a. **Medical care.** Many patients are identified because they either seek medical care for symptoms of tuberculosis or for other unrelated medical problems.
   b. **Contact investigation.** Some cases are identified because of contact investigation around known cases. Since positive culture results may take 8 weeks, contact investigation should begin if the history, sputum smear, and chest x-rays are suggestive of tuberculosis and should be performed in widening concentric circles (starting with household contacts) until the level of infection detected (as determined by a tuberculin skin test) approximates the level of infection within the local community. The decision to evaluate a contact should be based on characteristics of the case, the environment, and characteristics of the contact.
      (1) **Case characteristics** include an evaluation of the degree of infectiousness. Factors to consider include:
         (a) The duration of respiratory symptoms, such as cough
         (b) The type of disease, such as pulmonary cavitary disease or tuberculous laryngitis
         (c) The number of acid-fast bacilli in the sputum smear
         (d) The characteristics of the sputum; high volume and watery sputum are regarded as risk factors
      (2) **Environmental factors** consist mainly of the concentration of droplet nuclei in the air shared by the case and contacts.
         (a) The volume of air in the room
         (b) The ventilation of the room; in general, the concentration of infectious particles is increased in poorly ventilated rooms
         (c) Whether or not air is recirculated or subjected to ultraviolet radiation or filtration
      (3) **Contact characteristics** include:
         (a) The amount of time spent with the case; in general, high-risk contacts are normally household contacts or individuals who have had close contact over a prolonged period of time
         (b) The physical proximity to the case; transmission of tuberculous infection is unlikely with brief exposure to relatively small numbers of aerosolized particles

(c) Whether or not the contact had prior infection with tuberculosis or was taking antituberculosis therapy

c. **Screening programs.** A few cases are identified through screening programs. Routine screening of the general U.S. population is no longer recommended. Screening of some segments of the population is indicated to detect cases of tuberculosis so that further transmission can be prevented and so that chemoprophylaxis can be given.

(1) **Screening** consists of:

(a) The application of a two-step, intermediate-strength Mantoux test

(b) A chest x-ray for individuals who:

(i) Have a positive skin test

(ii) Are 65 years of age or older

(iii) Have signs or symptoms of tuberculosis

(2) **Screening** is indicated for:

(a) Close contacts with known or suspected tuberculosis

(b) Populations with a high rate of infection, such as immigrants from Asia, Latin America, and the Caribbean

(c) Institutions where transmission of tuberculosis is likely, such as health care facilities (i.e., nursing homes, mental hospitals), correctional institutions, or where a case of tuberculosis would pose a particular hazard to others (i.e., day-care centers, newborn nurseries)

(i) Initial screening of new personnel and clients should be done.

(ii) The need for repeat screening of nonreactors should be determined by the individual institutions and should be based on the risk of acquiring new infection.

(d) In all patients with positive HIV antibody tests

(e) Persons with medical risk factors known to increase the risk of disease

(f) Medically underserved populations

(g) Alcoholics and IV drug abusers

2. **Containment** refers to methods of stopping the spread of infection and disease. Containment activities consist of:

a. **Administration of proper antituberculosis chemotherapy for the proper duration of time.** Because of the duration of therapy and side effects of the drugs, the physician must work with the patient to make certain that he takes the medication. The patient can proceed normally as long as the prescribed medication is taken properly. More than 95% of cases can be cured with initial treatment.

(1) **Proper therapy** consists of two or more drugs, preferably drugs that the patient has never received before. Because of the emergence of drug-resistant organisms, the physician should never add one new drug at a time to a failing regimen or to a patient who has received previous therapy.

(2) Isoniazid (INH), rifampin (RMP), and pyrazinamide (PZA) for 2 months followed by INH and RMP for 4 additional months is the current recommendation for treating uncomplicated cases acquired in the United States. Over 90% of patients taking INH and RMP become sputum negative in 3 months.

(3) Ethambutol (EMB) should be added for patients who might have INH-resistant organisms or for patients with central nervous system or disseminated tuberculosis. Foreign-born Latin Americans and foreign-born Asians have resistant organisms in 12%–15% of cases. Drug therapy can be modified when sensitivity results become available.

(4) Drug sensitivity studies should be used when treating patients who might have drug-resistant organisms. Until drug sensitivities are available, the patient should be placed on two drugs that she has never had before. Intermittent regimens have been developed to treat patients who require close supervision.

b. **Administration of antituberculous chemoprophylaxis to infected individuals (those with a positive intermediate Mantoux skin test) who are at risk of developing clinical disease.** PHS trials have shown that INH preventive therapy can reduce the incidence of tuberculosis disease by 54%–88%. The level of protection exceeded 90% in patients who took their medication properly.

(1) **Groups that should benefit from preventive therapy** include:

(a) Individuals whose skin test has converted from negative to positive in the previous 2 years; many of these (5%–23%) may develop disease in a few years

(b) Close contacts of newly discovered cases of tuberculosis

(i) Tuberculin-positive reactors (≥ 5 mm induration) have a 1.6% incidence of developing tuberculosis during the first year after contact.

(ii) Tuberculin-negative contacts, especially infants, children under 6 years of age, or persons with impaired immunity should also be given preventive therapy.

(iii) For tuberculin-negative adults, other factors, such as degree of infectiousness of the index case, daily consumption of alcohol, and side effects of INH, should be considered.

(iv) All tuberculin-negative contacts should be retested 12 weeks later, and, if still negative and if exposure has ended, the preventive therapy can be discontinued. If positive, therapy should be continued for 6 months.

(c) Individuals with AIDS or HIV infection; an intermediate Mantoux is considered positive at 5 mm induration and preventive therapy should be given for at least 12 months

(d) Individuals with chest x-rays showing abnormalities suggestive of tuberculous parenchymal scarring (solitary calcified granulomas are excluded); the risk of developing disease ranges from 0.4%–3.5% each year

(e) Individuals with certain conditions, including hematologic or reticuloendothelial malignant neoplasm, silicosis, chronic renal insufficiency, and diabetes mellitus, and heroin addicts

(f) Individuals on immunosuppressive therapy or systemic corticosteroids in dosages greater than 15 mg prednisone per day

(g) Individuals with nutritional deficiency and substantial weight loss, including gastrectomy and intestinal bypass

(h) Intravenous drug abusers

(i) Tuberculin-positive individuals under 35 years of age; the rate of developing disease in this group is about 0%–1% per year and could yield a significant lifetime risk

(2) **INH** is the only drug proven to be effective preventive therapy. A dosage of 300 mg in adults and 20 mg/kg body weight (up to 300 mg) in children should be taken as a single daily oral dose. The duration of treatment is 6 months. The cost of the drug for 1 year is approximately $30.00.

(3) **Contraindications.** INH chemoprophylaxis should not be used:

(a) In the presence of clinical disease, in which case, two drugs are needed

(b) In individuals who were previously adequately treated

(c) In individuals who have had previous adverse reactions to INH

(d) In patients with unstable hepatic function

(e) In pregnant women until after delivery unless strongly indicated (i.e., close contact or recent converter)

(f) In individuals taking significant amounts of other hepatotoxins (i.e., alcohol)

(4) **Toxic effects** from INH include:

(a) **Hepatitis.** This occurs in 2.1% of individuals over 50 years of age and is rare in persons under 20. Patients who are over 35 years of age should be followed with transaminase levels at 1, 3, 6, and 9 months. Clinical symptoms should also be monitored, since enzyme elevations will occur.

(b) **Peripheral neuropathy, mood changes, and hypersensitivity reactions.** The peripheral neuropathy, which is more common in persons with diabetes, uremia, and alcoholism, can be prevented by daily administration of 10 mg of pyridoxine (vitamin B_6).

(5) Patients who have contacts with proven INH-resistant organisms and for whom the consequences of infection are likely to be severe may be given chemoprophylaxis with RMP at 10 mg/kg body weight up to 600 mg a day in a single oral dose. This regimen has not been shown to be effective in clinical trials, but it is believed to be effective on a theoretical basis. The cost of RMP for a year at this dosage is over $750.

3. **Control and eradication of tuberculosis** can only be accomplished by the combined efforts of both the private and public sectors of the medical community.

a. The **private medical community** should be aware of and implement current national recommendations for chemotherapy and for chemoprophylaxis. Reports submitted to the CDC by tuberculosis control programs in states and large cities indicate that less than 60%

of infected contacts of persons with newly diagnosed tuberculosis are being started on preventive therapy. The private physician also should report all cases of tuberculosis to the health department so that appropriate control procedures can be instituted.

b. **State and local health departments** have certain resources that can be helpful to physicians and that can be used to control tuberculosis.

(1) A **case registry** containing clinical and laboratory data on all reported cases, including:

(a) Duration of illness

(b) Type and extent of disease

(c) Hospitalizations

(d) Sputum smear and culture results

(e) Previous therapy and most recent sensitivity studies

(2) Consultants trained in the treatment of tuberculosis who can

(a) Help decide current therapy

(b) Resolve difficult clinical problems

(c) Advise on the feasibility of an intermittent therapy program

(3) Free antituberculosis drugs

(4) Free clinics where the patient can be followed on a regular basis

(5) An outreach program in which public health nurses or public health investigators can

(a) Conduct appropriate contact investigations

(b) Find patients who were lost to follow-up

(c) Administer therapy so that it is convenient for the patient

(6) A public health laboratory that can confirm the isolate and do appropriate sensitivity studies

VIII. MENINGITIS

VIII. MENINGITIS causes more concern among parents and officials of schools and day-care centers than any other disease. Since viral meningitis is rarely fatal, parental and public anxieties can be controlled by education and assurances. This section will discuss only bacterial meningitis, which is a serious public health problem that requires public health intervention. The three most common types of bacterial meningitis are *H. influenzae* meningitis, meningococcal meningitis, and pneumococcal meningitis. Almost 70% of the reported cases occur in children under age 5 years.

A. ***H. influenzae* meningitis.** *H. influenzae* is the most common cause of bacterial meningitis in children under age 5, with about 12,000 cases occurring each year.

1. Epidemiologic features

a. **Incidence.** *H. influenzae* type b (Hib) is a common infection of childhood. At least 50% of children have had at least one Hib infection during the first year of life. About two-thirds of the cases have occurred in infants and children under 15 months of age. Almost everyone has been infected by 3 years of age, with most of these occurring as middle-ear infections. **Peak incidence** is from age 3 months to 2 years. Before effective vaccines were developed, one in 200 children developed invasive Hib disease by age 5 years. Sixty percent of these children had meningitis.

b. **Morbidity and mortality of meningitis cases**

(1) Between 20%–30% of the survivors have permanent neurologic deficits ranging from mild hearing loss to mental retardation.

(2) It is one of the most preventable causes of mental retardation.

(3) The mortality rate is about 5%.

c. **Communicability.** Although the organism *H. influenzae* can be transmitted readily from one person to another, cases of meningitis occur primarily as isolated events with few secondary cases. Widespread outbreaks of Hib meningitis have not occurred.

d. **Secondary spread.** Secondary cases may occur in household contacts and in day-care contacts.

(1) Secondary spread within a month to household contacts is 0.3%, which is about 600 times higher than in the general population. Secondary household attack rate was 4% for children up to 2 years of age, 2% for children 2–3 years of age, 0.1% for children 4–5 years of age, and 0% for those over 6 years of age. Among household contacts, 64% of cases occurred within the first week, 20% during the second week, and 16% during the third and fourth weeks.

(2) Secondary spread to **day-care contacts** under 4 years of age is also high.

2. **Infectious disease process**
   a. **Agent.** The causative agent is *H. influenzae.*
      (1) *H. influenzae* exists in both the encapsulated and unencapsulated form. The encapsulated type can be subdivided into six capsular types—a, b, c, d, e, and f. The most invasive disease (i.e., meningitis and acute epiglottiditis) is caused by type b and is frequently called Hib.
      (2) Plasmid-mediated ampicillin-resistant strains have been occurring since 1974. Currently, about 12%–40% of isolates are resistant to ampicillin.
   b. **Reservoir.** Humans are the reservoir of infection. Nasopharyngeal carriage is common with colonization rates ranging from 0%–23% with a mean of 10%. During an 18-month period, 71% of toddlers and 48% of preschool children became colonized.
   c. **Mode of transmission** is by direct contact with respiratory droplets from the nose and throat of infected individuals more often carriers than cases.
   d. **Portal of entry** is the nasopharynx.
   e. **Susceptible host**
      (1) **Newborns** are protected by maternal antibodies during the first 3 months of life.
      (2) **Pharyngeal carriage** throughout infancy and childhood stimulates a naturally acquired immunity. Invasive disease caused by a capsular strain of *Hemophilus* is rare in adults.
      (3) Disease is more common in the following high-risk groups:
         (a) Native Americans and black Americans
         (b) Individuals of low socioeconomic status
         (c) Children who attend day-care centers
         (d) Patients with antibody-deficient syndromes, asplenia, sickle-cell disease, or malignancies associated with immunosuppression

3. **Control strategies for invasive Hib disease (i.e., meningitis, acute epiglottiditis)**
   a. **Immunization recommendation**
      (1) **Types of Hib conjugate vaccine**
         (a) Diphtheria CRM_{197} protein conjugate vaccine
         (b) Meningococcal protein conjugate vaccine
         (c) Diphtheria toxoid conjugate vaccine
      (2) **Recommendations for vaccine use**
         (a) Diphtheria CMR_{197} protein conjugate vaccine or meningococcal protein conjugate vaccine can be used in infants and children over 2 months of age. Diphtheria toxoid conjugate vaccine can be used in children 15 months of age and older.
         (b) All children should begin to be immunized at 2 months of age. Physicians should consult the package inserts in commercial products for appropriate immunization schedules. The same conjugate vaccine should be used throughout the entire vaccination series.
         (c) Unimmunized children 15–59 months of age can be given any of the three vaccines.
      (3) **Conferred immunity.** Children under 24 months of age who have had invasive Hib disease should still receive vaccine, since many children of that age fail to develop adequate immunity following natural disease.
   b. **Initial management** of a case of invasive Hib disease in a day-care center involves:
      (1) Verifying the diagnosis and treating the patient
      (2) Notifying the other parents that their child has had contact with a case of meningitis and that
         (a) Secondary spread to children over 6 years of age is uncommon
         (b) Their child should be monitored for signs of illness and if fever, rash, headache, or stiff neck develop, the child should be seen by a physician (This is a good practice to follow even if the child has not been exposed to a case of meningitis.)
         (c) In some instances, antimicrobial chemoprophylaxis and immunization with a polysaccharide vaccine might be indicated.
   c. **Antimicrobial chemoprophylaxis** is the most effective preventive measure for preventing immediate secondary cases. Hib vaccine cannot prevent immediate cases since it takes time for antibodies to develop.
      (1) Chemoprophylaxis should be offered to
         (a) All household contacts of a case of invasive Hib disease in which another child under 4 years of age resides

(b) All classmates and staff in a day-care center that has children under 2 years of age who have been exposed to invasive Hib disease; however, some authorities feel that this recommendation should not be implemented unless two cases have occurred

(c) All patients who were treated for invasive disease because antimicrobial therapy of invasive disease does not eradiacte nasopharyngeal carriage

(d) Children who have had the Hib vaccine or who have had previous Hib disease; although these groups are felt to be at decreased risk of disease, the Hib vaccine does not affect nasopharyngeal carriage of the organism, which may be passed on to susceptible classmates

(2) Nasopharyngeal cultures should not be done because they are not helpful in determining who should receive chemoprophylaxis.

(3) **RMP** is the drug of choice for chemoprophylaxis.

(a) The dosage is 20 mg/kg body weight by mouth once daily (maximum daily dose of 600 mg) for 4 days. In neonates under 1 year of age, the dosage is 10 mg/kg body weight once daily for 4 days.

(b) RMP is not recommended for pregnant women.

(c) RMP turns urine and tears orange. The patient should not wear contact lenses while taking chemoprophylaxis.

(4) To be effective in day-care centers, at least 75% of the children must receive RMP. All classroom contacts should receive RMP at the same time. In public health practice, this is difficult to achieve.

(5) For the pediatric population unable to swallow RMP capsules, the drug may be mixed with several teaspoons of applesauce immediately before administration or a suspension of RMP may be freshly prepared.

(6) Chemoprophylaxis should be offered as soon as possible after the index case is identified, but some benefit may be attained even if offered more than 14 days after the index case.

B. Meningococcal meningitis

1. Epidemiologic features

a. Incidence

(1) ***N. meningitidis*** is the second most common cause of bacterial meningitis in the United States, with 3000–4000 cases reported each year.

(2) The **peak incidence** is around age 6–12 months, with a smaller peak at age 15–24 years. It is more likely to occur in newly aggregated young adults who are living in crowded conditions such as institutions and barracks.

(3) **Seasonality.** Most cases occur in late winter and early spring.

b. Morbidity and mortality. The case fatality rate for meningitis and for meningococcemia is about 10%.

c. Communicability. Although the organism *N. meningitidis* can be transmitted readily from one person to another, cases of meningitis occur primarily as isolated cases or in small clusters. Large outbreaks due to serogroups A and C have occurred in recent years in the sub-Saharan region of Africa and in Brazil. The last major outbreak of group A meningitis in the United States was in 1945.

d. Secondary spread. Close contacts of confirmed cases are about 1000 times more likely to develop meningococcal illnesses than the general population. One-third of these secondary cases occur within 4 days of the index case.

2. Infectious disease process

a. Agent. The causative agent is *N. meningitidis*.

(1) Nine different serogroups—the most common of which are A, B, C, W-135, X, Y, and Z—have been identified on the basis of a specific capsular polysaccharide. Serogroup B accounts for 50%–55% of cases, serogroup C for 20%–25%, serogroup W-135 for 15%, serogroup Y for 10%, and serogroup A for 1%–2%.

(2) Some serogroups appear to be less virulent, although fatal infections and secondary spread have occurred with all types.

b. Reservoir of infection is humans. Pharyngeal carriage is high and ranges from 5%–70%, depending on the population, age, season, and living conditions.

c. Mode of transmission is by direct contact with respiratory droplets from the nose and throat of infected persons who are more often carriers than cases.

d. **Portal of entry** is the nasopharynx.
e. **Susceptible host**
   (1) **Newborns** are protected by maternal antibodies during the first 3 months of life.
   (2) **Pharyngeal carriage** throughout infancy, childhood, and early adulthood stimulates a naturally acquired immunity. Meningococcal disease in individuals over age 25 is uncommon.
   (3) **Individuals who are complement deficient** are at increased risk of disease and may actually have multiple episodes of infection. **Asplenic people** are at increased risk and also experience particularly severe infections.

3. **Control strategies**
   a. **Initial management of case**
      (1) Verify the diagnosis and treat the patient.
      (2) Notify the parents of other children exposed to the case [see VIII A 3 b (2) (b)].
   b. **Antimicrobial chemoprophylaxis** is the chief preventive measure in sporadic cases and should be offered to
      (1) Household contacts
      (2) Day-care center contacts
      (3) Medical personnel who resuscitated, intubated, or suctioned the patient before antibiotics were instituted
      (4) Individuals who had contact with the patient's oral secretions through intimate contact or through the sharing of food and beverages
      (5) All patients who were treated for meningococcal disease before discharge from the hospital, because antimicrobial therapy does not reliably eradicate nasopharyngeal carriage of *N. meningitidis*
   c. **RMP,** which has been shown to be 90% effective in eradicating nasopharyngeal carriage, is the drug of choice for chemoprophylaxis. RMP is given by mouth twice a day for 2 days. Dosage is 600 mg every 12 hours for adults, 10 mg/kg body weight every 12 hours for children age 1 month or older, and 5 mg/kg body weight every 12 hours for children under 1 month of age.
   d. **Meningococcal polysaccharide vaccine**
      (1) In the United States, there is a bivalent (serogroups A and C) vaccine and a quadrivalent (serogroups A, C, Y, and W-135) vaccine available.
      (2) Military recruits currently receive the quadrivalent vaccine.
      (3) Routine immunization of civilians in the United States is not recommended because
         (a) Risk of infection is low.
         (b) A vaccine against serogroup B, the major cause of disease, is not available.
      (4) Vaccines may be helpful
         (a) In certain high-risk groups
         (b) For international travel
         (c) In aborting communitywide outbreaks

C. **Pneumococcal meningitis** is caused by *S. pneumoniae* (see III D 7). Since pneumococcal meningitis only occurs as isolated endemic cases, vaccine administration or chemoprophylaxis to close contacts is not indicated.

BIBLIOGRAPHY

Advisory Committee on Immunization Practices (ACIP): Diphtheria, tetanus, and pertussis: guidelines for vaccine prophylaxis and other preventive measures. *MMWR* 34:405–414, 419–426, 1985.

ACIP: General recommendations on immunization. *MMWR* 38:205–214, 219–227, 1989.

ACIP: *Haemophilus* b conjugate vaccine for prevention of *Haemophilus influenzae* type b disease among infants and children two months of age and older. *MMWR* 40(RR-1):1–7, 1991.

ACIP: Measles prevention. *MMWR* 38(S-9):1–18, 1989.

ACIP: Meningococcal vaccines. *MMWR* 34:255–259, 1985.

ACIP: Mumps prevention. *MMWR* 38:388–392, 397–400, 1989.

ACIP: Pneumococcal polysaccharide vaccine. *MMWR* 38:64–68, 73–76, 1989.

ACIP: Poliomyelitis prevention. *MMWR* 31:22–26, 31–34, 1982.

ACIP: Poliomyelitis prevention: Enhanced-potency inactivated poliomyelitis vaccine—supplementary statement. *MMWR* 36:795–798, 1987.

ACIP: Prevention and control of influenza: Part 1, Vaccines. *MMWR* 38:297–298, 303–309, 1989.

ACIP: Prevention and control of influenza. *MMWR* 40(RR-6):1–15, 1991.

ACIP: Recommendations for protection against viral hepatitis. *MMWR* 39(RR-2):1–26, 1990.

ACIP: Rubella prevention. *MMWR* 33:301–310, 315–318, 1984.

ACIP: Update: Prevention of *Haemophilus influenzae* type b disease. *MMWR* 35:170–174, 179–180, 1986.

American College of Obstetricians and Gynecologists: Technical Bulletin, Washington, DC.

American College of Physicians Task Force on Adult Immunization and Infectious Disease Society of America: *Guide for Adult Immunization,* 2nd edition. Philadelphia, American College of Physicians, 1990.

American Academy of Pediatrics: *Report of the Committee on Infectious Diseases,* 21st edition. Evanston, IL, American Academy of Pediatrics, 1988.

American Thoracic Society: Control of tuberculosis. *Am Rev Respir Dis* 128:336–342, 1983.

American Thoracic Society: Diagnostic standards and classification of tuberculosis. *Am Rev Respir Dis* 142:725–735, 1990.

Benenson AS (ed): *Control of Communicable Diseases in Man,* 14th edition. Washington, DC, Official Report of the American Public Health Association, 1985.

Centers for Disease Control (CDC): Diagnosis and management of mycobacterial infection and disease in persons with human T-lymphotrophic virus type III/lymphadenopathy associated virus infection. *MMWR* 35:448–452, 1986.

CDC: Division of Sexually Transmitted Diseases and HIV Prevention Annual Report. Fiscal year 1990.

CDC: Guidelines for prevention of transmission of human immunodeficiency virus and hepatitis B virus to health-care and public-safety workers. *MMWR* 38(S-6):1–37, 1989.

CDC: Health Information for International Travel. Published annually.

CDC: The HIV/AIDS epidemic: The first 10 years. *MMWR* 40:357, 1991.

CDC: *HIV/AIDS Surveillance Report.* Atlanta, CDC, June 1991.

CDC: Increase in rubella and congenital rubella syndrome (CRS)—United States, 1988–1990. *MMWR* 40:93–98, 1991.

CDC: Measles—United States, 1990. *MMWR* 40:369–372, 1991.

CDC: Pertussis surveillance—United States, 1986–1988. *MMWR* 39:57–58, 63–66, 1990.

CDC: Racial differences in rates of hepatitis B virus infection—United States, 1976–1980. *MMWR* 38:818–821, 1989.

CDC: Recommendations for prevention of HIV transmission in health-care settings. *MMWR* 36(S-2): 15–175, 1987.

CDC: Screening for tuberculosis and tuberculous infection in high-risk populations and the use of preventive therapy for tuberculosis infection in the United States: Recommendations of the advisory committee for elimination of tuberculosis. *MMWR* 39(RR-8):1–12, 1990.

CDC: Second National Health and Nutrition Examination Survey (NHANES II). *MMWR* 38:818–821, 1989.

CDC: Second National Health and Nutrition Examination Survey (NHANES II). *MMWR* 39:9, 1990.

CDC: Tetanus—United States, 1987 and 1988. *MMWR* 39:37–41, 1990.

CDC: Update: Acquired immunodeficiency syndrome and human immunodeficiency virus infection among health care workers. *MMWR* 37:229–234, 239, 1988.

CDC: Update: Acquired immunodeficiency syndrome—United States, 1981–1990. *MMWR* 40: 358–363, 369, 1991.

CDC: Update: Transmission of HIV infection during invasive dental procedures—Florida. *MMWR* 40: 377–381, 1991.

CDC: Update: Universal Precaution for prevention of transmission of human immunodeficiency virus, hepatitis B virus and other bloodborne pathogens in health-care settings. *MMWR* 37:377–382, 387–388, 1988.

Farer LS: The current status of tuberculosis control efforts. *Am Rev Respir Dis* 134:402–407, 1986.

Francis DP, Maynard JE: The transmission and outcome of hepatitis A, B, and non-A, non-B: A review. *Epidemiol Rev* 1:17–31, 1979.

Garner JS, Favero MS: Guidelines for handwashing and hospital environmental control. Atlanta, Hospital Infections Program, Center for Infectious Diseases, CDC, US Public Health Service, US Department of Health and Human Services, 1985.

Garner JS, Simmons BP: Guidelines for isolation precautions in hospitals. *Infect Control* 4:245–325, 1983.

Holmes K, Mardh P, Sparling PF, et al: *Sexually Transmitted Diseases.* New York, McGraw-Hill, 1984.

Last JM (ed): *Maxcy-Rosenau Public Health and Preventive Medicine,* 12th edition. Norwalk, CT, Appleton & Lange, 1986.

Leman SM: Type A viral hepatitis: New developments in an old disease. *N Eng J Med* 313:1059–1065, 1985.

Mandell GL, Douglas JRG, Bennett JE: *Principles and Practice of Infectious Diseases.* New York, John Wiley, 1979.

Physicians' Desk Reference (PDR). Oradel, NJ, Medical Economics Company, Inc. published annually.

Stone KM, Grimes DA, Magder LS: Primary prevention of sexually transmitted diseases. A primer for clinicians. *JAMA* 255:1763–1766, 1986.

Williams WW: Guidelines for infection control in hospital personnel. *Infect Control* 4:326–349, 1983.

STUDY QUESTIONS

Directions: Each of the numbered items or incomplete statements in this section is followed by answers or by completions of the statement. Select the **one** lettered answer or completion that is **best** in each case.

1. All of the following statements about tuberculosis are true EXCEPT

(A) the risk of developing tuberculous disease is greatest within the first year following infection
(B) most cases of tuberculosis occur as a result of primary infection
(C) INH chemoprophylaxis may be given to selected high-risk patients over 35 years of age
(D) routine screening of the general U.S. population is no longer recommended
(E) most cases of tuberculosis can be successfully treated with a 6-month drug regimen

2. The most common cause of bacterial meningitis in children under 5 years of age is

(A) *Neisseria meningitidis*
(B) *Streptococcus pneumoniae*
(C) *Listeria monocytogenes*
(D) group B streptococci
(E) *Hemophilus influenzae* type B

3. Which of the following diseases confers natural immunity?

(A) Influenza
(B) Polio
(C) Tetanus
(D) Measles

4. Which of the following conditions contraindicates routine childhood immunization?

(A) Prematurity
(B) Acute illness with an oral temperature over 100° F
(C) Antibiotic therapy
(D) Living with a pregnant woman
(E) Allergy to penicillin

5. All of the following statements regarding the health status of HIV-infected individuals are true EXCEPT

(A) they are usually asymptomatic
(B) they have circulating HIV particles in their plasma and peripheral blood mononuclear cells
(C) they will ultimately develop AIDS
(D) they will be cured with AZT

Questions 6–8

A 27-year-old IV drug abuser presents with cough, fever, and an abnormal chest x-ray showing hilar and mediastinal adenopathy and bilateral lower lobe infiltrates. His intermediate Mantoux skin test shows a greater than 5 mm induration.

6. The most likely diagnosis is

(A) pneumococcal pneumonia
(B) pulmonary tuberculosis
(C) *Mycoplasma* pneumonia
(D) aspiration pneumonia
(E) viral pneumonia

7. The underlying condition associated with this illness is most likely

(A) sickle-cell disease
(B) alcoholism
(C) drug abuse
(D) HIV infection
(E) Hodgkin's disease

8. Initial treatment of this patient should include

(A) INH, RMP, and PZA
(B) penicillin
(C) erythromycin
(D) INH, RMP, PZA, and EMB

1-B	4-B	7-D
2-E	5-D	8-D
3-D	6-B	

Directions: Each item below contains four suggested answers of which **one or more** is correct. Choose the answer

A if **1, 2, and 3** are correct
B if **1 and 3** are correct
C if **2 and 4** are correct
D if **4** is correct
E if **1, 2, 3, and 4** are correct

9. The administrator of a day-care center reports that a child under his care has just been diagnosed as having meningitis. He is concerned about the other children in the center and wants to know what to do. Which of the following must be known in order that recommendations can be made?

(1) Number of children in the center
(2) Age range of the children
(3) Number of employees in the center
(4) Type of meningitis

10. HAV has which of the following epidemiologic characteristics?

(1) The virus is transmitted by poor personal hygiene, poor sanitation, and intimate household or sexual contacts
(2) The amount of virus shed in the stool appears to be related to the severity of clinical illness
(3) The administration of IG within 2 weeks of exposure can prevent or modify illness
(4) The existence of a chronic carrier state has been identified

11. The owner of a local restaurant reported that his short-order cook was just diagnosed as having HAV. The cook handled food only before it was cooked. Recommendations to prevent further spread of HAV should include which of the following?

(1) The short-order cook should not work until he is over his acute illness
(2) IG should be given to all restaurant employees
(3) IG should be given to all household contacts of the short-order cook
(4) IG should be given to all customers who ate in the restaurant during the previous 2 weeks

12. A nurse who works on a dialysis unit presents with jaundice. Her HBsAg is positive, and her IgM anti-HAV is negative. Recommendations to prevent further spread should include which of the following?

(1) Administer HBIG to her spouse
(2) Administer HBIG to her children
(3) Advise her not to share her toothbrush or razor
(4) Administer HBV vaccine to her spouse

13. A 2-year-old child is brought to the physician's office because of a broken arm. When a history is taken, it is discovered that she has had only two DTP and one OPV immunization during the first 6 months of life. The child has no illnesses, and the mother is in her first trimester of pregnancy. In regard to the immunizations, the physician should

(1) administer DTP, OPV, Hib, and MMR vaccines to the child
(2) tell the mother that the immunization series must be started all over again
(3) instruct the mother to bring the child back in 6 months for another DTP and OPV immunization
(4) instruct the mother that because of her pregnancy, she should avoid close contact with the child for 3 weeks after immunization

14. A 1-year-old child who attends a day-care center is diagnosed as having Hib meningitis. This day-care center has infants ranging from 6 months to 4 years of age. Thirty percent of the children over 2 months of age have already received some Hib vaccine. Control recommendations should consist of

(1) RMP prophylaxis for those unimmunized attendees under 18 months of age
(2) Hib vaccine for all attendees who are not properly immunized
(3) booster Hib immunizations for all children over 18 months of age
(4) RMP prophylaxis for all classmates and staff (except pregnant women) regardless of their immunization status

---

9-C
10-B
11-A
12-B
13-B
14-C

15. Documented spread of AIDS has occurred

(1) from mother to child in utero or at the time of birth
(2) in household contacts
(3) among heterosexual and homosexual contacts
(4) from eating food

16. Universal Precautions apply to

(1) saliva, nasal secretions, sputum, sweat, and tears
(2) blood and other body fluids containing visible blood
(3) feces, urine, and vomitus
(4) body fluids such as cerebrospinal, pleural, pericardial, peritoneal, amniotic, and synovial fluids

17. The National Gonococcal Isolate Surveillance Project, which was established to monitor trends in antimicrobial resistance, revealed that, of the 1989 gonococcal isolates, approximately

(1) 12% were resistant to penicillin
(2) 74% showed no resistance to commonly used antibiotics
(3) 17% were resistant to tetracycline
(4) none showed clinical resistance to ceftriaxone

Directions: Each group of items in this section consists of lettered options followed by a set of numbered items. For each item, select the **one** lettered option that is most closely associated with it. Each lettered option may be selected once, more than once, or not at all.

Questions 18–22

For each gonorrhea control strategy, select the characteristic of the disease that it is designed to prevent.

(A) Nonvenereal transmission
(B) Penicillin-resistant organisms
(C) Reinfection
(D) Asymptomatic infection

18. Multiple cultures should be taken on individuals being evaluated

19. All gonococcal isolates should be tested for β-lactamase production

20. Prophylactic eye drops should be instilled into the eyes c⁽ newborns to prevent gonococcal conjunctivitis

21. Contact tracing and epidemiologic treatment of all identified contacts should be performed

22. Gonorrhea cultures should be done on certain sexually active women

Questions 23–27

Match each characteristic of hepatitis with the type of hepatitis that is most appropriate.

(A) HAV
(B) HBV
(C) HCV
(D) HDV

23. It is the most common cause of post-transfusion hepatitis in the United States

24. Coinfection must take place for the clinical expression of the disease

25. It is a common problem in day-care centers and in families who have children attending day-care centers

26. Chronic infection may lead to cirrhosis or primary hepatocellular carcinoma

27. It can be prevented with a vaccine

15-B	18-D	21-C	24-D	27-B
16-C	19-B	22-D	25-A	
17-E	20-A	23-C	26-B	

ANSWERS AND EXPLANATIONS

1. The answer is B *[VII A 2, 3, B 6 b, C 2 a].*
Most individuals infected with the tubercle bacilli handle the disease quite well. Although they get over the primary infection, the organism remains viable inside the body. At any time in the future, the infection can reactivate causing tuberculous disease. Pediatric cases usually represent a primary infection, while most adult cases occur from the reactivation of a latent infection, one that was acquired many years previously. Of the 23,000 cases of tuberculosis that were reported in 1988, 90% occurred from reactivation of a latent infection, and only 10% represented new infections. This is why certain high-risk individuals should receive chemoprophylaxis with isoniazid (INH) to kill the viable organisms so that reactivation does not take place. The 6-month regimen consists of INH, rifampin (RMP), and pyrazinamide (PZA) for 2 months, followed by INH and RMP for an additional 4 months.

2. The answer is E *[VIII A].*
Hemophilus influenzae type B (Hib) is not only the most common cause of bacterial meningitis in children under 5 years of age, but also it is one of the most common causes of preventable mental retardation. Because of the severity of this disease, Hib conjugate vaccines have been developed to prevent infection. Immunization against Hib should begin at age 2 months.

3. The answer is D *[IV A 2 f (2)].*
Measles confers natural immunity, which eliminates the need for further immunizations against the disease. Although a case of measles confers lifelong immunity, it is important to document immunity since a measles-like illness can be caused by a number of other viral illnesses. A history of having had measles disease is not sufficient for a child to be permitted to attend school; a child must have serologic evidence of immunity or a documented measles immunization to attend school. Since the H and N component of the influenza A virus can undergo minor and major antigenic shifts, natural disease does not confer immunity. In fact, the composition of the vaccine must be updated continually to provide protection against the current strains. Clinical tetanus does not confer immunity, and it is possible to have this disease many times. Apparently, the amount of toxin necessary to cause disease is not sufficient to stimulate the immune response. Since there are three distinct types of poliovirus, it is possible to get polio on three separate occasions. Polio vaccine provides protection against all three types.

4. The answer is B *[III C 2 f (5)].*
Immunizations should not be given to an acutely ill patient with an oral temperature over 100° F. Otherwise, there are a very few contraindications for immunizing a child. Multiple vaccines can be given to any child. Prematurity, antibiotic therapy for bacterial infections, living with a pregnant woman, and penicillin allergies are common events and should never be used as excuses for not immunizing a patient. Every patient/physician encounter should be considered an opportunity for immunizations. The prevention of disease is more important than the treatment of disease. Most individuals who develop a vaccine-preventable illness have had contact with a physician who could have provided the necessary immunization.

5. The answer is D *[V D 3 b (5)].*
Azidothymidine (AZT) has been shown to lower plasma titers of human immunodeficiency virus (HIV), but it has little or no effect on cell-associated virus levels. Thus, treatment with AZT may slow the progression of the disease, but it will not cure it. The Centers for Disease Control (CDC) estimate that there are 1–2 million people infected with HIV. Most of them are asymptomatic individuals in the high-risk categories. Unfortunately, studies now show that most infected individuals have a chronic smoldering infection with viremia, and that most, if not all, will eventually develop acquired immune deficiency syndrome (AIDS).

6–8. The answers are: 6-B *[VII A 1 d, B 6 d],* **7-D** *[VII B 6 d],* **8-D** *[VII C 2 a (2), (3)].*
The most likely diagnosis is pulmonary tuberculosis, with human immunodeficiency virus (HIV) infection as the underlying condition. Since tuberculosis infection in an immunosuppressed individual is more likely to lead to disseminated disease, four-drug chemotherapy, isoniazid (INH), rifampin (RMP), pyrazinamide (PZA), and ethambutal (EMB), is recommended as initial treatment. Simultaneous infection with *Mycobacterium tuberculosis* and HIV occurs in certain segments of the population, such as intravenous drug abusers. Although the disease is a reactivation of previous infection, the clinical presentation may be atypical. A positive intermediate Mantoux skin test is read at 5 mm of induration.

9. The answer is C (2, 4) *[VIII A 3 a–c, B 3 a–c].*
The most important fact to determine before recommendations can be made to the administrator of the day-care center is the type of meningitis that the child contracted. Thus, the physician who made the initial diagnosis or the laboratory that isolated the organism must be contacted. The age-range of the children must be known to determine if antimicrobial chemoprophylaxis is required.

10. The answer is B (1, 3) *[VI A 2 b (2), (4), c (2), (3), d (1)–(3), 3 b].*
Hepatitis A virus (HAV) multiplies in the liver and, regardless of symptomatology, is excreted in the stool in large quantities. Consequently, it is transmitted by poor personal hygiene, poor sanitation, and intimate contact. Immune globulin (IG) can prevent or modify infection if given within 2 weeks of exposure. The chronic carrier state does not exist, and the infected person is only communicable from about 2 weeks before the onset of jaundice untii about 1 week later. The greatest period of infectivity is before the onset of jaundice.

11. The answer is A (1, 2, 3) *[VI A 3 b (3) (a)–(c)].*
The short-order cook should not work until he is over his acute illness, and immune serum globulin (IG) should be given to all restaurant employees and all household contacts of the cook. Hepatitis A virus (HAV) is excreted in the stools from about 1 to 2 weeks before the onset of illness until about 1 week after the onset of jaundice. An infected individual should not work in an occupation that prepares or serves food for public consumption during this interval of time. IG does not have to be administered to customers since the cook handled the food only before it was cooked. However, IG may be given to customers if the employee handled food that was not cooked before it was eaten, the hygienic practices of the food handler was deficient, and customers can be identified and treated within 2 weeks of exposure.

12. The answer is B (1, 3) *[VI B 2 a (3), 3 a, f (3), (4)].*
Hepatitis B immune globulin (HBIG) should be administered to the nurse's spouse, and she should be advised not to share her toothbrush or razor. Hepatitis B virus (HBV) is transmitted by sexual activity and by contaminated blood; therefore, HBIG should be administered to the spouse of the dialysis nurse because it gives immediate protection against HBV. HBV vaccine should only be given to all family members if the patient becomes a chronic carrier of the hepatitis B surface antigen (HBsAg). A chronic carrier of the HBsAg is defined as an individual with a positive blood test on two determinations separated by a 6-month period.

13. The answer is B (1, 3) *[III C 2 c (1), d (1)–(3), g (4)].*
The physician should administer diphtheria and tetanus toxoids and pertussis (DTP), oral poliovirus vaccine (OPV), *Hemophilus influenzae* type b (Hib) vaccine, and measles-mumps-rubella (MMR) immunizations to the child. The mother should be instructed to bring the child back in 6 months for another immunization of DTP and OPV. Children who are behind in their immunizations should be given multiple vaccines at the same time to catch up on their immunization schedule. The simultaneous administration of multiple antigens has been shown to produce effective immunity without any increase in adverse side reactions. Since the immune system can remember previous immunizations, there is never any need to start an immunization series all over again. Since persons immunized with MMR virus vaccines do not transmit these viruses, these vaccines may be given to children of pregnant women. Although the live polio vaccine strain is shed by recently immunized children, this immunization should not be delayed because of pregnancy in close adult contacts.

14. The answer is C (2, 4) *[VIII A 3 c].*
Rifampin (RMP) prophylaxis should be offered to all staff (except pregnant women) and classmates regardless of prior immunization. Although previously immunized individuals are at decreased risk of disease, *Hemophilus influenzae* type B (Hib) vaccine does not affect nasopharyngeal carriage of the organism, which may be passed to susceptible classmates. To be effective, RMP should be given to at least 75% of the contacts during one 4-day period. Because this is difficult to accomplish, some authorities would not implement these recommendations until a second case occurred. Although Hib vaccine cannot be used to prevent immediate secondary cases, the presence of a confirmed case should be used as an opportunity to update immunization levels in this population.

15. The answer is B (1, 3) *[V D 3 d].*
Epidemiologic data have clearly shown that acquired immune deficiency syndrome (AIDS) or human immunodeficiency virus (HIV) infection can only be transmitted by sexual contact, by percutaneous exposure to contaminated fluids, and from mother to child in utero or at the time of birth. A few documented cases have occurred from breast-feeding. AIDS or HIV infection has not been transmitted to nonsexual household contacts or to individuals eating food prepared by someone with AIDS or HIV infection.

16. The answer is C (2, 4) *[II D 1 b (2) (a), (c)].*
Universal Precautions, also called Universal Blood and Body Fluid Precautions, apply to blood and other body fluids containing blood and to body fluids such as cerebrospinal, pleural, pericardial, peritoneal, amniotic, and synovial fluids. Universal Precautions apply only to body fluids that are likely to transmit human immunodeficiency virus (HIV) infection or other biologic agents in a health care occupational setting. Since these bloodborne diseases can be transmitted by individuals who look and feel normal, and since these diseases cannot be determined by routine medical history or physical examination, Universal Precautions apply to everyone.

17. The answer is E (all) *[V C 1 f].*
A total of 12% of the recent gonococcal isolates were resistant to penicillin, 74% showed no resistance to commonly used antibiotics, 17% were resistant to tetracycline, and none showed clinical resistance to ceftriaxone. There are many different strains of *Neisseria gonorrhoeae,* and different strains circulate in different segments of the population in different geographic areas. To know how to treat gonorrhea in a particular geographic area, the physician needs to know the local sensitivity patterns, which can be obtained from the appropriate local state health department. *N. gonorrhoeae* organisms may be resistant to several antimicrobial agents. Resistance can be mediated by either plasmids or by chromosomal mutations.

18–22. The answers are: 18-D *[V C 3 a],* **19-B** *[V C 3 b (2)],* **20-A** *[V C 3 e],* **21-C** *[V C 3 d (2)],* **22-D** *[V C 3 c].*
Multiple cultures should be performed on individuals being evaluated in a sexually transmitted disease clinic. Women should have endocervical and rectal cultures taken, and homosexual men require urethral and rectal cultures. Pharyngeal cultures should be done on all individuals who have oral sex.

Testing gonococcal cultures for β-lactamase production determines whether or not the isolate is a penicillinase-producing *Neisseria gonorrhoeae* and, therefore, resistant to penicillin. However, the β-lactamase test will not pick up the organisms that have a chromosomally mediated penicillin resistance. Because of widespread resistance to penicillin in some areas of the United States, ceftriaxone is the treatment of choice.

Nonvenereal transmission of gonorrhea from mother to child at birth causes a neonatal ophthalmia. This can be prevented with prophylactic eye drops.

Although it is not possible to do contact tracing on all cases, it should be done on selected cases, such as individuals with repeated infections and women with pelvic inflammatory disease, to prevent reinfection. Since the organism may be difficult to isolate, all identified contacts should be treated epidemiologically. Screening certain sexually active women would identify asymptomatic carriers.

23–27. The answers are: 23-C *[VI C 1 a (1)],* **24-D** *[VI D 1 a (2)],* **25-A** *[VI A 1 b, 3 b (2)],* **26-B** *[VI B 1 e],* **27-B** *[VI B 3 d].*
Hepatitis C is the most common cause of post-transfusion hepatitis in the United States. Control strategies consist of good personal hygiene and not sharing intravenous needles. There are no vaccines, and immune globulin (IG) has no protective effect.

Hepatitis B (HBV) vaccine can prevent HBV infection as well as the clinical expression of delta hepatitis (HDV), which requires an HBV coinfection for synthesis. HDV usually has a severe clinical course.

Since hepatitis A (HAV) is transmitted by the fecal-oral route, HAV is a common problem in day-care centers, institutions, rural areas where sanitation may be poor, and where people are crowded together. Patients are communicable from about 2 weeks *before* the onset of clinical disease to about 1 week *after.* Although not currently available, an HAV vaccine will probably be marketed in the next couple of years.

Chronic HBV infection has been associated with cirrhosis and heptocellular carcinoma.

5 Epidemiology and Prevention of Selected Chronic Illnesses

Donald J. Balaban

I. INTRODUCTION. This chapter provides background on the prevalence and risk factors for selected chronic diseases in the U.S. population in the 1990s. Temporal trends in incidence, the financial burden to society, population subgroups who are particularly at risk, and recommended preventive activities are considered for each condition.

A. Prevention. Recommendations for screening and preventive measures constantly change. Specific recommendations for prevention will not be agreed upon by all clinicians, investigators, or administrative groups; thus, this chapter presents areas of general consensus and emphasizes preventive measures—whether primary, secondary, or tertiary—that are appropriate for primary care providers to consider. Recently, the U.S. Preventive Services Task Force, a blue ribbon committee formed by the U.S. Department of Health and Human Services (USDHHS), produced a *Guide to Clinical Preventive Services* (1989). The guide was the result of exhaustive literature reviews, formal debates, and multiple expert reviewers.

B. Statistics. Incidence and mortality rates for the diseases discussed in this chapter are summarized in Figures 5-1 and 5-2 and in Table 5-1.

II. HEART DISEASE

A. Epidemiology

1. **Mortality rate**
   a. **Coronary heart disease (CHD)** is the leading cause of death in the United States. There are over 500,000 deaths per year, constituting over 35% of all deaths in the United States.
   b. **The death rate from CHD** is more than 250 individuals per 100,000 population in the United States.
   c. Twenty-five percent of CHD deaths occur in individuals under the age of 65 years.
2. **Morbidity.** CHD accounts for about 1.5 million myocardial infarctions (MIs) each year.
3. **Prevalence**
   a. About 4.6 million Americans have CHD.
   b. The **gender differential** is much more prominent in white populations; white men are more likely than white women to suffer MI and sudden death. In general, women have a greater risk of angina pectoris; men have a greater risk of MI and sudden death.
4. **Time trends.** Age-adjusted CHD death rates in the United States for the decade ending in 1985 declined by more than 30% over the previous decade. This recent decline in CHD mortality is related to:
   a. Improvements in life-style and related CHD risk factor levels (e.g., reduced cholesterol, reduced smoking, possibly increased exercise)
   b. Better diagnosis and treatment (e.g., coronary care units, coronary artery bypass grafts, treatment of hypertension)

B. Costs. The cost of cardiac care for CHD, including lost productivity, was estimated to be $80 billion in 1986.

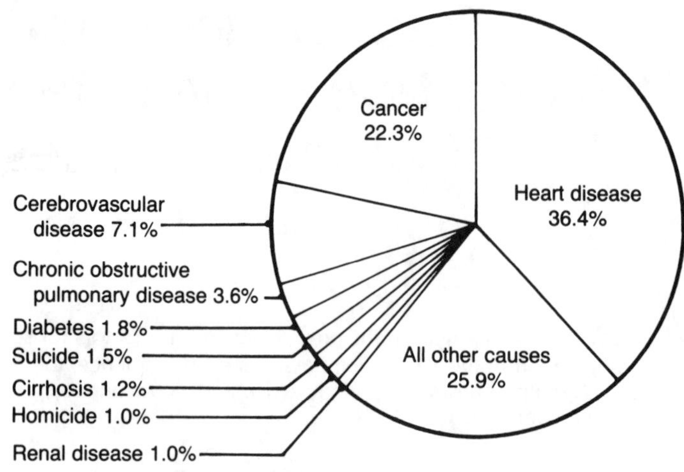

Figure 5-1. Mortality in the United States in 1986. (Adapted from American Cancer Society: Cancer statistics, 1990. *CA* 40:9–32, 1990.)

C. Causal and risk factors. Heredity, sex, and aging explain approximately 50% of cardiovascular deaths. Risk factors for cardiovascular disease modifiable by life-style change or drug treatment account for the remainder.

1. **Smoking** places individuals at an increased risk for developing and dying from CHD. The relative risk for CHD is increased by about 20% for smokers. Smoking kills almost as many individuals by cardiovascular deaths as by lung cancer deaths.

2. **High levels of serum cholesterol and low-density lipoprotein (LDL)** are tied to the frequency, mechanisms, and causation of CHD. Longitudinal studies of blood lipids in healthy adults show consistent and linear increases in individual risk of CHD, as indicated by high levels of total serum cholesterol and LDL, at least through middle age. Risk of coronary disease may be increased as much as 1% for each 1 mg/dl increase in cholesterol.

3. **Elevated blood pressure,** as indicated by increasing levels of systolic or diastolic blood pressure, is a major contributor to CHD risk. Over 37 million Americans have significant (moderate or severe) high blood pressure (blood pressures greater than 150/90 mm Hg recorded once a week at this level for at least 2 weeks in a row).
   a. **Race.** Blacks are almost twice as likely as whites to be hypertensive. Hypertension more frequently leads to congestive heart failure in blacks than in whites.
   b. **Age.** Hypertension is age-related. Approximately 50% of the geriatric population is hypertensive.

4. **Lack of moderate exercise** has been established as a risk factor for CHD deaths.

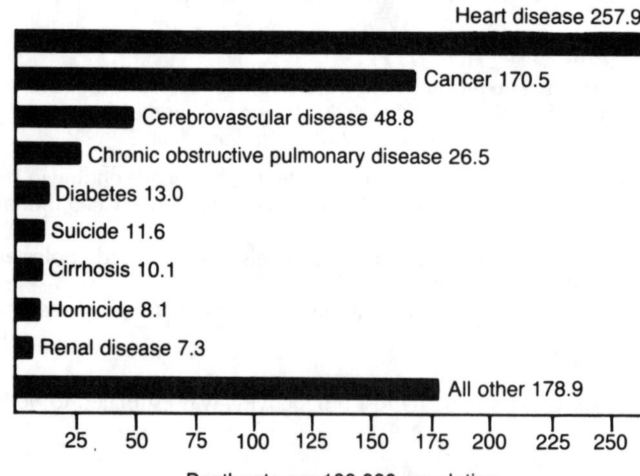

Figure 5-2. Leading causes of death in the United States in 1986, shown as percentages of all causes of death. (Adapted from American Cancer Society: Cancer statistics, 1990. *CA* 40:9–32, 1990.)

Table 5-1. Cancer Incidence and Mortality by Site and Sex

	Incidence*		Deaths*	
	Male	**Female**	**Male**	**Female**
Lung	20%	11%	34%	21%
Breast	. . .	29%	. . .	18%
Colon and rectum	15%	15%	11%	13%
Cervix/uterus	. . .	9%	. . .	4%
Prostate	20%	. . .	11%	. . .

Adapted from American Cancer Society: Cancer statistics, 1990. *CA* 40:9–32, 1990.
*Percentage of all cancers.

5. **Obesity,** especially among sedentary individuals, seems to be a minor independent contributory cause of heart disease.
6. **Oral contraceptive use,** especially among women who are over age 35 or who smoke, has been linked, although weakly, to an increased incidence of CHD.
7. **Family history of early CHD** is a well-known risk factor.

D. Prevention

1. **Primary prevention** should include screening for hypertension, high serum cholesterol, and behavioral factors (e.g., smoking, diet, exercise).
   a. **Blood pressure.** The Canadian Task Force (1979) recommends screening for hypertension at least every 5 years for men and women 16–64 years of age and every 2 years after age 65. The U.S. Preventive Services Task Force (1989) recommends testing yearly or every other year based on the most recent diastolic pressure. Hypertension control is believed to contribute greatly to the decline in cardiovascular mortality, particularly the mortality attributable to stroke and cardiac failure. For example, a 2 mm Hg decrease in diastolic blood pressure in a population can result in a decline of more than 5% in the population's risk of developing CHD. The cost-effectiveness of widespread screening for hypertension is not established.
   b. **Cholesterol.** Physicians should counsel all patients regarding the fat content of their diets. Decreased consumption of whole milk, butter, eggs, and animal fats results in lower cholesterol levels.
      (1) **Testing of serum blood cholesterol** is most important for middle-aged men, especially if there is evidence of CHD. Testing should be done at least every 5 years, using an accredited laboratory. Nonfasting blood may be used. Individuals with cholesterol above 200 mg/dl should be rechecked more frequently.
      (2) **Recommendations.** The U.S. Preventive Services Task Force (1989) recommends drug treatment if cholesterol is above 240 mg/dl with two other risk factors or if cholesterol is above 265 mg/dl without other factors.
   c. **Smoking.** Physicians must counsel their patients to stop smoking and must provide support and motivation through regularly scheduled visits. Early and complete cessation is associated with maximal effectiveness. However, the 20% decrease in smoking in the U.S. population has been estimated to have resulted in a 10.5% decline in the population's risk of developing CHD.
   d. **Physical exercise.** Epidemiologic evidence suggests a protective effect against CHD and coronary deaths from regular physical activity; even walking vigorously 30 minutes three times a week has a major effect on the conditioning associated with reduced coronary risks. The protective effects of regular physical activity are independent of the presence of other unfavorable risk factors, such as hypercholesterolemia, hypertension, smoking, and family history.
   e. **Education**
      (1) In the 1970s, the **National High Blood Pressure Education Program** formulated educational objectives to raise patients' awareness of hypertension. Programs were developed to keep hypertensive patients on appropriate therapy and to encourage them to follow their physician's advice. Results suggest that the percentage of hypertensive subjects controlling their blood pressure more than doubled, from 16.5% to 34.1%. Today, it is estimated that more than 40% of hypertensives are treated and controlled

and a similar percentage are treated but uncontrolled (i.e., they have the potential to be controlled if patient compliance or the proper mix of medication is achieved).

(2) Patient education should continue to be targeted to high-risk groups, such as black males, who have both higher rates of hypertension and lower control rates than other groups.

2. **Secondary prevention.** The U.S. Preventive Services Task Force (1989) recommends secondary prevention (screening) with electrocardiogram (EKG) only for men over age 40 who have more than two risk factors; who are about to begin a vigorous exercise program; or who are public safety risks, such as commercial pilots.

III. CANCER

A. Epidemiology. The death rate for all cancers was more than 190 individuals per 100,000 population; these deaths accounted for approximately 22% of all deaths in the United States, second only to CHD (see Table 5-1). Approximately 50% of cancers occur in persons over the age of 65. The elderly, who account for about 13% of the population, have increased risk for many cancers, especially lung, colon, and prostate cancer.

1. Lung

a. Mortality rate. Lung cancer is the number one cause of cancer death, accounting for 25% (140,000) of all cancer mortality and 5% of all deaths in the United States. It is the leading cause of cancer death in both men and women.

b. Incidence, time trends, and sex. The incidence of lung cancer has been increasing faster among American women than among American men. From 1950 to 1978, the age-adjusted lung cancer rate increased 192% for men and 263% for women.

(1) For **women,** between 1950 and 1957, the age-adjusted lung cancer rate increased an average of 1% per year, but from 1968 to 1977, the rate increased almost 7% per year.

(2) For **men,** between 1950 and 1957, the age-adjusted lung cancer rate climbed an average of 6.7% per year, but from 1968 to 1977, the rate climbed an average of 4% annually.

2. Breast

a. Mortality rate. Female breast cancer accounts for close to 10% (43,000) of all cancer deaths in the United States. The mortality rate is approximately 15 per 100,000 population.

b. Incidence. There are about 140,000 new cases each year in the United States, accounting for 28% of female cancers.

c. Time trends. There has been very little change in age-adjusted mortality rates since 1930.

d. Sex. Breast cancer is distinctly uncommon in males. The difference in incidence and mortality between males and females is believed to be related more to hormonal and genetic factors than to the amount of breast tissue.

3. Colon and rectum

a. Mortality rate. Colorectal cancer is the second most common cancer in the United States, accounting for approximately 12% (61,000) of all cancer deaths there. The mortality rate is approximately 25 per 100,000 population.

b. Incidence

(1) Age. The age-specific incidence rate of colorectal cancer begins to rise at age 10 years. The rate of increase in incidence continues until age 70–75 years, at which time rectal cancer incidence rates increase more slowly and then decline after age 85 years.

(2) Sex and race. Men and women are affected almost equally, although, among whites, the risk for men is somewhat higher than for women; among blacks, rates are nearly equal for men and women.

c. Time trends. There has been very little change in mortality rates since 1930.

4. Cervix

a. Mortality rate. Cervical cancer accounts for just under 1.5% (7000) of cancer deaths in the United States. The mortality rate is approximately 2.5 individuals per 100,000 population.

b. Incidence. The incidence among whites declined from 38.3 individuals per 100,000 population in 1947 to 11.3 per 100,000 in 1977. There are currently approximately 13,000 new cases each year.

c. Time trends. In the last 2 decades, there was a very slight increase in the incidence and mortality rates of cervical cancer observed in several western European countries and the

United States. These increases are considered to be due, in part, to changes in sexual practices, including increases in nonmonogamous sexual activity, oral contraceptive use, and the incidence of sexually transmitted diseases (STDs). The acquired immune deficiency syndrome (AIDS) epidemic has had an effect on sexual behavior; the magnitude is uncertain, and the behavior change appears to be distributed unevenly among the population.

5. Prostate

a. Mortality rate. Prostate cancer accounts for more than 5% (28,000) of cancer deaths in the United States. The mortality rate is approximately 9 per 100,000 population, a rate showing little change since 1930.

b. Incidence

(1) Prostate cancer is the **most common cancer in American men** (100,000 cases per year).

(2) Age. Prostate cancer primarily affects elderly men. The incidence increases with age more rapidly than for any other cancer.

(3) Race. American blacks have the highest prostate cancer incidence in the world.

B. Costs. The costs for the first year of treatment for all cancers was estimated to be $4.13 billion in 1975, compared to $1.39 billion for CHD, $2.86 billion for motor vehicle injuries, and $1.53 billion for stroke.

C. Causal and risk factors

1. Lung

a. Smoking. Case-control and prospective studies (see Ch 2 II D 1, E 1) have demonstrated consistently that cigarette smoking is the major causal factor in lung cancer.

(1) Sex. Several cohort studies have shown an average relative risk of 10.0 or more for men who smoke and 3.0 for women who smoke (compared to a relative risk of 1.0 for nonsmokers of both sexes). However, recent studies of women smokers are demonstrating that the gender gap in relative risk is ending. The lower risk for women is attributed to the fact that women:

(a) Began smoking later in this century than men

(b) Traditionally started to smoke at an older age than men

(c) Inhale less deeply than men

(2) Exposure. The relative risk for men ranges from approximately 5.0 for those smoking 1–9 cigarettes daily to approximately 20.0 for those smoking over 40 cigarettes daily. The relative risk for women ranges from approximately 1.3 for those smoking 1–9 cigarettes daily to more than 7.5 for those smoking over 40 cigarettes daily.

(3) Age. The risk of lung cancer is influenced by the age at which an individual begins to smoke. If smoking is not begun until the late teens or early adulthood, the risk of developing lung cancer at 60–70 years of age is reduced by as much as 20%.

(4) The **lifetime risk of developing lung cancer** in a male who is a heavy cigarette smoker and who began smoking at an early age approaches 25%. Lifetime risk of lung cancer in women who smoke is rising rapidly. The increased lung cancer rates in women may be attributable to the fact that the large number of women who smoke is a relatively recent occurrence.

(5) Environmental tobacco smoke (ETS) [i.e., involuntary, or passive, smoking] has been determined to be a cause of disease, including lung cancer, in healthy nonsmokers. The overall summary relative risk of lung cancer among nonsmokers in association with ETS exposure is 1.3. About one-third of the cases of lung cancer in nonsmokers living with smokers and about one-fourth of the cases of nonsmokers in general can be attributed to exposure to ETS. As much as 25%–46% and 13%–37% of lung cancer deaths among nonsmoking females and males, respectively, may be attributable to ETS.

b. Occupational exposure. Industrial exposure to substances such as asbestos, radon, nickel, chromium, mustard gas, and other industrial agents, especially in combination with cigarette smoking, leads to an increased risk of lung cancer. The increase in risk is dependent on the length and type of exposure.

c. Air pollution. Air pollution is suspected as a cause of lung cancer, but evaluation is difficult in part because the measurement of air pollution is inexact. Even in urban areas, it is unlikely to be a significant causal factor for lung cancer. Lung cancer in urban areas is still overwhelmingly attributed to cigarette smoking. Perhaps 10 cases per 100,000 cases of lung cancer in average smokers may be caused by air pollution.

d. **Radiation.** High radiation exposure (≥ 100 rads) increases the risk of lung cancer. It is an uncommon cause.

e. **Family history.** Some studies prior to 1970 demonstrated an increased familial pattern of lung cancer thought to be independent of smoking. Most recent studies suggest little or no independent familial association.

2. **Breast**

a. **Pregnancy.** Women who become pregnant for the first time after the age of 30 have an increased chance of developing breast cancer. For example, women with a first full-term pregnancy before age 20 have a relative risk of breast cancer that is one-third that of women whose first full-term pregnancy occurs after age 35. The protective effect is confirmed only for full-term births—that is, pregnancies ending in abortion or miscarriage have not been shown to reduce subsequent risk of breast cancer.

b. **Family history.** The risk to women whose mothers or sisters have had breast cancer is increased twofold, and the risk to women whose mother *and* sisters have had breast cancer is increased threefold.

c. **Diet.** Some studies have shown an association between consumption of fats and breast cancer. Other studies have shown associations of breast cancer rates with total fat and animal protein consumption. These studies are still controversial. Increased intake of fat and animal protein could influence endocrine metabolism and increase the risk of developing breast cancer by:

(1) Promoting growth, sexual development, and an early onset of menarche
(2) Increasing adiposity, leading to greater conversion of androstenedione to estrone
(3) Increasing prolactin release from the pituitary
(4) Increasing bile salt production in the gut, leading to altered bacterial flora and the production of carcinogenic substances

d. **Exogenous hormones**

(1) **Oral contraceptives.** The connection between oral contraceptive use and breast cancer is controversial; inconsistent findings have been reported. Some evidence suggests that oral contraceptive use of long duration at young ages leads to elevated risk of premenopausal breast cancer (i.e., cancer in women younger than age 45); relative risk has been estimated at 1.46. Also, some evidence suggests that women using oral contraceptives for progressively longer periods of time before their first term pregnancy are at increased risk—a risk independent of the "delay in first pregnancy" effect.

(2) **Postmenopausal hormone replacement therapy,** like oral contraceptive use, has been associated with breast cancer only inconclusively. Features of the therapy, such as the type (e.g., estradiol versus conjugated estrogens with or without progestins), the duration, and the dosage, may contribute to increased risk. Estradiol use, especially of long duration and at high daily doses (1.25 mg or more), may lead to increased risk, whereas low-dose therapy most likely will not.

e. **Radiation.** Exposure to ionizing radiation increases the incidence of breast cancer. Women in Hiroshima and Nagasaki who were exposed to 10 rads or more had a marked increase in breast cancer after a latent period of at least 10 years. The greatest risks were found at exposures of approximately 100 rads. The risk is significantly greater in women who were irradiated during adolescence.

f. **Other factors.** The development of breast cancer also is associated with:

(1) High socioeconomic status
(2) Age over 40 years
(3) An early menarche

3. **Colon and rectum**

a. **Diet.** Fiber deficiency and high dietary fat consumption have been related to colorectal cancer in many studies; however, no specific carcinogens associated with the production, preservation, and manufacture of food have been clearly identified.

b. **Physiologic factors.** Bacteria acting upon cholesterol and bile acids in the intestines may produce carcinogens that act either locally or elsewhere in the body. The mechanisms are poorly understood and are far from being established.

c. **Family predisposition.** Heredity is a factor in the development of colon cancer. The relative risk for first-degree relatives of someone with colon cancer is three times that of the general population.

d. **Alcohol consumption.** Per capita beer consumption correlates significantly with the colorectal cancer mortality of men 35–54 years of age. However, alcohol is not a confirmed causal factor for colon cancer.

e. **Socioeconomic and racial factors.** High socioeconomic group and white race are both independent risk factors for developing colorectal cancer. Diet or physiologic factors may explain the association.

4. **Cervix**

   a. **Sexual activity.** Multiple sexual partners and STDs, such as herpes, syphilis, and gonorrhea, increase a woman's risk of cervical cancer. It is not clear if these factors act independently or through similar pathophysiologic mechanisms (see also Ch 4 V A 4).

   b. **Oral contraceptives.** Use of oral contraceptives appears to be a risk factor, although it is not clear whether oral contraceptives increase the risk or whether barrier methods decrease it. Also, the statistical relationship between oral contraceptive use and increased numbers of sexual partners has linked pill use with an increase in cancer risk, due to the association between multiple sexual partners and STDs.

   c. **Coital history.** Age at first coital experience correlates highly with the risk for cervical cancer. Women who had first coitus before 20 years of age have a two- to threefold increase in risk for invasive cervical cancer, compared to women whose sexual activity began later. There appears to be a progressive increase in risk the earlier the age at first coitus, even if there are no other sexual partners after that (see also III C 4 g).

   d. **Smoking.** Women who smoke have a relative risk of 3.0 for developing cervical cancer compared to nonsmokers. The association is strongest in young age-groups (i.e., women 20–29 years of age) with a relative risk of 17.0. The risk for black women smokers is similar to that of white women smokers.

   e. **Racial and ethnic factors.** Blacks and Hispanics have an increased risk for cervical cancer, although it has not been absolutely established that these are independent factors.

   f. **Socioeconomic factors.** Cervical cancer has been associated with the socioeconomic class of the patient's husband, as indicated by his occupation. Studies suggest that men are a factor in cervical cancer, primarily due to penile hygiene or circumcision. Partners of noncircumcized males are at increased risk for cervical cancer, and cervical cancer rates are low among Jewish women.

   g. **Menarche and menopause.** Age at menarche, age at menopause, and the character of the menses do not appear to be risk factors for cervical cancer. The interval between menarche and first coitus may be a better predictor of risk than age at first coitus (i.e., the smaller the interval, the greater the risk).

5. **Prostate.** Although the cause of prostate cancer is unknown, it has been associated with testosterone level and sexual activity. Geographic, occupational, and racial differences in incidence also have been reported.

   a. **Diet.** Dietary fat appears to be related to prostate cancer in much the same way that it is related to breast cancer and colorectal cancer (see III C 2 c, 3 a).

   b. **Occupational exposure.** Workers exposed to industrial carcinogens, such as cadmium oxide dust, reportedly have a higher incidence of prostate cancer than expected.

   c. **Age.** The risk of developing prostate cancer increases with age.

   d. **Religion.** The frequency of prostate cancer deaths is higher in Protestants (1.9) and in Catholics (1.5) than in Jews.

   e. **Family history.** One study found that fathers and brothers of prostate cancer patients were three times more likely to die from prostate cancer than the fathers and brothers of those without prostate cancer. Whether there is an environmental or genetic basis for this increased risk has not been determined.

   f. **Marriage.** Married men have higher frequencies of prostate cancer than single men. Rates are highest among widowed and divorced men and among married men with children.

D. **Prevention and screening.** With the exception of lung cancer, the major cancers are not amenable to primary prevention. However, secondary prevention, through appropriate screening, can identify and favorably influence the outcome in these other major cancers.

1. **Lung.** Screening for presymptomatic lung cancer is by either pulmonary cytology or chest x-ray, neither of which is cost-effective even for targeted populations. In addition, screening seems to have no beneficial effect on mortality from lung cancer, even when it helps detect the cancer at an earlier stage.

a. Results of randomized trials of sputum cytology in smokers have not shown reduction in mortality among those screened.
b. Individuals with early lung cancer detected by chest x-rays do not have a more favorable prognosis than individuals with lung cancer diagnosed soon after symptoms appear. Unfortunately, by the time a lung tumor is radiographically visible, it is usually inoperable and incurable.

2. **Breast.** Screening for breast cancer is by mammography and physical examination (palpation) of the breast. Monthly self-examinations are recommended for all women, and the current mammogram recommendations are every 2–3 years for women age 40–50 years and annually or more frequently for women over age 50 years. In the presence of risk factors for breast cancer, more frequent or earlier mammography may be appropriate.
   a. **Mammography** can help to differentiate a benign from a malignant growth before it becomes palpable and when it is most curable. Thus, mammography remains the most effective imaging method of detecting nonpalpable cancer. However, 10%–20% of breast cancers are not visualized by mammography; in those cases, a woman may detect the lesion through palpation several months after the mammogram.
   b. **High-risk, or target, populations for screening** include women who:
      (1) Are over age 40
      (2) Are of high socioeconomic status
      (3) Are white
      (4) Are nulliparous
      (5) Had their first child after 30 years of age
      (6) Have a family history of breast cancer
      (7) Have benign breast disease
      (8) Have had previous breast cancer

3. **Colon and rectum.** Screening for colorectal cancer is by testing the stool for occult blood. Testing, which is debatably cost-effective for high-risk target populations, should be done annually in men and women over 45 years of age. The tests, even the newly developed ones, are not very sensitive or specific.
   a. **Endoscopy** has been recommended as clinically prudent by the U.S. Preventive Services Task Force (1989) for high-risk individuals over 50 years of age.
   b. **Target populations for screening,** in addition to individuals over age 45, include those with a history of:
      (1) Colitis
      (2) Familial polyposis or villous adenomas
      (3) Familial cancer of the colon

4. **Cervix**
   a. **Screening** for cervical cancer, which is by **Pap smear** to detect cervical abnormalities, is cost-effective, especially for high-risk target populations. The Canadian Task Force (1979) recommends testing when a woman or girl first becomes sexually active, then every 1–3 years until age 35 years, and then every 5 years thereafter. The U.S. Preventive Services Task Force (1989) recommends screening every 1–3 years, depending on patient risk.
   b. **High-risk target populations** for screening include women who:
      (1) Are between the ages of 25 and 60 years old
      (2) Have low socioeconomic status
      (3) Are prison inmates or prostitutes
      (4) Have a history of STDs
      (5) Had first intercourse at an early age
      (6) Have had induced abortions
      (7) Have a history of cervical squamous dysplasia
      (8) Are unmarried mothers

5. **Prostate**
   a. **Screening** for prostate cancer is by:
      (1) Digital palpation of the rectum
      (2) Prostatic massage and cytologic examination
      (3) Determination of serum acid phosphatase concentration
   b. The **target population** for screening includes men over the age of 65.

IV. CEREBROVASCULAR DISEASE

A. Epidemiology

1. **Mortality rates.** The 1986 death rate from cerebrovascular disease was 48.8 individuals per 100,000 population; these deaths comprised 7.1% of all deaths in the United States. Cerebrovascular disease accounts for about 150,000 deaths per year in the United States.

2. **Incidence and prevalence**
   a. There are approximately 500,000 new episodes of cerebrovascular disease each year.
   b. The incidence of stroke doubles each successive decade after age 45; the chances of suffering a stroke before the age of 70 are 1 in 20.

3. **Time trends**
   a. Stroke mortality, which declined by 46% between 1968 and 1981, stabilized in the 1980s.
   b. The decline in the rates for deaths attributable to hypertension, as well as for those attributable to CHD (both rates declined sharply from 1972 to 1980), may reflect changes in disease classification, diagnostic practices, and coding rules. It is more likely that the decline is due to increased awareness, more frequent detection, and, especially, more effective treatment of hypertension and CHD.

B. Costs.
The cost for the first year of treatment of stroke was estimated to be $1.53 billion in 1975. Current yearly cost of stroke is estimated at $5 billion per year.

C. Causal and risk factors

1. **Old age** is the most important risk factor for stroke.

2. **Hypertension** markedly increases the risk of stroke. Epidemiologic evidence is strong that hypertension is a major cause of atherosclerosis, particularly in combination with hyperlipidemia. Hypertension is the most important modifiable risk factor for stroke (see II C 3).

3. **Smoking** increases the risk of stroke. Studies have shown increases in both stroke incidence and stroke mortality among smokers.

4. **CHD, atrial fibrillation,** and **diabetes mellitus** are all independent factors that have been demonstrated to increase the risk of stroke.

5. **Oral contraceptive use, particularly by women who smoke,** has been associated with an increased risk of stroke in several studies.

D. Prevention

1. **Primary prevention**
   a. **Behavior modification.** Clinicians should counsel patients regarding diet, exercise, and smoking behaviors as factors in stroke prevention.
   b. **Aspirin use** has been a suggested, but not proven, method of preventing stroke.
      (1) One study reported a reduction in risk for stroke and stroke death among men who used aspirin regularly; no effect was established for women.
      (2) Another study reported no reduction in deaths from stroke in middle-aged physicians who used aspirin regularly.

2. **Secondary prevention.** As noted in II D 1 a, **screening for hypertension** is recommended by the Canadian Task Force (1979) and U.S. Preventive Services Task Force (1989) at regular intervals for men and women 16–64 years of age. The U.S. Preventive Services Task Force found insufficient evidence to recommend for or against either auscultation for carotid bruits or noninvasive testing for carotid stenosis, except in high-risk or symptomatic patients.

V. CHRONIC OBSTRUCTIVE PULMONARY DISEASE (COPD)

A. Epidemiology

1. **Mortality rate**
   a. The 1986 death rate for COPD was 26.5 individuals per 100,000 population. Deaths from COPD and related conditions constituted 3.6% of all deaths in the United States.
   b. Approximately 60,000 deaths per year in the United States are due to bronchitis, emphysema, or asthma; these diseases are contributory causes to another 60,000 deaths.

2. **Prevalence**
   a. It has been estimated that 16 million Americans have chronic bronchitis, asthma, or emphysema.
   b. Approximately 14% of adult men and 8% of adult women have chronic bronchitis, obstructive airways disease, or both.

3. **Time trends.** Deaths attributed to COPD are increasing; the age-adjusted death rate rose 28% between 1968 and 1978, during which time the overall death rate declined by 22%.

B. Costs

1. The estimated cost of COPD to the national economy in 1979 was $6.5 billion. Of this amount, $2.3 billion was for health care, and the remainder was for the indirect costs of morbidity and premature mortality.

2. The total cost of respiratory disease in the United States has been estimated at $25 billion annually—that is, $7 billion for direct costs, $12 billion for the indirect costs of morbidity (e.g., loss of productivity), and $6 billion for the indirect costs of mortality.

C. Causal and risk factors

1. **Smoking.** It has been demonstrated repeatedly during the past 20 years that smoking, particularly cigarette smoking, is the most important cause of COPD. The risk is related to the number of cigarettes smoked daily and to the duration of the smoking.

2. **Occupational exposure,** especially among tin, copper, and coal miners; chemical workers; foundry workers; cotton textile workers; and others engaged in certain heavy industry, increases the risk of COPD. This is especially true for smokers. The effect is usually considered additive but is considered by some to be multiplicative.

3. **Air pollution, including indoor pollutants,** has been demonstrated to be harmful at high levels; whether or not exposure to low levels of pollutants has a significant health effect has not yet been determined.

4. **Chronic exposure to ETS in healthy nonsmokers** leads to a reduction of small airway lung function resembling that of light smokers. Among children, exposure leads to more respiratory infections, increases in incidence of bronchitis and pneumonia, and a smaller rate of increase in lung function. ETS seems to worsen the acute symptoms of individuals with preexisting chronic health conditions such as asthma.

5. **Sex.** Men are at a higher risk than women of developing emphysema and COPD, but not chronic bronchitis; risk differences between the sexes increase with age. Older men are at much greater risk than older women, possibly because of occupational exposures.

6. **Socioeconomic factors.** Morbidity and mortality from COPD generally are higher in blue-collar workers than in white-collar workers and in people with few years of formal education. These associations likely are related to smoking and occupational exposure.

7. **Family history.** Offspring of affected parents and brothers and sisters of affected siblings are more likely to develop COPD.

D. Prevention

1. **Primary prevention** appears to be the only effective approach to COPD. Cessation of smoking before symptoms and incapacitation develop reduces the risk of developing COPD. Abstinence from smoking is associated with absence or low frequency of airway obstruction and respiratory disease mortality.

2. **Secondary prevention, or early detection,** is useful only if associated with smoking cessation and with avoidance of additional pulmonary tissue damage.
   a. **Chest x-rays** have not proven to be cost-effective as a screening method for identification of individuals with COPD.
   b. The most useful screening test is the **forced expiratory volume (FEV),** usually measured over 1 second (**FEV_1**).

VI. CIRRHOSIS of the liver, a scarring of tissue and malfunction in the liver that can lead to death, is the most serious of several liver problems brought on by excessive alcohol consumption.

A. Epidemiology. The 1986 death rate from cirrhosis was 10.9 individuals per 100,000 population. These deaths constituted 1.2% of all deaths in the United States.

B. Causal and risk factors. Excessive regular, if not daily, consumption of alcohol for many years places certain individuals who consume alcohol at increased risk for developing cirrhosis. In the United States, excessive consumption of alcohol is the primary cause of cirrhosis; in other countries, especially nonindustrialized countries, chronic hepatitis is also a cause.

1. **Sex**
   a. **Men** who consume more than 40 ml/day of ethanol for many years have an increased chance of developing cirrhosis.
   b. **Women** who consume more than 20 ml/day of ethanol for many years have an increased chance of developing cirrhosis.

2. **Genetics.** Evidence suggests that many aspects of alcoholism—which is linked with heavy drinking and thus cirrhosis—are inherited (see Ch 11 III A). Rates of alcohol elimination can vary as much as threefold among individuals.

3. **Nutrition.** Nutritional deficiencies, especially of proteins, may promote the toxic effects of alcohol by depleting hepatic amino acids and enzymes. Lack of dietary protein hinders proper liver function, whether alcohol is present or not.

C. Prevention

1. **Primary prevention**
   a. **Health protection measures** are recommended by alcoholism researchers and, thus, are not specific for cirrhosis. Those measures, which are not of proven value, include legislative and regulatory controls on:
      (1) Prices of alcoholic beverages
      (2) Types and locations of liquor outlets
      (3) Hours and days of liquor sales
      (4) Drinking age
      (5) Alcohol content of beverages
      (6) Differential taxation of various beverages
      (7) Alcohol distribution systems
   b. **Health promotion measures** include:
      (1) Public education programs
      (2) Specifically targeted preventive programs
      (3) Beverage substitution initiatives
      (4) Antialcohol promotion and marketing measures

2. **Secondary prevention** for alcoholism, which is being used increasingly by business and industry, entails the early identification of alcohol abusers through the administration of brief questionnaires to high-risk individuals and periodic unscheduled testing of blood and urine among certain groups of workers.

3. **Tertiary prevention** entails intensive treatment to aid the drinker with either moderating intake or total abstinence. Results have not been very encouraging; dropout, treatment failure, and recidivism are all high.

VII. DIABETES is a primary disorder of carbohydrate metabolism with multiple etiologic factors that generally involve absolute or relative insulin deficiency, insulin resistance, or both. All causes lead to **hyperglycemia,** the hallmark of the disease. The different types of diabetes are: insulin-dependent (type I) diabetes mellitus (IDDM) [formerly known as juvenile onset or ketosis prone diabetes]; noninsulin-dependent (type II) diabetes mellitus (NIDDM) [formerly known as adult-onset, maturity-onset, or nonketotic diabetes]; secondary diabetes (e.g., due to pancreatic disease); impaired glucose tolerance (formerly subclinical diabetes); and gestational diabetes (i.e., glucose intolerance with onset during pregnancy).

A. Epidemiology

1. **Mortality rate**
   a. The 1986 death rate for diabetes was 15.4 individuals per 100,000 population. These deaths (38,000) comprise 1.8% of all deaths in the United States.

b. Of those diagnosed with diabetes before the age of 30, median survival age is 10–15 years less than that of the general population; end-stage renal disease (see VIII) develops in 40% of these patients, and in the remainder, early death usually results from CHD.

2. **Morbidity.** Secondary problems associated with diabetes include:
   a. **Blindness** (approximately 6000 new cases every year) due to **retinopathy**. Diabetes is the leading cause of blindness in the United States.
   b. **Cardiovascular disease.** Diabetes is an important risk factor for CHD and peripheral vascular disease. Diabetic vascular disease is the major cause of amputations (50,000 per year).
   c. **Nephropathy.** Diabetic nephropathy occurs in approximately 10% of diabetics and accounts for 25% of dialysis patients. Hypertensive nephropathy is also a risk.

3. **Prevalence.** There are approximately 11 million diabetics in the United States, 90% of which have NIDDM. Prevalence in the U.S. population is estimated at 6.7%.

B. **Costs.** The cost of diabetes is estimated to be $10 billion per year, including medical care and lost productivity.

C. **Causal and risk factors**

1. **Deficiency in the action of the hormone insulin**—which may result from a quantitative deficiency of insulin, an abnormal insulin resistance to its action, or a combination of deficits—is believed to be the cause of diabetes.

2. **Obesity.** Although the etiology of both IDDM and NIDDM is poorly understood, studies have shown that approximately 80% of people with NIDDM are obese.

3. **Family history.** A family history predisposes individuals to diabetes. This predisposition is related to the gene loci HLA DR3/DR4.

4. **Sex.** Males and females have about the same risk for developing IDDM.

5. **Racial and ethnic factors**
   a. The incidence rate for IDDM among whites is about 1.5 times the rate for blacks.
   b. The incidence of NIDDM is very high among Native Americans, black women, Mexican Americans, and indigenous Micronesians and Polynesians.

6. **Socioeconomic factors.** Changes in socioeconomic status have been shown to lead to a marked and rapid increase in the incidence of NIDDM. The reasons for this interesting phenomenon are speculated to be:
   a. **More plentiful food sources** may lead to rapid rise in body weight and corresponding increased risk for developing NIDDM
   b. Increase in socioeconomic status is generally associated with a **decline in the overall level of physical activity**.

D. **Prevention.** Currently, there is no **primary prevention. Secondary prevention** is possible and may be cost-effective in high-risk groups.

1. **Routine screening for diabetes** by use of urine tests for glucose after fasting and by postprandial blood glucose tests can lead to early treatment, which may help to reduce secondary complications. Screening is recommended for those who:
   a. Have a family history of diabetes
   b. Have glucose abnormalities associated with pregnancy
   c. Have physical abnormalities, such as circulatory dysfunction and frank vascular impairment
   d. Are markedly obese

2. **Treatment of asymptomatic individuals with abnormal blood sugar** has not been shown to be effective in controlling complications. Diabetes itself is not preventable, but secondary complications such as neuropathy and nephropathy may be preventable.

3. **Modification of cardiovascular risk factors** such as weight, blood pressure, cholesterol, and smoking are the recommended approaches to prevention of complications.

4. **Home health aides to assist patients with diet, medication assistance and instruction, urine testing, and monitoring of vital signs** have been reported to lead to modest improvements in blood sugar levels for low-income and poorly educated patients.

VIII. RENAL DISEASE

A. Epidemiology

1. **Mortality rate.** The 1983 death rate for renal disease was 9.0 individuals per 100,000 population. These deaths accounted for 1.0% of all deaths in the United States in 1983.

2. **Incidence.** Annual incidence rates of end-stage renal disease ranging from 50–95 individuals per 1 million population have been reported. In one study, the annual incidence rate increased from 35 cases per 1 million population in 1973 to 59 cases per 1 million in 1979.
   a. **Race**
      (1) Black men have the largest increase in the incidence of end-stage renal disease; the incidence for black women has also increased dramatically over the past 20 years.
      (2) White men and women showed an increased incidence from 1973 and 1977 and then stabilized.
   b. **Age.** Individuals 65 years of age or over experienced the greatest increase in incidence, increasing tenfold in the past 20 years, with no indication of stabilization or decline.

B. Costs.

The cost of end-stage renal disease, including dialysis programs and transplantations, is estimated to be over $4 billion. Medicare coverage, which pays for the end-stage renal disease programs, has greatly increased both the availability of dialysis programs and their total cost.

C. Causal and risk factors

1. **Immune injury,** predominantly as a result of previous streptococcal infection, is the most frequent cause of glomerulonephritis.

2. **Occupational exposure.** Exposure to industrial solvents and gasoline by certain occupational groups (e.g., painters) is a much less frequent cause of renal disease.

3. **Race.** Black adults are more likely to develop renal diseases, in particular hypertensive nephropathy.

4. **Sex.** Men are 20%–30% more likely than women to develop renal disease.

5. **Age.** Individuals over 45 years of age are more likely to develop renal disease than those under age 45 years.

6. **Diabetes.** Diabetic nephropathy and hypertensive nephropathy are major causes of morbidity and mortality among diabetics.

D. Prevention

1. **Primary prevention**
   a. **Control of hypertension.** Antihypertensive drugs have been shown by clinical trials to be effective in reducing morbidity and mortality due to renal failure.
   b. **Routine screening for bacteriuria.** Pyelonephritis (bacterial infection of the kidney), bacteriuria (bacteria in the urine), and other urinary tract infections can lead to chronic pyelonephritis, although this is uncommon in the absence of structural or neurologic abnormalities or states, such as diabetes or pregnancy.
   c. **Avoidance of improper exposure to hydrocarbons, industrial solvents, paints, and gasoline** can help to prevent renal disease.

2. **Secondary prevention.** Better understanding of the immune process and of methods to arrest the progression of glomerulonephritis are both major areas of research.
   a. **Drug treatment of hypertension in diabetic patients** may reduce the progression of renal failure. It is unclear whether vigorous control of blood sugar in diabetics also reduces the probability of developing renal failure.
   b. **Dialysis and transplantation** are the only ways to prevent imminent death once end-stage renal disease develops.

IX. SUICIDE

A. Epidemiology.

It has been estimated that over 200,000 individuals in the United States attempt suicide each year. Approximately 30,000 died from suicide in 1986. The 1986 death rate was 11.6 individuals per 100,000 population. Deaths from suicide constituted 1.5% of all deaths in the United States in 1986; guns and poison are the most common means. Suicides are generally considered to be associated with chronic emotional disturbance.

B. Risk factors

1. **Conditions** associated with increased risk for suicide include:
   a. Chronic mental illness
   b. Substance abuse
   c. Feelings of helplessness and hopelessness associated with divorce, separation, living alone, and grief
   d. Socioeconomic factors, especially unemployment
   e. Serious physical illness or handicap

2. **People** with increased risk for suicidal intent include:
   a. Males
   b. Divorced, separated, and widowed individuals (married individuals have the lowest suicide rates)
   c. Whites (however, the rate among nonwhites is rising faster than that among whites)
   d. Protestants (suicide rates are lower for Catholics and Jews than for Protestants)
   e. Unemployed individuals
   f. Individuals who have been under the care of a psychiatrist for any reason
   g. Individuals who have already attempted and failed at suicide (this group is at the highest risk to complete suicide)
   h. Alcohol abusers
   i. Teenagers

C. Prevention

1. **Physician- and community-based programs** to control suicide through treatment of potential victims include:
   a. **Guidance and referral of high-risk individuals** for psychiatric evaluation and consultation
   b. **Provision of adequate and financially acceptable psychiatric, medical, legal, and social services** to those with evidence of serious suicidal intent

2. **Education** of the public, of physicians, and of other therapists about the warning signs of suicide may be an effective preventive measure.

3. **Better control of the agents used in suicide,** such as guns and drugs, may be an effective preventive measure.

X. HOMICIDE

A. Epidemiology

1. **Mortality rate**
   a. More than 20,000 Americans were murdered in 1987. The death rate was approximately 8.1 individuals per 100,000 population and constituted 1.0% of all deaths in the United States. Homicide may be a result of chronic social and societal problems.
   b. Homicide is the leading cause of death for black American men 15–24 years, approximately 5% of black men die from homicide.
   c. Of homicides reported to the Federal Bureau of Investigation (FBI):
      (1) Forty percent were committed by friends (9%) and acquaintances (31%)
      (2) Sixteen percent were committed by a member of the victim's family
      (3) Thirteen percent were committed by strangers
      (4) Thirty-one percent were labeled "relationship unknown"

2. **Time trends.** Homicide rates have increased gradually from low levels early in the century. They reached a peak during the Depression, then declined rapidly through the mid-1940s. Following World War II, rates rose steadily until 1962. In recent years, rates have been relatively stable and, for most age-groups of both sexes, are as high as or higher than any previously recorded in the United States.

B. Causal and risk factors*

1. **Age.** Individuals age 25–34 years are most likely to be victims of homicide, followed by those age 35–44 years, and then those age 15–24 years.
2. **Sex.** Men are four times more likely to be victims of homicide than women.
3. **Racial and ethnic factors**
   a. Blacks are eight to fifteen times more likely to be victims of homicide than whites.
   b. Hispanic men are two to three times more likely than white men to be victims of homicide.
4. **Substance abuse.** Excessive use of alcohol or other drugs by either the victim or the offender has been documented in approximately 50% of homicides.
5. **Socioeconomic factors.** There is evidence that individuals who feel unable to cope with unemployment, poverty, inadequate housing, and discrimination are a higher risk group for either committing or being a victim of homicide.
6. **Lack of traditional support systems** (such as family and religious institutions), **moral consciousness,** and a **sense of identity** have each been associated with an increased risk for committing or of being the victim of homicide.

C. Prevention

1. **Education.** Individuals under 18 years of age may be considered a primary target group for efforts to prevent homicide. Low academic achievement and high truancy rates are strongly associated with delinquency, and appropriate educational intervention may be indicated to counteract these patterns.
2. **Incarcerating criminals** decreases homicide rates, primarily by removing the criminal from society; however, it has not been established whether or not the threat of incarceration or execution deters criminals from murdering.

XI. PEPTIC ULCER DISEASE

A. Epidemiology

1. **Mortality rate.** The death rate for peptic ulcer disease is approximately 2.0 individuals per 100,000 population (1.1 gastric ulcer and 0.9 for duodenal ulcer). Approximately 6000 deaths per year (0.3%) are due to peptic ulcer disease (3000 gastric ulcers and 3000 duodenal ulcers) in the United States. Death can result from bleeding, perforation with rupture of gastric contents into the peritoneal cavity, or obstruction of the gastric outlet.
2. **Incidence and prevalence**
   a. An **annual incidence rate** of 3 per 1000 population leads to approximately 350,000 new cases per year.
   b. The **lifetime prevalence** of peptic ulcer disease is 5%–10%. The 1-year prevalence of self-reported peptic ulcer disease in the United States was about 1.7%–9% between 1961 and 1981. About 4 million Americans suffer from active peptic ulcers during any given year.
3. **Time trends**
   a. Although overall prevalence has remained stable, rates for men and women show opposite patterns; rates for men have decreased from 2.3% to 1.8%, while rates for women have increased from 1.1% to 1.7%. The reason is not established but may be due to changed smoking habits and stress associated with increased involvement in the workplace.
   b. The death rate for peptic ulcer disease has decreased by 30% since 1950.

B. Costs. It has been estimated that, in 1975, the cost of ulcer disease in the United States was $1.3–$2.6 billion.

---

*The causal and risk factors listed, which are due to socioeconomic, psychosocial, ethnic, or racial circumstances, are generally accepted as true but are based on weak evidence. Similarly, the preventive measures recommended have not been rigorously established.

C. Causal and risk factors. Factors such as cigarette smoking, regular use of aspirin, prolonged use of large doses of steroids, and family history have been associated with ulcer disease. Less conclusive associations have been reported for alcohol, caffeine, diet, and stress.

1. **Smoking.** Men who smoke cigarettes have higher peptic ulcer mortality rates than nonsmokers; strong conclusions cannot be made for women smokers.
   a. **Prospective studies** show that smokers of cigarettes, pipes, or cigars have a 33% increased risk of developing an ulcer later in life when compared with nonsmokers of similar socioeconomic status.
   b. **Retrospective studies** show that cigarette smokers are about twice as likely to have ulcers as nonsmokers. Men who smoke have a 2.1 times greater percentage of peptic ulcer disease, and the prevalence in women who smoke is 1.6 times greater than in nonsmokers. The percentage of people with ulcers increased significantly with the number of cigarettes smoked per day.
   c. **Recurrence of ulcers** is markedly increased for smokers.

2. **Aspirin or acetaminophen use** is associated with a three to six times higher prevalence of gastric ulcer disease. There is not a clear association with ibuprofen.

3. **Family history.** Family studies have shown that peptic ulcers occur 2–2.5 times as frequently among first-degree relatives of patients with ulcer disease as compared to relatives of those without ulcer disease. The increased risk is only for the same kind of ulcer.

4. **Individuals with blood type O,** regardless of Rh factor, are about 37% more likely to develop a duodenal ulcer than people with other blood types.

D. Prevention

1. **Primary prevention.** Avoidance of the agents known to increase the risk of ulcer disease is the basis for prevention.
   a. **Initial occurrence.** A nutritious diet, avoidance of nicotine, and temperance in the use of caffeine and alcohol will decrease the risk of developing duodenal ulcer disease.
   b. **Recurrence of gastric ulcer** may be avoided through avoidance of mucosal-disrupting substances, such as salicylates, nonsteroidal anti-inflammatory drugs, and oral corticosteroids, and, most importantly, by the cessation of smoking.

2. **Secondary prevention.** There are no current tests for determining a pre-ulcerous condition in asymptomatic individuals.

3. **Tertiary prevention**
   a. **Treatment** entails:
      (1) Neutralization of gastric acid
      (2) Reduction of gastric acid output
      (3) Increasing the integrity of the gastric and duodenal mucosa
   b. **Intensive antacid therapy and parenteral cimetidine** given intravenously or intramuscularly have been shown to be effective in preventing *recurrence* of stress ulcerations. Cimetidine is also effective in preventing *recurrences* of duodenal ulcer when given in a dose of 300–400 mg at bedtime for 3 months.

XII. ANEMIA is a reduction in either the volume of red blood cells or the concentration of hemoglobin in a sample of peripheral venous blood when compared with similar values from a reference population. There are four broad classifications: **hypoproliferative anemias** (e.g., marrow aplasias, myelophthisic anemias, anemias with blood dyscrasias), **maturation defects** (e.g., cytoplasmic, nuclear), **hyperproliferative** (e.g., hemorrhagic, hemolytic), and **dilutional** (pregnancy, splenomegaly).

A. Epidemiology

1. **Mortality rate.** Anemias were the thirteenth leading cause of death of children under the age of 15 in the United States in 1983, accounting for 0.8% of all deaths in that age-group, with a mortality rate of 0.3 per 100,000 population of individuals age 1–14 years. Death often results due to compromised oxygen delivery to tissues, especially in cases of compromised cardiac output, such as underlying vascular and cardiac disease states. Anemia accounts for less than 0.05% of deaths overall, with a mortality rate of 0.1 per 100,000 population.

2. **Prevalence.** The prevalence of anemia from 1976 to 1980 ranged from 2.3% to 5.9% in a study conducted by the Second National Health and Nutrition Examination Survey.
   a. Prevalence rates in children ranged from 5.7% in infants 1–2 years of age to 2.8% in children 9–11 years of age, including girls and boys of all races.
   b. Children 6–8 years of age and boys and men 12–44 years of age had the **lowest prevalence** rates (2.3% and 2.9% respectively).
   c. The **highest prevalence** rates, aside from infants, were experienced by girls 15–17 years of age (5.9%), young women (4.5%), and elderly men (4.8%).

B. Causal and risk factors

1. **Familial predisposition**
   a. **Sickle-cell anemia** is caused by a lack of hemoglobin A; a deprivation of oxygen results in crescent-shaped red cells. This disorder is almost entirely confined to blacks.
   b. **Thalassemia** is a type of anemia caused by partial or complete interference in synthesis of one of the normal hemoglobin peptide chains. Characteristics include unusually thin red corpuscles. This anemia occurs primarily in individuals of Italian, Greek, Syrian, or Armenian heritage, although there is also high incidence in Thailand and the rest of the Far East.

2. **Iron deficiency**
   a. **Children** may experience iron deficiency anemia at a time when increased iron is required for rapid growth.
   b. **Women** are susceptible to iron deficiency due to menstrual blood loss and the iron losses associated with pregnancy.
   c. **Individuals of low socioeconomic status** are more likely to develop anemia due to the absence of an iron-rich diet because of poverty or ignorance.

3. **Vitamin B_{12} deficiency. Pernicious anemia** is caused by insufficient intestinal absorption of vitamin B_{12}. It primarily affects individuals over the age of 30, and incidence increases with age. Individuals of northern European descent are more likely to develop pernicious anemia; it is less common among Asians and blacks.

4. **Sex and age.** In elderly men, anemia may be linked to a decrease in the androgen stimulation of erythropoiesis that began during puberty; in otherwise healthy subjects, anemia may indicate an overall reduction in hematopoietic reserve.

C. Prevention

1. **Screening by hematocrit** is considered cost-effective for target populations and, thus, is recommended for the following high-risk groups:
   a. Premature infants
   b. Infants born of a multiple pregnancy or an iron-deficient woman
   c. Individuals in low socioeconomic circumstances

2. **Iron supplements in foods,** primarily cereal products, have been shown to decrease the prevalence of anemia among women in Sweden from 30% in 1965 to 7% in 1975.

3. **Dietary iron and vitamin B_{12}.** Consumption of foods that are high in iron [e.g., red meats, organ meats (especially liver)] and leafy green vegetables that are high in B vitamins is recommended for those at high risk and those previously diagnosed with anemia.

BIBLIOGRAPHY

American Cancer Society: Cancer statistics. *CA* 40:9–32, 1990.

Battista RN, Lawrence RS (eds): *Implementing Preventive Services.* New York, Oxford University Press, 1988.

Canadian Task Force on the Periodic Health Examination: The periodic health examination. *Can Med Assoc J* 121:1194–1254, 1979.

Centers for Disease Control: Second National Health and Nutrition Examination Survey (NHANES II).

Dupont WD, Page DL: Menopausal estrogen replacement therapy and breast cancer. *Arch Intern Med* 151:67–72, 1991.

Eriksen MP, LeMaistre CA, Newell GR: Health hazards of passive smoking. *Annu Rev Public Health* 9:47–70, 1988.

Last JM (ed): *Maxcy-Rosenau Public Health and Preventive Medicine,* 12th edition. Norwalk, CT, Appleton & Lange, 1986.

National Cancer Institute, Division of Cancer Prevention and Control: *Working Guidelines for Early Cancer Detection: Rationale and Supporting Evidence to Decrease Mortality.* Bethesda, MD, National Cancer Institute, 1987.

National Cancer Institute: *1987 Annual Cancer Statistics Review, Including Cancer Trends, 1950–1985.* DHHS pub no (NIH) 88-2789 Washington, DC, US Department of Health and Human Services, 1988.

National Center for Health Statistics: Advance report of final mortality statistics, 1986. *Monthly Vital Statistics Report* (suppl) 37(6), 1988.

Office of Disease Prevention and Health Promotion: *Disease Prevention/Health Promotion.* Palo Alto, CA, Bull Publishing Company, 1988.

Romieu I, Berlin JA, Colditz G: Oral contraceptives and breast cancer: review and meta-analysis. *Cancer* 66:2253–2263, 1990.

Schottenfeld D, Fraumeni JF (eds): *Cancer Epidemiology and Prevention.* Philadelphia, WB Saunders, 1982.

Sherlock S (ed): *Alcohol and the Liver in Diseases of the Liver and the Biliary System,* 8th edition. Oxford, Blackwell Scientific Publications, 1989.

US Department of Health and Human Services: *The Health Consequences of Involuntary Smoking: A Report of the Surgeon General.* Rockville, MD, DHHS, 1986.

US Preventive Services Task Force: *Guide to Clinical Preventive Services. Report of the US Preventive Services Task Force.* Washington, DC, US Department of Health and Human Services, 1989.

Wald NJ, Nanchahal K, Thompson SG, et al: Does breathing other people's tobacco smoke cause lung cancer? *Br Med J* 293:1217–1222, 1986.

Woolf CM: A genetic study of cancer of the large intestine. *Am J Hum Genet* 10:42–52, 1958.

Wyngaarden JB, Smith LH (eds): *Cecil's Textbook of Medicine,* 18th edition, Philadelphia, WB Saunders, 1988.

STUDY QUESTIONS

Directions: Each of the numbered items or incomplete statements in this section is followed by answers or by completions of the statement. Select the **one** lettered answer or completion that is **best** in each case.

1. High levels of serum cholesterol are associated with an increased risk of CHD. However, decreasing daily cholesterol intake by 5 mg results in a decline in the risk of CHD by

(A) 5%
(B) 10%
(C) 15%
(D) 20%
(E) 25%

2. All of the following have been identified as major risk factors for CHD EXCEPT

(A) high serum cholesterol
(B) uncontrolled elevation in blood pressure
(C) lack of daily vigorous exercise
(D) cigarette smoking
(E) family history

3. According to the U.S. Preventive Services Task Force, which of the following individuals should be screened by EKG for evidence of CHD?

(A) A 45-year-old man with a cholesterol level of 242 mg/dl and blood pressure measuring 150/95 mm Hg
(B) A 65-year-old woman who wishes to start a vigorous regular exercise program
(C) A 35-year-old man who is an airline pilot and whose father died of CHD at the age of 40
(D) A 50-year-old paraplegic man who smokes and has blood pressure of 155/98 mm Hg
(E) A 70-year-old man who smokes and has blood pressure measuring 110/80 mm Hg and a cholesterol level of 189 mg/dl

4. The risk factors for peptic ulcer disease include all of the following EXCEPT

(A) familial predisposition
(B) regular use of aspirin, acetaminophen, or steroids
(C) tobacco smoking
(D) dietary habits
(E) type AB blood

1-A
2-C
3-D
4-E

Directions: Each item below contains four suggested answers of which **one or more** is correct. Choose the answer

A if **1, 2, and 3** are correct
B if **1 and 3** are correct
C if **2 and 4** are correct
D if **4** is correct
E if **1, 2, 3, and 4** are correct

5. Population subgroups that are at increased risk of developing anemias include

(1) children
(2) women
(3) elderly men
(4) blacks

6. Uncontrolled hypertension increases the risk of developing which of the following?

(1) Cerebrovascular disease
(2) CHD
(3) Renal disease
(4) Diabetes

Directions: The group of items in this section consists of lettered options followed by a set of numbered items. For each item, select the **one** lettered option that is most closely associated with it. Each lettered option may be selected once, more than once, or not at all.

Questions 7–10

For each type of cancer listed below, select the risk factors most likely to be associated with it.

(A) Family history
(B) Cigarette smoking
(C) Both
(D) Neither

7. Lung cancer
8. Breast cancer
9. Colorectal cancer
10. Cervical cancer

5-E 8-A
6-A 9-A
7-B 10-B

ANSWERS AND EXPLANATIONS

1. The answer is A *[II C 2, D 1 b].*
Studies of blood lipids in healthy adults show consistent and linear increases in individual risk of coronary heart disease (CHD), according to levels of total serum cholesterol and low-density lipoprotein (LDL). Studies have shown that a daily decrease of 5 mg of cholesterol in a population will result in an estimated 5% decline in the population's risk of developing CHD. Individually, lower cholesterol levels can usually be achieved by decreasing the consumption of milk, butter, eggs, and animal fat.

2. The answer is C *[II C 1–7].*
There is evidence of an increased risk for coronary heart disease (CHD) for sedentary individuals compared to vigorous exercisers, but lack of daily vigorous exercise has not been identified as a major risk factor for CHD. Instead, investigations increasingly demonstrate that moderate exercise three times a week markedly reduces the risk for individuals compared to others who are completely sedentary. Thus, middle-aged and elderly individuals need to be encouraged to be walkers rather than marathoners. Evidence has shown that cholesterol, blood pressure, smoking, and family history all independently increase a person's risk of CHD.

3. The answer is D *[II C, D 2].*
The U.S. Preventive Services Task Force recommends screening by electrocardiogram (EKG) to check for coronary heart disease (CHD) only for men over age 40 who have two or more risk factors for CHD, who are about to start a vigorous exercise program, or who are public safety risks. The known risk factors for CHD are high blood pressure (150/90 mm Hg recorded 2 weeks in a row is considered high), smoking, high cholesterol levels (anything over 200 mg/dl should be checked regularly), family history of early CHD, oral contraceptive use, and lack of at least moderate exercise. The 50-year-old paraplegic man is a candidate for EKG screening because he is male, over 40 years of age, and has more than two risk factors—that is, he is sedentary, he smokes, and he has very high blood pressure (155/98 mm Hg). The woman who wants to start exercising is not considered to be at as great a risk as a man in the same situation. Although the 70-year-old man smokes, his cholesterol level is good (under 200 mg/dl) and his blood pressure is very good (110/80 mm Hg). The 45-year-old man, while he is male and over age 40, has only two risk factors—high blood pressure (150/95 mm Hg) and high cholesterol (240 mg/dl). He does not need to be screened by EKG, but his blood pressure and cholesterol levels should be monitored and treated. The U.S. Preventive Services Task Force recommends drug treatment for cholesterol levels higher than 240 mg/dl. The 35-year-old male airline pilot is in an occupation that makes him a public safety risk, but since he is not yet age 40, he is not considered a candidate for EKG screening. Nonetheless, his family has a history of early CHD, so he may want to monitor his risk factors carefully, regardless of his age.

4. The answer is E *[XI C 1–4].*
Type AB blood is not a risk factor for peptic ulcer disease. However, individuals with type O blood are about 37% more likely to develop a duodenal ulcer than people with other blood types. Factors such as cigarette smoking, regular use of aspirin, and prolonged use of steroids in large doses have been closely associated with ulcer disease. Less conclusive associations have been reported for alcohol, caffeine, diet, and psychologic stress. Family studies have shown that peptic ulcer disease occurs 2–2.5 times more frequently among first-degree relatives of patients with ulcer disease as compared to relatives of those without ulcer disease. The increased risk is only for the same kind of ulcer.

5. The answer is E (all) *[XII B 1 a, 2, 4].*
Children are at an increased risk for anemia because increased iron is required for rapid growth. In women, menstrual blood loss and the iron losses associated with pregnancy can result in anemia. In elderly men, anemia may be linked to a decrease in androgen stimulation of erythropoiesis that began during puberty; in otherwise healthy subjects, anemia may indicate an overall reduction in hematopoietic reserve. Sickle-cell anemia is almost entirely confined to blacks.

6. The answer is A (1, 2, 3) *[II C 3; IV C 2; VIII C 6, D 1].*
Hypertension is a strong and independent risk factor for coronary heart disease (CHD) that is well established by descriptive studies. Hypertension increases the risk of stroke, and epidemiologic evidence is strong that hypertension is one of the causes of atherosclerosis, particularly in combination with hyperlipidemia. Controlling hypertension is one of the most effective ways of preventing morbidity and mortality due to renal failure. While hypertensive nephropathy is a major cause of morbidity and mortality among diabetics, hypertension itself does not increase the risk of developing diabetes.

7–10. The answers are: 7-B *[III C 1 a–e],* **8-A** *[III C 2 a–f],* **9-A** *[III C 3 a–e],* **10-B** *[III C 4 a–g].* Although studies done before 1970 indicated a tendency for lung cancer to aggregate in families, most recent studies suggest little or no independent familial association. Most studies consistently demonstrate that cigarette smoking is a major risk factor in the development of lung cancer. The earlier the age at onset of smoking and the higher the number of cigarettes smoked, the greater the risk. In addition, exposure to industrial carcinogens, air pollution, and radiation are considered risk factors.

Risk factors for the development of breast cancer include a family history of breast cancer, a first pregnancy after age 30, exposure to radiation, an early menarche, age over 40 years, and high socioeconomic status. Smoking does not appear to be a risk factor for breast cancer. Some studies have shown high intake of fat and animal protein to increase the risk of developing breast cancer, but these findings are still controversial. The risk of breast cancer to women whose mother or sisters had breast cancer is twofold, and the risk to those whose mothers *and* sisters had breast cancer is threefold.

The relative risk that first-degree relatives of people with colon cancer will develop colon cancer is three times the risk of the general population. Thus, there appears to be a familial predisposition for colon cancer. Other risk factors include fiber deficiency, high-fat dietary consumption, alcohol consumption, high socioeconomic status, and white race. Smoking does not appear to be a risk factor for colon cancer.

Smoking is considered an important risk factor for cervical cancer. Other risk factors include early age at first coitus; sexual activity with multiple partners, often leading to infections and other sexually transmitted diseases (STDs); and oral contraceptive use (which has been statistically associated with sexual activity with multiple partners). Although black women and Hispanic women are at increased risk for cervical cancer, family predisposition has not been found to be a risk factor.

6
Maternal Health Issues

Sally Faith Dorfman

I. DEFINITIONS

A. Maternal mortality consists of deaths attributed to complications of pregnancy, childbirth, and the puerperium, often within a fixed time (42 days, 6 months, or 1 year) of the pregnancy's termination.

1. **Direct maternal mortality** consists of deaths resulting from obstetric complications, omissions, interventions, and their sequelae.
2. **Indirect maternal mortality** consists of deaths resulting from preexisting conditions or conditions aggravated by the pregnancy.
3. **The maternal mortality rate** is the ratio of pregnancy-related deaths to live births over a specified time for a particular geographic area, usually per 100,000 live births.

B. Preterm terminations of pregnancy

1. **Abortion.** The abortion rate is the number of abortions per 1000 women who are 15–44 years of age. The abortion ratio is the number of abortions per 1000 live births.
   a. **Induced abortion** is a procedure that terminates a pregnancy, producing a nonviable fetus.
   b. **Spontaneous abortion** includes failure of embryonic development, fetal death in utero, and expulsion of all (complete) or any part (incomplete) of the products of conception before 20 weeks' gestation or expulsion of a fetus weighing less than 500 g.
2. **Ectopic pregnancy** is a pregnancy located outside the normal implantation area in the body of a normally shaped uterus. Continued growth may result in hemorrhagic rupture. In the United States during recent years approximately 1 of every 100 reported pregnancies has been ectopic in location, and 1 of every 1000 ectopic pregnancies resulted in the woman's death. Many factors have been *associated* with increased risk, but *causation* has not been established. Putative risk factors include:
   a. A history of ectopic pregnancy
   b. Tubal surgery
   c. A history of pelvic inflammatory disease (PID)
   d. Progestin exposure
   e. Infertility
   f. Smoking
3. **Stillbirth** is fetal death occurring after 20 weeks' gestation or spontaneous death of a fetus weighing more than 500 g.

C. Fetal and infant mortality

1. **Perinatal mortality** consists of fetal and infant deaths occurring between 28 weeks' gestation and 1 week postnatal, with fetal or infant weight $\geq$ 500 g.
2. **Neonatal mortality** consists of deaths of liveborn infants within 28 days of age (see Ch 7 I C 1).
3. **Infant mortality** consists of deaths of children less than 1 year of age.

II. MATERNAL MORTALITY

A. Statistics. Maternal mortality overall has decreased in the United States, particularly after the legalization of induced abortion in the early 1970s (Figure 6-1).

1. Analysis of U.S. maternal mortality rates by race reveals consistently lower rates for white women than for black women and women of other races (Table 6-1).
2. Analysis of international rates by age reveals a J-shaped curve, with somewhat higher maternal mortality rates for younger and older women; U.S. rates are higher primarily for older women (see Table 6-1).

B. Causes. Embolism, hypertensive diseases of pregnancy, hemorrhage, cardiovascular accidents, anesthesia complications, and infection are the major causes of maternal mortality. Ectopic pregnancy has emerged as another leading cause, despite declining death-to-case rates (Figures 6-2 and 6-3).

III. METHODS OF FAMILY PLANNING

A. Contraceptive methods (Table 6-2). Criteria for a good contraceptive include efficacy, safety, accessibility, acceptability, and reversibility. Risk-benefit analysis may be done for each method using these criteria. The absence of a method and the resultant unwanted pregnancy should also be included in the risk analysis.

1. **Abstinence from sex**
   a. **Advantages**
      (1) Accessible, safe, and reversible
      (2) Acceptable to most religious groups
   b. **Disadvantages**
      (1) Requires strong motivation
      (2) Not always desirable or acceptable

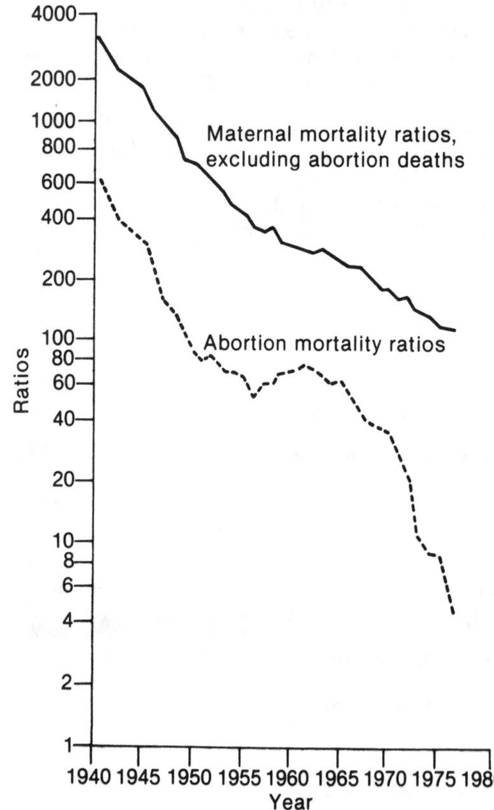

Figure 6-1. Number of women who died giving birth (excluding abortions) per 1 million live births (maternal mortality ratios) and number of women who died during abortion per 1 million live births (abortion mortality ratios) in the United States, 1940–1977. (Reprinted from Cates W Jr, Rochat RW, Grimes DA, et al: Legalized abortion: effect on national trends of maternal and abortion-related mortality (1940–1976). *Am J Obstet Gynecol* 132:211–214, 1978.)

Table 6-1. Maternal Death-to-Case Rates for Legal Abortions and for Childbirth by Year, Age, and Race (1972–1978)

	Maternal Death Rate (per 100,000 Abortions)		Maternal Death Rate (per 100,000 Live Births)		Relative Risk*
	Crude	Standardized	Crude	Standardized	
Year					
1972	4.1	4.1	15.2	16.8	4.1
1973	3.4	3.2	12.6	13.9	4.3
1974	2.8	2.6	12.1	13.9	5.3
1975	2.8	2.6	10.4	12.0	4.6
1976	0.9	0.8	10.5	11.7	14.6
1977	1.3	1.2	9.3	10.4	8.7
1978	0.5	0.4	8.0	9.1	22.8
Age					
≤19	1.3	1.3	8.5	7.7	5.9
20–24	2.1	2.1	7.4	7.9	3.8
25–29	2.0	2.0	9.4	11.6	5.8
30–34	2.5	2.3	17.1	20.1	8.7
≥35	3.4	3.2	43.7	46.3	14.5
Race					
White	1.3	1.3	8.3	8.2	6.3
Black and other	3.3	3.5	23.1	23.1	6.6
Overall	1.9	1.8	11.1	12.5	6.9

Adapted from LeBolt SA, Grimes DA, Cates W Jr: Mortality from abortion and childbirth: Are the populations comparable? *JAMA* 248(2):188–191, 1982.

*Ratio of standardized childbearing rate to standardized abortion rate.

2. **Natural family planning** includes calendar, temperature, and cervical mucus analyses. Combinations of the methods sometimes are referred to as the rhythm, Billings, or cervicothermal methods.
   a. **Advantages**
      (1) Safe and accessible
      (2) Acceptable to most religious groups

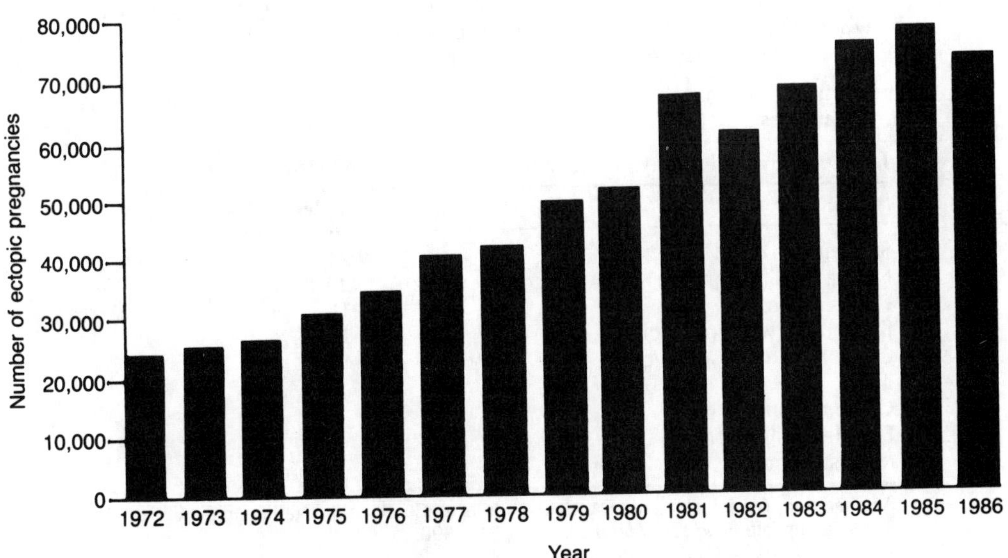

Figure 6-2. Number of ectopic pregnancies in the United States, 1972–1986. [Adapted from Lawson HW, Atrash HK, Saftlas AF, et al: Ectopic pregnancy in the United States, 1970–1986. *MMWR* 38(SS-2):1–10, 1989.]

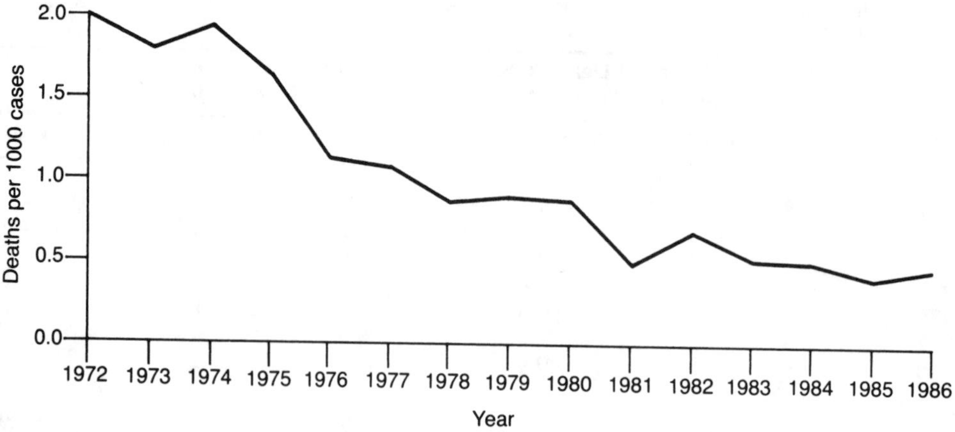

Figure 6-3. Death-to-case rates for women with ectopic pregnancies in the United States, 1972–1986. [Adapted from Lawson HW, Atrash HK, Saftlas AF, et al: Ectopic pregnancy in the United States, 1970–1986. *MMWR* 38(SS-2):1–10, 1989.]

b. Disadvantages

(1) Requires extensive education

(2) Requires strong motivation

(3) Variable efficacy according to individual motivation and physiologic and pathologic variables

3. **Coitus interruptus.** The efficacy and acceptability of coitus interruptus may be marginal.

a. **Advantage.** Coitus interruptus is available to everyone.

b. **Disadvantages**

(1) Ineffective for pre-ejaculate sperm

(2) Requires great motivation and control, which may not be attainable

4. **Lactation.** The efficacy of lactation in reducing populations, as studied by demographics, is significant on a worldwide basis, but it is unreliable for individual couples, since not all women can breast-feed, and some women ovulate and conceive even during early breast-feeding when protection is thought to be greatest.

a. **Advantages**

(1) Enhances infant nutrition and health as well as maternal-infant bonding

(2) Prolongs the interval between pregnancies from an overall demographic perspective

b. **Disadvantage.** Lactation is an undependable means of contraception for an individual, since ovulation may resume quickly in some breast-feeding women.

5. **Spermicides.** To enhance efficacy, spermicides can be used with other methods.

a. **Advantages**

Table 6-2. Typical Birth Control Failure Rate During the First Year of Use

Method	Percentage of Accidental Pregnancies*
Spermicides only	21
Natural family planning	20
Coitus interruptus	18
Diaphragm with spermicide	18
Condom without spermicide	12
IUD	3
Combination pill	3
Female sterilization	0.4
Male sterilization	0.15

Adapted from Trussel J, Hatcher RA, Cates W Jr, et al: Contraceptive failure in the United States: an update. *Stud Fam Plann* 21(1):51–54, 1990.

*These percentages represent the number of typical couples expected to experience an accidental pregnancy during the first year of using a birth control method, given that the method is used consistently and correctly and the couple does not stop using it.

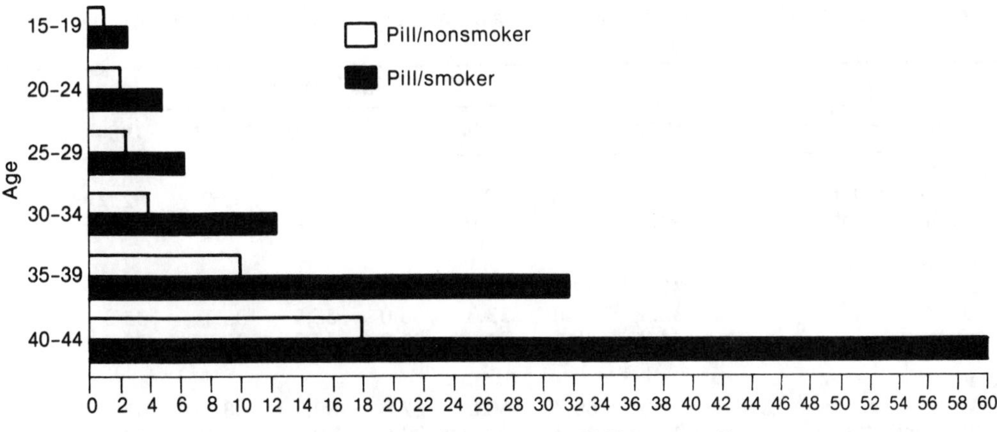

Figure 6-4. Annual death rate of smoking and nonsmoking women taking oral contraceptives (i.e., the *pill*), by age. Although women over 40 years of age are at greatest risk of death from simultaneous smoking and taking oral contraceptives, smoking increases the risk of death for *all* women of any age who use oral contraceptives. (Adapted from Teitze C: New estimates of mortality associated with fertility control. *Fam Plan Perspect* 2:74–76, 1977.)

- **(1)** Available without prescriptions or office visits
- **(2)** Generally safe (some allergic reactions have been reported, and there is some concern, which is difficult to support epidemiologically, regarding teratogenesis)

b. Disadvantage. Use of spermicides requires motivation and planning.

6. Barriers (e.g., sponge, cervical cap, diaphragm, condom)

a. Advantages

- **(1)** Provide some protection against sexually transmitted diseases (STDs), including human immunodeficiency virus (HIV) infection and PID
- **(2)** May be combined with other methods to enhance efficacy

b. Disadvantages

- **(1)** Require awareness of optimal method of use and consistent motivation and planning to be effective, as well as a certain amount of physical dexterity and anatomic knowledge by at least one partner
- **(2)** Minimal risk of toxic shock syndrome from sponge, diaphragm, or cervical cap, especially during menses
- **(3)** May require partner's cooperation and motivation (e.g., the condom)

7. Intrauterine device (IUD)

a. Advantage. The single insertion of an IUD gives protection for a year or more.

b. Disadvantages

- **(1)** Significant risks (especially if coupling is not mutually monogamous), including:
  - **(a)** PID
  - **(b)** Ectopic pregnancy
  - **(c)** Infertility; not recommended for those who have not completed childbearing
- **(2)** Heavier menstrual flow and cramping
- **(3)** Limited access and availability including:
  - **(a)** High initial cost
  - **(b)** Lengthy informed consent
  - **(c)** Medicolegal impediments

8. Pills (fixed combinations and phasics, both of which are estrogen-progestin pills)

a. Advantages

- **(1)** Highly effective
- **(2)** Not coitally related
- **(3)** Generally safe and reversible
- **(4)** Thought to be protective against such conditions as anemia, dysmenorrhea, ovarian cysts, and endometrial cancer
- **(5)** Possibly protective against breast and ovarian cancers

Table 6-3. Characteristics of Women Obtaining Legal Abortions in the United States (Selected Years, 1972–1986)

	Percentage Distribution*							
Characteristics	**1972**	**1974**	**1976**	**1978**	**1980**	**1982**	**1984**	**1986**
Residence								
Abortion in-state	56.2	86.6	90.0	89.3	92.6	92.9	92.0	92.4
Abortion out-of-state	43.8	13.4	10.0	10.7	7.4	7.1	8.0	7.6
Age (years)								
≤19	32.6	32.7	32.1	30.0	29.2	27.1	26.4	25.3
20–24	32.5	31.8	33.3	35.0	35.5	35.1	35.3	34.0
≥25	34.9	35.6	34.6	34.9	35.3	37.8	38.3	40.7
Race								
White	77.0	69.7	66.6	67.0	69.9	68.5	67.4	67.0
Black and other	23.0	30.3	33.4	33.0	30.1	31.5	32.6	33.0
Marital status								
Married	29.7	27.4	24.6	26.4	23.1	22.0	20.5	20.2
Unmarried	70.3	72.6	75.4	73.6	76.9	78.0	79.5	79.8
Number of live births†								
0	49.4	47.8	47.7	56.6	58.4	57.8	57.0	55.1
1	18.2	19.6	20.7	19.2	19.5	20.3	20.9	22.1
2	13.3	14.8	15.4	14.1	13.7	13.9	14.4	14.9
3	8.7	8.7	8.3	5.9	5.3	5.1	5.1	5.3
≥4	10.4	9.0	7.9	4.2	3.2	2.9	2.6	2.6
Type of procedure								
Curettage	88.6	89.7	92.8	94.6	95.5	96.4	96.8	97.0
Intrauterine instillation	10.4	7.8	6.0	3.9	3.1	2.5	1.9	1.4
Hysterotomy/hysterectomy	0.6	0.6	0.2	0.1	0.1	<0.05	<0.05	<0.05
Other	0.5	1.9	0.9	1.4	1.3	1.0	1.3	1.6
Weeks of gestation								
≤8	34.0	42.6	47.0	52.2	51.7	50.6	50.5	51.0
9–10	30.7	28.7	28.0	26.9	26.2	26.7	26.4	25.8
11–12	17.5	15.4	14.4	12.3	12.2	12.4	12.6	12.2
13–15	8.4	5.5	4.5	4.0	5.2	5.3	5.8	6.1
16–20	8.2	6.5	5.1	3.7	3.9	3.9	3.9	4.1
≥21	1.3	1.2	0.9	0.9	0.9	1.1	0.8	0.8

Adapted from Koonin LM, Atrash HK, Smith JC, et al: Abortion surveillance, 1986–1987. *MMWR* 39(SS-2):28–29, 1990.

*Excludes unknowns. Since the number of states reporting each characteristic varies from year to year, temporal comparisons should be made with caution.

†For years 1972–1976, data indicate number of living children.

b. Disadvantages

(1) Increased risk of cardiovascular and thromboembolic diseases among

(a) Women over 35 years of age who smoke (Figure 6-4)

(b) Women over 40 years of age who do not smoke

(c) Women taking high-dose pills

(2) The necessity of a prescription and regular office visits

(3) Possible major and minor side effects (e.g., hypertension, migraines, breakthrough bleeding, phlebitis, nausea, weight gain, mastalgia, bloating, emotional lability)

(4) Recurrent concerns regarding future risk of breast cancer, which, though currently not considered significant enough to warrant alterations in Food and Drug Administration (FDA) recommendations, need to be addressed with each candidate and reviewed periodically in light of future findings

9. Progestin-only minipills, injectables, and implants

a. Advantages

(1) Effective

(2) Can be used when estrogens are contraindicated (e.g., in postpartum lactating women)

3. **Maternal health status.** Ideally, the woman should be in good health prior to conception, for her own sake and the sake of her infant. Chronic illness (e.g., diabetes, hypertension) should be well controlled, and all medications should be reviewed for teratogenic potential.

B. Routine well-woman care during pregnancy

1. Perform a **Pap smear** and **breast and pelvic examinations** at the first visit and as indicated thereafter.
2. Give special attention to **nutrition,** particularly those areas most likely to be marginal, including dietary intake of calcium, folate, and iron. An overall weight gain of 25–30 lbs should be the goal.
3. Check **hematocrit** and **hemoglobin levels** to screen for anemia.
4. Stress the importance of **good hygiene**.
5. Advise sensible exercise levels.
6. Screen for and treat **STDs,** as indicated, including syphilis, gonorrhea, HIV, and herpes (HSV). Drug users and others at high risk for STDs should be screened repeatedly throughout pregnancy and thereafter. Counseling regarding STDs should be part of patient care.
7. Advise **abstinence from hazardous substances,** such as cigarettes, drugs, and alcohol.
8. Routinely **check weight, blood pressure, reflexes, extremities, and urine**. Other screening (e.g., testing for tuberculosis) should be performed as indicated.

C. Special pregnancy screening

1. **Infections**
   a. Screen for the **TORCH diseases** that may affect the fetus or neonate: toxoplasmosis, rubella, cytomegalovirus (CMV), HSV, hepatitis, and others.
   b. Screen for **rubella** and give rubella vaccine to susceptible individuals postpartum. Ideally, the vaccine should be administered at least 3 months prior to conception to women without documentation of immunity.
2. **Rh testing.** Follow special screening protocols for Rh-negative individuals.
3. **Sonography.** Screen for structural abnormalities, multiple gestation, and placental location as indicated.
4. **Amniocentesis and chorionic villus biopsy.** Test for congenital defects by direct sampling of the products of conception as indicated.
5. **α-Fetoprotein testing.** Detect some neural tube defects and other conditions (e.g., Down syndrome) by sampling maternal serum and amniotic fluid as indicated.

D. Continuous monitoring of maternal well-being. At a minimum, check blood pressure, weight, extremities, reflexes, and urine at each visit to identify:

1. **Hypertensive diseases of pregnancy** [i.e., preeclampsia or eclampsia (formerly referred to as toxemia) indicated by hypertension, edema, weight gain, hyperreflexia, and proteinuria]
2. **Gestational diabetes.** Many physicians advise routine midpregnancy screening, using a measured glucose load and timed serum sampling in addition to routine urine testing.

E. Continuous monitoring of fetal development is accomplished by comparing maternal weight and uterine size at each visit relative to the estimated date of conception in conjunction with other tests (e.g., sonography, monitoring of fetal heart rate, biophysical profile).

F. Avoidance of potentially hazardous substances, including possible teratogens (Barlow, 1982; Hunt, 1979; Shepard, 1989) that are otherwise relatively innocuous (e.g., tetracycline, other antibiotics, alcohol), should be advised.

1. **Substance abuse**
   a. **Tobacco** is associated with low birth weight and premature delivery.
   b. **Alcohol** is associated with teratogenic effects, including fetal alcohol syndrome.
   c. **Illegal or "recreational" drugs** may lead to teratogenic symptoms (e.g., from cocaine) or withdrawal symptoms (e.g., from heroin) in neonates, or to long-term behavioral problems

and learning disabilities. Even single doses of crack cocaine have been shown to cause deleterious effects (e.g., congenital malformations, long-term behavioral changes, developmental delays) on the offspring (see also IV B 6). The frequently used phrase "sex for drugs" explains the link between crack cocaine and STDs.

2. **Diethylstilbestrol (DES) and prescription drugs** (e.g., tetracycline, sulfonamides) may result in assorted teratogenic, structural, functional, or carcinogenic effects on offspring.

3. **Radiation**—either diagnostic, occupational, or environmental—may cause spontaneous abortion, birth defects, or childhood leukemia (Barlow, 1982; Hunt, 1979; Shepard, 1989).

4. **Occupational and environmental hazards,** including chemicals, pollutants, and radioactive substances that workers may carry home on skin or clothing to their pregnant partners, may cause reproductive problems (Barlow, 1982; Hunt, 1979; Shepard, 1989).

5. **Infectious agents** (e.g., syphilis, HIV, toxoplasmosis, rubella, CMV) are associated with assorted negative effects on the fetus.

G. **Low birth weight** (see also Ch 7 I C 1 a, E) can result from many maternal conditions (e.g., malnutrition, anemia, diabetes) and is a major cause of neonatal mortality. Low birth weight may be minimized by attention to all factors listed in this section, as well as to socioeconomic support, good health education, family planning, and proper obstetric management.

H. **Cervical testing later in pregnancy** is somewhat controversial regarding frequency and cost and benefit.

V. OBSTETRIC CONCERNS AT THE TIME OF DELIVERY

A. Infectious diseases of the birth canal

1. **HSV** may be an indication for cesarean section, as HSV of the genital tract may lead to encephalitis or disseminated HSV in the infant, either of which may be fatal to the infant.

2. **Gonorrhea,** if untreated, may cause blindness in infants.

3. **Chlamydial infection** may result in ophthalmologic and other damage.

4. **Candidiasis** can cause oral thrush.

5. **Streptococcal infection** may be transmitted to the infant.

6. **Hepatitis** may be transmitted during or prior to birth.

7. **HIV infection,** which leads to acquired immune deficiency syndrome (AIDS), can be transmitted during delivery, as well as during pregnancy or breast-feeding. An HIV-positive woman has a 30%–60% or greater chance of transmitting the virus to her offspring, with greater risk if she has already given birth to an HIV-positive child.

B. **Type of delivery** (i.e., spontaneous vaginal delivery, forceps, vacuum extraction, cesarean section, vaginal birth after previous cesarean) sometimes is a source of controversy among public health professionals and consumers (i.e., lay groups, including patients, partners, and self-appointed consumer advocates), as well as obstetricians, midwives, and pediatricians.

C. **Perinatal health care providers, alternative birthing centers, and home births.** Aspects of contemporary hospital-based care, such as the use of electronic fetal monitoring and ultrasound and the credentials of obstetric attendants, have polarized physicians, certified nurse midwives, public health professionals, lay midwives, and consumer groups.

1. Throughout most of the world, and until recently in the United States and other developed countries, most births occur at home, with laboring women assisted by lay midwives. Around the time of World War I, care of pregnant women in the United States shifted to physicians, and home births gradually were replaced by hospital deliveries. In the 1960s, a counterculture trend toward family-centered, midwife-assisted deliveries increased in popularity. **Most births in the United States currently occur in hospitals attended by physicians.** Many of these physicians are obstetric specialists, and others are family practitioners who have had training in obstetrics.

2. **Certified nurse midwives,** working in conjunction with physicians, have provided an increasing amount of prenatal and obstetric care in the United States over the past 2 decades. They often work in hospital-affiliated "home-like" birthing rooms, or in freestanding family-oriented birthing centers.

3. **Lay midwives** continue to function outside the realm of the regulatory agencies, providing care of variable quality for those unable or unwilling to use established services.

D. Access to care

1. Accessibility, acceptability, affordability, and coordination of adequate perinatal services remain spotty in the United States. Regionalization efforts have been designed to improve access to comprehensive, quality care for patients at all levels of medical risk by defined geographic areas.

2. Financial barriers to perinatal care and a healthy pregnancy remain a problem, despite local, state, federal, and private efforts such as private insurance, Medicaid, and Women, Infants, and Children (WIC) programs.

3. Medical liability issues and other factors have decreased the availability of obstetric care providers, as physicians choose to avoid or drop obstetrics from their practices.

4. Besides access to acceptable services, women must have an appropriate psychosocial attitude to avail themselves of the benefits of perinatal care.

VI. POSTPARTUM PREVENTIVE MEDICINE AND PUBLIC HEALTH CONCERNS

A. **Breast-feeding** usually enhances infant nutrition, immune defenses, bonding, and contraception, but it is contraindicated in HIV-positive women.

B. **Good parenting and bonding** help to ensure optimal development.

C. **Rh immune globulin and rubella vaccines** should be administered when indicated for the safety of future pregnancies. Specialist consultation should be obtained before live vaccines are given to immunocompromised women.

D. Contraception allows women to recuperate physiologically from pregnancy, adjust to the demands imposed by the new infant, and exercise some control over the timing of any future pregnancy. Too many pregnancies (defined in terms of a woman's baseline physical and emotional status and her environment) before maternal reserves can be replenished can have detrimental effects on maternal health and on the health of both the newborn and older children in the family.

BIBLIOGRAPHY

Alan Guttmacher Institute: *Blessed Events and the Bottom Line: Financing Maternity Care in the United States.* New York, Alan Guttmacher Institute, 1987.

Barlow S: *Reproductive Hazards of Industrial Chemicals.* New York, Academic Press, 1982.

Cherry SH, Berkowitz RL, Kase NG (eds): *Rovinsky and Guttmacher's Medical, Surgical, and Gynecologic Complications of Pregnancy,* 3rd edition. Baltimore, Williams & Wilkins, 1985.

Cunningham FG, MacDonald PC, Gant NF: *Williams Obstetrics,* 18th edition. Norwalk, Appleton & Lange, 1989.

Hatcher RA, Guest F, Stewart F, et al: *Contraceptive Technology 1990–1992,* 15th edition. Manchester, NH, Irvington, 1990.

Hern WM: *Abortion Practice.* Philadelphia, Lippincott, 1984.

Hodgson JE: *Abortion and Sterilization: Medical and Social Aspects.* New York, Grune and Stratton, 1981.

Hunt VT: *Work and the Health of Women.* Boca Raton, CRC Press, 1979.

Institute of Medicine: *Prenatal Care: Reaching Mothers, Reaching Infants.* Washington, DC, National Academy Press, 1988.

Institute of Medicine: *Preventing Low Birthweight.* Washington, DC, National Academy Press, 1985.

Koonin LM, Atrash HK, Smith JC, et al: Abortion surveillance, 1986–1987. *MMWR* 39(SS-2):23–56, 1990.

Last JM: *A Dictionary of Epidemiology.* New York, Oxford University Press, 1983.

Lawson HW, Atrash HK, Saftlas AF, et al: Ectopic pregnancy in the United States, 1970–1986. *MMWR* 38(SS-2):1–10, 1989.

Lawson HW, Atrash HK, Saftlas AF, et al: Abortion surveillance in the United States, 1984–1985. *MMWR* 38(SS-2):11–45, 1989.

LeBolt SA, Grimes DA, Cates W Jr: Mortality from abortion and childbirth: are the populations comparable? *JAMA* 248(2):188–191, 1982.

Ory HW, Forrest JD, Lincoln R: *Making Choices: Evaluating the Health Risks and Benefits of Birth Control Methods.* New York, Alan Guttmacher Institute, 1983.

Shepard TH: *Catalog of Teratogenic Agents,* 6th edition. Baltimore, Johns Hopkins University Press, 1989.

Trussel J, Hatcher RA, Cates W Jr, et al: Contraceptive failure in the United States: an update. *Stud Fam Plann* 21(1):51–54, 1990.

STUDY QUESTIONS

Directions: Each of the numbered items or incomplete statements in this section is followed by answers or by completions of the statement. Select the **one** lettered answer or completion that is **best** in each case.

1. In the United States, the number of ectopic pregnancies that result in death is closest to

(A) 1 in 10
(B) 1 in 100
(C) 1 in 1000
(D) 1 in 10,000

2. Which of the following statements describing the risk of death from simultaneous smoking and the use of oral contraceptives is true?

(A) A 39-year-old nonsmoker taking oral contraceptives is at greater risk than a 30-year-old smoker taking the same contraceptives
(B) Smoking increases the risk of death for all women of any age who are using oral contraceptives
(C) Smoking does not increase the risk of death in a woman taking oral contraceptives unless she is older than 35 years of age
(D) Women under age 20 years and those over age 40 years who smoke and take oral contraceptives are the two groups at the greatest risk

3. All of the factors listed below may increase a woman's risk of ectopic pregnancy EXCEPT

(A) infertility
(B) progestin exposure
(C) PID
(D) smoking
(E) alcohol consumption

Directions: Each item below contains four suggested answers of which **one or more** is correct. Choose the answer

A if **1, 2, and 3** are correct
B if **1 and 3** are correct
C if **2 and 4** are correct
D if **4** is correct
E if **1, 2, 3, and 4** are correct

4. Which of the following situations can be accurately described as a stillbirth?

(1) Dead fetus of unknown weight spontaneously expelled at 19 weeks' gestation
(2) Dead fetus weighing 501 g spontaneously expelled at 19 weeks' gestation
(3) Dead fetus weighing 499 g spontaneously expelled at 19 weeks' gestation
(4) Dead fetus weighing 499 g spontaneously expelled at 21 weeks' gestation

5. Breast-feeding usually improves which of the following?

(1) Bonding
(2) Infant nutrition
(3) Infant immune defenses
(4) Prevention of HIV infection

1-C
2-B
3-E
4-C
5-A

SUMMARY OF DIRECTIONS

A	B	C	D	E
1, 2, 3 only	1, 3 only	2, 4 only	4 only	All are correct

6. Leading causes of maternal mortality in the United States include

(1) embolism
(2) anesthesia complications
(3) hemorrhage
(4) ectopic pregnancy

7. Routine prenatal well-woman care should include

(1) weight checks
(2) urine testing
(3) blood pressure checks
(4) electronic fetal monitoring

8. Maternal exposure to which of the following substances or conditions is thought to harm the developing fetus?

(1) Alcohol
(2) Tetracycline
(3) Rubella
(4) Herpes

Directions: Each group of items in this section consists of lettered options followed by a set of numbered items. For each item, select the **one** lettered option that is most closely associated with it. Each lettered option may be selected once, more than once, or not at all.

Questions 9–11

For each case history below, select the classification that it most closely represents.

(A) Direct maternal mortality
(B) Perinatal mortality
(C) Both
(D) Neither

9. A woman whose ectopic pregnancy has ruptured at 18 weeks' gestation hemorrhages internally, goes into shock, and eventually dies

10. A woman with congenital heart disease and labile diabetes has a stillbirth 5 days after her due date, develops ketoacidosis and cardiac arrest during the labor, and dies

11. A woman dies of septic shock 4 days after an unsuccessful self-induced abortion attempt at 30 weeks' gestation; the male infant is born alive but dies 2 days later in a neonatal intensive care unit

Questions 12–15

For each description that follows, select the method of contraception that it best describes.

(A) Estrogen-progestin pills
(B) IUDs
(C) Injectables
(D) Barriers
(E) Lactation

12. Risks are increased for older women and smokers

13. PID, ectopic pregnancy, and infertility may be sequelae

14. A variety of STDs may be prevented with its use

15. It carries a very slight increased risk of toxic shock syndrome

6-E
7-A
8-A
9-A
10-B
11-C
12-A
13-B
14-D
15-D

ANSWERS AND EXPLANATIONS

1. The answer is C *[I B 2].*
In the United States during the past decade, approximately 1 of every 100 reported pregnancies has been ectopic, and about 1 of every 1000 ectopic pregnancies has resulted in the woman's death.

2. The answer is B *[III A 8 b (1) (a), (b); Figure 6-4].*
Although women age 40 and older are at the greatest risk of death from simultaneous smoking and taking oral contraceptives (i.e., the pill), smoking increases the risk of death for *all* women of *any* age who are using oral contraceptives. Smoking also increases the risk of death for women not using oral contraceptives and for men of all ages.

3. The answer is E *[I B 2; IV B 7, F].*
Alcohol consumption by pregnant women presents a prenatal risk because alcohol is a possible teratogen that can lead to fetal alcohol syndrome in newborns. However, consuming alcohol has not been found to increase a woman's risk of ectopic pregnancy. Infertility, progestin exposure, pelvic inflammatory disease (PID), and smoking all have been associated with increased risk of ectopic pregnancy, although no clear causal connection between any of the risk factors and ectopic pregnancy has been established.

4. The answer is C (2, 4) *[I B 3].*
Both a dead fetus weighing 501 g spontaneously expelled at 19 weeks' gestation and a dead fetus weighing 499 g spontaneously expelled at 21 weeks' gestation would be considered stillbirths. A stillbirth is defined as a fetal death occurring after the twentieth week of gestation or spontaneous death of a fetus weighing more than 500 g.

5. The answer is A (1, 2, 3) *[VI A].*
Breast-feeding usually enhances bonding and infant nutrition and immune defenses, particularly in the developing world. However, breast-feeding is contraindicated when the mother tests positive for the human immunodeficiency virus (HIV) because of the possibility of transmitting the infection to the infant.

6. The answer is E (all) *[II B].*
Embolism, anesthesia complications, hemorrhage, ectopic pregnancy, hypertensive diseases of pregnancy, cardiovascular accidents, and infections are major causes of maternal mortality. Despite declining death-to-case rates, ectopic pregnancy has emerged as a leading cause of death among pregnancies with abortive outcome as other causes become less prominent in this category.

7. The answer is A (1, 2, 3) *[IV B].*
Weight, urine, and blood pressure should be checked routinely at every well-woman prenatal visit. Each visit also should include a Pap smear; a breast examination; advice on nutrition, exercise, and hygiene; and screening for sexually transmitted diseases (STDs). Electronic fetal monitoring is an option that has specific indications during pregnancy and labor but is not always an essential component of prenatal care.

8. The answer is A (1, 2, 3) *[IV F 1, 2; V A 1].*
Excessive alcohol intake during pregnancy can result in fetal alcohol syndrome, which consists of excessive irritability, delayed mental and physical growth, and particular facial characteristics. Tetracycline exposure can cause discolored teeth in the child. Rubella exposure can result in mental retardation, deafness, and blindness. While a herpes simplex virus (HSV) infection in the mother during delivery can be fatal to a new infant, the harm is done during the birthing process not during gestation.

9–11. The answers are: 9-A, 10-B, 11-C *[I A 1, 2, C 1–3].*
The death of the woman with a ruptured ectopic pregnancy at 18 weeks' gestation is classified as direct maternal mortality. Her death was a direct result of the complications of an ectopic implantation; it did not result from a preexisting illness. Although the ectopic pregnancy itself may be categorized as a spontaneous abortion, the question refers to the death of the woman and not the product of conception.

The stillborn child is classified as perinatal mortality—that is, death of a fetus or infant between 28 weeks' gestation and 1 week postnatal with a fetal weight $\geq$ 500 g. The death of the woman who delivered the stillborn child is classified as indirect maternal mortality. Her death resulted from preexisting conditions—heart disease and diabetes—that were aggravated by the pregnancy. Although optimal medical and obstetric management may have altered both maternal and fetal outcome, the major factors contributing to her death preceded the pregnancy.

The death of the woman who died of septic shock is classified as direct maternal mortality. There is no evidence of illness preceding the pregnancy, and her death seems to be the result of the self-induced abortion. The death of the infant can be classified as a neonatal mortality—that is, death of a liveborn infant within 28 days of age—or perinatal mortality.

12–15. The answers are: 12-A, 13-B, 14-D, 15-D *[III A 4–9].*
Although birth control pills are highly effective, they carry significant risks of cardiovascular and embolic diseases for older women, especially women who also smoke. Oral contraceptives are also thought to be protective against certain conditions such as anemia, dysmenorrhea, ovarian cysts, and endometrial cancer.

The use of an intrauterine device (IUD) has been associated with increased risk of ectopic pregnancy, which may be due in part to the IUD's ability to prevent pregnancy in utero. IUDs are also associated with an increased risk of pelvic inflammatory disease (PID), which, along with ectopic pregnancy, may contribute to infertility.

Barrier methods of contraception may prevent the transmission of a variety of sexually transmitted diseases (STDs). Although protection is not absolute for every infection and every individual episode, the results are significant when large numbers of cases are reviewed. There is a slight increased risk of toxic shock syndrome from the barrier methods used by women (e.g., sponge, cervical cap, diaphragm), especially during the menses.

7
Health Care of the Young

Marie C. McCormick

I. HEALTH OF THE NEWBORN

A. Mortality rates. Several different rates are used to indicate health problems in infancy.

1. **Definitions**
   a. **Infant mortality rate (IMR)** is defined as the number of deaths among infants less than 1 year of age per 1000 live births in a given time period, usually 1 year. The IMR traditionally is divided into two segments: the **neonatal mortality rate (NMR)** and the **postneonatal mortality rate (PNMR)**.
      (1) The NMR is calculated as the number of deaths among infants less than 28 days old per 1000 live births.
      (2) The PNMR is calculated as the number of deaths among infants aged 28 days to 11 months per 1000 live births.
   b. **Fetal mortality rate (FMR)** refers to fetal loss in the third trimester of pregnancy, which results in stillbirth. This rate is defined as the number of stillbirths per 1000 births of gestational age greater than 28 weeks. The gestational age cutoff is meant to indicate that the fetuses are potentially viable. Some fetuses of lower gestational ages currently are surviving; a 20-week cutoff sometimes is used in calculating the FMR.
   c. **Perinatal mortality rate (PMR).** Since it may be difficult to determine what constitutes viability, especially in very tiny infants, the PMR is used to indicate infant loss around the time of the birth event. This rate is calculated as the number of deaths of fetuses of gestational age greater than 28 weeks (sometimes 20 weeks) plus the number of deaths of infants less than 7 days old per 1000 total births.

2. **Use of terms.** These mortality rates and the changes in them can be used to assess the type and volume of health problems in infancy because the causes of infant death also result in morbidity among surviving infants.
   a. **Neonatal mortality and perinatal mortality generally reflect causes of death related to maternal health** prior to pregnancy, as well as events during pregnancy, delivery, and the early neonatal period. These could include congenital anomalies, asphyxia, birth trauma, and immaturity.
   b. **Postneonatal mortality is more closely linked to environmental factors,** especially socioeconomic disadvantage. The major causes are infection, especially respiratory and gastrointestinal, sudden infant death syndrome, injury, and congenital anomalies.

B. Current trends in mortality. Mortality in infants is higher than that in any group of individuals under the age of 55 and accounts for the majority of deaths among individuals less than 18 years old. Current trends in infant, neonatal, and postneonatal mortality are summarized in Figure 7-1.

1. In 1989, the provisional IMR in the United States was 9.73 deaths per 1000 live births, which is a high figure for a developed country. (The United States ranks twenty-first among developed countries in infant mortality.) The 1989 IMR represents a major decline in infant mortality since the turn of the century, when it was about 100 in 1000 live births. The decrease has resulted from decreases in both postneonatal and neonatal mortality.
   a. Most of the decline in the PNMR occurred prior to 1950.
      (1) This decrease is attributed largely to changes in the environment, including improved sanitation and improved nutrition.
      (2) Little of this change is thought to have resulted from changes in medical care, including the introduction of immunization and antibiotics.

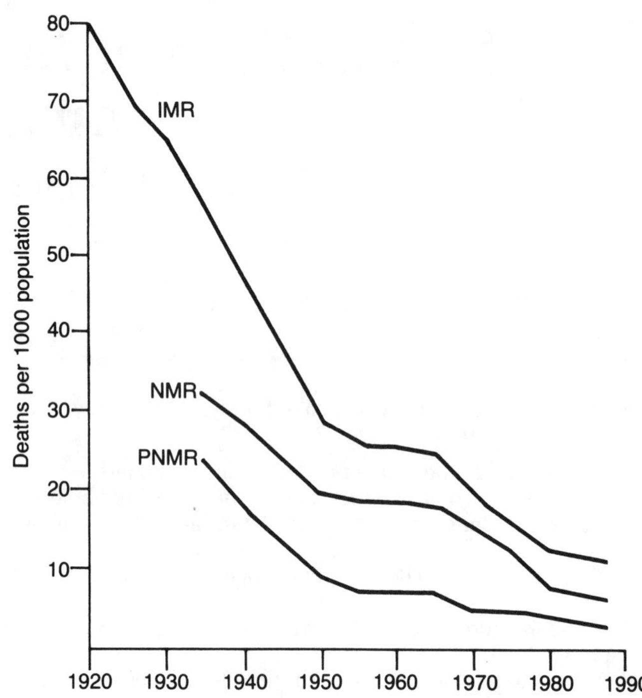

Figure 7-1. Infant mortality rate (*IMR*), neonatal mortality rate (*NMR*), and postneonatal mortality rate (*PNMR*) per 1000 population in the United States between 1920 and 1987. (Reprinted from US Department of Health and Human Services: *Health United States and Prevention Profile, 1988.* Hyattsville, MD, DHHS pub no (PHS) 90-1232, 1989.)

b. Although the NMR also decreased early in the twentieth century, a dramatic change has been seen over the past 20 years, when the NMR has been halved.
   - (1) In contrast to the decrease in PNMR, much of the decrease in the NMR is attributed to medical techniques aimed at increasing the survival of high-risk infants.
   - (2) Despite this decrease, deaths in the neonatal period account for two-thirds of infant deaths.

2. Since the early 1980s, however, the rate of decrease in infant mortality has slowed. The underlying reasons for this slowing include a lack of education about contraceptives and prenatal care, inaccessible prenatal services for disadvantaged groups, and the inability of technology to alter infant mortality in the absence of greater preventive successes.

C. Causes of mortality

1. **Neonatal mortality.** Most neonatal deaths are due to intrauterine growth failure, congenital anomalies, or birth injury.
   - a. **Intrauterine growth failure** is the major cause of neonatal mortality. This failure can occur in two ways.
     - (1) **Prematurity** refers to birth that occurs too soon. By definition, prematurity is gestation of less than 37 weeks since the last menstrual period.
     - (2) **Intrauterine growth retardation** refers to a lesser weight gain than appropriate for the duration of gestation. Because gestational age sometimes is difficult to determine, birth weight is used to designate the high-risk infant. A birth weight of 2500 g (5.5 lb) or less is believed to increase the risk of neonatal mortality, even if the infant is full-term or of gestational age of at least 37 weeks.
       - (a) Infants with a birth weight of 2500 g or less account for 6%–7% of births but more than 66% of neonatal deaths.
       - (b) As birth weight decreases, the NMR increases sharply, such that one-quarter to one-third of infants with a birth weight of 1500 g or less die in the neonatal period.
   - b. **Congenital anomalies and birth injury.** While low-birth-weight infants also may die from these causes, congenital anomalies and birth injury are the primary reasons for death among full-term and normal-birth-weight infants.
     - (1) **Birth injury and asphyxia** have declined as causes of death in the past 15 years. This is particularly true for infants weighing 4000 g or more at birth.

(2) In contrast, the NMR due to **congenital anomalies** has shown less change, remaining relatively constant at about 2 per 1000 live births. While prenatal screening may detect some types of anomalies and genetic disorders, two-thirds of these conditions cannot be anticipated or prevented with current techniques.

2. **Postneonatal mortality**
   a. **Lower respiratory tract infection** (e.g., bronchitis, pneumonia), diarrheal disease, and other infections are the major causes of postneonatal death. Most cases are manageable with current medical techniques, and many are preventable with good nutrition and hygiene.
   b. **Congenital anomalies** account for about 2 in 1000 postneonatal deaths. PNMRs above this level are considered to be related directly to socioeconomic disadvantage and lack of access to medical care.
   c. **Sudden infant death syndrome (SIDS)** also is a major cause of mortality and may include a heterogeneous set of conditions. While some of these deaths are not preventable, linking SIDS to a disadvantaged environment and linking the reduction of SIDS-related deaths to services for disadvantaged mothers suggest that some SIDS deaths are preventable.
   d. **Injury** is another cause of postneonatal death. In particular, infants are at much greater risk of dying in **motor vehicle accidents** than older children and adults because of their relatively large heads. The American Academy of Pediatrics (1990) recommends that infant car safety seats "designed to safely transport healthy newborns, premature infants, or infants with special needs" be used, starting with the first trip home from the hospital.

D. **Risk factors associated with infant mortality and morbidity** can be divided into those reflecting socioeconomic disadvantage and those reflecting biologic vulnerability of the mother.

1. **Socioeconomic disadvantage** can increase infant mortality in two ways: by increasing the risk of low birth weight and by increasing the risk of postneonatal death regardless of birth weight (e.g., due to infectious causes). The effects of socioeconomic disadvantage are believed to account for the increased risk of mortality among black infants, infants born to teenage mothers, and infants born to mothers of low educational attainment.

2. **Biologic vulnerabilities** are reflected primarily in neonatal loss, with an increased risk of low birth weight, as well as neonatal mortality regardless of birth weight (e.g., due to conditions secondary to immaturity and congenital anomalies). Biologic vulnerabilities may account for the increased risk of mortality among infants born to mothers aged 35 years and older and mothers with previous obstetric problems.

E. **Management and prevention of infant health problems**

1. **Identification of high-risk parents**
   a. **Maternal age**
      (1) Mothers younger than 18 have an increased risk of delivering a low-birth-weight infant.
      (2) Mothers older than 34 in the past presented an increased risk of delivering low-birth-weight infants but currently account for an insignificant percentage of such births.
   b. **Intrauterine infections.** Several organisms can produce congenital anomalies as well as increase the risk of low-birth-weight infants.
      (1) **Rubella** and **syphilis** are preventable.
      (2) **Other infections** [e.g., toxoplasmosis, herpes (HSV), cytomegalovirus (CMV)] can be detected by routine antibody screening of pregnant women.
   c. **Preexisting maternal illnesses.** Such conditions include heart, kidney, and thyroid disease; diabetes mellitus; hypertension; and substance abuse. Early detection and aggressive management of maternal illnesses can reduce the toll of infant loss.
   d. **Maternal history of reproductive problems.** Women who have experienced adverse conditions during prior pregnancies (e.g., premature labor, vaginal bleeding, hypertension, miscarriage, delivery of a low-birth-weight or stillborn infant) have an increased risk of adverse outcomes in subsequent pregnancies.
   e. **Family history of hereditary disease.** The presence of such a disease may suggest the need for screening and special management.

2. **Prevention of unwanted pregnancies among high-risk parents** may involve genetic counseling, sex education, and family planning.

3. **Management of high-risk pregnancies** includes:
   a. Early start of prenatal care, including preconceptional care and prenatal care recommended by the recent Public Health Service Expert Panel (1989)
   b. Identification of obstetric risk and referral to the appropriate level of obstetric care until resolution of the risk or delivery in a hospital equipped to manage potential problems related to complications of pregnancy
   c. A regionalized system of obstetric and neonatal services to coordinate and assure movement of patients and information among providers at various levels of care
   d. Monitoring and treatment of the newborn for problems related to obstetric and neonatal risk factors

4. **Management of high-risk newborns** includes:
   a. Immediate access to an intensive care nursery
   b. Continued medical, social, and nutritional monitoring following discharge from the intensive care nursery, including referral to early intervention programs (EIPs), mandated under PL 99-457 [see IV C 2 a (3) (f)]

II. HEALTH OF PRESCHOOLERS AND SCHOOLCHILDREN

A. Mortality

1. **Mortality rates**
   a. Mortality rates for children aged 1–14 years continue to decline.
      (1) Rates have declined from 870 per 100,000 children in 1900 to 30–40 per 100,000 as of 1987.
      (2) The declining mortality rates are attributed to improvements in sanitation, nutrition, and housing and to the availability of immunization and antibiotics.
   b. Despite the declining trend, childhood mortality remains a cause for concern.
      (1) Mortality among black children is twice that among white children.
      (2) Mortality rates for children in the United States are higher than those for children in other Western nations.
      (3) Over the past 10 years, childhood mortality rates have decreased very little.

2. **Causes of mortality**
   a. **Acquired immune deficiency syndrome (AIDS)** is an emerging cause of mortality in children between 1 and 4 years of age. In the United States as of August 1989, 1125 deaths due to AIDS were reported in children younger than 13 years. This figure is believed to underestimate the true extent of the disease.
      (1) **Transmission.** Most pediatric AIDS is acquired by transmission of human immunodeficiency virus (HIV) from the mother to the fetus around the time of birth, although transmission may also occur by transfusion, especially among hemophiliacs. Intrafamilial spread of HIV under routine conditions of care has not been documented.
      (2) Management of pediatric AIDS is complicated by the fact that the disease currently is concentrated in areas where the spread of AIDS is related to intravenous drug abuse. The mothers of pediatric AIDS patients may themselves be affected by both AIDS and drug addiction and may die before their children or may abandon them. Since these problems are currently concentrated in minority communities, management is further complicated by disadvantage and the risks of further stigmatization of minority groups.
   b. **Other causes** include:
      (1) Injuries (e.g., accidents, homicide), which account for 50% of all deaths
      (2) Congenital anomalies
      (3) Malignancies
      (4) Infections (e.g., influenza, pneumonia)
      (5) Gastroenteritis

B. Morbidity

1. **Morbidity rates**
   a. Morbidity rates are higher among children than adults. Children average 10 days of restricted activity and 5 days in bed per year, whereas adults 17–64 years of age average 9 days of restricted activity and 3–4 days in bed.

b. Morbidity rates generally are higher among children less than 6 years old and among those from lower income families. Acute conditions that are more common among poor individuals include *Hemophilus influenzae* meningitis, gastroenteritis, and parasitic disease.

2. Causes of morbidity

a. Acute physical conditions. Most acute conditions in children are attributable to three types of problems:

(1) Respiratory illnesses

(2) Infections and parasitic conditions

(3) Injuries

b. Chronic physical conditions. Although most childhood illnesses are self-limited, serious chronic illnesses affect 5%–10% of children.

(1) Congenital anomalies are the most frequently reported conditions among infants. **Asthma** is the most common chronic illness among older children, affecting 5% of schoolchildren.

(2) The current prevalence of serious chronic illness in children is directly related to the successful management of medical problems that previously resulted in early death.

3. "The new morbidity." There is recent concern for conditions that impede a child's achieving his or her full developmental potential. These conditions, referred to as "the new morbidity," include behavioral disorders, emotional problems, and specific learning disorders. Up to 15%–20% of children may experience one or more of these conditions.

C. Management and prevention of childhood mortality and morbidity

1. Immunization. Routine immunization of children has been shown repeatedly to be one of the most cost-effective means of preventing mortality and morbidity.

a. Recommended immunization schedules are detailed in Tables 7-1 and 7-2.

b. While vaccines are of demonstrated efficacy, access to immunizations may be limited by access to providers (e.g., public health clinics, pediatricians) and the high cost of vaccines as a result of liability concerns. Thus, attention to the mechanisms for delivering immunizations is required to assure that those children most vulnerable to morbidity due to disadvantage receive needed vaccines.

2. Screening for occult treatable conditions (see Ch 3 IV)

a. Criteria for screening

(1) The condition must represent an important health problem and have a recognizable latent or early symptomatic stage.

(2) Suitable screening tests and accepted treatment for the condition must exist, and diagnostic and treatment facilities must be available.

(3) The natural history of the condition should be understood.

(4) Case finding should be a continuing process, the cost of which should be balanced against the potential expenditures for treatment of symptomatic disease.

(5) There must be a policy dictating who should be treated.

b. Conditions for which screening has proven cost-effective follow, with the appropriate timing of the screening noted in parentheses.

(1) Phenylketonuria (PKU) [in the neonatal period]

(2) Congenital hypothyroidism (in the neonatal period)

(3) Iron deficiency anemia (at 9 months in high-risk populations)

(4) Lead poisoning (at preschool age in areas where the positive yield is greater than 6% of those screened)

(5) Tuberculosis (regularly during childhood in high-risk populations)

(6) Vision impairment (at 3–4 years)

c. Additional screening procedures that should be considered include:

(1) Assessment of physical growth and developmental status

(2) Measurement of blood pressure (in children 3 years of age and older)

(3) Hearing assessment

(4) Identification of sickle cell disease (in the neonatal period)

3. Prevention of specific health problems

a. Injuries are the major cause of death in preschoolers and school-age children. Two major approaches to prevention have been identified.

(1) Modification of hazards to reduce their potential to cause injury, such as:

(a) Use of products with child-proof caps

Table 7-1. Recommended Schedule for Active Immunization of Healthy Infants and Children

Recommended Age*	Immunizations	Comments
2 months	DTP, OPV, HbCV†	DTP and OPV can be initiated as early as age 4 weeks in areas of high endemicity or during epidemics
4 months	DTP, OPV, HbCV†	A 2-month interval (minimum of 6 weeks) is desired for OPV to avoid interference from previous dose
6 months	DTP, HbCV†	A third dose of OPV is not indicated in the United States but is desirable in geographic areas where polio is endemic
15 months	MMR,‡ HbCV§	Tuberculin testing may be done at the same visit
15–18 months	DTP,‖ OPV#	
4–6 years	DTP,** OPV	DTP and OPV can be given at or before school entry
11–12 years	MMR	MMR can be given at entry to middle school or junior high school unless a second dose was previously given
14–16 years	Td	Repeat every 10 years throughout life

DTP = diphtheria and tetanus toxoids with pertussis vaccine; *OPV* = oral poliovirus vaccine containing attenuated poliovirus types 1, 2, and 3; *MMR* = live measles, mumps, and rubella viruses in a combined vaccine; *HbCV* = *Hemophilus influenzae* type B (Hib) conjugate vaccine; *Td* = adult tetanus toxoid (full dose) and diphtheria toxoid (reduced dose) for adult use.

For all products used, the manufacturer's package insert should be consulted for instructions on storage, handling, dosage, and administration. Biologics prepared by different manufacturers may vary, and package inserts of the same manufacturer may change from time to time. (Reprinted from American Academy of Pediatrics: *Report of the Committee on Infectious Diseases,* 22nd edition. Elk Grove Village, IL, American Academy of Pediatrics, 1991, pp 17–18.)

*These recommended ages should not be construed as absolute (e.g., 2 months can be 6–10 weeks). However, MMR should not be given to children younger than age 12 months.
†As of October 1990, only one HbCV has been approved for use in children younger than age 15 months.
‡MMR may be given at 12 months of age in areas with recurrent measles transmission.
§Any licensed HbCV may be given.
‖DTP should be given 6–12 months after the third dose; it may be given simultaneously with MMR at age 15 months.
#OPV may be given simultaneously with MMR and HbCV at age 15 months or at any time between 12 and 24 months of age; priority should be given to administering MMR at the recommended age.
**DTP can be given up to the seventh birthday.

(b) Lowering the temperature of hot water heaters
(c) Installation of window guards

(2) **Modification of behavior** to reduce exposure to hazards, including the use of:
(a) Motorcycle and bicycle helmets
(b) Infant car seats

b. **Psychosocial problems** are more prevalent among children from socioeconomically disadvantaged families. Early intervention may prevent these problems in targeted groups of children.

(1) **High-risk groups** include:
(a) Children with an increased risk of morbidity and mortality by virtue of the circumstances of their birth (e.g., low birth weight, congenital malformations)
(b) Disadvantaged children whose development is hampered by lack of environmental stimulation
(c) Children with established problems known to result in severe developmental delay, such as Down syndrome

(2) **Preventive strategies**
(a) **Screening and monitoring** to detect the emergence of problems can be conducted as part of well-child care. Formal instruments have been developed for office use to screen for developmental delay, behavioral problems, school readiness, learning disabilities, and sports readiness. Problems discovered in such screening efforts require further diagnostic evaluation before recommendations can be made.
(b) Increasingly, the literature suggests that **more extensive preventive efforts** are successful in high-risk groups, especially those who are socioeconomically disadvantaged. Such efforts include the provision of child and maternal education to foster

Table 7-2. Recommended Immunization Schedules for Children Not Immunized in First Year of Life

Recommended Time Interval or Age	Immunizations	Comments
	Younger Than Age 7 Years	
First visit	DTP, OPV, MMR	MMR is given to children age 15 months or older; tuberculin testing may be done at same visit
	HbCV*	For children 15–59 months of age, HbCV can be given simultaneously with DTP and other vaccines (at separate sites)†
Interval after first visit		
2 months	DTP, OPV (HbCV)	A second dose of HbCV is indicated only in children whose first dose was received when younger than 15 months
4 months	DTP	A third dose of OPV is not indicated in the United States but is desirable in geographic areas where polio is endemic
10–16 months	DTP, OPV	OPV is not given if third dose was given earlier
4–6 years (should be at or before school entry)	DTP, OPV	DTP is not necessary if the fourth dose was given after the fourth birthday; OPV is not necessary if the third dose was given after the fourth birthday
11–12 years	MMR	MMR is given at entry to middle school or junior high
10 years later	Td	Repeat every 10 years throughout life
	7 Years of Age and Older‡§	
First visit	Td, OPV, MMR	
Interval after first visit		
2 months	Td, OPV	
8–14 months	Td, OPV	
11–12 years	MMR	MMR is given at entry to middle school or junior high
10 years later	Td	Repeat every 10 years throughout life

DTP = diphtheria and tetanus toxoids with pertussis vaccine; *OPV* = oral poliovirus vaccine containing attenuated poliovirus types 1, 2, and 3; *MMR* = live measles, mumps, and rubella viruses in a combined vaccine; *HbCV* = *Hemophilus influenzae* type B (Hib) conjugate vaccine; *Td* = adult tetanus toxoid (full dose) and diphtheria toxoid (reduced dose) for adult use. (Reprinted from American Academy of Pediatrics: *Report of the Committee on Infectious Diseases,* 22nd edition. Elk Grove Village, IL, American Academy of Pediatrics, 1991, pp 17–18.)

*As of October 1990, only one HbCV has been approved for use in children younger than 15 months.
†The initial three doses of DTP can be given at 1- to 2-month intervals; HbCV, MMR, DTP, and OPV can be given simultaneously at separate sites if return of the patient for future immunizations is doubtful.
‡If a person is age 18 years or older, routine OPV is not indicated in the United States.
§The minimal interval between doses of MMR is 1 month.

normal development through intensive schedules of home- and center-based physical therapy and educational services.

c. **Dental caries** remain a source of morbidity. Preventive techniques include:
   (1) Reduction of sugar in food, drink, and medicines
   (2) Community fluoridation of water supply
   (3) Topical fluoride applications and fluoride supplementation

d. **Strategies to prevent adult diseases.** Increasing attention is being paid to encouraging health behaviors in childhood to prevent adult chronic illness. Caution should be exercised, however, in the recommendations being made, as the long-term consequences of a lifetime commitment to special diets and other habits in a developing child are often unknown. Current recommendations include:
   (1) Routine measurement of blood pressure after age 3 years

(2) A prudent, balanced diet appropriate to the growth needs of the child
(3) An active exercise program appropriate to the child's age and coordination

III. HEALTH OF THE ADOLESCENT

A. General considerations

1. **Adolescence** is the period of life between puberty and full maturity, which is roughly from **12 to 17 years** of age. This period is characterized by rapid growth and change in anatomy and physiology as well as shifting values and allegiances. Approximately 11% of the population of the United States falls within this age-group.

2. **General health status of adolescents.** Using traditional morbidity and mortality measures, the health status of the adolescent in the United States is good. Most adolescents fall within a health category bounded by the categories of acute illnesses of childhood and the chronic conditions of later life.

B. Mortality

1. **Mortality rates.** Although mortality rates are relatively low (i.e., 35.1 per 100,000 adolescents 10–14 years of age and 101.6 per 100,000 adolescents 15–19 years of age), they are increasing—the only age-group for which this is true.

2. **Causes of mortality**
   a. **Injuries** represent the leading cause of death among adolescents; 36% of adolescent deaths are motor vehicle–related.
   b. Other traumatic causes of death include **homicide, suicide,** and **drowning**.
   c. **Cancer** is the only major cause of adolescent death that is not related to injury.
   d. **Use of alcohol and drugs and emotional problems** account for a substantial portion of adolescent deaths.

C. Morbidity

1. **Physical and mental problems**
   a. One in five adolescents has some form of **chronic illness, deformity,** or **physical handicap**.
   b. **Dental problems** affect two-thirds of the adolescent population, and **vision problems** affect one-third.
   c. **Skin pathology,** which includes acne, affects more than one-third of the adolescent population.
   d. **Mental health problems** are the fourth leading reason for short-term hospitalization, accounting for 11% of all adolescent hospital stays.

2. **Behavioral problems**
   a. **Alcohol use** is decreasing among adolescents, but still close to one-half (42%) of adolescents aged 16–17 years report some alcohol use in the past month.
   b. **Cigarette smoking** is reported by more than 10% of the population. Teenage girls smoke more than their male counterparts. Most adult smokers begin in adolescence.
   c. **Drug abuse,** including the use of marijuana, inhalants, hallucinogens, and cocaine, is increasing among this population.
   d. **Pregnancy and sexually transmitted diseases (STDs)** become important concerns as the teenager becomes sexually active. By age 19, 55.5% of the adolescent population has had sexual intercourse. Problems associated with adolescent pregnancy include the following.
      (1) There is a higher incidence of infant mortality among those infants born to adolescent mothers.
      (2) Adolescent mothers usually are unprepared psychologically, economically, and educationally for parenthood.
      (3) Adolescent parents are at increased risk for failure to complete their education and to find employment, thereby limiting their future economic well-being.
   e. **Eating behavior**
      (1) Preoccupation with body image and adult sexual roles has led to an increase in **anorexia nervosa** and **bulimia**—conditions with potentially severe metabolic side effects, including death.
      (2) The incidence of **obesity** also increases in adolescence, especially among adolescent girls.

D. Management and prevention of adolescent health problems

1. **Sex-related problems**
   a. **Sex education** is intended to increase the use of contraceptives by adolescents and thereby reduce the risk of unwanted pregnancy. The same is true for the provision of free contraceptive services.
   b. **Intensive management of adolescent pregnancies** may reduce the risk of low-birth-weight infants and, with follow-up, the risk of postneonatal death.
   c. **Routine adolescent care** should also include Pap smears and vaginal cultures for sexually active adolescent girls to screen for STDs and early cervical changes indicative of cancer.
   d. **Reproductive health services** for adolescents should be incorporated into routine well-person care in a setting that provides continuity of care sensitive to the needs of adolescents. School-based clinics have proven successful models of such care.

2. **Smoking and substance abuse**
   a. **Educational campaigns** meet with limited success, but intensive school-based efforts may limit cigarette smoking among adolescents.
   b. Potential **methods for prevention** of substance abuse include:
      (1) Enforcement of drinking-age laws
      (2) Parental monitoring

3. **Injuries**
   a. **Regulatory activities** have proven more effective than educational campaigns. Such activities include the establishment of
      (1) Drinking-age laws
      (2) Motorcycle and bicycle helmet laws
      (3) Requirements for protective gear in athletic programs
      (4) Regulations concerning access to firearms
   b. **Management** of injuries is an essential component of an adolescent health program, which should also include prompt access to emergency services and careful assessment of psychologic status. Management of injuries and drug ingestion in adolescents also may require referral to mental health services if suicidal intent is indicated.

IV. ORGANIZATION AND FINANCING OF CHILDREN'S HEALTH SERVICES

A. Health care providers

1. **Pediatricians**
   a. Visits to pediatricians account for 35% of physician visits by children who are 19 years of age or younger. Remaining visits are primarily to family and general practitioners.
   b. Visits to pediatricians account for the majority of physician visits by children who are less than 10 years of age, and by children in urban areas under 19 years of age.

2. **Specialists.** Children with chronic problems (e.g., diabetes, seizure disorders, arthritis) may have to rely on adult specialists because pediatric specialists may not be available.

3. **Nurse practitioners and child health associates** constitute the major health care providers in certain settings, such as:
   a. Schools
   b. Jails
   c. Specific populations, such as disadvantaged high-risk groups

4. **Dentists and dental hygienists** are widely available to children of middle-class families but, because of cost considerations, are less frequently visited by children of low-income families.

B. Sources of care

1. Most children (65%) receive care from private practitioners in office-based practices.

2. Other sources of care include hospital emergency and outpatient departments (12%), school health services (13%), public health clinics (5%), special government programs (3%), and special volunteer agencies (2%).

3. Minority and disadvantaged children are more likely to rely on hospital and public health facilities. Children with more health problems rely on hospital clinics.

C. Financing care

1. **Insurance.** In 1988, 73% of children under 21 years of age had private insurance coverage; 14% were without any coverage, public or private.
   a. Even with insurance, the payment for much of child health care is provided out-of-pocket by the parents.
   b. Most children's health services occur in the ambulatory setting and may not be covered by insurance.
   c. Insurance packages may not cover catastrophic situations (e.g., neonatal intensive care, treatment of cancer).
   d. The proportion of the general population without insurance has risen in the past few years. Children are disproportionately affected for the following reasons:
      (1) They are more likely to be in poor families, and the proportion of poor families with public insurance for health services has decreased since the mid-1970s.
      (2) Young adults in the childbearing age-range are the group least likely to have health insurance, due to shifts in the job market.
      (3) Increasingly, even insured working adults may not have dependent coverage, or coverage may be lost with divorce.
2. **Government services.** Several mechanisms for health care financing are available to disadvantaged children and children with special health problems.
   a. **Federal services**
      (1) **Medicaid,** which is both state and federally funded, pays for the health care of adults (and their children) who are on welfare **(Aid to Dependent Children)**.
      (2) **Social Security Act**
         (a) **Title V** of this act provides services for maternal and child health, crippled children's services, child welfare, and aid to dependent children.
         (b) **Title XX** provides payment for social services related to child neglect and abuse.
      (3) **Other child services** financed through the federal government include:
         (a) Special Supplemental Food Program for Women, Infants, and Children **(WIC)**
         (b) **PL-142,** which provides for the education of all handicapped children
         (c) **Centers for Disease Control programs** (e.g., immunization services, screening for lead poisoning)
         (d) Office of Adolescent Pregnancy Program
         (e) Sudden Infant Death Program
         (f) **PL99-457,** which provides support for the provision and coordination of early intervention programs (EIPs) for children 0–3 years of age.
   b. **State and local services.** State and local governments also have major funding responsibilities, including matching funds for federal programs as well as direct funding of health services. For example, routine pregnancy and well-child care and screening and therapy for lead poisoning and tuberculosis are provided by city and county health departments.

BIBLIOGRAPHY

American Academy of Pediatrics: *Pediatrics* 86:486–487, 1990.

Committee on Prenatal and Newborn Screening for HIV Infection: *HIV Screening of Pregnant Women and Newborns.* Washington, DC, National Academy Press, 1991.

Furstenberg FF, Brooks-Gunn J: Teen-age childbearing: causes, consequences and remedies. In *Applications of Social Science to Clinical Medicine and Health Policy.* Edited by Aiken CH, Mechanic D. New Brunswick, NJ, Rutgers University Press, 1988.

Kalter H, Warkany J: Congenital malformations: etiologic factors and the role in prevention. *N Engl J Med* 308:424–431, 491–497, 1983.

Kramer MS: Intrauterine growth and gestational duration determinants. *Pediatrics* 80:502–511, 1987.

McCormick MC: The contribution of low birth weight to infant mortality and childhood morbidity. *N Engl J Med* 312:82–90, 1985.

McCormick MC, Brooks-Gunn J: The health of children and adolescents. In *Handbook of Medical Sociology,* 4th edition. Edited by Freeman HE, Levine S. Englewood Cliffs, NJ, Prentice Hall, 1989.

Newacheck PN: Improving access to health care for children, youth, and pregnant women. *Pediatrics* 86:626–635, 1990.

Novello AC, Wise PH, Willoughby A, Pizzo PA: Final report of the United States Department of Health and Human Services secretary's work group in pediatric human immunodeficiency virus infection and disease: content and implications. *Pediatrics* 84:547–555, 1989.

Pharoah POD, Morris JN: Postneonatal mortality. *Epidemiol Rev* 1:170–183, 1978.

Renner C, Navarro V: Why is our population of uninsured and underinsured persons growing? The consequences of the "deindustrialization" of America. *Ann Rev Public Health* 10:85–94, 1989.

Rivara FP: Traumatic deaths in children in the United States: currently available prevention strategies. *Pediatrics* 75:450–462, 1985.

Shapiro S, Schlesinger ER, Nesbitt REL: *Infant, Prenatal, Maternal and Childhood Mortality in the United States.* Cambridge, MA: Harvard University Press, 1963.

US Department of Health and Human Services: *Health United States and Prevention Profile, 1988.* Hyattsville, MD, DHHS pub no (PHS) 90-1232, 1989.

US Public Health Service Panel on The Content of Prenatal Care: *Caring for Our Future: The Content of Prenatal Care.* Washington, DC, US Department of Health and Human Services, US Public Health Service, 1989.

Wegman ME: Annual summary of vital statistics—1989. *Pediatrics* 86:835–847, 1990. (The annual summary of vital statistics appears each year in the December issue.)

STUDY QUESTIONS

Directions: Each of the numbered items or incomplete statements in this section is followed by answers or by completions of the statement. Select the **one** lettered answer or completion that is **best** in each case.

1. All of the following statements concerning the IMR in the United States are true EXCEPT

(A) the IMR in the United States is considered high for a developed country
(B) the United States ranks about twenty-first among developed countries in infant mortality
(C) the decline in the IMR over the past century has resulted from decreases in only the NMR
(D) the IMR accounts for the majority of deaths among individuals less than 18 years of age
(E) the decline in the IMR is closely linked to both advances in medical care and changes in the environment

2. The PNMR has been most closely linked to

(A) maternal health prior to pregnancy
(B) events during delivery
(C) environmental factors
(D) maternal health during pregnancy
(E) events during the early neonatal period

3. All of the following are criteria for screening a population for a given condition EXCEPT

(A) the natural history of the condition should be understood
(B) the condition must represent an important health problem
(C) suitable screening tests for the condition must exist
(D) screening should be available to and used by the entire population
(E) accepted treatment for the condition must be available

4. Screening of children has been proven cost-effective for all of the following EXCEPT

(A) tuberculosis
(B) iron deficiency anemia
(C) hypertension
(D) vision impairment
(E) PKU

5. Most physician visits by children 19 years of age or younger are to

(A) pediatricians
(B) family and general practitioners
(C) subspecialty physicians
(D) internists
(E) emergency room physicians

1-C
2-C
3-D
4-C
5-B

Directions: Each item below contains four suggested answers of which **one or more** is correct. Choose the answer

A if **1, 2, and 3** are correct
B if **1 and 3** are correct
C if **2 and 4** are correct
D if **4** is correct
E if **1, 2, 3, and 4** are correct

6. Measures taken in the management and prevention of infant health problems include

(1) managing high-risk pregnancies
(2) managing high-risk newborns
(3) preventing unwanted pregnancies among high-risk parents
(4) providing neonatal intensive care units at all hospitals offering obstetric services

7. Mortality rates in the United States are increasing for

(1) infants
(2) preschoolers
(3) schoolchildren
(4) adolescents

8. The recommended immunization schedule for children includes vaccination against

(1) polio
(2) pertussis
(3) tetanus
(4) smallpox

9. At each well-child visit for a child up to 24 months of age, the pediatrician will measure

(1) height
(2) weight
(3) head circumference
(4) blood pressure

10. Motor vehicle safety, especially the use of appropriate restraining devices, should be discussed at routine visits for which of the following age-groups?

(1) Infants under 1 year of age
(2) Toddlers 1–4 years of age
(3) School-age children 5–13 years of age
(4) Adolescents older than 13

11. Reproductive care for sexually active adolescent girls should include

(1) prescription for an acceptable method of birth control
(2) HIV screening
(3) routine pelvic examinations and Pap smear
(4) recommendations of abstinence

12. Children who may receive inadequate well-child care include

(1) children on Medicaid
(2) children with chronic health problems
(3) children of mothers who started receiving prenatal care late in the second trimester
(4) children whose parents work at jobs that do not provide health insurance

13. Children are at greater risk now than 10 years ago for no health insurance or for underinsurance because

(1) Medicaid, the major public health insurance for the poor, now covers a lower percentage of those below the federal poverty level
(2) young adults are more likely to work at jobs that do not offer health insurance as a benefit or do not offer coverage for dependents
(3) more children live in poverty
(4) more children live in single-parent families due to divorce

---

6-A
7-D
8-A
9-A
10-E
11-B
12-E
13-E

ANSWERS AND EXPLANATIONS

1. The answer is C *[I B 1].*
The decline in the infant mortality rate (IMR) in the United States over the past century has resulted not only from decreases in the neonatal mortality rate (NMR) but also from decreases in the postneonatal mortality rate (PNMR). (The IMR is traditionally divided into two segments, NMR and PNMR.) Most of the decline in PNMR occurred prior to 1950 and can be attributed to environmental changes (e.g., improved sanitation, improved nutrition). The more dramatic decreases in NMR have occurred over the past 20 years and are attributed to the development of medical techniques aimed at increasing the survival rate of high-risk infants. Despite these decreases, the United States has a high IMR for a developed country, ranking about twenty-first in the world.

2. The answer is C *[I A 2 b, D 1].*
Postneonatal mortality (PNMR) has been most closely linked to environmental factors, especially economic disadvantage. Maternal health prior to pregnancy as well as events during pregnancy, delivery, and the early neonatal period are most closely linked to neonatal and perinatal mortality.

3. The answer is D *[II C 2 a].*
Screening does not need to be available to nor used by the entire population to be effective. Screening procedures have been found to be most effective when there are policies dictating who should be treated. In general, all screening tests may not be warranted or cost-effective for the entire population. Screening should be used only when the natural history of the condition is understood, the condition represents an important health problem, suitable screening tests exist, and an accepted treatment for the condition is available.

4. The answer is C *[II C 2 b, c].*
Targeted screening among children has been proven cost-effective for tuberculosis, iron deficiency anemia, vision impairment, and phenylketonuria (PKU). Although screening for hypertension (i.e., blood pressure measurement in children 3 years of age and older) should be considered, this technique may not be cost-effective because the natural history of hypertension in this age-group is not well understood, and blood pressure measurement is difficult.

5. The answer is B *[IV A 1].*
Most physician visits by children 19 years of age or younger are to family and general practitioners. Visits to pediatricians account for only 35% of physician visits by children in this age-group. However, visits to pediatricians account for the majority of physician visits by children who are younger than 10 and by children in urban areas.

6. The answer is A (1, 2, 3) *[I E].*
Measures taken in the management and prevention of infant health problems include managing high-risk pregnancies and high-risk newborns and preventing unwanted pregnancies among high-risk parents. It is not necessary to have neonatal intensive care units at all hospitals offering obstetric services. Rather, these services should be effectively regionalized, guaranteeing accessibility to those in need of the services.

7. The answer is D (4) *[III B 1].*
Although mortality rates for adolescents are relatively low, they are increasing. This is the only age-group in the United States exhibiting increasing mortality rates. Conversely, the mortality rates for infants in this country is quite high but is decreasing. Mortality among infants is higher than that among any other group of individuals under the age of 55 years. Mortality rates for children 1–14 years of age continue to decline in the United States but remain a cause for concern. Childhood mortality rates in this country are higher than those in other Western nations and, over the last 10 years, have decreased very little.

8. The answer is A (1, 2, 3) *[Tables 7-1, 7-2].*
The recommended immunization schedule for children includes vaccination against polio, diphtheria, pertussis, tetanus, measles, mumps, *Hemophilus influenzae* type B, and rubella; a schedule for their administration is well established. Smallpox vaccine is no longer recommended for the general population. Routine immunization of children has been shown repeatedly to be one of the most cost-effective means of preventing childhood mortality and morbidity.

9. The answer is A (1, 2, 3) *[II C 2 c].*
At each well-child visit up to 24 months of age, the pediatrician measures height, weight, and head circumference. Routine monitoring of growth parameters is an important screen for a variety of health problems, and failure to attain expected physical growth along one or more of these measures may be the first sign of hereditary problems or acquired disease. Obtaining blood pressure measurements in infants is difficult and may require special equipment. Also, normal values are less well established for infants than for other age-groups. Current recommendations are for routine blood pressure measurements to begin at age 3 years.

10. The answer is E (all) *[II C 3 a; III B 2 a].*
Motor vehicle accidents are a major cause of death due to injuries in all age ranges. For infants and toddlers, discussion should focus on the use of car seats and when to start using regular seat belts, appropriate to all ages. Modeling of behavior by reinforcing parental use of seatbelts is also important.

11. The answer is B (1, 3) *[III C 2 d, D 1 c, d].*
If the adolescent girl is already sexually active, the preventive services are aimed at preventing pregnancy and detecting sex-related problems such as infection or dysplasia. Human immunodeficiency virus (HIV) testing should not be routine unless there is a history of contact with an HIV-positive sexual partner, prostitution, or intravenous drug abuse. Recommendations of abstinence may reinforce a later start of intercourse in the adolescent who has not initiated such behavior, but it is not likely to influence the sexually active girl, and it may reduce the effectiveness of the physician as a resource in her care.

12. The answer is E (all) *[IV B, C].*
Children on Medicaid, children with chronic health problems, children of mothers who started receiving prenatal care late in the second trimester, and children whose parents work at jobs that do not supply health insurance are at risk for not receiving adequate preventive care. Although poor children on Medicaid have their medical care paid for, alterations in eligibility and a history of inadequate care may predispose to an emphasis on care related only to illness. While children with chronic illnesses may be seen frequently for their health problems, routine preventive services may be forgotten, although often of greater importance to children who are compromised by other health conditions. The working parent may or may not be able to afford medical care in the absence of insurance and may have less flexibility in scheduling routine care for their child. Finally, failure to use one preventive service is a risk factor for failure to use other such services. Thus, the mother with inadequate prenatal care should be a red flag with regard to well-child care.

13. The answer is E (all) *[IV C 1–2].*
More children live in poverty than 10 years ago, in part because of the increase in the number of single-parent families. Welfare eligibility requirements have been tightened; hence, fewer such families are eligible for Medicaid coverage, the major source of medical coverage for poor families. Health insurance coverage may also be lost with divorce in cases where the insurance was obtained through the noncaretaking parent's job. Even with employment, the job structure has changed so that fewer industries offer health insurance as a benefit or as a benefit for dependents.

8
Injuries

Lawrence D. Budnick

I. INTRODUCTION

A. Definition

1. The term **injury** is derived from the Latin term *in juris* meaning "not right."
2. An injury is the physical damage to a person that occurs as a result of exposure to physical or chemical agents at rates greater than the body can tolerate or the absence of such essentials as heat or oxygen. An injury is generally considered to occur acutely after exposure. Injury and **trauma** are synonymous.
3. Injuries are often considered separately from diseases, although they are part of the spectrum of diseases. The difference between an injury and a disease may be only one of the dose of the causal factor, the time course during which the causal factor operates, or the body's adaptation and response to the causal factor.
   a. Injuries and diseases are often caused by the same factors, although the amount or the rate of exposure may differ.
      (1) Radiation can cause a burn (injury) and cancer (disease).
      (2) Carbon monoxide can cause brain damage and encephalopathy (injury) and secondary polycythemia (disease).
      (3) Kinetic energy can cause a fracture (injury) and arthritis (disease).
   b. Although the symptoms of an injury are usually immediately obvious as compared to the symptoms of disease, the duration of latency periods for injuries and diseases overlap.
      (1) Whiplash, an acceleration extension injury of the cervical spine, may not cause symptoms until days after the injury occurred.
      (2) Lead poisoning damage may not be evident until long after the exposure, but once evident, may progress rapidly.
      (3) Foodborne *Bacillus cereus* disease has an incubation period as short as 1 hour.
      (4) Altitude decompression sickness, or caisson disease (the "bends"), which is due to nitrogen bubbles forming in the blood and tissues, occurs immediately after a too rapid decompression from a high pressure environment.

B. Accidents

1. Injuries, especially unintentional injuries (see IV A 2) have often been referred to as "accidents." The term "accident," however, inappropriately implies chance misfortune and lack of predictability, which inaccurately describe the epidemiology of injuries (see II). The convention of describing the injury and the injury-causing event should be followed rather than using the term "accident," which is imprecise and unscientific.
2. The term "accident proneness," first used in 1926, is also inappropriate because hidden psychological impulses or motives have little to do with the cause of injuries.
3. Although the term "accident" generally is not used in scientific communications, it continues to be used in some classification and surveillance systems.
   a. The International Classification of Diseases (ICD) from the U.S. Department of Health and Human Services (DHHS) [Table 8-1] still uses the term.
   b. The U.S. National Center for Health Statistics classifies unintentional injuries as "accidents and adverse effects."
   c. Statistics Canada classifies injuries as "accidents, poisonings, and violence."

Table 8-1. International Classification of Diseases (ICD): Supplementary Classification of External Causes of Injury and Poisoning (E Code Classification)

Transport accidents*
Accidental poisonings†
Surgical and medical procedures‡
Accidental falls
Accidents caused by fire and flames
Accidents due to natural and environmental factors
Accidents caused by submersion, suffocation, and foreign bodies
Other accidents
Late effects of accidental injury
Drugs, medicinal and biologic substances causing adverse effects in therapeutic use
Suicide and self-inflicted injury
Homicide and injury purposely inflicted by other individuals
Legal intervention
Injury undetermined whether accidentally or purposely inflicted
Injury resulting from operations of war

Adapted from US Department of Health and Human Services: *International Classification of Diseases,* 9th revision, clinical modification, vol 1. Washington, DC, DHHS pub no (PHS) 80-1260, 1982.

*Include railway, motor vehicle traffic, motor vehicle nontraffic, other road vehicle, water transport, air and space transport, and vehicle accidents not classifiable elsewhere.

†Include by drugs, medicinal and biologic substances, and by other solid and liquid substances, gases, and vapors.

‡As the cause of an abnormal reaction of a patient or later complication, with or without mention of misadventure at the time of the procedure.

C. **Injury control and public health.** As the scientific base of information concerning injuries, their causes, and their prevention expands, public health and preventive and clinical medicine practitioners are applying increasing attention and resources to the field of injury prevention and control (see V; VI D).

1. The five principal **areas of study in injury control** are
   a. **Epidemiology** (see II), including surveillance (see V)
   b. **Prevention** (see VI)
   c. **Injury biomechanics,** which applies the principles of mechanics in studying the physical and functional responses of the human body to the traumatic impact of energy
   d. **Treatment,** including emergency response
   e. **Rehabilitation,** the process by which an injured person's functional capacities are restored or developed to the fullest extent possible, consistent with irreversible impairments and environmental limitations
2. The **public health model of injury prevention and control** offers opportunities for decreasing the incidence of injuries using the following approaches:
   a. **Surveillance,** including feedback from those conducting surveillance to those being studied and to those with a need to know
   b. Interdisciplinary **education** and **prevention** programs
   c. **Environmental** modifications
   d. **Regulatory** action
   e. The support of **clinical** interventions

II. EPIDEMIOLOGIC CONSTRUCTS.

An injury is a problem of medical ecology—that is, it is a problem in the relationship between one or more individuals and the surrounding environment, related to time. An epidemiologic web consisting of factors relating to the host or individual, the physical and social environments, the agent, and the vector can be delineated for injuries, as well as for infectious and chronic diseases (see Ch 1 IV A).

A. Host

1. The host, or **affected individual,** has been the principal focus of the research related to injuries and preventive measures aimed at decreasing injury rates.

2. An injury may result when the requirements of a task being performed exceed an individual's performance capacity, which varies with the individual's physical, psychological, and cognitive abilities. **Ergonomics, or human factors,** research focuses on the interface between the host's capabilities and the environmental and task demands.

3. A **risk factor** is an attribute, determinant, or exposure that is associated with an increased probability of a condition or outcome. **Host factors** that affect the risk of injuries differ according to the type of injury, as do some **risk indicators**. According to Clark (1981), characteristics that are associated with a condition but are neither causal nor controllable, such as age, sex, and race, are more appropriately called risk indicators, not risk factors.
   - **a. Age.** Figure 8-1 shows the mortality rates due to injuries in the United States in 1988 by age-group.
     - **(1)** Young children have less control over their environment. For example, suffocation or asphyxiation is the leading cause of fatal infant injuries.
     - **(2)** Young adults have less experience in responding to dangerous situations and are more likely to engage in high-risk behaviors. Homicide and motor vehicle–related injury rates are highest in young adults.
     - **(3)** Adults 65 years of age or older are most susceptible to complications when injured.
       - **(a)** The case-fatality rate for injuries is increased for older adults, compared to younger persons.
       - **(b)** Older adults have increased mortality rates due to suicide, motor vehicle–related injuries, and falls.
   - **b. Sex.** Table 8-2 summarizes the ratios of age-standardized death rates for injuries in the United States in 1988 by sex. Males are more prone to violent behavior and are at an increased risk of injury.
   - **c. Race**
     - **(1)** American blacks have over a sixfold higher rate of homicide (rates are especially high among young adult males) and a lower rate of suicide than whites (see Table 8-2).
     - **(2)** Native Americans and Alaskan Natives have a threefold higher rate of fatal injuries compared to other Americans (e.g., childhood poisonings, drownings, firearms-related injuries, homicide, motor vehicle–related injuries).
     - **(3)** Asian Americans have a lower rate of firearms-related injuries than other Americans.
   - **d. Alcohol use.** The use of alcohol increases the risk of injuries.
     - **(1) Motor vehicle–related injuries**
       - **(a)** Almost 50% of all motor vehicle–related fatalities are alcohol-related in either the driver, pedestrian, or bicyclist (the rate increases during holiday periods). In 1988, Congress urged the Surgeon General to declare drunk driving a national crisis.
       - **(b) Blood alcohol concentration.** As alcohol consumption increases, the risk of, and severity of, injury increases.
         - **(i)** A blood alcohol concentration of **0.10 g/dl** is used in most states as the legal limit for evidence of impaired driving due to alcohol.
         - **(ii)** Five states—California, Maine, Oregon, Utah, and Vermont—currently use a blood alcohol concentration of 0.08 g/dl as the legal limit.
         - **(iii)** A number of federal agencies have proposed using a blood alcohol concentration of 0.05 g/dl as the legal limit.
     - **(2) Other injuries.** Alcohol use is associated with other injuries, including burns, drownings, falls, firearms-related injuries, homicide, hypothermia, occupational injuries, poisonings, suicide, and injuries related to sports and aviation.
   - **e. Drug use** also can increase the risk of injuries.
     - **(1) Medications,** such as tranquilizers and barbiturates, increase the rate of injuries when they interfere with adaptive performance.
     - **(2) Illegal drugs.** The use of cocaine and other illegal drugs has been associated with fatal motor vehicle–related injuries. In addition, these drugs often are used in association with alcohol.
   - **f. Physical condition**
     - **(1) Chronic medical conditions.** Some chronic medical conditions, such as poor vision and uncontrolled seizure disorders, increase the risk of injuries.
     - **(2) Physiologic status.** Osteoporosis, which is often related to endocrine status, increases the risk of fall-related injuries.

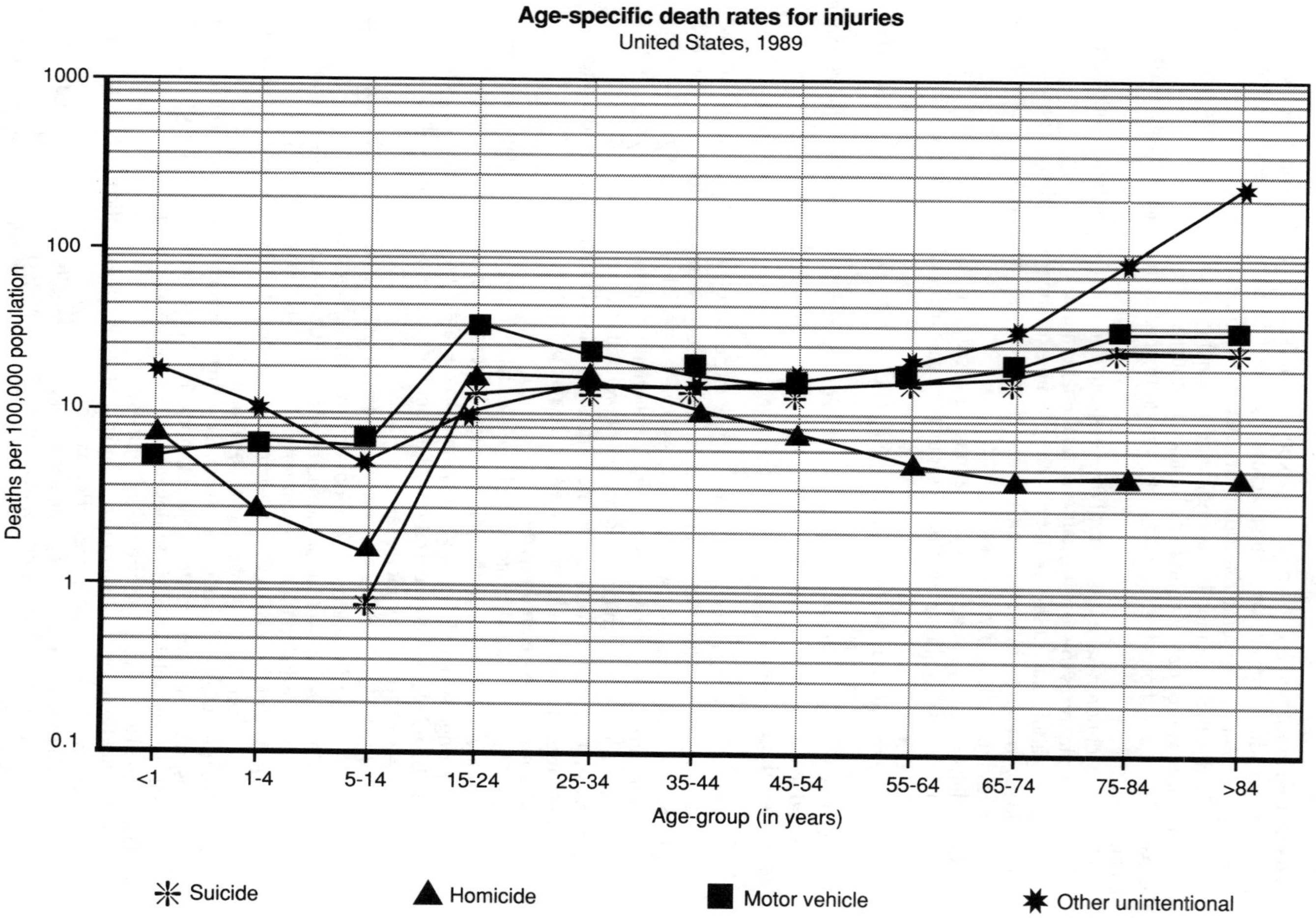

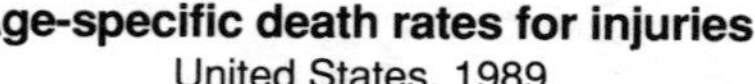

Figure 8-1. Age-specific death rates for injuries and all causes in the United States, 1988. [Adapted from National Center for Health Statistics: Advance report of final mortality statistics, 1988. *Monthly Vital Statistics Report* 39(7):24–25, 1990.]

Table 8-2. The Ratio of Age-Adjusted Death Rates for Injuries in the United States in 1988 by Sex and Race

Injury Type	Male:Female	Black:White
Unintentional motor vehicle–related	2.50	0.94
Other unintentional	2.95	1.77
Homicide and legal intervention	3.31	6.43
Suicide	3.98	0.56
All causes of death	1.72	1.55

Adapted from National Center for Health Statistics: Advance report of final mortality statistics, 1988. *Monthly Vital Statistics Report* 39(7):7, 1990.

B. Environment

1. **Physical environment** is the location at which the injury occurs. Examples of alterations made in the physical environment that can increase or reduce the risk of injuries include the following.
   a. Road design can decrease or increase the risk of injuries. A road barrier can assist an automobile to come to a safe stop or can become a hazard by functioning as a spear and piercing an occupant of an automobile.
   b. Homes can be built or equipped with safety features, such as smoke detectors and automatic sprinkler systems, in which case a fire is less likely to result in fire and flame-related injuries than a fire in a home without such devices.
   c. Swimming pools with fences are safer than pools without fences.

2. **Social environment** consists of societal attitudes, laws, and regulations that control or tolerate the occurrence of events that can lead to injuries. Examples of social environmental factors that increase the risk of injuries include:
   a. Tolerance of violent behavior
   b. Acceptance of the use of alcohol and other drugs
   c. Economic deprivation
   d. Racism
   e. Sexism

C. Agent. The injury-causing agent is **energy**. As noted in I A 3, a large amount of energy quickly transmitted may result in injury, while a small amount of energy transmitted over a long period of time may result in disease. There are five types of energy that cause injuries.

1. **Kinetic, or mechanical, energy** is the most common cause of injuries.
   a. In an automobile crash, the energy transferred by the motor vehicle that injures a person is kinetic energy. The energy imparted is proportional to the square of the speed of the vehicle. Thus, if the speed doubles, the amount of energy transmitted to the occupant quadruples.
   b. The energy resulting from a fall that injures a person also is kinetic energy.

2. **Thermal energy,** when excessive, is the most common cause of burns. A marked lack of thermal energy results in hypothermia and frostbite.

3. **Electrical energy** causes electrocutions and burns.

4. **Radiation energy** causes burns.

5. **Chemical energy,** by interfering with the body's energy metabolism, can cause injuries.
   a. Inhaled water interferes with pulmonary function, which can result in drowning.
   b. Carbon monoxide interferes with the oxygen-carrying capacity of blood, which can result in acute brain injury.

D. Vector. The vectors, or vehicles of injury, are the carriers of the energy. The design of the vector markedly alters the amount of energy available to cause an injury. Examples of vector factors that alter the occurrence of injuries follow.

1. **Weapons** are vectors of kinetic energy. Firearm design can decrease or increase the risk of injuries.
   a. Firearms with safety locks discharge unintentionally less frequently than firearms without safety locks.
   b. Small, easily concealed firearms can increase the risk of aggravated assault.

2. **Automobiles** are vectors of kinetic energy. Automobile design can decrease or increase the risk of injuries.
   a. **Safety features.** Automobiles with **air bags** and **automatic safety belts** can protect occupants from many potentially fatal or injury-causing crashes.
      (1) The National Highway Traffic Safety Administration estimates that safety belts saved the lives of almost 11,000 front-seat occupants between 1983 and 1987.
      (2) As of 1990, all new cars in the United States were required to have the following:
         (a) Either a driver-side air bag and manually operated safety belts or automatic safety belts for front-seat occupants
         (b) Lap and shoulder safety belts for rear-seat occupants
   b. **Small automobiles** are associated with an increased risk of fatal injuries.
3. **Electric wires** are vectors of electrical energy. Insulated electric wire is safer than noninsulated wire.

III. MEASURES OF IMPACT

A. Morbidity

1. **United States.** The total incidence of injuries and disability prevalence due to injuries in the United States in 1985, as recently reported in a major cost-estimate study, are summarized in Figure 8-2, which is a pyramid showing the distribution of injuries by hospitalization and death.
   a. **Incidence.** About **57 million people** were injured in 1985, which is almost one-fourth of the population.
      (1) Injuries account for about 16% of all **acute conditions,** ranking second after respiratory conditions.
      (2) **Falls** are the leading cause of nonfatal injury, causing about 12 million injuries annually and about 800,000 hospitalizations. Falls resulting in hospitalization are especially prevalent among individuals 65 years of age and older.
   b. **Host factors**
      (1) **Age.** Overall, the incidence rates of most nonfatal injuries decrease with age. The hospitalization rates increase with age, because the risks of complications resulting from an injury increase with age.
      (2) **Sex.** The incidence rate of injuries is greater among males than females, except among individuals 65 years of age and older (see Table 8-2).
2. **Canada**
   a. The injury pyramid is similar in Canada. For example, 300 children are injured for every 1 hospitalized, and 40 children are hospitalized for an injury for every 1 injury death.
   b. The risk of firearms-related injuries is markedly decreased in Canada compared with the United States.

B. Mortality

1. **United States.** The incidence of fatal injuries and the years of life lost due to injuries in the United States in 1985 are summarized in Figure 8-2. The patterns of fatal and nonfatal injuries are not necessarily similar.
   a. **Incidence**
      (1) **Fatal injuries,** which constitute the most widely available data base for surveillance, make up only a small percentage of injuries. In addition to the 143,000 who died in 1985 due to injuries, an estimated 13,000 more will die sometime after 1985 as a result of injuries sustained in that year.
      (2) In 1988, all injuries caused about 152,600 deaths and were the **third leading cause of death**. The leading cause of death was diseases of the heart (765,000 deaths), followed by malignant neoplasms (485,000 deaths).
   b. **Host factors.** Injury mortality rates vary by host factors (see II A). For example, injuries cause about 50% or more of all deaths among people 1–34 years of age. For people 1–44 years of age, injuries are the leading cause of death.
   c. **Environmental factors.** Mortality rates of unintentional injuries are higher in rural areas, and mortality rates of intentional injuries are higher in urban areas.

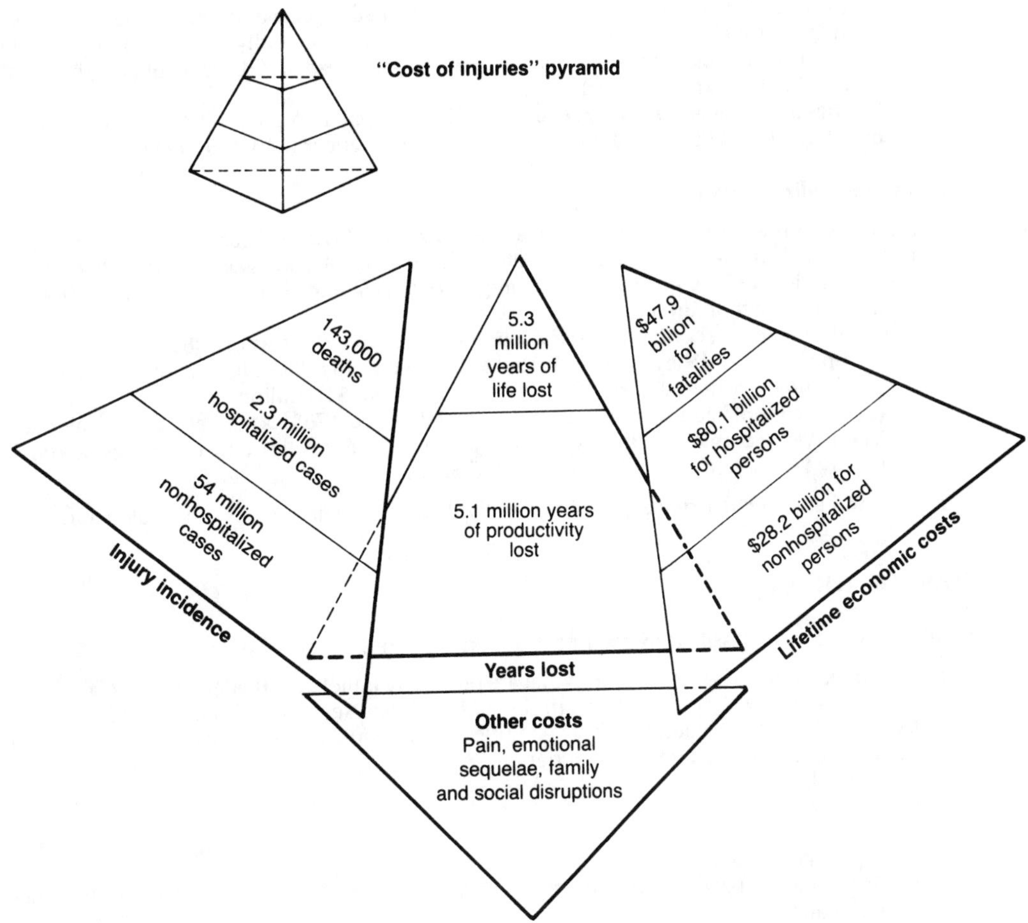

Figure 8-2. A pyramid conceptualizing the estimated costs of injuries in the United States in 1985. The *back triangle side* represents the years of productive life lost, the *right triangle side* represents the amount of money spent on injuries (lifetime economic costs), and the *left triangle side* represents the number of people suffering from injuries (injury incidence). The three horizontal levels on the sides of the pyramid correspond to nonhospitalized people with injuries (*bottom level*), hospitalized people with injuries (*middle level*), and injury deaths (*top level*), respectively. On the back triangle side, the *top level* is years of life lost (YLL) and the *bottom level* is years of productivity lost due to injuries. The *base* of the pyramid represents other, less quantifiable costs of injury (e.g., pain, emotional sequelae, family and social disruptions). (Reprinted from Rice DP, MacKenzie EJ, et al: *Cost of Injury in the United States: A Report to Congress*. San Francisco, Institute for Health & Aging, University of California and Injury Prevention Center, Johns Hopkins University, 1989, pp 13, 38, 58, 59.)

2. **Canada**
   a. **Incidence.** Injuries cause approximately 12,500 deaths among males (15% of all deaths) and 6100 deaths among females (7% of all deaths) annually.
   b. **Host factors.** Injuries are the leading cause of death for persons less than 40 years of age.
3. **Years of life lost (YLL)** is a measure of premature death; it is the difference between the age at death and the age of life expectancy. If the difference between age at death and an arbitrary cutoff for productive or potential age (generally taken as either 65, 70, or 75 years) is measured, it is called the **years of productive (or potential) life lost (YPLL)**.
   a. The **constant endpoint methods** generally emphasize the causes of death that have a greater impact on younger people, while the methods based on remaining life expectancy resemble the patterns of crude mortality.
   b. The **impact of mortality** is based on the age at death, with the YPLL varying inversely with the age at death. For example, three individuals die; they are 20, 35, and 50 years of age. If the arbitrary cutoff for productive life is 65 years, then the YPLLs for the three are 45, 30, and 15 years, respectively. Note that the YPLL for the 20-year-old person is three times the YPLL for the individual who is 50 years old.

c. **Injuries** cause about 5.3 million YLL and **are the leading cause of YPLL** (to age 65 years), accounting for about 3.7 million YPLL (to age 65 years) annually in the **United States**. In comparison, malignant neoplasms, the next leading cause of YPLL, account for about 1.8 million YPLL (to age 65 years) annually.

d. **Injuries** are the **second leading cause of YPLL** in **Canada** (to age 75 years), accounting for about 420,000 YPLL in 1989; the leading cause is cancer (440,000 YPLL).

C. Direct and indirect costs

1. **Economic costs** include medical and related expenses, wage losses, insurance administration costs, indirect work losses (e.g., long-term disability, premature death), and associated property damage.
   a. The **lifetime economic cost** is the aggregate of the estimated cost due to an injury for the lifetime of each injured person.
      (1) The lifetime economic costs of injuries in the United States in 1985 are summarized in Figure 8-2. They were estimated to be over $156 billion. In Canada, the estimated lifetime economic costs of injuries in 1986 were $10 billion.
      (2) The **costs of injuries** in the actual year of injury are about 75% of the lifetime economic costs.
   b. **Motor vehicle–related injuries** account for the single greatest cost of injuries, approximately $48 billion annually in the United States.

2. **Pain and emotional sequelae** of injured individuals and their families are incalculable.

IV. CLASSIFICATIONS

A. Intent. Injuries are classified by the intent or purposefulness of occurrence.

1. **Intentional injuries**—that is, injuries that are purposely inflicted and often are associated with violence—caused about 52,400 deaths in 1988 and represent about 1.4 million YPLL (to age 65) annually in the United States. The injuries can be inflicted by one person on another or can be self-directed. Examples include:
   a. Child abuse
   b. Domestic violence
   c. Sexual assault
   d. Aggravated assault
   e. Homicide and legal intervention (the tenth leading cause of death—fifth among Hispanics and blacks)
   f. Suicide (the eighth leading cause of death)*
   g. Abuse of the elderly

2. **Unintentional injuries**—that is, injuries that are not purposely inflicted—caused about 97,100 deaths in 1988 and represent about 2.3 million YPLL (to age 65) annually in the United States. During the past decade, the death rate due to unintentional injuries decreased by about 15%. The five leading causes of unintentional death, in order of frequency are
   a. Motor vehicle mishaps
   b. Falls
   c. Poisonings
   d. Drownings
   e. Fires and burns

3. **Distinction between intentional and unintentional injuries.** It is often difficult to define the intent of an injury; thus, the distinction between intentional and unintentional injuries can be tenuous and artificial, as in the following examples.
   a. Although motor vehicle–related injuries are generally classified as unintentional, vehicular assault is not uncommon.
   b. Automobiles intentionally built without certain safety features (i.e., without air bags) could result in injury to the occupants during a crash, and while the crash may be unintentional, the resultant injuries could be considered preventable, and, conceivably, intentional.
   c. The decrease in carbon monoxide levels in domestic gas has been accompanied by decreases in both unintentional poisonings and suicides due to domestic gas.

---

*Recently, operational criteria for determining suicide were developed, including evidence that the death was self-inflicted and that the deceased intended to die.

B. Place of occurrence. Injuries are classified by the place of occurrence. There are four principal locations at which injuries occur.

1. **Motor vehicles.** Motor vehicle–related injuries involve all transport vehicles in motion. The most common cause of motor vehicle–related injuries and deaths are automobile collisions. Some risk factors for motor vehicle–related injuries include alcohol use, decreased vehicle size, increased vehicle speed, night driving, poor road design, and vehicle instability.
   a. **Morbidity.** About 5 million people sustain motor vehicle–related injuries annually in the United States. Of these injuries, about 1.7 million are disabling, of which about 140,000 result in permanent impairment.
   b. **Mortality.** Motor vehicle–related injuries cause about 49,000 deaths and represent about 1.7 million YPLL (to age 65) annually in the United States. Motor vehicle–related injury mortality rates are greatest for individuals 15–24 years of age.

2. **Workplace.** Occupational injuries occur at the work site or result from incidents in the work environment. The risk of an injury is greatest during the first year on the job (see also Ch 12).
   a. **Morbidity**
      (1) **Incidence.** About 11 million people sustain occupational injuries annually in the United States. Of these injuries, about 1.8 million are disabling, of which about 60,000 result in permanent impairment.
      (2) **Musculoskeletal injuries** have been the most common type of occupational injury and low back injuries the most costly.
      (3) The incidence of **repetitive motion injuries,** especially carpal tunnel syndrome, is increasing rapidly.
      (4) **Manufacturing jobs** were associated with the greatest number of injuries.
   b. **Mortality**
      (1) **Incidence.** Occupational injuries cause about 11,000 deaths and represent about 300,000 YPLL (to age 65) annually in the United States.
      (2) About one-third of all fatal occupational injuries are **motor vehicle–related**. Falls and homicides each account for over 10% of the fatal occupational injuries.
      (3) **Agriculture, mining, and quarrying jobs** are associated with the highest rates of fatal work-related injuries.

3. **Home.** Home injuries occur in the house and the surrounding premises, including swimming pools. Causes of home injuries include fires, drownings, suffocation, falls, firearms, and poisoning.
   a. **Morbidity.** About 25 million people sustain injuries at home annually in the United States. Of these injuries, about 3.4 million are disabling, of which about 90,000 result in permanent impairment.
   b. **Mortality.** Home injuries cause about 22,500 deaths annually in the United States. Falls are the most common cause of home injury deaths.

4. **Public places.** About 29 million injuries occur in public places (e.g., parks, lakes, rivers, golf courses, athletic stadiums) in the United States annually. These injuries include recreational injuries and injuries occurring from natural events, such as lightning and floods.
   a. **Morbidity.** Of the injuries sustained in public places, about 2.4 million are disabling and, of these, about 60,000 result in permanent impairment.
   b. **Mortality.** About 19,000 deaths occur annually in public places in the United States. The most common cause of death from injury in a public place is drowning in a natural body of water.

C. Nature of injury

1. The International Classification of Diseases (ICD) is the principal classification scheme that defines the nature of injuries (**N codes**).
   a. The ICD code is the **primary** coding mechanism for diseases and conditions and the **secondary** coding mechanism for injuries after classification by external cause (see IV D).
   b. The ICD code provides information concerning necessary health care resources and services.
   c. It is most useful when accompanied by the classifications by external cause (see IV D) and by severity of injury. Examples of severity classifications include the following:
      (1) Abbreviated Injury Scale
      (2) Injury Severity Score
      (3) Consumer Product Safety Commission Hazard Index
      (4) Revised Trauma Score
      (5) Pediatric Trauma Score

2. Injuries classified by the nature of the injury are classified by the part of the body that was injured and the type of damage that occurred, including injuries resulting from infectious or parasitic agents. For example, the ICD code for head injuries includes all causes, such as motor vehicles (primary cause in young people), falls (primary cause in older people), and firearms, whether intentionally or unintentionally inflicted.

D. External cause of injury

1. The ICD Supplementary Classification of External Causes of Injuries and Poisonings (**E codes**) is the principal classification scheme that
   a. Defines the external cause of injuries
   b. Classifies the injuries by apparent intent
   c. Provides information concerning etiology
   d. Is used in conjunction with the nature of injury codes
2. Injuries classified by external cause, regardless of the resultant body damage, are classified by the etiologic environmental events and circumstances.
3. The most important external causes of injury are listed in Table 8-1.
   a. Injuries by motor vehicle are the leading cause of injury mortality.
   b. Falls are the leading cause of injury morbidity for all age-groups and of injury mortality among people over 75 years of age.
   c. Suffocation is the leading cause of injury mortality among children less than 1 year of age.
   d. Firearms cause 60% of all homicides and suicides and result in about 30,000 deaths each year in the United States. Almost half of all deaths among young black males are firearms-related. In Canada, firearms cause about one-third of all suicides and homicides.

E. Other classifications are dependent upon the purposes for which the injury data are used.

1. **Product.** The United States Consumer Product Safety Commission classifies and studies injuries by the type of consumer product associated with the injury (see V A 2).
2. **Criminality.** Police departments often classify injuries by the criminal nature of the event that caused the injury.

V. SURVEILLANCE SYSTEMS for injuries (the quality of which varies greatly) measure the incidence of various injuries and their severity, describe the risk factors and indicators involved, and may measure the effectiveness of interventions (see Ch 1 IV D).

A. Federal agencies. Table 8-3 lists some of the federal agencies that conduct national injury surveillance. For example, the Centers for Disease Control (CDC) and the Consumer Product Safety Commission are discussed in detail. In addition, the National Highway Traffic Safety Administration and the Bureau of Maternal and Child Health of the U.S. Public Health Service (PHS) play a major role in federal support for injury prevention activities.

1. The **CDC of the PHS** was designated by Congress in 1986 as the primary federal focus for injury prevention and control activities. The **Division of Injury Epidemiology and Control** was created to accomplish this mission. Its functions include:
   a. Providing epidemiologic assistance
   b. Improving surveillance systems
   c. Assisting state and local health departments to develop injury control programs
   d. Supporting university-based injury prevention research centers, epidemiologic research, and demonstration projects.
2. The **Consumer Product Safety Commission** was created in 1972 to protect the public from unreasonable risks of injuries associated with consumer products.
   a. Although the commission has general regulatory responsibility and legislated responsibility for some specific products (e.g., flammable fabric), it is required by statute to rely on voluntary industry standards rather than on government rule-making authority, whenever possible.
   b. The commission maintains the **National Injury Information Clearinghouse** as a repository for product-related injury information.

Table 8-3. Selected Federal Agencies That Conduct National Injury Surveillance

Agency	Surveillance System
Consumer Product Safety Commission	Medical Examiners' and Coroners' Alert Program National Electronic Injury Surveillance System
Federal Bureau of Investigation	Uniform Crime Reports
Food and Drug Administration	Poison Control Case Reports
National Center for Health Statistics, Centers for Disease Control	Vital Statistics Surveillance National Ambulatory Medical Care Survey National Health Interview Survey National Hospital Discharge Survey
National Fire Data Center, Federal Emergency Management Agency	National Fire Incident Reporting System
National Highway Traffic Safety Administration	Fatal Accident Reporting System National Accident Sampling System
National Institute for Occupational Safety and Health, Centers for Disease Control	National Traumatic Occupational Fatality Database
National Institute of Justice	National Crime Survey
National Institute on Drug Abuse	Drug Abuse Warning Network
National Transportation Safety Board	Transportation Safety Reports
Office of Record Keeping and Data Analysis, Occupational Safety and Health Administration	Occupational Injury and Statistics Program
U.S. Coast Guard	Boating Accident Reporting System

c. The commission runs the **National Electronic Injury Surveillance System,** which obtains data from 91 hospital emergency departments that were chosen as a national probability sample of all United States hospital emergency departments. Estimates of national product-related injury incidence are derived from the system.

B. State and local agencies

1. **Departments of health**
   a. Health departments conduct surveillance of fatal injuries as part of their vital statistics function (see Ch 3 I A 1 c)
   b. An increasing number of state and local departments of health are conducting surveillance of nonfatal injuries and developing injury prevention and control programs.
   c. The **Council of State and Territorial Epidemiologists** recommended in 1987 that traumatic spinal cord injuries, which were legally reportable in 10 states, be designated the first injury condition reportable to all state health departments. In support of this, the CDC currently maintains surveillance for spinal cord injuries using a uniform clinical case definition.*
2. **Transportation departments** conduct surveillance of motor vehicle crashes and injuries.
3. **Police departments** conduct surveillance of violent and intentional injuries and motor vehicle crashes and injuries.
4. **Departments of labor** conduct surveillance of occupational injuries.
5. **Fire departments** conduct surveillance of fire and flame-related injuries.

*A spinal cord injury is an acute traumatic lesion of the neural elements in the spinal canal, resulting in temporary or permanent sensory deficit, motor deficit, or bowel or bladder dysfunction.

C. Other organizations

1. The **National Safety Council,** a nongovernmental, nonprofit, public service organization chartered by an act of Congress, annually compiles data from many sources on injury morbidity, mortality, and costs and conducts injury prevention programs. It publishes a yearly update of data.

2. **Researchers** in public health and medical schools, universities, hospitals, corporations, and unions conduct studies on injury epidemiology and prevention. For example, hospital trauma registries, initially established to monitor the quality of clinical care, are increasingly being used to support prevention activities.

3. Numerous public health and clinical **professional and voluntary organizations** (e.g., the American Public Health Association, the Insurance Institute for Highway Safety, Mothers Against Drunk Driving, the National Committee for Injury Prevention and Control) provide support for the study and prevention of injuries, conduct injury prevention programs and campaigns, and educate professionals and the public.

VI. MODELS OF PREVENTION.

The practical approach to the prevention and control of injuries should involve strategies chosen on the basis of their actual effectiveness in reducing injuries, not on the relative importance or the time of occurrence of the causal or contributing factors they influence. Usually a combination of strategies and interventions are most effective. For example, the safest automobile restraint system incorporates both air bags and seat belts.

A. Passive and active strategies

1. **Passive strategies** are automatic, require no individual or repetitive action to be protective, and are generally the most effective. For example, the installation of air bags in motor vehicles is a passive strategy because the occupants of the automobile will be protected in a crash regardless of their individual actions.

2. **Active strategies** are voluntary, require repetitive, individual action to be protective, and are generally less effective than passive strategies. For example, seat belts in most motor vehicles must be buckled by the occupant every time the vehicle is used in order to be effective.

B. The four Es of intervention

1. **Engineering interventions** are aimed at the vectors and physical environments that promote or support the occurrence of injuries. These interventions, which are often passive, are among the most effective in decreasing the occurrence of injuries. For example, medicine containers were redesigned to be child-proof.

2. **Economic interventions** are aimed at influencing behavior based on monetary incentives and rewards or penalties. For example, many insurance companies have lower rates for residences equipped with smoke detectors and sprinkler systems.

3. **Enforcement interventions** are aimed at influencing behavior by laws and regulations that may only be effective when enforced. For example, since 1978, every state has made the use of federally approved child safety seats mandatory for children who ride in automobiles. The enforcement of these laws, however, is variable.

4. **Educational interventions** are aimed at influencing behavior through reasoning and knowledge. These interventions are usually the least effective, especially when used alone without other interventions. Educational interventions could be more effective if they were directed toward societal leaders and decision-makers. For example, because high school driver education programs are often accompanied by licensure at younger ages and by an increase in the proportion of young people who drive, populations with these programs have relatively *more* motor vehicle crashes among young people than populations that do not have such programs.

C. The **Haddon Models,** formulated by Dr. William H. Haddon, Jr., are useful for determining possible interventions and prevention measures for particular injuries.

1. The **Haddon Matrix,** or multifactorial approach, arranges intervention and prevention strategies by agent, vector, host, and physical and social environmental factors, according to the time at which the strategy would be effective in relation to the occurrence of the injury event.

Table 8-4. The Haddon Matrix

Strategies	Agent and Vector	Host	Environment: Physical	Environment: Social
Pre-event phase	Install improved braking systems	Have good vision	Groove pavements	Revoke driver's licenses of intoxicated drivers
Event phase	Install airbags	Use motorcycle helmets	Use roadside poles that break away	Mandate the use of safety glass in windows
Post-event phase	Use burn-resistant fabrics	Obtain emergency medical care	Have a rapid emergency transportation system	Support medical and rehabilitation services

This model emphasizes the time of action in reference to the injury event. Table 8-4 depicts the Haddon Matrix and provides examples of each factor- and phase-specific strategy concerning motor vehicle–related injuries.

a. **Pre-event strategies** are designed to prevent the agent from reaching the susceptible host and, therefore, prevent the occurrence of the injury-producing event.
b. **Event strategies** are effective at the time the injury could occur and are designed to minimize the interaction between the agent and the host to prevent or minimize the damage.
c. **Post-event strategies** are designed to limit or repair the damage already incurred.

2. The **Ten Countermeasure Strategies** (Table 8-5) evolved from the Haddon Matrix. They are injury prevention strategies based on the energy exchanges that result in injuries and the need to minimize injuries that have occurred. The strategies are generic descriptions of the prevention methods that would interfere with the harmful impact of energy on people. The table lists the strategies and gives examples concerning the prevention of injuries among people 65 years of age and older.

D. Clinical prevention

1. The U.S. Preventive Services Task Force (1989) evaluated health promotion and disease and injury prevention activities applicable to primary care practitioners.
2. Figure 8-3 summarizes the specific injury prevention counseling and screening activities and the signs and symptoms of which practitioners should be aware, by patient age-group.
3. Some injury prevention activities should be undertaken for all patients in the age-group (e.g., counseling concerning the use of safety belts) while others are for patients at high risk (e.g., a patient who has a child or an elderly person at home).

Table 8-5. The Ten Countermeasure Strategies

Countermeasure Strategies	Examples for Persons Aged 65 Years and Older
1. Prevent the marshalling of potentially injurious agents	1. Store medicine in the original container, which should be clearly labeled
2. Reduce the amount of the agent	2. Hot water temperature ≤120° F
3. Prevent the inappropriate release of the agent	3. Apply textured strips on the floors of bathtubs and showers
4. Modify release of the agent	4. Use safety belts in a car
5. Separate the host from the agent by time or space	5. Provide sufficient time to cross the street at intersections
6. Separate the host from the agent by physical barriers	6. Use a heating pad only with additional covering pads
7. Modify surfaces and basic structures	7. Use carpeting
8. Increase resistance to injury	8. Prevent or treat osteoporosis
9. Improve emergency responses	9. Provide good emergency medical services
10. Improve medical care and rehabilitation	10. Provide good clinical services

Type of Injury	Prevention Topics for Patient Counseling	Other Recommended Actions	<2	2–6	7–12	13–18	19–39	40–64	≥65
Motor vehicle-related injuries	Child safety seats		■						
	Safety belts			■	■	■	■	■	■
	Bicycle safety helmets			■	■	■	■	■	■
	Motorcycle safety helmets					■	■	■	■
Poisonings	Syrup of ipecac		■	■					
	Poison control telephone number		■	■					
	Storage of drugs and toxic chemicals		■	■	■				
		Screen for erythrocyte protoporphyrin*	■	■					
Falls	Stairway gates		■						
	Window guards		■	■					
	Caregiving for the elderly**						■	■	
	Danger of falls								■
Burns and fire-related injuries	Smoke detectors		■	■	■	■	■	■	■
	Hot water temperature (<120 ° F)		■	■					■
	Storage of matches			■	■				
	Smoking near bedding and upholstery					■	■	■	■
Drownings	Pool fences		■	■					
Intentional injuries	Use of firearms (especially men)					■	■		
	Storage of firearms			■	■				
	Violent behavior (especially men)					■	■		
		Remain alert for child abuse or neglect	■	■	■	■			
		Remain alert for physical abuse or neglect					■	■	■
		Remain alert for depressive symptoms				■	■	■	■
		Remain alert for suicide risk factors*				■	■	■	■
Other	Driving and other dangerous activities while under the influence of alcohol or other drugs					■	■	■	■
	Occupational illness and injury					■	■	■	
	Back conditioning exercises*						■	■	

*For those at risk. **For those with elderly in the home.

Figure 8-3. Injury prevention activities for primary care clinicians. When the patient is under 2 years of age, the parent or guardian is counseled. For patients 2–12 years of age, the parent or guardian and the patient are counseled. For patients over 12 years of age, only the patient is counseled. (Adapted from US Preventive Services Task Force: *Guide To Clinical Preventive Services: An Assessment of the Effectiveness of 169 Interventions.* Baltimore, Williams & Wilkins, 1989.)

BIBLIOGRAPHY

Baker SP, O'Neill B, Grinsburg MJ, et al: *The Injury Fact Book,* 2nd edition. New York, Oxford University Press, 1991.

Brown ST, Foege WH, Bender TR, et al. Injury prevention and control: prospects for the 1990s. *Annu Rev Public Health* 11:251–266, 1990.

Centers for Disease Control: 1987 conference on injury in America. *Public Health Reports* 102:574–676, 1987.

Centers for Disease Control: Case definitions for public health surveillance. *MMWR* 39(RR-13):2, 33–34, 1990.

Centers for Disease Control: Childhood injuries in the United States. *Am J Dis Child* 144:627–646, 1990.

Centers for Disease Control: *The Public Health Consequences of Disasters 1989.* Atlanta, CDC, 1989.

Centers for Disease Control: Public health surveillance of 1990 injury control objectives for the nation. *MMWR* 37(SS-1), 1988.

Chapdelaine A, Rochette L: Goal: reduce mortality due to traffic injuries by 35% by the year 2000. *Chron Dis Canada* 11:91–94, 1990.

Clark DW: A vocabulary for preventive and community medicine. In *Preventive and Community Medicine,* 2nd edition. Edited by Clark DW, MacMahon B. Boston, Little Brown, 1981, pp 3–15.

Committee on Trauma Research, Commission on Life Sciences, National Research Council and the Institute of Medicine: *Injury in America: A Continuing Public Health Problem.* Washington, DC, National Academy Press, 1985.

Haddon W Jr: On the escape of tigers: an ecologic note. *Am J Public Health* 60:2229–2234, 1970.

Haddon W Jr, Baker SP: Injury control. In *Preventive and Community Medicine,* 2nd edition. Edited by Clark DW, MacMahon B. Boston, Little Brown, 1981, pp 109–140.

Last JM, Wallace RB (eds): *Public Health and Preventive Medicine,* 13th edition. Norwalk, CT, Appleton & Lange, 1992.

National Committee for Injury Prevention and Control: Injury prevention: meeting the challenge. *Am J Prev Med* 5(Suppl 3):1–303, 1989.

National Institute for Occupational Safety and Health: Surveillance in occupational safety and health. *Am J Public Health* 79(Suppl):1–63, December 1989.

National Safety Council: *Accident Facts,* 1990 edition. Chicago, National Safety Council, 1990.

Rice DP, Mackenzie EJ, et al: *Cost of Injury in the United States. A Report to Congress.* San Francisco, Institute for Health & Aging, University of California and Injury Prevention Center, Johns Hopkins University, 1989.

Robertson LS: *Epidemiology.* New York, Oxford University Press, 1992.

US Preventive Services Task Force: *Guide to Clinical Preventive Services: An Assessment of the Effectiveness of 169 Interventions.* Baltimore, Williams & Wilkins, 1989.

Waller JA: *Injury Control: A Guide to the Causes and Prevention of Trauma.* Lexington, MA, DC Heath, 1985.

STUDY QUESTIONS

Directions: Each of the numbered items or incomplete statements in this section is followed by answers or by completions of the statement. Select the **one** lettered answer or completion that is **best** in each case.

1. All of the following factors have been found to contribute to an increased risk of fall-related injuries among the elderly EXCEPT

(A) poor vision
(B) slippery bathtubs
(C) osteoporosis
(D) poorly lit stairways
(E) carpeted floors

2. All of the following statements concerning fatal motor vehicle–related injuries in the United States are true EXCEPT

(A) motor vehicles are the leading cause of all fatal injuries
(B) motor vehicles are the leading cause of fatal occupational injuries
(C) motor vehicles are the leading cause of fatal injuries among people ages 15–24 years
(D) motor vehicles are the leading cause of fatal injuries among people age 75 years and older
(E) motor vehicle–related fatal injuries are two to three times greater among men than women

3. Four people—ages 40, 45, 50, and 60 years—die in a car crash. The total YPLL (to age 65 years) for this group is

(A) 16.25 years
(B) 47.5 years
(C) 48.75 years
(D) 65 years
(E) 195 years

4. The correct rank order for the three leading causes of YPLL (to age 65 years) in the United States is

(A) injuries, cancer, heart disease
(B) cancer, injuries, heart disease
(C) cancer, heart disease, injuries
(D) heart disease, injuries, cancer
(E) injuries, heart disease, cancer

5. All of the following increase the risk of fatal motor vehicle–related injuries EXCEPT

(A) alcohol use
(B) high school driver education
(C) break-away roadside poles
(D) compact cars
(E) night driving

1-E
2-D
3-D
4-A
5-C

Directions: Each item below contains four suggested answers of which **one or more** is correct. Choose the answer

A if **1, 2, and 3** are correct
B if **1 and 3** are correct
C if **2 and 4** are correct
D if **4** is correct
E if **1, 2, 3, and 4** are correct

6. The Ten Countermeasure Strategies are

(1) based on the transfer of energy
(2) host-factor specific
(3) used to define interventions for many injuries
(4) used to enforce interventions for many injuries

7. Individuals who have an increased risk of injuries include

(1) Native Americans
(2) men
(3) individuals with osteoporosis
(4) the poor

8. The ICD E codes classify causes of injuries and poisonings by

(1) body part affected
(2) apparent intent
(3) nature of injury
(4) cause of injury

9. The Haddon Matrix is based on the

(1) surveillance of injuries
(2) factors associated with injuries
(3) ICD
(4) time course of the injury event

10. Vectors that are associated with injuries include

(1) electric wires
(2) electricity
(3) bullets
(4) carbon monoxide

11. True statements concerning firearms-related injuries in the United States include which of the following?

(1) Firearms are the leading cause of death among children
(2) Firearms result in about 30,000 deaths each year
(3) Firearms-related injuries occur more frequently among females
(4) Firearms cause about 60% of all homicides and suicides

6-B
7-E
8-C
9-C
10-B
11-C

Directions: The group of items in this section consists of lettered options followed by a set of numbered items. For each item, select the **one** lettered option that is most closely associated with it. Each lettered option may be selected once, more than once, or not at all.

Questions 12–16

For each injury ranking listed below, select the type of injury that is described by the ranking.

(A) Motor vehicle–related injuries
(B) Fall-related injuries
(C) Suffocation-related injuries
(D) Knife-related injuries
(E) Firearm-related injuries

12. Leading cause of injury morbidity

13. Leading cause of injury mortality

14. Leading cause of homicide

15. Leading cause of injury mortality among the elderly

16. Leading cause of injury mortality among infants less than 1 year old

---

12-B
13-A
14-E
15-B
16-C

ANSWERS AND EXPLANATIONS

1. The answer is E *[II A 3 f; VI C 2; Table 9-5].*
Poor vision, slippery bathtubs, osteoporosis, and poorly lit stairwells are factors that have been found to contribute to an increased risk of fall-related injuries among the elderly. Carpeted floors have been suggested as a countermeasure against slippery floors. About one-third of people age 65 years and older fall each year, with almost half of the falls resulting in injury. Almost one-third of admissions to nursing homes or long-term care facilities are for persons with a fall-related injury, usually hip fracture. Over 12,000 persons die each year from fall-related injuries, and about 75% are at least 65 years of age. Fall-related injuries are the leading cause of fatal injury among persons 75 years of age and older. Poor vision, osteoporosis, Parkinson's disease, osteoarthritis, and peripheral neuropathy are among the host factors that increase the risk of fall-related injuries. Environmental factors include slippery surfaces, poorly lit areas, and lack of handrails.

2. The answer is D *[IV B 1 b, 2 b (2), D 3; Figure 8-1; Table 8-2].*
Among people 75 years of age and older, falls cause about 7600 deaths annually, which is about twice as many deaths as are caused by motor vehicles. Fatal motor vehicle–related injuries account for about one-third of all fatal injuries, half of all fatal unintentional injuries, and one-third of all fatal occupational injuries. Among people 15–24 years old, motor vehicle–related injuries account for about half of all fatal injuries.

3. The answer is D *[III B 3].*
The total years of productive life lost (YPLL) is 65 years. YPLL is a measure of premature mortality that emphasizes causes of death among younger people. YPLL (to age 65 years) for an individual is calculated by subtracting the age at death from 65 years. A 40-year-old person who dies has lost 25 YPLL to age 65. The total YPLL is the sum of the individual YPLL's and, in this example, is 65 (25 + 20 + 15 + 5). The mean YPLL is 16.25, the median age at death is 47.5 years, and the mean age of death is 48.75 years. Altogether, these four people have lived 195 years.

4. The answer is A *[III B 3 c].*
Injuries are the leading cause of years of productive (or potential) life lost (YPLL) to age 65 years, with unintentional injuries accounting for about 2.3 million and intentional injuries about 1.4 million YPLL each year. Malignant neoplasms, the second leading cause of YPLL, account for about 1.8 million YPLL. Heart disease accounts for about 1.5 million YPLL each year.

5. The answer is C *[II A 3 d, D 2 b; IV B 1; VI B 4, C 1; Table 8-4].*
The use of break-away roadside poles *decreases* the risk of fatal motor vehicle–related injuries. The risks of motor vehicle–related injuries are increased by many factors, including alcohol use, high school driver education, compact cars, and night driving. About half of all drivers who die in motor vehicle crashes have elevated blood alcohol concentrations. Although driver education programs are aimed at influencing and improving driving behavior, populations with these programs have relatively more vehicle-related injuries among young drivers than populations without these programs. This is no doubt a result of licensure at young ages and an increase in the proportion of young people who drive. Night driving (from 10:00 P.M. to 3:59 A.M.) is associated with over one-third of all fatalities although less than one-fifth of crashes occur during that time.

6. The answer is B (1, 3) *[VI C 2; Table 8-5].*
The Ten Countermeasure Strategies are based on the transfer of energy that results in injuries and on the need to minimize injuries. These strategies are used to define interventions. The strategies relate to all factors and do not emphasize host factors. Enforcement of the interventions, however, depends on society.

7. The answer is E (all) *[II A 3 a–c, f, B 2 c].*
Individuals who have an increased risk of injuries include Native Americans, men, individuals with osteoporosis, and the poor. The host, or the individual affected, has been the principal focus of research related to injuries and preventive measures aimed at decreasing injury rates. Host factors that affect the risk of injuries differ according to the type of injury; for example, Native Americans have a higher rate of all injuries than other racial groups, even when income is controlled. Men have an increased incidence of almost all injuries and mortality resulting from these injuries as compared to women. Osteoporosis increases the risk of fall-related injuries such as hip fractures. Social environmental factors that increase the risk of injuries include violent behavior, alcohol and drug use, economic deprivation, racism, and sexism.

8. The answer is C (2, 4) *[IV D 1].*
The International Classification of Diseases (ICD) E codes classify injuries by apparent intent and by external environmental cause. ICD is the principal classification scheme that defines the nature of injuries (N codes) and the external cause of injuries (E codes). The N codes classify injuries by the part of the body that was injured, the type of damage that occurred, and the infectious or parasitic etiology (if applicable).

9. The answer is C (2, 4) *[VI C 1; Table 8-4].*
The Haddon Matrix is based on the factors associated with injuries and the time course of the injury event. It arranges intervention and prevention strategies by agent, vector, host, and physical and social environmental factors, according to the time course of the injury event. Pre-event strategies are designed to prevent the agent from reaching the susceptible host and thus prevent the injury-producing event. Event strategies are effective at the time the injury could occur; they are designed to minimize the interaction between the agent and the host to prevent or minimize the damage. Post-event strategies are designed to limit or repair the damage already incurred. The Haddon Matrix is not associated with the surveillance of injuries or the International Classification of Diseases (ICD).

10. The answer is B (1, 3) *[II D].*
Vectors that are associated with injuries include electric wires and bullets. Vectors are the carriers of the injury agents, or energy. The design of the vector markedly alters the amount of energy available to cause an injury. Electric wires are vectors of electrical energy (electricity). Bullets are vectors of kinetic energy. Carbon monoxide and electricity are injury-causing agents, not vectors.

11. The answer is C (2, 4) *[II A 3 a; IV D 3 d; Figure 8-1; Table 8-2].*
Firearms result in 30,000 deaths each year and cause about 60% of all homicides and suicides. Injuries due to the use of firearms are the second leading cause of death due to injury in the United States, after motor vehicles. They account for over 10% of all deaths among children 1–19 years old. Blacks are at an increased risk of firearms-related injuries, and males have a greater risk than females.

12–16. The answers are: 12-B *[IV D 3 b],* **13-A** *[IV D 3 a],* **14-E** *[IV D 3 d],* **15-B** *[IV D 3 b],* **16-C** *[IV D 3 c].*
The leading cause of injury morbidity is falls, which account for 20% of all injuries. Each year, about 5% of the population receive emergency treatment for fall-related injuries.

The leading cause of injury mortality is motor vehicles. Overall, motor vehicles account for about half of the unintentional injury deaths that occur each year. Among people 15–24 years of age, motor vehicles account for about 75% of unintentional injury deaths that occur.

The leading cause of homicides is firearms. Firearms are the cause of about 60% of all homicides and suicides and are also the sixth leading cause of fatal unintentional injuries for all ages. They cause about 20% of all deaths for people 15–29 years of age.

The leading cause of injury mortality among the elderly is falls. There are about 12,000 fatal falls yearly, and almost three-fourths occur among the elderly.

The leading cause of injury mortality among infants is mechanical suffocation or asphyxiation due to food or a foreign object. Suffocation is the cause of death for about 35% of the 950 children less than 1 year of age who die yearly from unintentional injuries. Homicide is the second leading cause of fatal injuries in infants and results in over 300 deaths per year.

9
Mental Health

Christina L. Herring

I. DEFINITIONS

A. Mental health. A comprehensive definition of mental health is that given by Ginsburg (1955), who stresses the relationship of mental health to mastery of the environment as manifested in three crucial areas of living—love, work, and play. Per Ginsburg, mental health is "the ability to hold a job, have a family, keep out of trouble with the law, and enjoy the usual opportunities for pleasure."

B. Mental disorder. Defining mental disorder is problematic because the consensus that exists regarding the undesirability of a somatic disorder (i.e., pain, disability, death) does not always exist for the symptoms of a mental disorder.

1. **Lack of consensus** over a definition of mental disorder concerns:
   a. Whether or not a given condition should be regarded as undesirable
   b. The degree to which the condition should be considered undesirable in order to be designated as an illness
   c. Whether or not the condition should be regarded as within the domain of psychiatry or some other discipline
2. **Approaches to defining mental disorder**
   a. Mental disorder can be viewed as any significant deviation from an ideal state of positive mental health. This approach, which accepts the basic psychoanalytic principles, is characteristic of the approach taken by most psychiatrists in the United States.
   b. Mental disorder also can be viewed as a part of a continuum of conditions ranging from highly desirable to highly undesirable, placing the cutoff point for mental disorder close to the highly undesirable end of the continuum; thus, only conditions unequivocally associated with suffering and disability are designated as illness or disorder. This approach is characteristic of European psychiatrists and may explain why epidemiologic studies conducted in the United States report a much higher incidence of mental disorder than European studies.
3. **The most comprehensive definition of mental disorder** is that proposed by Spitzer (1973), who states the following.
   a. The manifestations of the condition are primarily psychological and involve alterations in behavior.
   b. The condition in its full-blown state is regularly and intrinsically associated with subjective distress, generalized impairment in social effectiveness or functioning, or voluntary behavior that the subject wishes he could stop because it is regularly associated with physical disability or illness.
   c. The condition is distinct clinically from other conditions, and ideally, follow-up studies, family studies, and response to treatment are also distinct.

II. APPLICATION OF EPIDEMIOLOGY TO MENTAL ILLNESS

A. Types of case definitions. To define a case of mental disorder, studies have used the following sources:

1. Hospital admissions and discharges

2. Physicians' examinations and diagnoses
3. Register statistics, which are a central listing of every individual who makes use of either outpatient or inpatient psychiatric services

B. **Problems of case definitions** are greatest in chronic diseases of unknown etiology (e.g., schizophrenia, bipolar disorder). Since the disease persists over the patient's lifetime, the symptoms usually wax and wane, and not all physicians would agree on a diagnosis every time the patient is examined.

1. **Schizophrenia** is a disorder or group of disorders with a variety of symptoms, including delusions, hallucinations, agitation, affective flattening, social withdrawal, apathy, anhedonia, and poverty of thought and content of speech. While the course of these symptoms varies widely in individuals, current criteria for the diagnosis of schizophrenia require that the symptoms be present for at least several months. The **two major types of schizophrenia** are **acute** and **insidious onset**.
   a. **Incidence and prevalence.** Although the incidence of schizophrenia is comparatively low, its prevalence and lifetime risk of just over 1% indicate that it is by no means a rare disease. In most populations, and at any given time, at least 5 out of every 1000 adults would meet the clinical diagnostic criteria for schizophrenia, and the disorder accounts for about 20% of all chronic and severe disability. In the World Health Organization (WHO) Program for Cross-Cultural Research in Schizophrenia (1967–1985), acute onset cases amounted to less than 15% of cases in the follow-up period, while, in the majority of cases with insidious onset, the patients tended to remain psychotic for over 75% of the follow-up period. Relatively few cases were of an intermediate type (WHO, 1979).
      (1) **Age and sex.** There is a marked gender effect of the age-specific incidence rate of schizophrenia.
         (a) The **cumulative risk of developing schizophrenia** is identical in males and females up to age 54 years. The risk after age 54 is almost zero for both males and females.
         (b) The **mean age of onset,** however, is higher in females. This could mean that, in the critical age period of reproduction, the speed of onset of schizophrenia is either slowed down in females or speeded up in males.
      (2) **Cultural, geographic, and social factors**
         (a) The WHO Program found that the **syndrome of schizophrenia is universal** and that the incidence rates of schizophrenia are similar across cultures. Culture and the social environment do, however, have a significant effect on the outcome of schizophrenia. A striking finding of the WHO studies was that schizophrenic patients in nonindustrialized cultures had a significantly better 2- and 5-year course and outcome than patients in the industrialized world (WHO, 1973).
         (b) **Seasonality.** There is a consistent seasonal effect on the distribution of births of individuals who develop schizophrenia. Schizophrenics are more likely to be born in the season with the lowest average temperatures, regardless of the latitude.
   b. **Risk factors.** Kraepelin (1921), who introduced the concept of schizophrenia (then called **dementia praecox**) considered that the causes included both **heredity** and **organic brain damage**. Improved twin and adoption studies emphasize the role of aberrant genes, and the subsequent computed tomography (CT) scan has revealed neuropathology in the brains of schizophrenics.
      (1) An individual's risk of being schizophrenic rises the more closely she is related to a schizophrenic. The maximum risk is almost 50% for the identical co-twin of a schizophrenic.
      (2) Kety (1983) demonstrated that the crucial factor in determining the risk for schizophrenia is not the type of upbringing an adopted child receives but whether a biologic parent was schizophrenic.
      (3) Another area of impressive advance has been neuroimaging. Over 50 CT scan studies of schizophrenics have been carried out. Agreement has been reached that **enlargement of the lateral ventricles** is observed in many cases (Shelton, 1986). Ventricular enlargement appears to be present at the outset of schizophrenia and shows no evidence of progression on follow-up after several years (Illowsky et al, 1988).
      (4) The clinical characteristics that have been found to correlate most frequently with structural changes are poor premorbid personality, cognitive impairment, neurologic "soft signs," and vegetative symptoms. Crow (1985) characterized this constellation as the **type II syndrome**.

(5) A **history of adverse events during fetal and neonatal life** is obtained more frequently regarding schizophrenic patients than normal subjects. Obstetric complications are noted particularly in schizophrenics without a positive history for psychosis (Lewis and Murray, 1988). A number of studies have shown that obstetric complications predict ventricular enlargement in adult schizophrenics (Owen, 1989).

c. Relation to other diseases

(1) Schizophrenia can occur as a symptomatic disorder in association with a variety of cerebral and physical diseases, of which **epilepsy** is the most notable example.

(2) Schizophrenia shows both positive and negative associations with other conditions.

(a) The Oxford Record Linkage Study (Baldwin, 1979) has demonstrated an increased risk in schizophrenics for arteriosclerotic disease, malabsorption syndrome associated with celiac disease, and myxedema.

(b) In a recent WHO study (Dupont, 1986), there was a significant reduction of the relative risk for cancer found in schizophrenic patients. Data analyses indicated that cancer risk reduction was positively correlated with the length of neuroleptic treatment, which suggests a protective effect of phenothiazines with regard to cancer.

2. Bipolar disorder (formerly manic-depressive illness)

a. The concept of manic-depressive illness was proposed by Kraepelin in 1895 (published in 1921). There were three criteria:

(1) The intense emotion during the acute episode

(2) The tendency to return to premorbid functioning

(3) The tendency to recur, with multiple episodes during the patient's lifetime

b. In 1962, Leonhard proposed separating patients with Kraepelin's manic-depressive illness into two groups; patients with a history of both depressive and manic episodes, which Leonhard called **bipolar disorder,** and those with only depressive episodes or only manic episodes, which he called **unipolar**.

c. In the early 1960s, three research groups (i.e., Perris; Angst; Winokur, Clayton, and Reich) undertook family studies of patients with affective disorder (depression, mania) and separated probands into unipolar and bipolar illness. The three studies confirmed the usefulness of Leonhard's separation and indicated a greater degree of family aggregation in bipolar than in unipolar patients. There were very few patients with unipolar manic illness.

d. The *Diagnostic and Statistical Manual of Mental Disorders,* third edition, revised (*DSM-III-R*) lists three types of bipolar disorders. The essential feature of bipolar disorder is one or more manic episodes usually accompanied by one or more major depressive episodes.

(1) Organic mood disorders, which are secondary to drugs (i.e., the side effects of drugs, not necessarily drug abuse) and to medical and especially central nervous system (CNS) diseases

(2) Major affective disorders, which are primary bipolar disorders

(3) Schizoaffective disorders, which are also called schizoaffective-manic psychoses

e. Incidence and prevalence. Akiskal (1983) estimates that 4%–5% of the population are at risk for developing a bipolar disorder. Some of these patients do not manifest full-blown bipolar disorder but are seen as outpatients and often are misdiagnosed.

(1) Sex. In patients admitted to the hospital with a diagnosis of bipolar disorder, women are likely to outnumber men.

(2) Social. In sharp contrast to schizophrenia, the upper classes are more likely to be represented than the lower classes.

(3) Age. With respect to individual episodes of either unipolar or bipolar disorder, the manic form of the disorder occurs primarily in younger individuals, and the depressive disorder occurs primarily in the older age-group.

(4) Marital status. Bipolar patients are more likely to be married than schizophrenic patients, but, in bipolar illness, marital status is not related to prognosis.

III. EXTENT AND COST OF MENTAL ILLNESS

A. Extent of mental illness. At least 10% of the population of the United States (about 25 million Americans) have some form of mental disorder that could benefit from professional help. The extent of mental illness is often estimated by the **number of hospitalizations for mental disorder**.

1. There are more patients in hospitals with mental disorders at any time than all other diseases combined, including cancer and heart disease.

2. Horgan (1985) indicated that 360,000 individuals are receiving psychiatric care in public and private mental hospitals, psychiatric wards of general hospitals, and Veterans Administration (VA) psychiatric facilities on any given day of the year and that 1.75 million individuals receive treatment at these institutions annually.

3. Readmissions to mental hospitals are common; of the 972,000 patients admitted to mental hospitals and psychiatric services of general hospitals annually, more than one-third are readmissions.

B. **Professional services for mental disorders** are carried out by a number of different practitioners.

1. There are 30,000 practicing psychiatrists in the United States (1300 are psychoanalysts), but the distribution is very uneven: five states (New York, New Jersey, Pennsylvania, Massachusetts, California) have more than one-half of all psychiatrists.

2. There are 20,000 psychologists, 19,000 psychiatric social workers, and 30,000 psychiatric nurses, resulting in a ratio of 35 mental health workers for every 100,000 people in the United States.

C. **The cost of mental illness** is quite high.

1. Mental health costs have risen from 6% of the nation's total health care spending in 1955 to 15% in 1982 (Sharfstein, 1988). Approximately 70% of these costs are spent for inpatient care. Less than 25% of the population with mental illness ever receive treatment (Horgan, 1985).

2. About 25% of the nation's total mental health costs are paid by federal funds, 28% by state and local governments, and 12% by private health insurers. The percentage of mental health care costs paid by governmental sources (53%) is higher than the percentage of total U.S. health care costs paid by governmental sources (43%). The percentage of mental health care costs paid by private insurers (12%) is less than half the percentage of total health care costs paid by this source (30%). In 1983, 40% of a private psychiatrist's gross income came from patients' out-of-pocket payments, while only 25% of a general medical physician's income came from that source.

3. Nearly 60% of the nation's total spending for chronic mental illness are paid by the federal government. Approximately 1.7 million chronically mentally ill individuals in this country—less than 5% of the nation's mentally ill—consume 37% of the overall spending.

4. Psychiatric care represents a very small part of total Medicare expenditures: approximately 2.4% in 1981, with inpatient services accounting for 83% of that amount.

5. Medicaid limits the number of inpatient psychiatric days to 30 or fewer per year in most states and does not pay for adult care in state mental hospitals.

6. Only 39% of employer health insurance plans provided inpatient mental illness coverage comparable to that for other medical illnesses in 1986. Only 6% of plans provided the same outpatient coverage for mental illness that they did for other medical conditions in 1986. These limitations significantly increase referrals to public mental health facilities.

D. **The burden of mental illness on industry** is impressive.

1. The National Association for Mental Health (Joint Commission on Mental Illness and Health, 1981) estimates that individuals hospitalized for mental illness lost nearly $2 billion per year in purchasing power.

2. Mental disorders account for at least 50% of all absenteeism, which costs industry $5 billion annually.

3. Mental disorders are important factors in the etiology of 75% of all injuries, which cost industry $3 billion annually in injury to workers and damage to their machines.

IV. **CARE OF THE MENTALLY ILL.** The history of care of the mentally ill in the United States is not a record to be viewed with pride. It was once widely believed that individuals suffering from mental illness were possessed by demons and should be put away in jails, poorhouses, or kennels, or punished in stocks or at whipping posts.

A. **State-supported mental hospitals** were established in most states by the end of the nineteenth century.

1. There are presently about 250 state and county mental hospitals in the United States.
2. The number of patients in these mental hospitals increased steadily until around 1955, after which the population of the institutions dropped continually as a result of:
   a. The use of psychotropic drugs
   b. Advanced methods of intensive therapy, including group therapy and milieu therapy
   c. The development of community mental health centers in the 1960s

B. Private psychiatric hospitals

1. Although there are about 450 private psychiatric hospitals in the United States, 16 states have no private facilities, and 10 states have only one.
2. Whereas 20 years ago, 95% of the beds were in the public sector, today less than 50% are government-owned.
3. Private psychiatric hospitals offer many obvious advantages to mental patients who can afford to pay, since these patients are more likely to receive individual psychotherapy; the private hospitals are unevenly distributed: 40% of the hospitals and 25% of the beds are found in California and New York.

C. Community hospitals. Approximately 1500 community hospitals, or one out of every four, have separate units for treating psychiatric patients.

1. Approximately 22,000 beds are reserved for treating the mentally ill in these institutions, and the average stay is about 18 days.
2. The admissions for psychiatric services in community hospitals are approximately equal to those of state mental hospitals.

D. For-profit psychiatric systems

1. Since the introduction of Medicare prospective hospital payment in the early 1980s, inpatient psychiatric services have become more profitable than general medical hospital care.
2. In the mid-1980s, there was an 8%–10% growth in the number of for-profit psychiatric hospitals, especially those for the treatment of adolescents and substance abuse.
3. In 1986, 43% of the psychiatric hospitals in states with mandated psychiatric inpatient coverage operated under for-profit auspices; in states without such mandates, only 13% of the psychiatric hospitals were under for-profit control.

V. CHANGING CONCEPTS AND ATTITUDES

A. The development of psychotropic agents, one of the most outstanding changes in the field of mental health, has had the following effects.

1. It has allowed mental patients to return to the community and, in some cases, to their families and jobs.
2. It has had a profound impact upon public acceptance of mental illness. As a result of increased public and private awareness, federal grants from the Hospital Improvement Program and the Hospital Staff Development Program have helped to provide better facilities and better trained personnel than ever before.
3. Prior to the availability of these drugs, there was little chance for a short hospital stay or rapid recovery. The period of hospitalization has been reduced from years to months and even weeks for some patients [see also V C 2 b (1)].

B. Insurance coverage of mental illness

1. **Mandates for psychiatric care.** In 1986, the U.S. Supreme Court decided that states have the right to stipulate a minimum level of mental health coverage for individuals insured under general insurance policies or employee benefit plans.
   a. Fifteen states had enacted minimal levels of mental health benefits by 1987.
   b. Laws requiring health maintenance organizations (HMOs) to provide a certain level of mental health coverage have been enacted in 24 states, and laws regulating HMO levels of alcohol and substance abuse services have been enacted in 23 states.

c. HMOs in states with mandated coverage cannot exclude patients with chronic mental conditions.
d. Nursing home care became the primary alternative to hospitalization for older chronically mentally ill patients in the 1980s. One-half to two-thirds of nursing home residents have mental problems. By April 1, 1990, states were required to screen current nursing home residents for mental illness and determine whether or not they need active treatment; those who do must be discharged to mental health facilities.

2. **Psychiatric practice settings**
   a. By the mid-1990s, 75% of all Americans will be receiving their health care from various types of managed care systems. The majority of psychiatric practice settings will be within such systems.
   b. Psychiatrists who remain in private practice in the 1990s will be faced with delivering 80%–90% of the care they render through managed care contracts offered by Medicare, Medicaid, Blue Cross/Blue Shield, physician provider organizations, and HMOs at approximately 60% of their usual and customary charges.
   c. Only 30% of HMO mental health visits are to psychiatrists. Forty percent of HMO mental health visits are to nondoctoral level therapists. Psychiatrists will constitute only 20%–30% of mental health personnel in larger managed care organizations.

C. **Community mental health centers** have had a lasting effect on the care of the mentally ill in this country.

1. The Joint Commission on Mental Illness and Health established by Congress in 1955 issued a report in 1961 titled *Action for Mental Health*. This report revealed the deficiencies that existed in the public mental health system and called for a number of significant changes, including:
   a. A need for more community clinics for outpatient treatment
   b. A recommendation to increase the use of general hospitals for the inpatient treatment of psychiatric illness
   c. A need for a change in the nature of the public mental hospital

2. President John F. Kennedy, in his now historic special message of 1961, "Mental Illness and Mental Retardation," proposed a new approach to the care of the mentally ill.
   a. This new approach was designed and implemented to do the following:
      (1) To use federal resources to stimulate state, local, and private action to create, at the community level, a significant number and range of mental health services
      (2) To reduce patient populations in state mental hospitals
   b. Although the establishment of community mental health centers has provided needed services, disastrous consequences have resulted from reliance on these services.
      (1) Although the population of patients in state mental hospitals has been markedly reduced, the number of readmissions has risen so sharply that the state hospital system has become a "revolving door." Psychiatrists now agree that they have been overly optimistic about the efficacy of psychotropic drugs.
      (2) Community resources have proven inadequate to handle the large number of former state hospital patients, resulting in an extraordinary number of homeless mentally ill people.
      (3) Because federal funding has not provided sufficient impetus to state, local, or private sources of funding, reductions in federal funding usually lead to reductions in services.

D. The ***Diagnostic and Statistical Manual of Mental Disorders* (*DSM*)** has provided a significant change in the diagnosis of mental disorders.

1. The *DSM-I* was the first publication to contain a glossary of diagnostic categories.

2. The *DSM-II* (second edition) based the classification of mental disorders on the eighth edition of the *International Classification of Diseases* (*ICD-8*).

3. The *DSM-III* (third edition) provides a classification of mental disorders based on the *ICD-9*. The approach taken is atheoretical with regard to etiology. It attempts to describe disorders comprehensively and to provide specific diagnostic criteria as guides for making each diagnosis, unlike the *DSM-I, DSM-II,* and *ICD-9*.

a. Each of the mental disorders is conceptualized as a clinically significant behavioral or psychological syndrome that occurs in an individual and typically is associated with either a painful symptom (**distress**) or an impairment in one or more important areas of functioning (**disability**).
b. There is no assumption that each mental disorder is a discrete entity with distinct boundaries between it and other mental disorders or between it and no mental disorder.

4. The *DSM-III-R* (revised) recently has been published. The main change has to do with substance abuse and is explained in Chapter 11 I C.

VI. PREVENTION OF MENTAL DISORDERS

A. **Primary prevention** involves the promotion of general mental health and the protection against the occurrence of specific diseases.

1. **Promoting mental health** is a perplexing problem.
   a. There must be a definition of mental health.
   b. It must be assumed that mental health can be affected by measures undertaken during the lifetime of the individual who is the target of the measures.

2. **Specific diseases** are the aim of primary prevention.
   a. **Organic brain syndrome,** resulting from diseases such as syphilis and vitamin deficiencies, was the leading cause of mental hospital admissions 50–75 years ago (i.e., 1900–1920), but it is unusual to find cases in the United States today.
   b. **Crisis or situational reaction** is a condition that currently is receiving much attention in terms of preventive efforts.
      (1) Caplan (1964) developed a theory and techniques for **preparing** individuals in advance to deal with crises in the hope of avoiding the distress that usually results.
      (2) There are two aspects to crisis preparation
         (a) **Anticipatory guidance** (the **cognitive aspect**) consists of a group discussion of the crisis situation that the individual will potentially face, of techniques others have found effective, and of the individual's own experiences in mastering previous crises.
         (b) **Functional inoculation** (the **emotional aspect**) involves putting an individual through a series of increasingly stressful experiences to the point at which he is almost overwhelmed.
   c. **Schizophrenia** is a disease for which preventive efforts have received considerable attention.
      (1) Unfortunately, all evidence suggests that the rate of schizophrenic breakdown has remained stable for many years in spite of preventive efforts.
      (2) There also seems to be an inherited tendency toward schizophrenia (see II B 1 b), but the precise mechanism of inheritance presently is unknown.
   d. **Senility** has become a serious problem in our society as the number of people over 65 years of age increases. There has been a strong trend to classify elderly people with problems of living as psychiatric patients and admit them to mental hospitals.
      (1) Effective prevention probably requires changes in life-style and attitudes in society, especially among young individuals, so that elderly people have a respected niche.
      (2) Young people can be prepared in advance with the skills, resources, and attitudes necessary to combat the disengagement common to old age.
   e. **Personality disorders** result from distorted relationships in childhood. Bowlby (1955) has shown that raising infants in institutions leads to disturbed development in childhood. These findings imply that preventive efforts for orphaned or abandoned children should include not allowing them to be raised in institutions or shifted among foster homes.

B. **Secondary prevention** encompasses early diagnosis and prompt and adequate treatment to prevent sequelae and limit disability. The value of secondary prevention is untested with regard to most mental disorders. Current efforts at early diagnosis and treatment of mental disorders are in four major areas.

1. **Screening large population groups** to find mentally ill people who may then be directed into treatment has been done only as part of research projects. Although most studies have methodologic problems, it seems fair to say that a minimum of 10% of the general American population reports significant psychiatric disability at any one time and, therefore, is in need of treatment. Schools are an obvious setting in which screening procedures followed by treatment would be logical and effective.

2. **Crisis intervention** offers service immediately. Service is brief and focuses on the presenting problem. Rather than attempt to bring about major personality changes, the mental health worker focuses on returning the individual to her previous level of functioning. Because of the vulnerability of the individual in crisis, the mental health worker who intervenes is in a very powerful position.
   a. Crisis intervention has its roots in the work of two investigators.
      (1) Lindemann (1944) studied survivors of the famous Coconut Grove fire and members of several other bereaved and distressed groups during World War II and found that a normal grief reaction is expected. In fact, if this reaction does not occur, other, more disabling manifestations are likely to occur.
      (2) Tyhurst (1958) included grief reactions in a group he called "transition states—circumstances representing significant change, often sudden or intense, in the life situations of individuals."
   b. The treatment of post-traumatic stress disorder is a hallmark for crisis intervention. In the recent Gulf War, treatment was immediate, focused, and carried out on the front lines so that soldiers knew they would be returned to battle.
   c. Terr (1979) did crisis intervention in a group of schoolchildren who were kidnapped and has studied the effectiveness of that crisis intervention as the children have matured. Terr found that the effectiveness of the intervention depended on premorbid functioning.
3. **Educating the public to recognize mental illness in the early stages and then to seek help early** seems to be a useful but unproven approach.
   a. Davis (1965) has done an extensive review of mental health education efforts. He suggests that when mental health education aims only to provide education, it is likely to succeed; when it aims to change behavior, it is likely to fail.
   b. Avnet (1962) found that the use of mental health services was surprisingly low, even after intensive efforts to educate insured people about the availability of their coverage.

C. **Tertiary prevention** encompasses rehabilitation after the occurrence of defect and disability, in an attempt to reduce the disability.

1. Despite major reductions in hospital use, there are over 400,000 patients in state and VA psychiatric hospitals, many of whom suffer from schizophrenia. Pasamanick and colleagues (1967) demonstrated that, for most schizophrenics, hospitalization was not necessary. Such patients could be handled as well at home with regular visits from public health nurses and with medication. Obstacles to this approach include the patients' inability to maintain a home and the difficulty of getting funds to carry out treatment in the community.

2. The general objective of psychiatric rehabilitation is to produce behavior in the patient that will enable him to function in society. It is obvious that the institution should encourage behavior appropriate for life outside.

3. The aged mentally disabled differ in that they previously had a full range of social skills but have lost these through a combination of lack of use, depression, and apathy either in response to change in life circumstances or due to CNS damage. **Reality orientation**—a technique resembling remotivation as practiced with the mentally ill—is advised. Reality orientation starts with simple social interaction and progresses to more complicated skills.

BIBLIOGRAPHY

Akiskal HS: Diagnosis and classification of affective disorders: new insights from clinical and laboratory approaches. *Psychiatr Dev* 1:123–160, 1983.

Angst J, Felder W, Lohmeyer E: Course of schizoaffective psychoses: Results of a follow-up study. *Schizophr Bull* 6:579–584, 1980.

Avnet H: *Psychiatric Insurance: Financing Short-Term Ambulatory Treatment—A Research Project Report.* New York, Group Health Insurance, 1962.

Baldwin JA: Schizophrenia and physical disease. *Psychol Med* 9:611–618, 1979.

Bowlby J: *Attachment and Loss.* New York, Basic Books, 1955.

Caplan G: *Principles of Preventive Psychiatry.* New York, Basic Books, 1964.

Crow TJ: The two-syndrome concept: origins and current status. *Schizophr Bull* 11:471–485, 1985.

Davis JA: *Education for Positive Mental Health: A Review of Existing Research and Recommendation for Future Studies.* Chicago, Aldine, 1965.

Diagnostic and Statistical Manual of Mental Disorders (*DSM-I*). Washington, DC, American Psychiatric Association, 1952.

Diagnostic and Statistical Manual of Mental Disorders, 2nd edition (*DSM-II*). Washington, DC, American Psychiatric Association, 1968.

Diagnostic and Statistical Manual of Mental Disorders, 3rd edition (*DSM-III*). Washington, DC, American Psychiatric Association, 1980.

Diagnostic and Statistical Manual of Mental Disorders, 3rd edition, revised (*DSM-III-R*). Washington, DC, American Psychiatric Association, 1987.

Dorwart RA, Schlesinger M: Privatization of psychiatric services. *Am J Psychiatry* 145:543–553, 1988.

Dorwart RA, Schlesinger M, Davidson H, et al: A national study of psychiatric hospital care. *Am J Psychiatry* 148:204–210, 1991.

Dupont A, Moeller-Jensen O, Stromgren E, et al: Incidence of cancer in patients diagnosed as schizophrenic in Denmark. In *Psychiatric Case Registers in Public Health.* Edited by ten Horn GHMM, Giel R, Gulbinat W, et al. Amsterdam, Netherlands, Elsevier, 1986, pp 229–239.

Ellis RP, McGuire TG: Cost sharing and patterns of mental health care utilization. *Human Resources* 21:359–379, 1986.

Ginsburg SW: The mental health movement and its theoretical assumptions. In *Community Programs for Mental Health.* Edited by Kotinsky R, Witmer H. Cambridge, Harvard University Press, 1955.

Goldman HH: Financing the mental health system. *Psychiatric Annals* 17:580–585, 1987.

Horgan CM: Specialty and general ambulatory mental health services. *Arch Gen Psychiatry* 42:556–572, 1985.

Illowsky BP, Juliano DM, Bigelow LB, et al: Stability of CT scan findings in schizophrenia: results of an 8 year follow-up study. *J Neurol Neurosurg Psychiatry* 51:209–213, 1988.

International Classification of Diseases, 9th edition (*ICD-9*). Washington, DC, World Health Organization, 1988.

Jablensky A: Multicultural studies and the nature of schizophrenia: a review. *J R Soc Med* 80:162–167, 1987.

Joint Commission on Mental Illness and Health: *Action for Mental Health.* New York, Basic Books, 1961.

Kety SS: Mental illness in the biological and adoptive relatives of schizophrenic adoptees. *Am J Psychiatry* 140:720–727, 1983.

Kraepelin E: *Manic-Depressive Insanity and Paranoia.* Edited by Robertson GM. Edinburgh, Scotland, Livingstone, 1921.

Leonhard K, Korf I, Schulz H: Die temperamente in den familien der monopolare und bipolare phasischen psychoses. *Psych Neurol Med Psychol* 143:416–434, 1962.

Lewis SW, Murray RM: Obstetric complications, neurodevelopmental deviance, and risk of schizophrenia. *J Psychiatr Res* 21:373–421, 1988.

Lindemann E: Symptomatology and management of acute grief. *Am J Psychiatry* 101:141, 1944.

Loranger AW: Sex difference in age at onset of schizophrenia. *Arch Gen Psychiatry* 41:157–161, 1984.

Mortensen PB: Environmental factors modifying cancer risk in schizophrenia. Presented at the World Psychiatric Association Symposium. Copenhagen, Denmark, August 1986.

Muszynski S, Brady J, Sharfstein SS: Paying for psychiatric care. *Psychiatric Annals* 14:861–869, 1984.

Owen MJ, Lewis SW, Murray RM: Obstetric complications and schizophrenia: a CT scan study. *Psychol Med* 18:332–340, 1989.

Pasamanick B, Scarpitti FP, Dinitz S: *Schizophrenics in the Community.* New York, Appleton-Century-Crofts, 1967.

Perris C: Study of cycloid psychosis. *Acta Psychiatr Scand* (Suppl):253, 1974.

Sartorius N, Jablensky A, Korten A, et al: Early manifestations and first-contact incidence of schizophrenia in different cultures. *Psychol Med* 16:909–928, 1986.

Sharfstein SS, Dunn L, Kent JJ: The clinical consequences of payment limitations: the experience of a private psychiatric hospital. *Psychiatr Hosp* 19:63–66, 1988.

Shelton RC, Weinberger DR: X-ray computerized tomography studies in schizophrenia: a review and synthesis. In *The Neurology of Schizophrenias.* Edited by Nasrallah HA, Weinberger DR. Amsterdam, Netherlands, Elsevier, 1986, pp 207–250.

Spitzer RL, Endicott J: Computer diagnosis in an automated record keeping system: a study of clinical acceptability. In *Progress in Psychiatric Information Systems: Computer Application.* Edited by Crawford JL, Morgan DW, Grantinco DT. Cambridge, England, Ballinger Books, 1973, p 103.

Terr L: Children of Chowchilla. *Psychoanal Study Child* 34:547–623, 1979.

Tyhurst JS: The role of transition states—including disasters—in mental illness. In *Symposium on Social and Preventive Psychiatry.* Washington, DC, Walter Reed Army Institute of Research, US Government Printing Office, 1958, pp 149–169.

Winokur G, Clayton P, Reich T: *Manic Depressive Illness.* St. Louis, CV Mosby, 1969.

World Health Organization: *Report of the International Pilot Study of Schizophrenia, vol I.* Geneva, Switzerland, WHO, 1973.

World Health Organization: *Schizophrenia. An International Follow-up Study.* Chichester, England, John Wiley, 1979.

STUDY QUESTIONS

Directions: Each of the numbered items or incomplete statements in this section is followed by answers or by completions of the statement. Select the **one** lettered answer or completion that is **best** in each case.

1. Which of the following statements concerning the definition of a mental disorder is correct?

(A) There is general consensus regarding the undesirability of the symptoms of a mental disorder
(B) Only conditions unequivocally associated with suffering and disability are characterized as mental illness by American psychiatrists
(C) The distinction among mental disorders is usually not clinically apparent
(D) Mental disorder is associated with subjective distress and impairment in social functioning

2. Which of the following is a correct statement concerning schizophrenia?

(A) The incidence of schizophrenia is comparatively high, appearing in 10 out of every 1000 adults
(B) Schizophrenic patients in industrialized countries have a better course and outcome than those in undeveloped countries due to advances in medical treatment
(C) There is a consistent seasonality in the distribution of births of individuals who develop schizophrenia
(D) There is a higher mean age of onset in males

3. Organic disease in schizophrenics has which of the following risks?

(A) An increased risk of malabsorption syndrome
(B) An increased risk of cancer
(C) A decreased risk of arteriosclerotic heart disease
(D) A decreased risk of hypothyroidism

4. Which of the following statements is correct regarding the etiology of schizophrenia?

(A) Familial risk for schizophrenia cannot be conclusively predicted
(B) The crucial factor in determining the risk of schizophrenia is not the upbringing an adopted child receives but whether the biologic parent was schizophrenic
(C) The lateral ventricles in the brains of schizophrenics are much smaller than normal
(D) A relationship between an adverse event in pregnancy and the risk of schizophrenia has not been definitively established

5. Which of the following is true regarding the community mental health movement?

(A) Federal funding has, for the most part, established the impetus to state funding so that when federal funds run out, the state has been able to take over
(B) The population of state mental hospitals has been sharply reduced, but the community resources have been inadequate to care for these patients
(C) Community mental health centers have done an enormous service by providing counseling to the homeless mentally ill
(D) The use of psychotropic drugs has made it easy to treat the chronic mental patient in the community

---

1-D
2-C
3-A
4-B
5-B

Directions: Each item below contains four suggested answers of which **one or more** is correct. Choose the answer

- **A** if **1, 2, and 3** are correct
- **B** if **1 and 3** are correct
- **C** if **2 and 4** are correct
- **D** if **4** is correct
- **E** if **1, 2, 3, and 4** are correct

6. Bipolar disorder is associated with which of the following characteristics?

(1) A tendency to return to premorbid functioning in between episodes
(2) A lack of emotionality during episodes
(3) A large percentage of patients being married as contrasted with schizophrenics
(4) A diagnostic requirement of having both manic and depressive episodes

7. Recent studies of bipolar illness have shown that

(1) there is a greater degree of family aggregation in unipolar than in bipolar patients
(2) five percent of the population is at risk for developing bipolar disorder
(3) the manic form occurs at an older age than the depressive form, which may occur in adolescence
(4) women with bipolar illness are more likely to outnumber men with this disease

8. The third edition of the *Diagnostic and Statistical Manual of Mental Disorders* (*DSM-III*) is characterized by

(1) the assumption that each mental disorder is a discrete entity
(2) an atheoretical approach with regard to the etiology of syndromes
(3) the use of the term "reaction" throughout to reflect a psychobiologic view
(4) the conceptualization of each mental disorder as a clinically significant behavioral or psychologic syndrome

9. True statements regarding expenditures for mental health include which of the following?

(1) Psychiatric care represents a sizable portion of the total Medicare budget—over 30%
(2) Medicaid limits the number of inpatient days to 30/year
(3) Over 80% of employer health insurance plans provide for mental health coverage
(4) Nearly 60% of the United States total spending for chronic mental illness is paid for by the federal government

---

6-B
7-C
8-C
9-C

Directions: The group of items in this section consists of lettered options followed by a set of numbered items. For each item, select the **one** lettered option that is most closely associated with it. Each lettered option may be selected once, more than once, or not at all.

Questions 10–13

Match the type of research with the researcher who conducted it.

(A) Spitzer
(B) Lindemann
(C) Kraepelin
(D) Caplan

10. Crisis preparation as primary prevention
11. The definition of mental disorder
12. Crisis intervention as secondary prevention
13. Description of schizophrenia and manic-depressive illness

---

10-D
11-A
12-B
13-C

ANSWERS AND EXPLANATIONS

1. The answer is D *[I B 3 b].*
The most comprehensive definition of mental disorder describes it as a condition that is associated with subjective distress, impairment in social functioning, and voluntary behavior that the patient wishes he could stop because it is regularly associated with physical disability or illness. The problem of defining a mental disorder is that consensus does not always exist for the symptoms. European psychiatrists characterize only conditions unequivocally associated with suffering and disability as mental disorders. Pain and disability associated with a somatic disorder make it easy to form a consensus on definition, but they are not always associated with mental disorders.

2. The answer is C *[II B 1 a].*
A consistent seasonality exists in the distribution of births of people who develop schizophrenia. That is, individuals who will develop schizophrenia are more often born in the season with the lowest average temperatures, regardless of latitude. There are two major types of schizophrenia—acute and insidious onset. The World Health Organization (WHO) Program for Cross-Cultural Research in Schizophrenia found that the syndrome is universal, although its incidence is comparatively low (e.g., 5/1000). The mean age at onset is higher in females than in males. Schizophrenic patients in nonindustrialized cultures have a significantly better 2- to 5-year outcome than patients in industrialized cultures.

3. The answer is A *[II B 1 c (2)].*
In schizophrenics, there is an increased risk of malabsorption syndrome, arteriosclerotic heart disease, and myxedema (hypothyroidism). The cancer risk is decreased in schizophrenics, which has been positively correlated with the length of neuroleptic treatment.

4. The answer is B *[II B 1 b (2)].*
Kety (1983) demonstrated that the crucial factor in determining the risk for schizophrenia is not the type of upbringing an adopted child receives but whether a biologic parent was schizophrenic. As found in adoption studies, an individual's risk rises the more closely related she is to a schizophrenic. Enlargement of the lateral ventricles has been found in computed tomography (CT) scan studies of schizophrenics. A history of adverse events during fetal and neonatal life is obtained more frequently regarding schizophrenic patients than normal subjects.

5. The answer is B *[V C 2 b (1)–(3)].*
Community resources have not been adequate, and, when federal funds have run out, so have services. There are no services for the homeless mentally ill, and the use of psychotropic drugs has been vastly overrated in the treatment of the mentally ill in the community, as is witnessed by the sharp rise in the number of readmissions to state hospitals.

6. The answer is B (1, 3) *[II B 2 a–e].*
Kraepelin (1921) stated that one of the three criteria in what was then called manic-depressive illness was the tendency to return to premorbid functioning. Although marital status is not related to prognosis in bipolar illness, epidemiologic studies have found that bipolar patients are more likely to be married than schizophrenic patients. Kraepelin reported the pressure of intense emotion during acute episodes in manic-depressive illness. Leonhard (1962) separated manic-depressive illnesses into two groups, bipolar disorder and unipolar disorder (i.e., only depressive or manic episodes).

7. The answer is C (2, 4) *[II B 2 a–e].*
Akiskal (1983) estimates that 4%–5% of the population are at risk for developing bipolar disorder. In patients admitted to hospitals with this diagnosis, women are likely to outnumber men. Recent studies (i.e., Perris; Angst; Winokur, Clayton, and Reich) have indicated a greater degree of family aggregation in bipolar than in unipolar patients. Akiskal has found that the manic form occurs primarily in younger individuals, and the depressive disorder occurs in the older age-group.

8. The answer is C (2, 4) *[V D 1–3].*
The third edition of the *Diagnostic and Statistical Manual of Mental Disorder* (*DSM-III*) uses an atheoretical approach with regard to etiology. It attempts to describe disorders comprehensively and to provide specific diagnostic criteria as guides for making each diagnosis. Each mental disorder is conceptualized as a clinically significant behavioral or psychologic syndrome. However, there is no assumption that each mental disorder is a discrete entity with sharp boundaries. The term "reaction" was used throughout the

10
Mental Retardation

Robert A. Velin
Christina L. Herring

I. DEFINITION.

I. DEFINITION. Mental retardation is not a single entity but a group of syndromes resulting from many causes; thus, it is not classified as a disease or an illness. The American Psychiatric Association (APA) and the American Association on Mental Retardation (AAMR; formerly the American Association on Mental Deficiency—AAMD) have set forth the following clinical definition of mental retardation.

A. A **diagnosis of mental retardation** requires the concurrent presence—before the age of 18 years—of significant impairment in intellectual functioning, as well as deficits in general adaptation and social function.

1. In more than 90% of cases, mental retardation exists at birth or occurs within the first 2 years of life.
2. In more than 95% of cases, mental retardation occurs before the age of 5 years.

B. Exclusions. This definition excludes mental retardation acquired in adulthood and conditions in which intelligence may be masked by illness or by emotional, drug-induced, or epileptic syndromes.

II. CLASSIFICATION

A. Classification by AAMR criteria

1. **Definitions.** The classification of mental retardation is appropriate only when an individual falls into the retarded category in both intellectual (intelligence) and adaptive behavior functioning, according to the AAMR's definition of mental retardation (see I A, B).
   a. **Intelligence** is assessed by objective measurement using standardized tests with well-established reliability and validity. Classification by **intelligence quotient (IQ)** level is the result of performance on these standardized tests. Two of the most commonly used tests of intelligence are the **Wechsler Intelligence Scale for Children-Revised (WISC-R)** and the **Stanford-Binet Intelligence Test (form L-M)**.
   b. **Adaptive behavior** can be assessed clinically or with an objective scale (e.g., Vineland Social Maturity Scale, AAMR Adaptive Behavior Scale). Even with objective measures, the quantification of adaptive behavior is less precise than the assessment of intelligence, and even the best tests serve only as guidelines.
2. **Classification levels** for severity of mental retardation generally are based on IQ score ranges. However, due to differences in psychometric properties of the various tests used to assess intelligence, standard deviations (SD) of an IQ score from the mean also must be considered.
   a. **Mild mental retardation** (IQ level 2–3 SD below average; IQ range about 50–70)
      (1) **Distribution.** This group makes up about 80%–85% of the population of mentally retarded individuals.
      (2) **Skills and impairments.** Mildly retarded individuals have minimal impairments in sensorimotor areas and often are not distinguishable from normal children until a later age.
         (a) During the **preschool period,** these individuals can develop social and communication skills.
         (b) By **late teens,** they can learn academic skills up to a sixth-grade level.

(c) During **adulthood,** they usually can achieve social and vocational skills adequate for minimum self-support; they may require assistance in financial planning and situations requiring more complex problem solving.

(d) Mildly retarded persons can usually live successfully in the community, independently or in supervised homes.

b. **Moderate mental retardation** (IQ level 3–4 SD below average; IQ score range about 35–50)

(1) **Distribution.** This group makes up roughly 10%–15% of the mentally retarded population.

(2) **Skills and impairments.** Moderately retarded individuals have only poor awareness of social conventions, and this may especially interfere with peer relationships during adolescence.

(a) During the **preschool period,** they can talk or learn to communicate.

(b) During the **school-age years,** they can profit from training in social and occupational skills and may function up to a fourth-grade level by the late teens if given special education.

(c) During **adulthood,** they may be able to contribute to their own support by performing unskilled or semiskilled work under close supervision.

(d) This group of individuals needs guidance and supervision even when under just mild stress. Their poor awareness of social conventions, combined with impaired general problem-solving skills, can lead to low frustration tolerance.

(e) They generally adapt well to life in the community but usually in structured and supervised group homes.

c. **Severe mental retardation** (IQ levels 4–5 SD below average; IQ score range about 20–35)

(1) **Distribution.** This group makes up 3%–4% of individuals who are mentally retarded.

(2) **Skills and impairments.** Up to age 5 years, there is poor motor development and minimal speech.

(a) During the **school-age period,** they may learn to talk and wash themselves. They may learn to be toilet-trained.

(b) During the **preschool and school-age periods,** they generally profit only minimally from instruction in pre-academic subjects, but they can learn to recognize some important and essential words such as "men," "women," and "stop."

(c) **Adults** are unable to benefit from vocational training but may be able to perform simple, repetitive work tasks under close supervision.

(d) Most severely retarded people generally adapt well to life in the community, in group homes or with their families, provided that they do not have associated handicaps that require specialized nursing or medical care.

d. **Profound mental retardation** (IQ level 5 or more SD below average; IQ score below 20)

(1) **Distribution.** This group constitutes only 1%–2% of individuals with mental retardation.

(2) **Skills and impairments**

(a) During the **preschool period,** these children display minimal capacity for sensorimotor functioning.

(b) **School-age children** may respond to minimal or limited training in self-care, and communication and motor skills may improve with appropriate training.

(c) During **adulthood,** very limited self-care may occur in a structured environment with constant supervision.

(d) In general, an individualized relationship with a caregiver and constant aid and supervision are necessary for optimal development.

B. **Etiologic classification** often is based on whether the condition is acquired prenatally, at birth, or postnatally. It can be difficult to determine prenatal and natal causes; thus, these two etiologic groups sometimes are combined as congenital causes of mental retardation.

1. **Prenatal causes of mental retardation**

a. **Genetic transmission** is reported to be a common cause of mental retardation, accounting for about 50% of cases not classified as mild. The etiology is more difficult to determine in cases of mild retardation, and multiple factors are likely involved.

b. **Conditions acquired in utero** include maternal infections [e.g., rubella, acquired immune deficiency syndrome (AIDS)], maternal metabolic diseases (e.g., diabetes, toxemia of pregnancy), and maternal ingestion of alcohol or other drugs (e.g., fetal alcohol syndrome).

2. **Natal causes of mental retardation** primarily are traumatic and anoxic, resulting from abnormal fetal presentation, accidents of delivery, and maternal oversedation. Although fetal monitoring has reduced the incidence of severe neurologic impairment by indicating the need for emergency cesarean section, it is still impossible to predict the need for cesarean section from gestational history. Recent studies have reported a combined rate of neonatal death and severe neurologic impairment to be in the range of 1%–2% of all births.

3. **Postnatal causes of mental retardation** include lead and mercury ingestion, infections (e.g., encephalitis, meningitis), and severe trauma (e.g., skull fractures, cerebral hemorrhage). It is important to note that although closed-head injuries are relatively common in children, these injuries rarely result in mental retardation.

III. EPIDEMIOLOGY.

The incidence of mental retardation is determined by the number of new cases documented per year and is estimated to be approximately 1 in 100 births.

A. **Profound, severe, and moderate mental retardation** usually are caused by a genetic or prenatal condition. These conditions often are obvious at birth or in the immediate postnatal period because of particular physical or biochemical characteristics recognized by health professionals [e.g., the physical characteristics associated with Down syndrome; abnormal thyroxine (T_4), or thyroid-stimulating hormone (TSH) levels in infants with congenital hypothyroidism].

1. **The incidence of some genetic disorders,** such as Down syndrome, has gradually decreased since World War II, primarily as a result of changing fertility patterns and, perhaps because of prenatal diagnosis.

2. **The incidence of most infectious disorders** and their sequelae have declined sharply over the last 3–4 decades with the widespread use of antibiotics and immunization. However, some infectious disorders appear to be increasing despite modern treatment protocols and increased public awareness (e.g., syphilis, AIDS).

B. **Mild mental retardation** accounts for the vast majority of all cases of mental retardation, but it often is not recognized until the preschool years or when a child enters school. It usually is thought to be a result of multiple factors (environmental and genetic) and is overly represented in families from lower socioeconomic brackets.

IV. GENETIC CAUSES OF MENTAL RETARDATION

A. Disorders of amino acid metabolism

1. **Classic phenylketonuria (PKU)** is a rare autosomal recessive disease of amino acid metabolism. It is one of the milestone diseases of medicine because it was the first disease in which a biochemical cause of mental retardation was discovered and a dietary treatment was effective.

   a. The **incidence** of PKU ranges from 1 in 5000 live births in individuals of Irish and Scottish ancestry, to 1 in 300,000 in blacks, Ashkenazi Jews (Jews of eastern European ancestry), and Finns. Before screening was instituted, the prevalence of PKU-related retardation was 1% of all institutionalized mentally retarded individuals.

   b. **Cause.** The biochemical defect responsible is a deficiency of **phenylalanine hydroxylase,** the enzyme complex essential for the breakdown of phenylalanine to tyrosine.

   (1) The fetus is not affected since the mother has the essential enzyme for the breakdown of phenylalanine, or (if she is affected) is controlling circulating phenylalanine levels through diet or other treatment. The problem arises when the infant must break down the protein postnatally.

   (2) Since an infant with PKU cannot break down phenylalanine, it accumulates in the blood and the resulting hyperphenylalanemia adversely affects the developing infant's brain, leading to irreversible mental retardation if left unchecked.

   (3) Reduction of phenylalanine levels in the blood will not reverse existing mental retardation, but if treatment is instituted prior to the age of 1–2 months, the child has a statistically significant chance of attaining normal intelligence.

   c. **Genetics.** Classic PKU is transmitted by an autosomal recessive gene. Thus, if both parents carry this gene, the statistical chances of their children having PKU are as follows.

(1) One in four offspring will be unaffected and not be a carrier.
(2) Two in four offspring will be unaffected carriers.
(3) One in four offspring will have PKU.

d. **Clinical features** of PKU include:
(1) Increased levels of phenylalanine in the blood and increased levels of phenylalanine and its by-products in urine
(2) Severe or profound mental retardation if not treated early
(3) A tendency for seizures
(4) Eczema

e. **Prevention** of PKU-related mental retardation involves protecting affected children from high levels of circulating phenylalanine, especially during the developmentally critical first 5 years of life. Therefore, **the key to prevention is to identify affected newborns as soon as possible** by such methods as:
(1) **Screening.** All newborns should be screened at birth with a blood test for the presence of PKU. Plasma phenylalanine levels may be normal at birth, but rise rapidly after the initiation of protein feedings, and are usually abnormal by day 4. The **Guthrie bacterial inhibition assay** generally is used for initial screening.
(2) **Identification.** A family at risk can be detected either after an affected child has been identified or by genetic testing of prospective parents. Once at-risk individuals are identified, the entire family and any subsequent offspring should be checked for PKU and undergo genetic counseling.
(3) **Prenatal diagnosis** of classic PKU is feasible using restriction length polymorphisms identified by **DNA-DNA blot hybridization.**

f. **Successful dietary treatment** of PKU with a low-phenylalanine diet has created a new problem—there are now women who are capable of reproduction, but who, as adults, lack the appropriate enzyme to break down phenylalanine.
(1) An affected mother can bear a normal infant, but there is an increase both in the rate of spontaneous abortion and in the risk of bearing offspring with nonphenylketonuric mental retardation, microcephaly, and congenital heart disease.
(2) Although high levels of phenylalanine may be not so dangerous to adults, affected pregnant women should have phenylalanine levels monitored so that the fetus is not adversely affected. Current evidence suggests that dietary restriction in classic PKU should be continued indefinitely, as there is not yet convincing evidence that the dietary restriction can be terminated safely.

g. **Deficiency of tetrahydrobiopterin.** If an affected child develops progressive neurologic impairment despite prompt diagnosis and dietary treatment, deficiency of tetrahydrobiopterin must be considered.
(1) This deficiency is a variant of PKU (as opposed to classic PKU) and, along with **transient hyperphenylalaninemia** and **benign hyperphenylalaninemia,** accounts for 1%–5% of all PKU children.
(2) Dietary treatment alone is generally not sufficient for PKU resulting from tetrahydrobiopterin deficiency, and pteridine cofactor replacement is under study for this disorder.

2. **Homocystinuria** is the second most common inborn error of amino acid metabolism.
a. The **incidence** is roughly 1 in 200,000 live births.
b. **Cause.** Most cases are due to a deficiency of the liver enzyme **cystathionine β-synthase,** which is essential to the metabolism of homocystine to cystine. Two other, less common forms of the disease are the result of impaired conversion of homocystine to methionine.
c. **Genetics.** Homocystinuria is an **autosomal recessive** disorder.
d. **Clinical signs and symptoms** are due to defective collagen formation. They occur in the eye, skeletal system, central nervous system (CNS), and cardiovascular system, and include:
(1) Lens ectopia, which is the clinical hallmark
(2) Osteoporosis and genu valgum, and frequent chest, vertebral, and foot deformities
(3) Mental retardation in approximately one-half of cases
(4) A predisposition for major seizures
(5) A propensity for arterial and venous thromboses as a result of enhanced platelet stickiness
(6) Liver disease

(b) Prenatal diagnosis for type II disease has been reported, but the relative unreliability of the methods warrants caution when attempting to use results for decisions regarding parental counseling.

d. Treatment for the Niemann-Pick group of diseases is not available, except for supportive care.

3. **Gaucher's disease** is a lysosomal storage disease with three specific clinical forms (two neuronopathic and one non-neuronopathic).

   a. The **incidence** of the **non-neuronopathic** form (the so-called **adult form**) of this disease is highest in Ashkenazi Jews (about 30 times higher than in other ethnic groups), and estimates vary from 1 in 600 to 1 in 2500 births. For the **acute neuronopathic** forms, there does not appear to be an ethnic predilection.

   b. **Cause.** The disease is caused by a diminution of the enzyme activity of glucocerebrosidase, which leads to accumulation of cerebrosides in the neurons and cells of the reticuloendothelial system.

   c. **Genetics.** The disease is an autosomal recessive disorder.

   d. **Clinical features**

      (1) The **chronic non-neuronopathic form** may appear at any age and is most common.

         (a) This type is associated with a normal IQ, but hepatosplenomegaly and bone pain are common. Fractures often result from minor trauma.

         (b) The course is variable, but slowly progressive splenomegaly is typical. Some severe cases may involve liver failure and portal hypertension.

      (2) An **acute neuronopathic form** (the so-called **infantile form**) manifests in infancy.

         (a) This type is associated with hepatosplenomegaly and strabismus. The head is retroflexed, and the limbs are spastic.

         (b) The course is rapidly fatal; about 80% of affected infants die within the first year.

      (3) A **subacute neuronopathic form** (the so-called **juvenile form**) may begin any time during childhood. This type usually is associated with neurologic abnormalities that cause behavior problems, low IQ, seizures, tremors, and dysmetrias.

   e. **Prevention** is best accomplished by identifying families at risk and providing genetic counseling.

   f. **Treatment** is supportive.

C. **Down syndrome** occurs when there is an excess of chromosomal material relating to chromosome 21.

1. **Types**

   a. **Trisomy 21,** the most common type, involves three members of chromosome 21; the extra chromosome is acquired due to a failure in chromosomal pairing of one of the parental germ cells.

   b. **Translocation** occurs when the long arm of chromosome 21 attaches to another chromosome (13, 18, or another 21). Unlike trisomy 21, this disorder usually is inherited. The translocation chromosome may be found in unaffected parents and siblings; these asymptomatic carriers have only 45 chromosomes.

   c. **Trisomy mosaic 21** is the rarest form; only some of the cells are trisomic while others are normal.

2. The **incidence** of Down syndrome in the United States is about 1 in 650 births, and it accounts for roughly 25% of all cases of mental retardation not classified as mild. The incidence of affected fetuses rises steeply with increased maternal age to about 1 in 40 births among mothers over 40 years of age.

3. **Characteristic pathologic findings** include:

   a. Embryonic convolutional patterns of the brain

   b. Small cerebellum and brain stem

   c. Abnormalities of the pituitary gland

   d. Cardiac abnormalities (particularly septal defects)

4. **Cardinal clinical and physical features** include:

   a. Mental retardation (most affected individuals are moderately or severely retarded, with only a minority having an IQ above 50)

   b. Hypotonia

   c. Oblique palpebral fissures

   d. Epicanthal folds

e. Small flattened skull
f. High cheek bones
g. Broad, thick hands with a transverse palmar crease
h. Fissured and thickened tongue

5. **Prenatal detection** of Down syndrome can be attempted with **amniocentesis** or **chorionic villus sampling**. However, these methods have drawbacks.
   a. There is risk to the fetus (fetal injury, miscarriage), albeit quite small.
   b. Because these methods are performed primarily on women over 35 years of age, they do not address the issue of Down syndrome births among young women.

6. **Prevention** (except in cases due to translocation) is possible only by abortion, which raises ethical and religious concerns. Genetic counseling is useful for preventive purposes when a translocation in a parent is present.

7. **Treatment.** There is no treatment for Down syndrome, although some of the concomitant defects respond to treatment (e.g., cardiac defects).

D. **Spina bifida** is a congenital neurologic defect in which part of one (or more) vertebrae fail to develop completely, leaving a portion of the spinal cord exposed. It can occur anywhere in the spine but is most common in the lower back. The severity of the condition depends on how much of the cord is exposed.

1. The **incidence** is variable among different ethnic groups but generally is about 1 in 1000 births. The incidence is highest for those of Irish ancestry. Overall, there is evidence that the incidence increases with very young or old maternal age, and a woman who has had one affected child is ten times more likely than average of having another.

2. The **cause** of spina bifida remains unknown. It is thought that many factors are involved.

3. **Genetics.** Although no one cause has been identified, a genetic factor is implicated because there is some ethnic predilection and because the familial risk of recurrence is approximately 5%.

4. **Types**
   a. **Spina bifida occulta.** This is the most common and the least serious form. It often goes unnoticed in otherwise healthy children, and unlike the other forms, there is little external evidence of the defect (aside from a dimple or tuft of hair over the area of the underlying abnormality).
   b. **Meningocele.** This form is more severe than spina bifida occulta, but less severe than other forms. There is a bulging sac over the spine, but the nerve tissue of the spinal cord itself is usually intact.
   c. **Encephalocele.** This is a rare type in which the protrusion occurs through the skull. There usually is severe brain damage.
   d. **Myelocele.** This is the most severe form and is associated with changes in the spinal cord itself. Clinical features include:
      (1) Mental retardation
      (2) Paraplegia
      (3) Incontinence
      (4) Hydrocephalus
      (5) Seizures
      (6) Obvious raw swelling over the spine

5. **Prenatal detection**
   a. **Amniocentesis at midgestation** can be used to detect **elevated α-fetoprotein (AFP)** levels consistent with a neural tube defect. However, as with most tests, its sensitivity and specificity are not perfect. That is, false-positives and false-negatives are possible.
   b. **Ultrasound scanning** may allow for the detection of some defects.

6. **Prevention,** as in Down syndrome, primarily depends on induced abortion after detection of the abnormality. However, counseling is also important for those who have already had a child with a neural tube defect, since the probability of having additional affected infants is increased.

7. **Treatment** of spina bifida generally requires surgery to close the defect and prevent further damage to the cord. Ideally, this should occur within the first few days of life. If the defect is severe, surgery may allow the child to survive, but the likelihood of serious physical and mental handicaps is high. If hydrocephalus develops, the placement of a shunt may be necessary.

V. NONGENETIC CAUSES OF MENTAL RETARDATION

A. Infections

1. **Syphilis.** When this preventable disorder occurs in pregnant women, it can result in congenital syphilis. If left untreated, CNS complications can occur, resulting in mental retardation as well as general paralysis.
   a. The **incidence** of syphilis in the United States increased during the late 1970s and early 1980s, especially in homosexual men. Although there was a general decrease in incidence during the mid-1980s, recently the incidence has risen dramatically, particularly in black women and crack cocaine users. During the past decade, the number of reported cases of congenital syphilis (i.e., acquired in utero) has remained at about 2 per 100 reported cases of primary and secondary syphilis in women.
   b. **Cause.** The disease is caused by infection with *Treponema pallidum,* and transmission to a fetus can occur across the placenta at any stage of pregnancy; however, lesions develop only after the fourth month of gestation, when immunologic competence begins to develop. The risk of fetal infection during untreated early maternal syphilis is estimated to be 75%–95%. The risk decreases to about 35% for maternal syphilis lasting 2 years or longer.
   c. **Types of congenital syphilis**
      (1) **Early congenital syphilis** (within the first 2 years of life) is characterized by the following clinical signs.
         (a) The most severely affected fetuses are stillborn.
         (b) Of the live-born syphilitic infants, most have no lesions at birth but develop papular skin rashes, rhinitis, osteochondritis, and jaundice.
         (c) Invasion of the CNS usually is asymptomatic at this early stage.
      (2) **Late congenital syphilis** is defined as congenital syphilis that remains untreated after 2 years of age and is characterized by the following features:
         (a) Hutchison's teeth (notched or peg-shaped central incisors)
         (b) Mulberry molars—sixth-year molars with multiple and poorly developed cusps, rather than the usual four
         (c) Interstitial keratitis, which often leads to blindness
         (d) CNS involvement, which can result in mental retardation and paresis
   d. **Prevention** of congenital syphilis involves:
      (1) Preventing the transmission of syphilis to women of childbearing age through safe sex practices
      (2) Identifying syphilitic pregnant women via a nontreponemal test at the first prenatal visit and repeating the test in the third trimester in women at high-risk for acquiring sexually transmitted diseases (STDs)
      (3) Providing adequate treatment of the mother before the sixteenth week of pregnancy, which should prevent fetal damage in utero
      (4) Identifying and treating syphilitic infants as soon as possible
   e. **Treatment**
      (1) **Penicillin G** is the drug of choice for the treatment of syphilis, although penicillin-resistant strains have been reported. Other effective antibiotics are the tetracyclines, erythromycin, and the cephalosporins.
      (2) The fetus may be treated successfully in utero via medication given to the mother.

2. **Rubella (German measles)** seriously affects the fetus only if it is contracted during the first trimester, although well-documented cases have resulted from infection several days prior to conception. The earlier in the pregnancy infection occurs, the more likely the fetus is to be affected and the more serious the abnormalities tend to be. About 20% of affected infants die in early infancy.
   a. The **incidence** of rubella, although once very high, had been reduced to only 225 reported cases in 1988. During the period from 1988 to 1990, there had been a small but significant increase in reported cases of both rubella and congenital rubella. One estimate of rubella infection for 1990 placed the incidence at roughly 0.4 cases per 100,000 persons. Ten confirmed cases of congenital rubella syndrome (CRS) among infants born in the United States were reported for 1990. This represents an increase from 1989 figures. Thus, although rising, the absolute rate of CRS remains quite low.
   b. **Cause.** The disease is caused by the rubella virus, which is spread from person to person in airborne droplets. Symptoms generally develop after a 2- to 3-week incubation period.
   c. **Clinical features** in the affected infant, in order of frequency, include:
      (1) Deafness

(2) Congenital heart disease
(3) Mental retardation
(4) Cataract and other eye disorders
(5) Purpura
(6) Cerebral palsy
(7) Bone abnormalities

d. Prevention of rubella-related mental retardation is best addressed by:

(1) **Immunization** of all children and adults who do not already demonstrate immunity, since rubella vaccine is highly effective (antibodies are induced in roughly 95% of recipients) and appears to provide long-lasting immunity

(2) Immunization of all females of childbearing age

(3) Administration of gamma globulin soon after exposure to nonimmune pregnant women who become infected (which *may* prevent infection of the fetus)

e. Treatment. There is no treatment for CRS.

3. Human immunodeficiency virus type-1 (HIV-1) infection is a new and increasing cause of encephalopathy and other CNS complications in the fetus and newborn. Given the asymptomatic course of the disease in adults during its early stages [Centers for Disease Control (CDC) stage II and possibly III], the infant may show signs of infection prior to the mother. However, unlike many other prenatal infections, HIV manifests itself over time and, thus, may not be clinically apparent at birth.

a. The **incidence of AIDS**—the disease caused by HIV-1 infection in its late stages—varies widely from region to region in the United States, with Washington, D.C., having an annual rate of 111.9 per 100,000 population as compared to only 0.3 per 100,000 in the state of North Dakota.

(1) Overall, the rate of AIDS cases was roughly 16.7 per 100,000 persons in the United States during the period December 1989–November 1990. This represents a slight increase from the previous year.

(2) In the United States, women now constitute the fastest growing group of persons with AIDS. The annual incidence of AIDS among children and women of childbearing age in the United States has been increasing yearly for most racial and ethnic groups, but rates are especially high among black and Hispanic women.

(3) If a woman with HIV becomes pregnant, there is a 30%–50% chance that the fetus will become infected in utero or during delivery.

(4) By the first year of life, about 60% of HIV-infected infants will have developed AIDS.

(5) The United States Public Health Service (USPHS) projected that there would be roughly 3000 cases of pediatric AIDS in the United States by the end of 1991, and most of these infants would have acquired the virus by transmission from their mother.

b. Cause. Almost all cases of AIDS in the world are caused by infection with the retrovirus HIV-1. Other retroviruses similar to HIV-1 have been discovered, one of which has been shown to cause a similar immunodeficiency syndrome in Africa (HIV-2), but there is no evidence of spread of HIV-2 in the United States.

c. Clinical features. In addition to the classic clinical features associated with immunocompromise, an HIV-infected child may have signs that include:

(1) Microcephaly

(2) Cerebral atrophy on magnetic resonance imaging (MRI) or computed tomography (CT) scan

(3) Mental retardation—a failure to meet developmental milestones

d. Prevention of AIDS-related mental retardation and pediatric AIDS requires that women of childbearing age remain uninfected. This is best accomplished by:

(1) Educating individuals regarding transmission of the disease and ways to protect oneself (e.g., safe sex practices, intravenous drug abusers not sharing needles)

(2) Rehabilitation of intravenous drug abusers

e. Treatment. There is no cure for AIDS, but the use of therapeutic drugs such as azidothymidine (AZT) and dideoxyinosine (ddI) appear to slow progression to AIDS. In addition, they appear to improve cognitive functioning to some degree in both children and adults. Data necessary for firm conclusions regarding the efficacy of AZT and ddI in treating the cognitive sequelae of HIV are still being gathered.

B. Environmental factors leading to mental retardation

1. Lead exposure can result in damage to the brain, nerves, red blood cells, and digestive system. Acute poisoning, which is quite rare but sometimes fatal, occurs when a large amount of lead is taken into the body over a short period. Chronic poisoning is less rare, and results from small amounts being taken in over a longer period. The body excretes lead very slowly, and thus, it accumulates in body tissues, especially the bones.

a. Incidence. Chronic lead poisoning is most common in children who have licked or eaten old paint that contains high levels of lead. The clinical syndrome (**plumbism**) associated with lead ingestion affects roughly 2 million preschool children annually in the United States. Lead poisoning also can occur through either occupational exposure (e.g., workers in lead mining and smelting industries) or ingestion of food or drink stored or cooked in lead-glazed or lead-soldered containers. Lead also is emitted in the exhaust of vehicles using leaded gasoline.

b. Cause. Lead is a poison of enzymes. In high concentrations, it alters the structure of intracellular proteins, resulting in cell death and tissue inflammation.

c. The **toxic effects of lead** differ between adults and children. Since lead is an enzymatic poison it has a greater impact on developing tissue, which is more vulnerable than tissue with stable metabolism.

(1) In **adults,** poisoning is generally characterized by:

(a) Abdominal pain
(b) Anemia
(c) Renal disease
(d) Headache
(e) Peripheral neuropathy with demyelination of long neurons
(f) Ataxia
(g) Memory loss

(2) In **children,** the clinical features of acute poisoning include anemia and abdominal pain, but the CNS effects are most important. **Subclinical poisoning** of children is of great importance, because physical symptoms generally are not sufficiently severe to bring the child to the attention of medical professionals, yet there can be irreversible CNS effects. These include (depending on the age at exposure):

(a) Mental retardation
(b) Selective deficits in language and cognitive functions (e.g., attention, psychomotor functioning)

d. Prevention of mental retardation related to lead ingestion is best addressed by:

(1) Assuring that children are not in contact with paints containing lead (currently, there is a legal limit to the amount of lead that paints may contain)
(2) Removing children from (or renovating) dilapidated housing or surroundings where paint is peeling from surfaces and, thus, is more likely to be ingested (regardless of amount of lead in the paint)
(3) Not using lead-glazed or lead-soldered containers for food/beverage storage or cooking
(4) In adults, minimizing and monitoring occupational exposure to lead, which is particularly important for pregnant women, as maternal exposure may affect the developing fetus.

e. Treatment. The first and most obvious step in treatment is removal from the source of exposure. Once this is accomplished, reduction of lead levels in the body is best facilitated by the use of chelating agents, primarily the calcium salts of ethylenediaminetetraacetic acid (EDTA), dimercaprol, and penicillamine, which bind to the lead and aid the body in excreting it.

2. Fetal alcohol syndrome, associated with maternal alcohol use, may result in mental retardation. Even small amounts of alcohol consumption may be harmful in pregnancy (since some proportion of ingested alcohol will reach the developing fetus, and alcohol appears to affect fetal growth), but the syndrome appears to occur primarily with persistent alcohol use during pregnancy. Fetal alcohol syndrome has been reported in infants of women who consistently consumed 30 ml of alcohol per day (roughly 2 mixed drinks, or 2–3 bottles of beer or glasses of wine) through the course of their pregnancy. Binge drinking also leads to a higher risk for fetal alcohol syndrome.

a. The **incidence** of fetal alcohol syndrome has been suggested to be at least 0.02%.

b. Mortality rate. Almost 20% of affected infants will die during the first few weeks of life.

c. Clinical features. Many of those who survive will show some of the following clinical features:

(1) Low birth weight

(2) Microcephaly
(3) Mild to moderate mental retardation
(4) Cleft palate
(5) Cardiac atrial or ventricular septal defects
(6) Poorly formed concha
(7) Joint deformities, such as dislocated hip

d. **Prevention** of fetal alcohol syndrome–related mental retardation is best addressed by:
(1) Maternal abstinence from alcohol ingestion during gestation
(2) At the very least, *strict* moderation of maternal alcohol consumption (reduction in consumption only decreases the relative risk; abstinence is still the safest recommendation)
(3) Identification of women most at risk (i.e., those with a significant drinking history) so that education and treatment can be provided
(4) Information to the general public regarding the dangers of drinking (even in moderation) during pregnancy

e. **Treatment.** Once the syndrome is present, treatment focuses on the various physical manifestations of the syndrome (i.e., treatment of cardiac defects, cleft palate). Resultant mental retardation is irreversible.

3. **Nutritional deficiencies.** Maternal **iodine deficiency** (resulting in hypothyroidism) at conception or during early pregnancy or postnatal iodine deficiency in the infant can lead to **cretinism,** a chronic condition resulting from lack of thyroid secretion.

a. **Incidence.** Although there are not good estimates for maternal iodine deficiency per se, the incidence of hypothyroidism (regardless of etiology) in neonates is approximately 1 in 5000. Only a minority of these cases are due to maternal iodine deficiency. Depending on the severity of the deficiency, cretinism may or may not be present.

b. **Geography.** Iodine deficiency primarily occurs in noncoastal areas.

c. **Clinical and physical features** of cretinism include:
(1) Stunted growth
(2) Mental retardation
(3) Course, dry, brittle hair
(4) Rough, dry skin
(5) Large tongue
(6) Proneness to umbilical hernias

d. **Prevention and treatment** of maternal iodine deficiency and resulting cretinism in infants is best accomplished by providing dietary iodine supplementation to women who are deficient. In addition:
(1) **Dietary supplementation,** when indicated, should begin as soon as possible to prevent mental retardation.
(2) **All infants should be screened** for hypothyroidism with measurements of T_4 or TSH to test for proper thyroid functioning.

VI. PREVENTION OF MENTAL RETARDATION.

Primary measures of prevention involving the physician include the following.

A. **Continuing research** into the various causes of mental retardation, including the inborn errors of metabolism, storage diseases, and chromosomal abnormalities. Causes of milder forms of mental retardation are particularly poorly understood.

B. **Providing genetic counseling** if either prospective parent has relatives who have genetic or hereditary abnormalities. For many recessive disorders, this could substantially help reduce the number of affected offspring, either by identifying the need for immediate treatment (e.g., PKU) to avoid mental retardation or by assisting prospective parents in deciding whether or not to have children if there is risk for an abnormality.

C. **Preventing infections and parasitic diseases as well as monitoring the environment** to protect against chemical and physical hazards. Occupational exposure to poisonous agents should be reported to appropriate regulatory agencies, such as the Occupational Safety and Health Administration (OSHA).

D. **Encouraging improvement of social and economic conditions** that may lead to secondary phenomena, such as malnutrition, iodine deficiency, lack of prenatal care, or ingestion of lead-containing paint in run-down housing.

E. **Providing good obstetric, prenatal, and postnatal care,** including treatment of maternal illness; fetal monitoring; recognition of obstetric abnormalities; and prediction, prevention, and treatment of biochemical abnormalities.

VII. TREATMENT OF MENTAL RETARDATION. Unfortunately, if not prevented, mental retardation generally is irreversible. However, much can be done to improve the quality of life for the retarded person and to minimize the limitations resulting from the mental retardation. Although important for all mentally retarded individuals, the following treatment suggestions are particularly important for those with mild retardation (as this group, in particular, is most likely to benefit from intervention).

A. A **stimulating environment** should be provided for the child to encourage intellectual and mental development. Studies have shown that variables such as freedom to engage in verbal expression, language teaching, parental involvement, and provision of language development models are significantly related to intelligence. Given the fact that a disproportionate number of mildly retarded individuals come from families in the lower economic classes where a positive, stimulating environment may be less likely to exist, this consideration is particularly important.

B. **Suitable educational programs** need to be provided for infants and children who have isolated motor, sensory, perceptual, behavior, and intellectual difficulties.

C. When a mentally retarded child reaches school age, an **appropriate educational plan** must be developed [**individual educational plan (IEP)**]. This should be based partly on results from a battery of tests, including tests of intelligence and achievement, and one or more special ability tests. The IEP consists of five sections including:

1. A section containing identifying information on the child plus a detailed description of the child's present level of functioning
2. A section containing goals and short-term objectives for the child's school program
3. Two sections that serve as monitoring vehicles, which contain the types of services and programs the child needs to receive, when these should begin, how long they should last, and which professionals should be responsible for each of them
4. A final section containing the evaluation plan for the child's program and detailing which techniques will be used to measure progress

D. If mentally retarded children are to be assisted in reaching their potential, test scores should not be used for prohibiting a child from participating in programs that could be stimulating. Studies have shown that many children whose test scores fall into the mentally retarded range develop into self-sufficient adults.

E. **The physician plays an important role** in helping parents adapt to having a mentally retarded child and needs to be prepared to play the role of parental counselor.

1. **Early diagnosis of mental retardation** can improve the chances of harmonious parent-child relations, making it easier to meet goals such as creating a positive and stimulating environment.
2. **Parents' helplessness,** a common reaction following the identification of a mentally retarded child, is best handled by giving parents a specific task to do and stressing their role in helping the child to develop as normally as possible.
3. **In cases of severe mental retardation,** the most difficult decision to make is whether or not to institutionalize the child. In this event, it is essential that the physician help establish communication with appropriate community services for counseling and support in this decision.

BIBLIOGRAPHY

Belman AL, Diamond C, Dickson D, et al: Pediatric acquired immune deficiency syndrome. *Am J Dis Child* 142:29–55, 1988.

Centers for Disease Control: *HIV/AIDS Surveillance Report.* Atlanta, CDC, October 1990.

Centers for Disease Control: *HIV/AIDS Surveillance Report.* Atlanta, CDC, December 1990.

Centers for Disease Control: Increase in rubella and congenital rubella syndrome (CRS)—United States, 1988–1990. *MMWR* 40(6):93–98, 1991.

Clayman C (ed): *The American Medical Association Encyclopedia of Medicine.* New York, Random House, 1989.

Crandall B: Update on genetics and mental retardation. *Psychiatric Annals* 19(4):197–204, 1989.

Diagnostic and Statistical Manual of Mental Disorders, 3rd edition, revised (*DSM-III-R*). Washington, DC, American Psychiatric Association, 1987.

Forness SR, Macmillan DL: Mental retardation and the special education system. *Psychiatric Annals* 19(4):190–196, 1989.

Grossman HJ, Begab MJ, Cantwell DP, et al: *Classification in Mental Retardation.* Washington, DC, American Association on Mental Deficiency, 1983.

Pizzo PA, Eddy J, Falloon J, et al: Effect of continuous intravenous infusion of zidovudine (AZT) in children with asymptomatic HIV infection. *N Engl J Med* 319:889–896, 1988.

Scriver CR, Beaudet AL, Sly WS, et al (eds): *The Metabolic Basis of Inherited Disease,* 6th edition. New York, McGraw-Hill, 1989.

Tarjan G: Mental retardation revisited. *Psychiatric Annals* 19(4):176–178, 1989.

Valente M: Etiologic factors in mental retardation. *Psychiatric Annals 19(4):179–183, 1989.*

Wilson JD, Braunwald E, Isselbacher KJ, et al (eds): *Harrison's Principles of Internal Medicine,* 12th edition. New York, McGraw-Hill, 1991.

STUDY QUESTIONS

Directions: Each of the numbered items or incomplete statements in this section is followed by answers or by completions of the statement. Select the **one** lettered answer or completion that is **best** in each case.

1. A high maternal AFP level is present in most cases of

(A) spina bifida
(B) Gaucher's disease
(C) Tay-Sachs disease
(D) Down syndrome

2. A 2-month-old infant has lens ectopia, a history of major seizures, abnormal liver functions, and a demonstrated propensity for arterial and venous thromboses. Which of the following disorders that result in mental retardation most likely caused these findings?

(A) Tay-Sachs disease
(B) Homocystinuria
(C) Gaucher's disease
(D) Lead poisoning

3. Which of the following statements regarding the classification levels for mental retardation is true?

(A) Mild mental retardation accounts for 50% of all cases of mental retardation
(B) Less than 5% of all cases of mental retardation are classified as severe mental retardation
(C) Roughly 25% of all cases of mental retardation fall into the moderate classification
(D) Profound mental retardation accounts for over 5% of all cases of mental retardation

4. The most common prenatal cause of mental retardation is

(A) maternal infections
(B) maternal ingestion of alcohol or other drugs
(C) genetic transmission
(D) nutritional deficiencies

5. Niemann-Pick disease type I is a result of which of the following?

(A) A deficiency in cystathionine synthase
(B) A diminution of the enzyme activity of glucocerebrosidase
(C) Infection with *Treponema pallidum*
(D) An absence of sphingomyelinase

1-A
2-B
3-B
4-C
5-D

Directions: Each item below contains four suggested answers of which **one or more** is correct. Choose the answer

A if **1, 2, and 3** are correct
B if **1 and 3** are correct
C if **2 and 4** are correct
D if **4** is correct
E if **1, 2, 3, and 4** are correct

6. Which of the following statements regarding the assessment of mental retardation is true?

(1) The measurement of adaptive behavior functioning is more precise than intellectual assessment
(2) Deficits in either intellectual functioning or adaptive behavior functioning are sufficient to diagnose mental retardation
(3) Individuals who score 1 SD below average on an intelligence test but who are severely impaired in adaptive behavior functioning can be classified as mentally retarded
(4) Individuals who score 2–3 SD below average on an intelligence test but who have normal adaptive behaviors are not classified as mentally retarded

7. A diagnosis of mental retardation according to the AAMR requires which of the following functional impairments?

(1) Significant impairment in intellectual functioning
(2) Below average academic performance
(3) Deficits in general adaptation
(4) Limited speech ability

Directions: The group of items in this section consists of lettered options followed by a set of numbered items. For each item, select the **one** lettered option that is most closely associated with it. Each lettered option may be selected once, more than once, or not at all.

Questions 8–11

A variety of disorders—both genetic and nongenetic—may cause mental retardation. For each characteristic below, select the most appropriate disorder that may underlie mental retardation.

(A) Classic PKU
(B) Tay-Sachs disease
(C) Down syndrome
(D) Gaucher's disease

8. Diminution of the enzyme activity of glucocerebrosidase

9. Increased levels of phenylalanine in the blood

10. Lipid accumulation in ganglion cells as a result of hexosaminidase-A deficiency

11. Cardiac abnormalities, particularly septal defects

6-D
7-B
8-D
9-A
10-B
11-C

ANSWERS AND EXPLANATIONS

1. The answer is A *[IV D 5].*
A high maternal α-fetoprotein (AFP) level is present in most cases of open neural tube defect (spina bifida), which is a neurologic aberration that permits leakage of cerebrospinal fluid (CSF). Amniocentesis at midgestation can detect an AFP level consistent with this neural defect. Gaucher's disease is an autosomal recessive lysosomal storage disease associated with an accumulation of cerebrosides in the neurons and cells of the reticuloendothelial system due to a dimunition in the enzyme activity of glucocerebrosidase. It is not associated with elevated AFP levels. Tay-Sachs disease also is an autosomal recessive lysosomal storage disease, and amniocentesis or chorionic villus sampling is used to determine if there is a deficiency of the enzyme hexosaminidase A, which is the cause of this disease. Down syndrome is associated with an abnormality of chromosome 21; either there is an extra chromosome 21 (as in trisomy 21 and trisomy mosiac 21) or the long arm of chromosome 21 has attached to another chromosome.

2. The answer is B *[IV A 2 d].*
The cardinal signs and symptoms of homocystinuria include lens ectopia, osteoporosis, frequent physical deformities, liver disease, a propensity for seizures, and a propensity for arterial and venous thromboses as a result of enhanced platelet stickiness. Homocystinuria is an autosomal recessive disorder and is the second most common inborn error of amino acid metabolism. It is a result of a deficiency of the liver enzyme cystathionine β-synthase, which is necessary for the metabolism of homocystine. In contrast, Gaucher's and Tay-Sachs are lysosomal storage diseases. The acute neuronopathic form (so-called infantile form) of Gaucher's disease is generally associated with hepatosplenomegaly, strabismus, a retroflexed head, and spastic limbs. About 80% of affected infants die within the first year. The subacute form of Gaucher's disease may begin at any time during childhood and usually is associated with neurologic abnormalities resulting in low intelligence quotient (IQ), seizures, tremors and dysmetrias. A propensity for arterial and venous thromboses is not usual. There also is a non-neuronopathic form of Gaucher's disease (so-called adult form). All forms of Gaucher's disease are the result of a dimunition of the enzyme activity of glucocerebrosidase, which leads to accumulation of cerebrosides in the neurons and cells of the reticuloendothelial system. Tay-Sachs disease is caused by a deficiency of the enzyme hexosaminidase A, which results in a build-up of G_{M2} ganglioside in the ganglion cells. It is the most common of the lysosomal storage diseases. It is clinically apparent by 4–8 months of age, and invariably results in death by the age of 3–4 years. Its clinical features include blindness, dementia, deafness, seizures, and paralysis.

3. The answer is B *[II A 2 a–d].*
Whereas the majority (roughly 80%–85%) of all cases of mental retardation are classified as mild, only 3%–4% fall into the severe category. A total of 10%–15% fall into the moderate range. Those with mild mental retardation generally achieve social and vocational skills adequate for minimum self-support and usually can live successfully in the community independently or in supervised homes. Persons classified as moderately retarded make up the second largest group of all cases of retardation, and by adulthood, they often can perform unskilled or semiskilled work under close supervision. They generally adapt well to life in the community but usually in structured and supervised group homes. Those with severe mental retardation generally do not benefit from occupational or vocational training, but they may be able to perform simple, repetitive work tasks under close supervision. Persons with profound retardation constitute the smallest group of mentally retarded individuals (1%–2%). Although limited self-care may occur during adulthood in a structured environment with constant supervision, persons with profound mental retardation generally need an individualized relationship with a caregiver and constant aid and supervision. Genetic transmission is reported to account for approximately 50% of all cases of mental retardation not classified as mild.

4. The answer is C *[II B 1 a].*
The most common prenatal cause of mental retardation is genetic transmission. It accounts for about 50% of all cases not classified as mild and plays a strong role in most cases of mild retardation. In contrast, maternal infections, nutritional deficiencies, and ingestion of alcohol (i.e., fetal alcohol syndrome) account for a much smaller percentage of cases. In fact, nutritional deficiencies are rare in the United States.

5. The answer is D *[IV B 2 a].*
Niemann-Pick disease type I is due to an absence of sphingomyelinase, which leads to the excessive storage of phospholipids, especially sphingomyelin, in the reticuloendothelial system. Niemann-Pick disease type II includes patients for whom the nature of the metabolic defect is uncertain but who show elevation in one or more of sphingomyelin, cholesterol, glycolipid, or bis(monoacylglycero)-phosphate in spleen

or liver. Sphingomyelin storage is less marked than in type I disease, when it is present, and sphingomyelinase activity is often normal in solid tissues. Gaucher's disease is a result of diminution of the enzyme activity of glucocerebrosidase, which leads to accumulation of cerebrosides in the neurons and cells of the reticuloendothelial system. Homocystinuria is most commonly caused by a deficiency in cystathionine β-synthase, which is necessary for the metabolism of homocystine. It is the second most common inborn error of amino acid metabolism. Infection with *Treponema pallidum,* on the other hand, causes syphilis. If left untreated, syphilis can be passed from mother to fetus in utero and can result in numerous central nervous system (CNS) complications.

6. The answer is D (4) *[II A 1, 2].*
Individuals who score 2–3 standard deviations (SD) below average on an intelligence test but who have normal adaptive behaviors are not classified as mentally retarded; that is, one must show deficits *both* in intelligence and adaptive behavior before qualifying for a diagnosis of mental retardation. Furthermore, one must score *at least* 2 SD below average on a standardized test of intelligence to fall into the mentally retarded range. Measurements of adaptive behavior functioning are much less precise than the intelligence quotient (IQ) testing used to assess intellectual functioning.

7. The answer is B (1, 3) *[I A; II A 1].*
According to the American Association on Mental Retardation (AAMR) definition, a diagnosis of mental retardation requires that the individual show significant impairment in intellectual functioning (as measured by an individual intelligence test) and deficits in general adaptation. Although mentally retarded individuals may show limited speech ability (particularly in the more severe cases), speech ability can be multiply determined and is not part of the AAMR definition of mental retardation. Below average academic performance also is not included in the AAMR definition. Mentally retarded individuals may, in the standard classroom, perform below normal levels, but poor academic performance can and frequently does occur in the absence of mental retardation (i.e., it is multiply determined).

8–11. The answers are: 8-D *[IV B 3 b],* **9-A** *[IV A 1 b],* **10-B** *[IV B 1 b],* **11-C** *[IV C 3 d].*
Gaucher's disease is a lysosomal storage disease caused by a diminution of the activity of glucocerebrosidase. This leads to an accumulation of cerebrosides in the neurons and cells of the reticuloendothelial system. It is the most common lysosomal storage disorder, and there are three distinct clinical types of the disease. One (the so-called adult form) is non-neuronopathic and two (the so-called infantile and juvenile forms) are neuronopathic.

Classic phenylketonuria (PKU) is caused by a deficiency of enzymes necessary for the breakdown of phenylalanine. As a result of this deficiency, circulating phenylalanine levels rise and result in damage to the developing brain. If left untreated, severe mental retardation will result. Fortunately, PKU can be treated effectively with dietary modification and mental retardation avoided with prompt treatment. Newborn screening programs have been very effective at identifying affected infants. Protecting affected children from high levels of circulating phenylalanine is especially important during the developmentally critical first 5 years of life. Prenatal diagnosis of classic PKU also is feasible.

Tay-Sachs is an autosomal recessive disease caused by a deficiency of the enzyme hexosaminidase A, resulting in a buildup of G_{M2} ganglioside in the ganglion cells. It is clinically apparent within the first 4–8 months of age, and results in death by the age of 3–4 years.

Down syndrome is often associated with cardiac abnormalities, especially septal defects. There are three types of the syndrome, but all types involve an excess of material relating to chromosome 21. In trisomy 21 and trisomy mosaic 21, the abnormalities are the result of an extra chromosome 21. A third cause of the syndrome is a result of translocation, which occurs when the long arm of chromosome 21 attaches to the arm of another chromosome.

11
Psychoactive Substance Abuse

Christina L. Herring

I. DRUG ADDICTION VERSUS DRUG DEPENDENCE. Historically, there has been confusion between drug addiction and drug dependence.

A. The ***Diagnostic and Statistical Manual of Mental Disorders,* second edition (*DSM-II*)** used the term "drug dependence" instead of "drug addiction" and listed drug and alcohol abuse as distinct entities.

B. The ***DSM-III*** combines drug and alcohol abuse under **"substance abuse disorders**."

C. The ***DSM-III-R*** (revised) has made major revisions that include:

1. Removing the distinction between abuse and dependence and broadening the definition of dependence from symptoms to a syndrome of clinically significant behaviors that indicate a serious degree of involvement with psychoactive drugs
2. Creating a new category called "psychoactive substance neuroadaptation syndrome" for individuals whose physiologic adaptations to high doses of psychoactive substances do not arise from their own behaviors (i.e., iatrogenic drug dependence)
3. Using an identical set of symptoms and behaviors to determine dependence on all different classes of psychoactive substances
4. Providing a **system for rating severity of dependence,** which considers the following factors:
   a. **Degree of effort or persistent desire** to cut down or control substance abuse
   b. **Frequency of intoxication or impairment** by substance abuse when expected to fulfill social or occupational obligations or when substance abuse is hazardous
   c. **Tolerance**—the need for increased amounts of substance in order to achieve intoxication or desired effect, or diminished effect with continued use of the amount
   d. **Withdrawal**—substance-specific syndrome following reduction of intake of substance
   e. **Frequency of preoccupation** with seeking or taking the substance
   f. **Abandonment of important social, occupational, or recreational activity** in order to seek or take the substance
   g. **Regular use of psychoactive substance** to relieve or avoid withdrawal symptoms
   h. **Use of substance in larger doses** or over a longer period than user intended
   i. **Continuation of substance use** despite a physical or mental disorder or a significant social or legal problem that the individual knows is exacerbated by the use of the substance

II. EPIDEMIOLOGY OF SUBSTANCE ABUSE. Substances associated with abuse and physical dependence include alcohol, cocaine, barbiturates, opioids, amphetamines, tobacco, and cannabis. Phencyclidine (PCP) and most hallucinogens are not associated with physical dependence.

A. Alcohol. Alcohol dependence constitutes the most serious drug problem in the United States in terms of prevalence.

1. **Incidence**
   a. Nearly 100 million people in the United States drink alcohol, and although more than 90% do so without harm, an estimated 9 million Americans suffer from **alcoholism,** although a large number of these individuals would not describe themselves as alcoholics.

b. The most comprehensive survey of alcohol and other drug use among young people is conducted annually by the **National Institute on Drug Abuse (NIDA)**.
   (1) In their 1985 survey, NIDA found that 92% of high school seniors reported having used alcohol at least once in their lifetime, 66% had used alcohol within the last month, and 5% were daily users.
   (2) A startling 37% reported having five drinks on at least one occasion in the 2 weeks prior to being surveyed.

2. **Population surveys** indicate that 5%–8% of adult men and 1%–6% of adult women are alcoholic.

3. **Injuries.** Alcoholics are associated with an annual toll of 25,000 traffic fatalities, 15,000 homicides, and 20,000 deaths from alcohol-related diseases.

4. One-third of the arrests that occur each year are for public intoxication. If arrests for drunken driving, disorderly conduct, vagrancy, and other alcohol-related offenses are included, the proportion rises to 50% of arrests.

5. **Social profile.** One study showed that alcoholics tended to be:
   a. Men and women 45–49 years old
   b. Members of low socioeconomic groups
   c. Service workers
   d. Unmarried
   e. City dwellers
   f. Catholic or Protestant
   g. Native Americans

B. Drugs

1. **Cocaine**
   a. **Incidence**
      (1) The number of people who have tried cocaine at least once (**lifetime prevalence**) increased from 5.4 million in 1974 to 22.2 million in 1985 (NIDA, 1985).
      (2) The estimated number of current abusers (use in the past 30 days) increased from 1.6 million in 1977 to 4.3 million in 1979, remained stable in 1982, and increased to 6 million in 1985.
      (3) By 1985, 3 million Americans were considered dependent on cocaine.
      (4) Increased abuse of the drug leveled off substantially until 1984 when crack cocaine appeared. Crack is a cheap smokable form of cocaine that can produce a one-try addiction because of the incredibly unpleasant withdrawal symptoms.
   b. **Sex.** The prevalence of cocaine abuse is higher among males (19.3%) than females (11.9%).
   c. **Adverse effects.** A 1988 study (Herridge) selected 500 cocaine abusers who called a national telephone helpline.
      (1) The average caller reported 10 of a possible 21 items for adverse psychological effects: depression, anxiety, irritability, apathy, paranoia, difficulty concentrating, memory problems, sexual disinterest, panic attacks, and attempted suicide.
      (2) The average caller reported 10 of a possible 22 items for adverse physical effects: sleep problems, chronic fatigue, severe headaches, nasal sores, chronic cough, sore throat, nausea, vomiting, seizures, and loss of consciousness.
      (3) Callers reported numerous social, familial, financial, and employment problems associated with their cocaine abuse.
         (a) These included loss of job (25%), loss of spouse (26%), loss of friends (51%), and loss of all monetary assets (42%).
         (b) They also reported violent arguments (66%), threat of divorce (27%), and absenteeism coupled with reduced productivity at work (40%).
         (c) Eleven percent reported having an auto accident while high on cocaine.
         (d) Callers also reported selling cocaine (39%) or stealing from work, family, or friends (29%) to support their cocaine habit; 12% said they had been arrested for a cocaine-related crime.
   d. **Social profile**
      (1) Cocaine abuse is distributed throughout the population among all income groups, although the prevalence of use in the population earning over $50,000 is less than in other groups.
      (2) Abuse is greater among the unemployed.

(3) Abuse among homemakers and those who are married is lower than among other groups, and the highest prevalence is found among those who are cohabiting or living as married.

(4) Lifetime prevalence is higher among white males than among Hispanic or black adults of either sex.

(5) Abuse is greater in metropolitan areas.

(6) Other variables associated with high rates of cocaine abuse were the number of moves in the past 5 years, the number of jobs in the past 5 years, and early use of alcohol, cigarettes, and marijuana.

2. **Barbiturates.** Barbiturates, such as secobarbital and amobarbital, are legitimately manufactured in immense quantities and are readily available in numerous forms. Production is presently sufficient to supply every individual in the United States with 50 doses.
   a. The **incidence and prevalence** of barbiturate abuse are impossible to estimate.
   b. **Social profile.** Individuals with a dependence on barbiturates fall into one of three patterns of use.
      (1) **Chronic intoxication** occurs in 30- to 50-year-old individuals who obtain the drugs from their physicians rather than from illegal sources. They are members of the middle or upper classes, and their drug dependence may go unnoticed by family members or close friends for months or years.
      (2) **Episodic intoxication** occurs in teenagers or young adults who ingest barbiturates for the same purpose that they consume alcohol—to produce a high.
      (3) **Intravenous (IV) barbiturate abuse** occurs in young adults who are involved in the illegal drug culture. They may also abuse amphetamines and heroin and resort to barbiturates only when their money supply is low, since barbiturates are less expensive than other drugs. For the most part, IV barbiturate users make up a small group.

3. **Opioids.** Opioids consist of **opium, opium alkaloids,** and **synthetics**. Opium is produced from the poppy plant, *Papaver somniferum*. There are two classes of opium alkaloids, phenanthrene and benzylisoquinolone. The important class in drug dependence is phenanthrene, of which morphine and codeine are the most important. The synthetic opioids are heroin, methadone, and meperidine. Although opioids occur in forms that can be smoked, snorted, or taken orally, it is **opioids taken intravenously** (especially heroin) that are most frequently abused.
   a. **Incidence.** Most addiction rates are calculated according to the **Baden formula,** which assumes that the number of heroin deaths reported in New York City represents 1% of all addicts. According to a recent study by Hahn (1989), the number of current IV drug abusers has been estimated at between 900,000 and 1.2 million people in the United States.
   b. **Sex.** Among all IV drug abusers, men are primarily affected; the men-to-women ratio is approximately 5:1.
   c. **Social profile of heroin abusers**
      (1) In the 1950s, the typical heroin addict was an urban dweller, a member of a minority group (especially black or Hispanic), male, and 25–35 years old. In the latest survey done by NIDA (1985), this is still the case.
      (2) In 1985, 98% of the heroin addicts admitted to federally funded treatment programs were urban residents.
      (3) Among the **medical profession,** the heroin addiction rate is estimated to be 1%–2%, as contrasted with the overall rate of 0.3% for the U.S. population.
   d. **Acquired immune deficiency syndrome (AIDS)**
      (1) The **medical consequences of IV drug abuse** can be dire. The sharing of needles among drug abusers is a major mode of transmission of the human immunodeficiency virus (HIV), and thus of AIDS.
      (2) The **size of the HIV-infected population** in the United States was estimated to be between 945,000 and 1.41 million in 1989.
      (3) The **infected IV drug abuser population** was estimated to be about 226,000 in the United States in 1987 and represents 16%–24% of the total number of IV drug abusers. Although the rate of AIDS infection in the homosexual population has decreased, the number of infected IV drug abusers has continued to rise.
      (4) The **highest rates of infected drug abusers** continue to be concentrated in northeastern cities, with the highest rates in Baltimore (29%); Newark, N.J. (39%–50%); and New York City (33%–50%). Puerto Rico also has a high rate of infected drug abusers (45%–59%). There are low rates in Atlanta (10%), Denver (5%), Detroit (7%), and San Francisco (13%).

(5) **Median rates for black IV drug abusers** infected with AIDS exceeded those of white IV drug abusers by 4 to 1.
(6) **Median age-specific rates** increase with age to a maximum of 6% in the age range of 35–39 years.
(7) **Heroin abusers** had the highest rate of AIDS infection followed by cocaine abusers.

4. **Amphetamines.** Benzedrine was first available in an over-the-counter inhaler in 1932 and was to be used for narcolepsy, a rather uncommon condition. Since then, benzedrine ("speed") has become widely available. Recent surveys (Johnston, 1988) among student populations have revealed that, in some cities, significant amphetamine use occurs in children in the fifth and sixth grades and that 15%–25% of all high school students are regular speed users. There has been growth in black market production of injectable methamphetamine ("meth").
   a. The **incidence** of amphetamine abuse is impossible to determine. Most abusers do not come to the attention of the medical profession because the abstinence syndrome is not so severe as for other drugs.
   b. **Uses.** In the 1950s, amphetamines were popularly prescribed as a safe way to diet, since the addiction potential was not known. Today, the only legitimate uses are for attention deficit in children, narcolepsy, and to potentiate tricyclic antidepressants.

5. **Marijuana**
   a. **Social profile.** The **Commission on Marijuana and Drug Abuse** conducted the first large scale probability study of individuals over 12 years of age (Kandel, 1989) and found that:
      (1) Young adults 18–25 years of age are the heaviest abusers, with about 25% currently using marijuana.
      (2) Approximately 11% of high school seniors use marijuana daily.
      (3) There appears to be a sharp decline in use after the age of 25 years.
      (4) The demand for marijuana has not increased substantially over the past 10 years.
   b. The **predictors of cessation of marijuana use** also have been studied by Kandel (1989). Factors that predict cessation of abuse in adulthood parallel those that predict lack of initiation in adolescence: conventionality in social role performance, social context unfavorable to use of drugs, and good health. The degree of prior drug involvement remained the strongest predictor of drug cessation in marijuana abuse. Those who abuse drugs in response to social influences are more likely to stop than those who abuse drugs for psychological reasons.

6. **Benzodiazepines.** There are two classes of benzodiazepines: **anxiolytics** (e.g., diazepam, chlordiazepoxide, lorazepam, alprazolam) and **hypnotics** (e.g., triazolam, temazepam, flurazepam). Taken as a group, anxiolytics and hypnotics sometimes are known as **minor tranquilizers**.
   a. **Social profile.** It is impossible to obtain an accurate profile of the individual who abuses minor tranquilizers because they are so widely prescribed as well as available on the street. In fact, the elderly receive a great deal of benzodiazepine treatment. One survey (Schweizer, 1989) reported that 26% of prescriptions for benzodiazepine anxiolytics and 40% of prescriptions for benzodiazepine hypnotics had been written for patients 65 years of age and older. Another survey (Foy, 1986) found that 33% of long-term benzodiazepine abusers were elderly.
   b. **Uses.** General practitioners and internists are much more likely to prescribe benzodiazepines when an antidepressant might be more appropriate. Although these medications may be helpful for stress in the short run, there is great addiction potential, and chronic use should be avoided.

III. BIOLOGIC ETIOLOGY OF PSYCHOACTIVE SUBSTANCE ABUSE.

All of the research done in this area concerns the etiology of alcoholism, possibly because alcohol is a legally obtained psychoactive substance.

A. **Family studies** on alcoholism (e.g., Cotton, 1979) consistently emphasize the high prevalence of alcoholism among relatives of alcoholics. In most studies, at least 25% of male relatives are alcoholic. These studies also show a higher than expected frequency (5%–10%) of alcoholism among female relatives. Identification of hereditary factors in family studies involves twin, genetic marker, and adoption studies.

1. **Twin studies** examine identical and fraternal twins to determine concordance for alcoholism (Vesell, 1971). **Identical twins** are:
   a. More often concordant for alcoholism than are fraternal twins
   b. More often concordant for quantity and frequency of drinking but not for the adverse consequences of drinking than are fraternal twins
2. **Genetic marker studies** examine the relationship between a known inherited biologic trait and a familial disease, to establish whether the latter is genetically transmitted. Associations between a genetic marker and alcoholism have not been determined unequivocably.
3. **Adoption studies** involve interviewing children of alcoholics (Cloninger, 1983).
   a. **Biologic children of alcoholics** are particularly vulnerable to alcoholism whether they are raised by their alcoholic parents or by nonalcoholic foster parents. This vulnerability is specific for alcoholism and does not involve risk for other psychopathology.
   b. **Individuals raised apart from their biologic parents** were significantly more likely to have a drinking problem if a biologic parent was alcoholic than if an adoptive parent was alcoholic.
4. **Sex.** Although women are less often alcoholic than are men, among those who do drink heavily, an unusually high percentage become alcoholic (Bohman, 1981). Also, women from alcoholic families are prone to be depressed, while men in these families are prone to alcoholism. In the above study, 30% of daughters raised by alcoholics had been treated by age 32 for depression, compared to about 5% of controls.

B. **Familial alcoholism,** which is a useful subcategory of alcoholism, has been proposed and includes:

1. A family history of alcoholism
2. Early onset of alcoholism
3. Severe symptoms requiring treatment at an early age
4. Absence of other conspicuous psychopathology

IV. PSYCHOLOGICAL THEORIES OF ADDICTION

A. Psychoanalytic theories

1. **Freud** (1914, 1957), **Menninger** (1938), and **Adler** (1941) proposed theories that are inadequate and untestable.
2. **Rado** (1933) was the first psychoanalyst to suggest that drug abuse might represent an individual's attempt to cope with difficult emotional states. Rado argued that it was not the drug, but rather the individual's impulse to use it, that made him or her an addict.
3. **Chein, Gerard, Lee, and Rosenfeld** (1964) argued that not only depression but also states of anxiety, panic, and self-rejection fed the impulse to use drugs.
4. **Vaillant** (1966) urged practitioners to assess the addict's ego functions and then attempt to:
   a. Find a substitute for each immature defense
   b. Control self-destructive behavior
   c. Provide a context for involvement and acceptance
5. **Khantzian** (1975) focused on how specific drug effects—energizing (amphetamines and cocaine), relaxing (sedatives, hypnotics), and controlling (opiates)—interact with distinct personality factors and behavior patterns. He suggested that individuals select one drug over another in an attempt to cope with specific problems in their internal and external environments that would be unmanageable for these individuals without the particular drug effect.
6. Unfortunately, none of these theories is supported with hard data.

B. Sociological theories

1. **Horton** (1943) studied the consumption of alcohol, subsistence security, and accessibility of alcohol in 77 cultures. He found a high degree of correlation between subsistence insecurity and excessive drinking.

2. **Bales** (1946) relates social organization and cultural practice to alcoholism based on the following:
   a. The degree to which a culture influences the needs for adjustment or inner tensions in its members
   b. Attitudes toward drinking that the culture encourages in its members
   c. The degree to which the culture provides suitable substitute means of satisfaction
3. Although these theories may be valid for explaining some group behavior, they only go so far. A biopsychosocial model is needed for alcoholism.

V. PREVENTION OF PSYCHOACTIVE SUBSTANCE ABUSE.

Approaches to the prevention of alcohol and drug-related problems have been derived mainly from three important models.

A. Public health model. Although critics question whether the health field is capable of preventing alcohol and drug problems—given that these problems may be more social than medical in nature—the public health model (see Ch 1 IV A) proposes three points of intervention.

1. **Host.** The individual's knowledge about alcohol and drugs and the attitudes that influence abuse patterns must be considered.
2. **Agent.** The content, distribution, and availability of alcohol and drugs are important factors that influence abuse patterns.
3. **Environment.** The setting or context in which substance abuse occurs and the community mores that influence it must be examined.

B. Distribution of consumption model. A direct relationship appears to exist between per capita consumption and the prevalence of heavy use of alcohol and drugs.

1. **de Lint** (1976) reviewed research on control measures and concluded that minor variations in density, location, and type of outlet, hours and days of sales, or other regulations have no measurable effect on the rates of alcohol consumption.
2. **Popham and associates** (1953) noted that an increase in opportunities to drink results in increased drunkenness. However, they also found that widespread availability promoted moderate drinking. In addition, they reviewed the effect of the legal restraints on drinking and discovered the following.
   a. Highly restrictive controls on accessibility lead to lower consumption levels and fewer alcohol problems.
   b. Controls are unlikely to be implemented in the absence of substantial public support.
   c. Controls usually involve a variety of social and political costs that eventually are perceived to outweigh their benefits.
3. **Smart** (1976) concluded that lowering age limits for purchase and consumption of alcohol leads to increased alcohol consumption and alcohol problems among young people.
4. Reviews indicate that a rise in alcohol prices generally led to a decrease in alcohol consumption, and a rise in the income of consumers generally led to an increase in alcohol consumption.

C. The sociocultural model emphasizes the relationship between alcohol problems and the normal patterns of alcohol use within a society. Alcohol-related problems are likely to occur:

1. In the presence of personal ambivalence and anxiety about alcohol
2. In situations in which the juxtaposition of drinking events and social situations generate social conflict and problematic consequences
3. In the presence of norms that encourage excessive and problem drinking
4. As one set of problems in a cluster of other problems that occur in the individual's relationship to social structures

VI. TREATMENT AND REHABILITATION OF PSYCHOACTIVE SUBSTANCE ABUSERS.

Surveys of alcoholism treatment programs reveal a startlingly high prevalence of drug abuse among alcoholics. In a study of 17 New York City alcoholism rehabilitation centers, 46% of 1340 alcoholic patients had abused other psychoactive drugs in the 30 days before entering treatment, and approximately 20% of all patients reported abusing two or more drugs in addition to alcohol (Sokolow, 1981). The drugs most frequently abused included minor tranquilizers, marijuana, sedatives, amphetamines, hallucinogens, and opioids. Several studies have documented the growing prevalence of concurrent alcohol and cocaine addiction. Miller and associates (1988) found that the number of cocaine addicts with additional diagnoses of alcohol dependence may range from 70% to 90%. Alcohol abuse is also known to be a significant complication in heroin and methadone addicts, where prevalence rates range between 50% and 75%. Thus, psychoactive substance withdrawal may have to be aimed at several substances.

A. Alcohol treatment programs. Studies (Nace, 1987) indicate that recovery rates and improvement rates for alcoholics following treatment depend on a number of factors.

1. Alcoholics of **higher socioeconomic status and higher social stability** have significantly higher improvement rates than alcoholics of lower socioeconomic status and lower social stability.
2. Recent studies (Nace, 1987) of treatment outcome for socially stable middle-class alcoholics provide evidence that **alcoholism inpatient treatment is effective**.
3. A **multidisciplinary approach** was more effective than individual psychotherapy.
4. **Psychological problems.** Patients with few psychological problems improved in any treatment program, while patients with serious psychological problems showed virtually no improvement in any program.
5. For treatment to be effective, **abstention** remains the ideal goal.
6. The **environment** of a rehabilitation program for alcoholism is usually highly structured: Time is ordered, activities are tightly scheduled, and behavior is regulated by rules and regulations. Setting limits is a constant feature of such programs. A reality orientation based on the here and now is emphasized; coping behaviors are stressed, and regression is discouraged. Emphasis on recognition of feelings and tolerance of feelings, rather than avoidance of painful affect through use of alcohol, drugs, and acting out, serves as an integrating process essential to self-control.
7. The program of **Alcoholics Anonymous** focuses not only on alcohol but also extends its program of recovery to the alcoholic's relationships. As the alcoholic progresses through the **12-step program** he must accept the limitation of his relationship to alcohol and also examine his relationship to others and to a "higher power." The first three steps are **surrender steps**—the alcoholic begins to overcome helplessness and gains internal control. Steps 4 and 5 are **inventory steps** in that they encourage self-examination. Steps 6 and 7 are considered to be **personality treatment steps,** as they address defects of character. Steps 8 and 9 promote **honest relationships,** and the remaining steps are referred to as **"sharing one's knowledge with others."**

B. Drug treatment programs. The first step in drug-free treatment is withdrawal from the drug abused.

1. In the case of **opiate dependence,** the abuser is withdrawn gradually with the use of **clonidine** to suppress withdrawal symptoms. If the patient has been addicted to opiates for more than two years, **methadone** may be substituted for heroin or other opiates. Depending on the philosophy of the program, the patient may remain on methadone maintenance of up to 40 mg/day or be gradually withdrawn. When an addict has been abusing opiates for 2 or more years, methadone is the treatment of choice, not abstinence. Although methadone is addicting, it is thought to control the craving for heroin and eliminate the associated social problems (e.g., stealing to get money to buy heroin).
2. The problem of treatment programs for **cocaine addiction** is that there is no known substitute therapy, although many programs are using **desipramine**. This has not been very successful (Gawin, 1989) because, even though high doses of antidepressants do attenuate cocaine withdrawal craving, their efficacy is delayed 7–14 days. By that time, the abuser has gone back to crack. **Flupentixol** is a depot xanthene derivative that has rapid antidepressant activity at low doses and neuroleptic activity at high doses. Preliminary data show that it is well tolerated, appears to decrease cocaine craving, and produces a 260% increase in average time retained in treatment. **Bromocriptine** has also been used for withdrawal, but data on efficacy are not available yet.

BIBLIOGRAPHY

Adler A: Individual psychiatry of alcoholic patients. *J Crim Psychopathol* 3:74, 1941.

Bales RF: Cultural difference in rates of alcoholism. *Q J Stud Alcohol* 6:480, 1946.

Bohman M, Sigvardsson S, Cloninger CR: Maternal inheritance of alcohol abuse: cross-fostering analysis of adopted women. *Arch Gen Psychiatry* 38:965–969, 1981.

Chein I, Gerard DL, Lee RS, et al: *The Road to H: Narcotics, Delinquency and Social Policy.* New York, Basic Books, 1964.

Cloninger CR: Genetic and environmental factors in the development of alcoholism. *J Psychiatr Treat Eval* 5:487–496, 1983.

Cotton NS: The familial incidence of alcoholism. *J Stud Alcohol* 40:89–96, 1979.

de Lint J: Alcohol control policy as a strategy for prevention: a critical examination of the evidence. Presented at the International Conference on Alcoholism and Drug Dependence, Liverpool, England, 1976.

Diagnostic and Statistical Manual of Mental Disorders, 3rd edition, revised (*DSM-III-R*). Washington, DC, American Psychiatric Association, 1987.

Foy A, Drinkwater V, March S, et al: Confusion after admission to hospital in elderly patients using benzodiazepines. *Br Med J* 293:1072, 1986.

Freud S: On narcissism: an introduction. In *The Standard Edition of the Complete Psychological Works of Sigmund Freud,* vol 14. London, Hogarth Press, 1957 (original paper in German published in 1914).

Gawin FH, Kleber HD, Byck R, et al: Desipramine facilitation of initial cocaine abstinence. *Arch Gen Psychiatry* 46:117–121, 1989.

Goodwin DW: Is alcoholism hereditary? A review and critique. *Arch Gen Psychiatry* 25:545–549, 1971.

Hahn RA: Prevalence of HIV infection among IV drug users in the US. *JAMA* 18:2677–2688, 1989.

Herridge P, Gold MS: The new user of cocaine: evidence from 800-COCAINE. *Psychiatr Ann* 18:521–522, 1988.

Horton D: Function of alcohol in primitive societies: cross-cultural study. *Q J Stud Alcohol* 4:199, 1943.

Johnston L, O'Malley P, Bachman J: *Illicit Drug Use, Smoking and Drinking by American High School Students, College Students and Young Adults 1975–1987.* Washington, DC, US Department of Health and Human Services, 1988.

Kandel DB, Ravei S: Cessation of illicit drug use in young adulthood. *Arch Gen Psychiatry* 46:109–116, 1989.

Khantzian EJ: Self-selection and progression in drug dependence. *Psychiatry Digest* 36:19–22, 1975.

McLennan AT, O'Brien CP, Krou R, et al: Matching substance abuse patients to appropriate treatments: a conceptual and methodological approach. *Drug Alcohol Depend* 5:189–195, 1980.

Menninger KA: *Man Against Himself.* New York, Harcourt Brace, 1938.

Miller NS, Gold MS, Belken BM, et al: *National Survey on Drug Abuse: Main Findings 1982.* Rockville, MD, National Institute on Drug Abuse, 1983.

Mirin SM, Weiss GD: Genetic factors in the development of alcoholism. *Psychiatr Ann* 19:239–242, 1989.

Nace EP: *The Treatment of Alcoholism.* New York, Bruner/Mazel, 1987.

National Institute on Drug Abuse: *National Household Survey on Drug Abuse, 1985.* Rockville, MD, National Clearinghouse for Drug Abuse Information, 1985.

Popham RE: A critique of the genetotrophic theory of the etiology of alcoholism. *Q J Stud Alcohol* 14:228, 1953.

Rado A: The psychoanalysis of pharmacothymia. *Psychoanal Q* 2:1–23, 1933.

Rounsaville BJ, Spitzer RL, Williams JBW: Proposed changes in DSM-III substance use disorders: description and rationale. *Am J Psychiatry* 143:463–468, 1986.

Schweizer E, Case WG, Rickels K: Benzodiazepine dependence and withdrawal in elderly patients. *Am J Psychiatry* 146:529–531, 1989.

Siegel RK: Cocaine smoking disorders: diagnosis and treatment. *Psychiatr Ann* 14:728–732, 1984.

Smart RG: The relationship of availability of alcoholic beverages to per capita consumption and alcoholism rates. *Q J Stud Alcohol* 38:891–896, 1976.

Sokolow L, Welte J, Hynes G, et al: Multiple substance abuse by alcoholics. *Br J Addict* 76:147–158, 1981.

Vaillant GE: A 12 year follow-up of New York narcotic addicts (IV). *Am J Psychiatry* 123:573–584, 1966.

Vesell ES, Page JG, Passananti GT: Genetic and environmental factors affecting ethanol metabolism in man. *Clinical Pharmacol Ther* 12:192–201, 1971.

STUDY QUESTIONS

Directions: Each of the numbered items or incomplete statements in this section is followed by answers or by completions of the statement. Select the **one** lettered answer or completion that is **best** in each case.

1. Which of the following statements is true regarding alcohol treatment programs?

(A) Some alcoholics may resume controlled social drinking
(B) Limit-setting is de-emphasized because the alcoholic has had too many guilt provokers in the past
(C) Alcoholics Anonymous has been criticized because it does not take into account the patient's family
(D) Socioeconomic status has no relationship to the recovery of an alcoholic
(E) Patients with few psychological problems improve in any program, while patients with serious psychopathology show no improvement despite monumental efforts

2. Which of the following is true regarding drug treatment programs?

(A) Most drug abusers confine themselves to a single drug of choice
(B) The aim of every drug treatment program is abstinence, regardless of the length of time of addiction
(C) Cocaine addiction is becoming easy to treat because of the use of tricyclic antidepressants
(D) Clonidine is used to treat the physical effects of withdrawal from opiates
(E) Methadone is no longer used to treat heroin addiction because of its addiction potential

3. Studies on the epidemiology of barbiturate use have shown that

(A) because it is an expensive habit to maintain, users often resort to petty crime to finance their addiction
(B) chronic intoxication may go unnoticed for years, even by family members and close friends
(C) the incidence is relatively easy to compute since barbiturate prescriptions are controlled by the Food and Drug Administration
(D) most users engage in IV administration since that is the most intense high

4. Which of the following is a psychological effect of cocaine use?

(A) Sedation
(B) Schizophrenia
(C) Panic attacks
(D) Auditory hallucinations
(E) Illusions

5. All of the following statements regarding marijuana use are true EXCEPT

(A) the demand for marijuana has increased substantially over the past 10 years
(B) young adults are the heaviest users
(C) after the age of 25 there is a sharp decline in use
(D) those who use marijuana in response to peer group pressure are more likely to stop than those who use marijuana for psychological reasons
(E) the degree of prior drug involvement is the strongest predictor of cessation of marijuana use

---

1-E 4-C
2-D 5-A
3-B

Directions: Each item below contains four suggested answers of which **one or more** is correct. Choose the answer

A if **1, 2, and 3** are correct
B if **1 and 3** are correct
C if **2 and 4** are correct
D if **4** is correct
E if **1, 2, 3, and 4** are correct

6. Revisions concerning drug and alcohol abuse included in the *DSM-III-R* include

(1) strengthening the distinction between abuse and dependence
(2) provision of a system for rating severity of dependence
(3) separate criteria for dependence on alcohol and dependence on drugs
(4) creation of a new category that includes individuals with iatrogenic drug dependence

7. Findings regarding the biologic etiology of substance abuse include

(1) identical twins are more often concordant for alcoholism than fraternal twins
(2) identical twins are more concordant for the adverse consequences of drinking than fraternal twins
(3) there is no known genetic marker for alcoholism
(4) children of alcoholics are not vulnerable if raised by nonalcoholic foster parents

Directions: The group of items in this section consists of lettered options followed by a set of numbered items. For each item, select the **one** lettered option that is most closely associated with it. Each lettered option may be selected once, more than once, or not at all.

Questions 8–12

For each theory, select the investigator with whom it is most likely to be associated.

(A) Khantzian
(B) Horton
(C) de Lint
(D) Rado
(E) Smart

8. The distribution of consumption model, which showed that minor variations in availability of alcohol has no effect on consumption

9. A psychoanalytic theory that states that drug use might represent an attempt to cope with painful emotions

10. A theory that lowering the drinking age increases alcohol problems in young people

11. A sociological theory that there is a high correlation between subsistence insecurity and excessive drinking

12. A psychoanalytic theory that individuals select the drug of abuse because of personality factors

---

6-C
7-B
8-C
9-D
10-E
11-B
12-A

ANSWERS AND EXPLANATIONS

1. The answer is E *[VI A 1–7].*
According to studies of alcoholic treatment programs, patients with few psychological problems improved in any program, while patients with serious psychopathology showed no improvement despite monumental efforts. There is no evidence that an alcoholic can resume social drinking, and thus, abstention is the goal of all programs. Patients of higher socioeconomic status, as well as greater social stability, have a greater chance of recovery. Limit-setting is an important part of any treatment program. Alcoholics Anonymous extends its program to include the alcoholic's relationships.

2. The answer is D *[VI B 1, 2].*
Clonidine is used to treat the physical effects of withdrawal from opiates. Most drug abusers use several drugs, in addition to alcohol. If an addict has been using opiates for 2 years or more, methadone maintenance is the treatment of choice—not abstinence. Even though methadone is addicting, it is thought to control the craving for heroin and eliminate the social problems. Cocaine addiction is very difficult to treat with tricyclics because of the long period of time needed to build up to an effective level of a tricyclic antidepressant.

3. The answer is B *[II B 2].*
Chronic intoxication from barbiturates is not easily detected and may go unidentified even by family members for months or years. Barbiturate use is a habit that is relatively inexpensive to maintain since barbiturates are manufactured for a medical use. The incidence and prevalence are impossible to estimate because most abusers go undetected. Intravenous (IV) barbiturate use does occur, but it involves a small number of people—usually young adults involved in an illegal drug culture.

4. The answer is C *[II B 1 c (1), (2)].*
In a 1988 study (Herridge), cocaine users reported irritability and anxiety, as well as panic attacks, but not sedation. Schizophrenia, auditory hallucinations, and illusions were not mentioned.

5. The answer is A *[II B 5 a (1)–(4), b].*
The demand for marijuana has not increased substantially over the past 10 years. Young adults 18–25 years of age are the heaviest users, with about 25% currently using marijuana. There appears to be a sharp decline in use after the age of 25 years. Those who use drugs in response to social influences are more likely to stop than those who use drugs for psychological reasons. The degree of prior drug involvement is the strongest predictor of cessation of marijuana use.

6. The answer is C (2, 4) *[I C 1–4].*
Revisions in the *Diagnostic and Statistical Manual of Mental Disorders,* third edition, revised (*DSM-III-R*) include a rating scale for severity of drug or alcohol dependence and a new category called "psychoactive substance neuroadaptation syndrome" for individuals with iatrogenic drug dependence. The *DSM-III-R* has abolished the distinction between abuse and dependence. Drugs and alcohol are combined, and criteria for dependence are the same.

7. The answer is B (1, 3) *[III A 1–3].*
Studies have shown that identical twins are more often concordant for alcoholism than are fraternal twins. However, identical twins are not more concordant than fraternal twins for the adverse consequences of drinking. Children of alcoholics have been shown to be vulnerable to alcoholism even if they are raised by nonalcoholic foster parents. Although tests have been conducted to find a genetic marker for alcoholism (i.e., tests have tried to associate alcoholism, the suspected genetic trait, with a known genetic trait), no known genetic marker for alcoholism has been identified.

8–12. The answers are: 8-C *[V B 1],* **9-D** *[IV A 2],* **10-E** *[V B 3],* **11-B** *[IV B 1],* **12-A** *[IV A 5].*
de Lint (1976) showed that minor variations in liquor store hours had no effect on alcohol consumption. Rado (1933) said that drug abuse was an attempt to cope with painful emotions. Smart (1976) showed that lowering the drinking age increases alcoholism among young people. Horton (1943) was a sociologist who studied the correlation between alcohol consumption and subsistence insecurity. Khantzian (1975) said that certain drugs are selected by drug abusers based on certain personality factors. Both Rado and Khantzian proposed psychoanalytic theories, while de Lint and Smart did research on the distribution of consumption model.

12 Occupational Medicine

Anne Krantz
Peter Orris
Stephen Michael Hessl

I. INTRODUCTION

A. Labor force. In 1989, the labor force in the United States numbered 123,827,000 of a total population of 186,726,000 individuals who were age 16 years or older.

1. Approximately 54.6% of the labor force were men and 45.4% were women in 1989. The percentage of women in the labor force has increased by approximately 5.6% since 1980 and 9.6% since 1975.
2. Approximately 85.8% of the labor force were white and 10.8% were black in 1989.

B. Distribution of labor force. From 1979 to 1989, the percentage of the labor force engaged in manufacturing and agriculture declined, while those engaged in service and trade increased. See Table 12-1 for the distribution of the work force in 1979 and 1989.

C. Occupational diseases and injuries

1. Occupational injuries increased from 4.9 million in 1983 to 6.2 million in 1988. Nearly one-half of these were serious enough to cause lost work time, restricted work activity, or both.
2. The U.S. Bureau of Labor Statistics recorded 240,900 new cases of occupational illnesses in 1988, which represented an increase of 190,400 cases over 1987. Part of this increase may represent improved reporting systems.

D. Definitions

1. **Impairment** is the objective description of the loss of function of the human body.
2. **Disability** is the effect of an impairment on the ability of an individual to function in society.
3. **Toxin** is a substance in the environment with the potential for causing human disease or injury.
4. **Toxicology** is the study of external substances and their effects on humans.
5. **Epidemiology** is the study of disease in populations.
6. **Environmental epidemiology** is the study of environmental toxins and their effects on populations.
7. **Ergonomics** is the study of the mechanical interaction between people and their living or work environment for the purpose of tailoring tools, tasks, and workplace design for better overall efficiency and individual well-being.
8. **Occupational disease** is any disease caused in whole or in part by exposure in the work environment, usually excluding workplace trauma.
9. **Occupational medicine** is the diagnosis and treatment of human disease caused in whole or in part by an individual's work environment.
10. **Medical surveillance** is periodic medical testing designed to identify adverse health effects of environmental substances prior to the point at which they cause permanent disability.
11. **"Right to know"** refers to workers' legal or ethical right to unrestricted access to information regarding the workplace hazards to which they are potentially exposed.
12. **Workers' compensation** is a series of state laws that establishes a no-fault insurance system for workers disabled on the job.

Table 12-1. Distribution of the Work Force in 1979 and 1989 as Reported by the Labor Department

	Percentage of Labor Force	
	1979	**1989**
Manufacturing	21.1%	18%
Service	19.4%	32%
Agriculture	3.3%	2%
Trade	22.0%	20%

13. **Occupational Safety and Health Administration (OSHA)** is an agency of the U.S. Labor Department that was established in 1970 to "assure safe and healthful working conditions" for American workers (Occupational Safety and Health Act of 1970, Public Law 91-596, 1970). It is charged with establishing, enforcing, and educating the public concerning workplace health and safety standards. OSHA's jurisdiction includes all nongovernmental workplaces.
14. **National Institute for Occupational Safety and Health (NIOSH)** is an agency of the U.S. Department of Health and Human Services (DHHS) that was established in 1970 to provide research, professional training, and advice to OSHA concerning the science of occupational safety and health.
15. **American Conference of Governmental Industrial Hygienists (ACGIH)** is a voluntary independent association that publishes a set of recommended exposure limits for industrial toxins.
16. **Environmental Protection Agency (EPA)** is an agency established as a separate branch of the federal government in 1970 to provide research, standard setting, and enforcement related to protecting human health in the environment.
17. **Time-weighted average (TWA)** is an average concentration of airborne substances usually calculated on an 8- or 10-hour workday.
18. **Threshold limit value (TLV)** is the airborne concentration of substances established by the ACGIH to represent conditions under which nearly all workers may work without adverse effects.
19. **Permissible exposure limit (PEL)** is a term created by OSHA to identify the maximum legally allowable exposure of a toxic substance in the workplace.

II. OCCUPATIONAL HISTORY.

Occupational diseases frequently present as common medical conditions, such as asthma, lung cancer, atopic dermatitis, peripheral neuropathy, and psychiatric disorders. A key factor in a physician's ability to recognize an occupational disease is the occupational history.

A. Screening the patient. A schema that can be used routinely by all practicing physicians, regardless of specialty, to assist in the detection of occupational and environmental diseases follows. Screening questions related to work exposure should be asked of all patients and should include:

1. **A chronologic list of all jobs, focusing on work processes encountered.** This is important because work exposures in the past may be etiologic factors in diseases presenting years later.
2. **A description of any temporal relationships between a work exposure and a presenting illness.** This relationship may provide clues as to the etiology of disease. It is important to ascertain, for example, if the patient's condition improves on weekends or vacations.
3. **Known hazards in the workplace.** As part of a review of systems, the patient always should be asked questions about exposure to fumes, dusts, chemicals, loud noise, or radiation in the workplace.

B. Screening the employer. Additional information may be required to establish the degree of exposure when an occupational disease is suspected. In addition to seeking occupational information from the patient, it may be useful to obtain information from the employer, OSHA records, the labor union, or by a site visit to the workplace, remembering that **these activities must be**

E. Office workers. Occupational disorders that afflict office workers only recently have been recognized. These disorders can result from:

1. **Video display terminals.** Workers who must spend a large portion of their time working with video display terminals commonly complain of:
   a. Eye strain
   b. Musculoskeletal discomfort
2. **Repetitive trauma.** Repetitive tasks (e.g., mail sorting) may produce conditions such as:
   a. Carpal tunnel syndrome
   b. Tendonitis
3. **Indoor air pollution.** The **"sick building syndrome,"** which results from office work in modern, energy-efficient buildings with reduced outside air exchange, can produce:
   a. Headache
   b. Nausea
   c. Eye irritation
4. **Stress.** Isolation, confinement, overload, or an inability to control the work load or work conditions can produce stress, leading to:
   a. Anxiety
   b. Depression
   c. Drug and alcohol abuse
   d. Cardiovascular disease
   e. Peptic ulcer disease

F. Health care workers. There are more than 3 million health care workers in the United States. Due to the complexity of health care and the risks inherent in caring for sick patients, there are a great many health hazards to which health care workers are exposed, including the following.

1. **Safety hazards,** such as:
   a. Lifting heavy patients, which can cause back injury
   b. Electric shocks
   c. Needle sticks, which can lead to transmission of bloodborne infectious agents, such as human immunodeficiency virus (HIV) and hepatitis B virus (HBV)
   d. Accidents caused by long work hours
2. **Ethylene oxide.** This commonly used gas sterilant is mutagenic and a suspected human carcinogen and teratogen. It can cause:
   a. Skin and mucous membrane burns
   b. Neuropathy
   c. Leukemia
3. **Waste anesthetic gases.** In the United States, more than 50,000 operating room personnel are exposed to anesthetic gases in trace concentrations, which are associated with:
   a. Spontaneous abortion
   b. Teratogenesis
   c. Mutagenesis
   d. Carcinogenesis
   e. Liver disease
4. **Infectious agents,** such as:
   a. HBV and non-A, non-B hepatitis
   b. Tuberculosis
   c. Herpes simplex virus
   d. Acquired immune deficiency syndrome (AIDS)
5. **Cytotoxic agents.** Chemotherapeutic agents are administered to an estimated 200,000–400,000 people annually. Although undocumented as yet, chronic effects in workers who administer these agents may include:
   a. Reproductive abnormalities
   b. Cancer
   c. Irritation to mucous membranes, eyes, and skin (caused by the cytotoxic agent nitrogen mustard)

G. Machinists. Machine tools (e.g., drill presses, milling machines, lathes) are in general use in many workshops. Common hazards include:

1. **Noise,** which is associated with hearing loss and hypertension
2. **Safety hazards.** Injuries occur when hair or clothing becomes entangled in machines or when safety mechanisms have not been installed or used correctly. Common injuries include:
   - **a.** Finger loss
   - **b.** Lacerations
   - **c.** Musculoskeletal strain
3. **Cutting and cooling oils.** Conditions associated with use of these oils include:
   - **a.** Skin cancer
   - **b.** Oil acne
   - **c.** Eczematous dermatitis
   - **d.** Febrile illness (Pontiac fever), which is caused by oil contaminated with *Legionella pneumophila* and characterized by fever, chills, myalgia, and headache.

IV. POTENTIAL HAZARDS

A. Metals

1. **Arsenic**
   - **a. Uses.** Arsenic is used in metallurgy and pesticides and is produced as a by-product of smelting ores.
   - **b. Exposure**
     - **(1)** Inhalation
     - **(2)** Skin absorption (especially organic forms and arsenic trichloride)
     - **(3)** Ingestion
   - **c. Toxicity.** Exposure to arsenic fumes or dust may produce:
     - **(1)** Nasal septal ulceration and perforation
     - **(2)** Skin disorders (e.g., hyperpigmentation, hyperkeratosis, and gangrene of the fingers and toes)
     - **(3)** Lung cancer after chronic exposure in gold miners and others
     - **(4)** Peripheral neuropathy, particularly after repeated high-dose exposure
   - **d. Special tests** to aid in the diagnosis of toxicity include:
     - **(1)** Urinary arsenic levels
     - **(2)** Analysis of hair and nails for arsenic
2. **Beryllium**
   - **a. Uses.** Beryllium is used as a hardening agent in alloys.
   - **b. Exposure** is by inhalation.
   - **c. Toxicity**
     - **(1) Acute.** Exposure to the soluble salts of beryllium can cause acute cases of:
       - **(a)** Pneumonitis
       - **(b)** Conjunctivitis
       - **(c)** Nasal pharyngitis
       - **(d)** Tracheitis
       - **(e)** Bronchitis
     - **(2) Chronic.** Granulomas of the skin and lung may be accompanied by **berylliosis,** a chronic debilitating disease characterized by dyspnea, dry cough, anorexia, fatigue, malaise, and weight loss. Beryllium causes cancer in animals and may be linked to human lung cancer.
   - **d. Special tests** to aid in the diagnosis of toxicity include:
     - **(1)** Assay of tissue samples for beryllium levels
     - **(2)** Analysis of blood samples for lymphocyte blast transformation, indicating beryllium salt sensitization
3. **Cadmium**
   - **a. Uses.** Cadmium is used in electroplating, as an aluminum solder, and in nickel-cadmium batteries.
   - **b. Exposure** is by inhalation.

c. Toxicity

(1) Acute. Cadmium dust and fumes are severe pulmonary irritants, which may result in:

(a) Pneumonitis

(b) Pulmonary edema

(2) Chronic. Repeated exposure to low levels of cadmium may result in:

(a) Emphysema and chronic bronchitis

(b) Renal tubular damage

(c) Osteomalacia-like disease

(d) Prostate cancer

(e) Respiratory tract cancer (weak association)

d. Special tests

(1) Elevated urinary cadmium levels indicate exposure only and do not reveal degree of toxicity.

(2) Low molecular weight proteinuria may be an early sign of renal toxicity.

4. Chromium

a. Uses. Chromium is used in welding, electroplating, tanning, and textile processing.

b. Exposure

(1) Inhalation

(2) Skin absorption

(3) Ingestion

c. Toxicity. Exposure can result in:

(1) Pulmonary and skin sensitization

(2) Mucous membrane irritation and nasal perforation

(3) Increased incidence of lung cancer and cancer of the nasal sinuses (associated with hexavalent chromium only)

5. Lead

a. Uses. Lead is used in batteries, paint, ceramics, and ammunition.

b. Exposure

(1) Inhalation

(2) Ingestion

c. Toxicity, which is usually manifested in the adult after chronic exposure, results in:

(1) Nervous system abnormalities, such as:

(a) Central nervous system (CNS) effects (e.g., neurobehavioral abnormalities, chronic encephalopathy)

(b) Peripheral nervous system (PNS) effects (e.g., motor weakness, especially of the extensor muscles of the wrist; nerve conduction abnormalities)

(2) Hematologic abnormalities, such as anemia secondary to impaired heme synthesis

(3) Nephropathy, including chronic renal failure and hyperuricemia

(4) Reproductive abnormalities, such as:

(a) Fetal toxicity

(b) Abnormal sperm

d. Special tests to aid in the diagnosis of toxicity include:

(1) Analysis of whole blood for lead content

(2) Assay of free erythrocyte porphyrin or zinc protoporphyrin levels in blood to assess the body's burden of lead

(3) Injection of calcium disodium ethylenediaminetetraacetic (EDTA) and measurement of subsequent urinary lead excretion for further assessment of the body's burden of lead

6. Mercury

a. Uses. Mercury is used in industrial instruments, pesticides, electrical apparatus, and dental amalgams.

b. Exposure is by:

(1) Inhalation

(2) Ingestion

(3) Skin absorption

c. Toxicity

(1) Neurologic disturbances, including:

(a) Incoordination

(b) Tremor

(c) Psychic disturbances (e.g., insomnia, irritability, indecision)

(d) Visual field abnormalities

(2) Renal abnormalities (e.g., proteinuria)
(3) Skin and mucous membrane abnormalities
(a) Stomatitis
(b) Gingivitis
(c) Skin irritation
(4) Pulmonary disease
(a) Pneumonitis
(b) Bronchitis

d. **Special tests** to aid in the diagnosis of toxicity include assaying the amount of mercury in a 24-hour urine sample.

7. **Nickel**
a. **Uses.** Nickel is used in electroplating, in the production of catalysts, in nickel-cadmium batteries, and in alloys.
b. **Exposure** is by inhalation or skin contact.
c. **Toxicity**
(1) **"Nickel itch"** is a dermatitis that results from sensitization to nickel.
(2) **Asthma** has also been described from inhalation of nickel sulfate.
(3) **Cancer of the paranasal sinuses and lungs** has been associated with chronic exposure in workers in nickel refineries.
d. **Special tests.** Nickel may be monitored in the urine.

8. **Zinc**
a. **Uses.** Zinc chloride is used as a soldering flux in the welding process. Zinc oxide is produced when elemental zinc is heated at high temperatures, such as in the manufacturing of bronze and in galvanizing.
b. **Exposure** is by inhalation and skin contact.
c. **Toxicity**
(1) Zinc is an essential element in human metabolism; however, inhalation of zinc oxide fumes may cause an influenza-like illness called **metal fume fever**. (Metal fume fever also may be caused by other metals.)
(2) Zinc chloride may produce eczematous or allergic **dermatitis**.
d. **Special tests** include patch testing for the diagnosis of zinc chloride skin allergy.

B. **Solvents** are a very large and heterogeneous group of chemical substances that are used to dissolve other materials. In general, common usage refers to **organic and inorganic solvents,** which cause both acute and chronic health effects, including toxicity to the CNS and PNS, as well as to the dermatologic, renal, hepatic, cardiovascular, and hematologic systems. Common organic solvents are listed below.

1. **Aliphatic hydrocarbons** (e.g., *n*-hexane, which should not be confused with common hexane)
a. **Uses.** Aliphatic hydrocarbons are solvents that are used in quick-drying rubber cements and inks as well as in oil extraction processes.
b. **Exposure** is by inhalation.
c. **Toxicity of *n*-hexane**
(1) Upper respiratory irritation
(2) CNS depression
(3) Peripheral neuropathy
d. **Special tests.** Urine testing can detect 2,5-hexanedione.

2. **Aromatic hydrocarbons** (e.g., benzene)
a. **Uses.** Aromatic hydrocarbons are used as chemical intermediates in the production of other organic chemicals. They are used in solvents, unleaded gasoline, and paint removers.
b. **Exposure** is by:
(1) Inhalation
(2) Skin absorption
c. **Toxicity.** There is clinical and epidemiologic data linking benzene with:
(1) Leukemia, especially the acute myeloblastic type
(2) CNS depression
(3) Bone marrow depression and aplastic anemia
d. **Special tests.** Total phenols can be detected in the urine.

3. **Cyclic hydrocarbons** (e.g., cyclohexane)
   a. **Uses.** Cyclic hydrocarbons are used as chemical intermediates and in solvents for rubber, waxes, resins, oils, and fats.
   b. **Exposure** is by inhalation.
   c. **Toxicity**
      (1) Irritation of the skin and mucous membranes
      (2) CNS depression
      (3) Possible liver and kidney damage
   d. **Special tests.** Cyclohexanol can be detected in the urine.

4. **Alcohols** (e.g., methanol)
   a. **Uses.** Alcohols are used in paints, varnishes, cements, and in the production of formaldehyde, inks, and dyes.
   b. **Exposure** is by:
      (1) Inhalation
      (2) Skin absorption
   c. **Toxicity**
      (1) Optic neuropathy
      (2) Metabolic acidosis
   d. **Special tests**
      (1) Measurement of formic acid (a metabolite of methanol) levels in urine
      (2) Measurement of acid-base balance, such as arterial blood gas determinations

5. **Nitrohydrocarbons** (e.g., nitroethane)
   a. **Uses.** Nitrohydrocarbons are used for organic chemical synthesis and as solvents.
   b. **Exposure** is by inhalation.
   c. **Toxicity**
      (1) Irritation of the mucous membranes and respiratory system
      (2) Possible CNS depression
      (3) Liver toxicity (associated with high-dose exposure)
   d. **Special tests.** Biologic monitoring is not generally useful.

6. **Glycols** (e.g., ethylene glycol)
   a. **Uses.** Glycols are used in antifreeze and hydraulic fluids.
   b. **Exposure** is by ingestion. Respiratory exposures are not considered to be toxic.
   c. **Toxicity**
      (1) CNS depression
      (2) Renal failure related to the formation of glycolic and oxalic acids after ingestion
   d. **Special tests.** Ethylene glycol can be measured in the blood.

7. **Esters** (e.g., ethyl acetate)
   a. **Uses.** Esters are used as lacquer solvents.
   b. **Exposure** is by inhalation.
   c. **Toxicity**
      (1) Mucous membrane irritation
      (2) Eczematous eruptions
      (3) Possible CNS depression
      (4) Anemia
      (5) Pulmonary irritation (associated with high exposures)
   d. **Special tests.** Biologic monitoring is not readily available.

8. **Ethers** (e.g., ethylene glycol monoethyl ether)
   a. **Uses.** Ethers are used as solvents for lacquers and alkyl resins in the dyeing of textiles and leather and as cleaners and varnish removers.
   b. **Exposure** is by:
      (1) Inhalation
      (2) Skin absorption
   c. **Toxicity**
      (1) Mucous membrane irritation
      (2) Possible bone marrow disorders
      (3) Lung and renal injuries (associated with high doses)
   d. **Special tests.** Biologic monitoring is not readily available.

9. **Ketones** (e.g., methyl ethyl ketone)
   a. **Uses.** Ketones are used as solvents for resins, gums, synthetic rubber, lacquers, varnishes, and lubricating oils.
   b. **Exposure** is by inhalation.
   c. **Toxicity**
      (1) Mucous membrane irritation
      (2) Possible CNS depression (associated with high exposure)
   d. **Special tests.** Acetone can be measured in the blood and urine.

10. **Aldehydes** (e.g., formaldehyde)
   a. **Uses.** Aldehydes are used in urea formaldehyde, phenol formaldehyde, and other plastics, as a disinfectant and a fumigant, and in paper, rubber, and dye manufacturing.
   b. **Exposure** is by inhalation.
   c. **Toxicity.** Formaldehyde is mutagenic and carcinogenic in animal species and is being investigated as a human carcinogen. Toxic effects of formaldehyde include:
      (1) Strong irritation to mucous membranes and the respiratory system
      (2) Skin irritation and allergic dermatitis
      (3) Possible asthma
   d. **Special tests.** Biologic monitoring is not generally useful.

11. **Halogenated hydrocarbons** (e.g., carbon tetrachloride)
   a. **Uses.** Halogenated hydrocarbons are used as solvents for lacquers, varnishes, waxes, resins, oils, and fats. Carbon tetrachloride has been used for degreasing, for cleaning, and in the past, as a fire extinguisher.
   b. **Exposure** is by:
      (1) Inhalation
      (2) Skin absorption
   c. **Toxicity**
      (1) CNS depression
      (2) Severe damage to the liver and kidneys, including necrosis of the liver and renal tubular necrosis
   d. **Special tests.** Biologic monitoring is not generally useful.

C. Dusts

1. **Inorganic dusts**
   a. **Asbestos**
      (1) **Uses.** Asbestos is used as insulation; in fireproofing and roofing materials; and in automotive parts.
      (2) **Exposure** is by inhalation; however, ingestion may be a factor in malignancy.
      (3) **Toxicity**
         (a) Interstitial lung disease (e.g., asbestosis)
         (b) Benign pleural effusion
         (c) Pleural thickening and calcification
         (d) Malignant mesothelioma
         (e) Lung cancer
         (f) Laryngeal cancer
         (g) Gastrointestinal cancer
      (4) **Special tests.** Screening of asbestos-exposed people should include periodic chest x-rays, pulmonary function testing, and testing for occult blood in the stool.
   b. **Coal**
      (1) **Uses.** Coal is used as a heating fuel and in the manufacture of coke.
      (2) **Exposure** is by inhalation.
      (3) **Toxicity**
         (a) Chronic exposure to coal dust can lead to **coal workers' pneumoconiosis** (**CWP,** or black lung disease), a condition characterized by progressive dyspnea on exertion, nodular lung opacities visible on chest x-rays, and soft, black, indurated nodules (coal macules) detectable by pathologic examination.
         (b) **Progressive massive fibrosis (PMF)**—that is, the coalescence of coal macules or silicotic lung nodules, causing massive obliteration of the underlying tissue—may develop as a result of CWP.
         (c) Coal workers may also have an increased risk of **gastric cancer**.

(b) Inhalation
(c) Ingestion
(2) **Toxicity**
(a) Irritation of the skin, eyes, and upper respiratory system
(b) Hyperpyrexia and heat stroke
(c) Chloracne, a condition characterized by comedones, straw-colored cysts, milia, and papules found typically on the malar portion of the face, neck, shoulders, abdomen, and genitals
(d) Cancers associated with certain phenols
(3) **Special tests** include urine testing for pentachlorophenol.

c. **Dimethyldithiocarbamate compounds**
(1) **Exposure** is by:
(a) Inhalation
(b) Skin absorption
(c) Ingestion
(2) **Toxicity**
(a) Irritation of the eyes and respiratory tract
(b) Skin irritation and allergic dermatitis
(c) Disulfiram-like effect after ethanol ingestion
(d) Mutagenesis, carcinogenesis, and teratogenesis

d. **Organotin compounds**
(1) **Exposure** is by:
(a) Inhalation
(b) Skin absorption
(c) Ingestion
(2) **Toxicity**
(a) Irritation of eyes, mucous membranes, and skin
(b) Hepatic necrosis
(c) Cerebral edema
(3) **Special tests.** Screening is not readily available.

3. **Herbicides**

a. **Chlorophenoxy compounds**
(1) **Exposure** is by:
(a) Inhalation
(b) Skin absorption
(c) Ingestion
(2) **Toxicity**
(a) Chloracne
(b) CNS dysfunction and peripheral neuropathy
(c) Liver dysfunction
(d) Adverse reproductive effects
(e) Soft tissue sarcoma and other cancers
(3) **Special tests.** These compounds can be measured in the blood and urine.

b. **Paraquat**
(1) **Exposure** is by:
(a) Inhalation
(b) Skin absorption
(c) Ingestion
(2) **Toxicity.** Ingestion has been associated with:
(a) Rapid progressive pulmonary fibrosis
(b) Myocardial, hepatic, and renal dysfunction
(c) Irritation of eyes, skin, and mucous membranes

4. **Vertebrate poisons. Rodenticides** will be used as an example, although many other genus-specific poisons exist.

a. **Warfarin**
(1) **Exposure** is by:
(a) Inhalation
(b) Skin absorption
(c) Ingestion

(2) **Toxicity**
(a) Hypoprothrombinemia
(b) Vascular injury resulting in hemorrhage
(3) **Special tests.** Blood prothrombin time will be prolonged.

b. **Yellow (white) phosphorus**
(1) **Exposure** is by:
(a) Inhalation
(b) Ingestion
(c) Skin absorption
(2) **Toxicity**
(a) **Direct contact** may result in deep thermal burns. Prolonged direct absorption may cause necrosis of the maxilla and mandible ("phossy jaw").
(b) **Ingestion** results in severe injury to the gut and peripheral zonal necrosis of the liver.
(c) **Inhalation** results in strong irritation to mucous membranes.
(3) **Special tests.** Specific testing for phosphorus is not useful.

5. **Nematocides**
a. **Dibromochloropropane (DBCP)**
(1) **Exposure** is by:
(a) Inhalation
(b) Skin absorption
(2) **Toxicity**
(a) Oligospermia
(b) Aspermia

b. **Ethylene dibromide**
(1) **Exposure** is by:
(a) Inhalation
(b) Skin absorption
(2) **Toxicity**
(a) Severe irritation of the mucous membranes and respiratory system
(b) CNS depression
(c) Central lobular necrosis of the liver
(d) Focal proximal tubular damage in the kidney
(e) Possibly cancer of the gut, skin, and lung
(3) **Special tests.** Exposed workers should be screened for cancer of the gut, skin, and lung.

E. **Irritant gases.** Several gases can produce acute and chronic damage to the air passages and pulmonary parenchyma.

1. **Water-soluble gases.** Gases that are highly water soluble, such as sulfur dioxide, ammonia, and chlorine, cause intense irritation to mucous membranes. Thus, unless workers are trapped, they should remove themselves immediately from exposure. Chlorine, an example of a soluble irritant gas, has the following characteristics.
a. **Uses.** Chlorine is used for water purification and in chemical manufacturing of pesticides, bleach, disinfectants, and household cleaners.
b. **Exposure** is by inhalation.
c. **Toxicity.** Severe irritation of mucous membranes, eyes, and skin at high concentrations may result in burns to these areas. Tracheobronchitis, pulmonary edema, and pneumonitis may occur after inhalation of high concentrations. Chronic effects include prolonged airflow obstruction and mild hypoxemia.

2. **Water-insoluble gases.** Gases that are less water soluble, such as phosgene, nitrogen dioxide, and ozone, may be inhaled deeply into the lungs without warning or a cough reflex. Nitrogen dioxide (NO_2), an example of an insoluble irritant gas, has the following characteristics.
a. **Uses.** NO_2 is a by-product of silo filling, welding, combustion of nitrogen-containing materials (e.g., explosives) chemical manufacturing, space flight, and nitric and sulfuric acid production.
b. **Exposure** is by inhalation.
c. **Toxicity.** Pulmonary edema may occur within 1–2 hours after heavy exposure. However, a late, recurrent pulmonary edema may occur as late as 2–3 weeks after exposure. In those who survive the acute injury, chronic pulmonary disease with bronchiolitis obliterans may develop.

3. **Other irritant gases** include:
   a. **Acetaldehyde,** which is used in the manufacture of plastics, synthetic rubber, acetic acid, and disinfectants
   b. **Acrolein,** which is used in the manufacture of pharmaceuticals, resins, and food supplements
   c. **Ammonia,** which is used in refrigeration and in the manufacture of fertilizers, nitric acid, plastics, and explosives
   d. **Hydrogen chloride,** which is used in pickling of steel, the manufacture of chlorinated organic chemicals, and in dyes
   e. **Hydrogen fluoride,** which is used in etching of glass, manufacturing of aluminum, fluorocarbons, and in alkylation processes
   f. **Ozone,** which is a by-product of photochemical smog, of welding, and of high-voltage electrical equipment
   g. **Phosgene,** which is a by-product of combustion of chlorinated compounds
   h. **Phosphine,** which is used in fumigation, acetylene gas production, and flares
   i. **Sulfur dioxide,** which is used in the manufacture of sulfuric acid, bleaches, fumigation, and refrigeration, and is a by-product of petroleum refining and of combustion of fossil fuels

F. **Asphyxiant gases.** Any gas in high enough concentrations can displace oxygen and cause asphyxiation due to oxygen deprivation. The gases listed below, however, are especially toxic and have caused many deaths because of the direct effect they have on oxygen transport or utilization processes within the body.

1. **Carbon monoxide (CO)**
   a. **Uses.** CO is a by-product of the incomplete combustion of carbonaceous substances.
   b. **Exposure** is by inhalation.
   c. **Toxicity.** CO has an affinity for hemoglobin that is about 240 times greater than that of oxygen. This binding with hemoglobin interferes with the release of oxygen from hemoglobin and affects such critical tissues as the myocardium and the CNS.
   d. **Special tests** include measurement of blood carboxyhemoglobin levels.

2. **Hydrogen cyanide**
   a. **Uses.** Hydrogen cyanide is used in fumigation, annealing of steel, and the purification of gold and silver. It is said to have a sweet almond-like odor, which 20%–40% of the general population is unable to smell.
   b. **Exposure** is by:
      (1) Inhalation
      (2) Skin absorption
      (3) Ingestion
   c. **Toxicity.** Cyanide ion inhibits many enzyme systems, particularly the cytochrome oxidase system, thereby inhibiting cellular respiration.
   d. **Special tests** include measurement of blood and tissue cyanide levels.

3. **Hydrogen sulfide**
   a. **Uses.** Hydrogen sulfide is used in leather tanning and is a by-product of sewage and petroleum. It has a characteristic "rotten egg" odor.
   b. **Exposure** is by inhalation.
   c. **Toxicity**
      (1) Disruption of oxygen transport via the cytochrome oxidase system
      (2) Irritation of the mucous membranes and eyes
      (3) Myocardial and respiratory depression and death

G. **Physical stressors**

1. **Noise**
   a. **Definitions**
      (1) **Decibel (db)** is a unit of measure of sound intensity measured on the logarithmic scale. Whispers occur at 20–30 db, normal conversation at 60 db, and a jet takeoff at 120–140 db.
      (2) **Hertz (Hz; cycles per second)** is a unit of measure of pitch or frequency.
   b. **Exposure** is by the auditory route. Exposure to noise occurs in a variety of industrial settings, including in foundries and forges.
   c. **Toxicity** to the auditory system usually is manifested after chronic exposure to at least **90 db**.

(1) **Acoustic trauma.** Bone or tissue damage can result from exposure to a high-pressure wave (e.g., an explosion).

(2) **Noise-induced hearing loss.** A sensorineuronal deficit involving the hair cells of the cochlea can be produced by loud, sustained noise.

(a) **Temporary threshold shift** is a loss of hearing that recovers within the first 24 hours after exposure but may also show further improvement over a 7-day period.

(b) **Permanent threshold shift** is a loss of hearing that occurs first in the 4000 Hz range, extending gradually with continued exposure through the higher frequencies and finally in the lower frequencies as well. These changes are irreversible.

(3) **Noise levels of 90 dbA** (a decibel scale reflecting the attenuation produced by the human ear) can be expected to produce a 25% hearing loss in the 1000–3000 Hz range in approximately 25% of individuals exposed over a 40-year period. A similar hearing loss would be produced in 10%–15% of individuals chronically exposed to 85 dbA, and in up to 5% of individuals chronically exposed to 80 dbA. Thus, there is a dose-response curve for hearing loss and noise exposure.

d. **Special tests** include audiometric hearing testing at intervals between 500 and 8000 Hz.

2. **Heat**

a. **Exposure.** The ACGIH recommends that for an 8-hour day, 40-hour week, light work should not be performed at ambient temperatures higher than 86° F in a humid environment and heavy work, at no more than 77° F.

b. **Toxicity**

(1) **Acute toxicity** can include the following:

(a) Heat fatigue

(b) Heat cramps characterized by muscle spasm

(c) Heat exhaustion characterized by:

(i) Volume depletion

(ii) Fatigue

(iii) Occasional emesis

(iv) Lightheadedness

(d) Heat stroke resulting in:

(i) Hyperthermia of over 106° F

(ii) Dry, flushed skin

(iii) Confusion progressing to coma

(2) **Chronic toxicity** is poorly defined by the literature.

c. **Treatment.** Heat stroke is treated with rapid cooling, intravenous fluids, and treatment of any electrolyte abnormalities. All other reactions can be treated with rest, removal from the hot environment, and oral fluids.

3. **Cold**

a. **Exposure.** Workers should not be exposed to environments that do not permit the body to maintain its core temperature.

b. **Toxicity**

(1) **Hypothermia** is characterized by:

(a) Decreased core temperature

(b) Confusion progressing to coma

(c) Cardiac arrhythmias on rewarming

(2) **Frostbite** is characterized by frozen tissue with irreversible cellular damage.

(3) **Chilblains** is characterized by swelling of exposed skin after prolonged damp, cold exposure.

4. **Acute trauma disorders,** the most common occupational health problem, include:

a. Fractures

b. Dislocations

c. Strains

d. Abrasions

e. Lacerations

5. **Cumulative trauma disorders,** a consequence of repetitive motions, include:

a. Bursitis

b. Tenosynovitis

c. Carpal tunnel syndrome

d. Degenerative joint disease

6. **Barotrauma**
   a. **Exposure.** Workers who are employed in occupations below sea level, such as divers, tunnel diggers, and others, may experience barotrauma.
   b. **Toxicity** derives from air emboli and nitrogen emboli in the tissues.
   c. **Clinical manifestations** include:
      (1) Acute, incapacitating pain, typically around a major joint ("the bends")
      (2) Complications of the CNS, the PNS, and the cardiac and pulmonary systems
      (3) Bone necrosis
   d. **Prevention** requires surfacing slowly.
   e. **Treatment** includes recompression in a hyperbaric chamber.

H. Radiation

1. **Ionizing radiation** includes x-rays, gamma rays, alpha particles, and beta particles.
   a. **Exposure.** The average annual dose equivalent for occupationally exposed workers in the United States is 0.3 rem; the maximum allowable dose is 5 rems. A chest x-ray produces gamma radiation equivalent to 0.017 rem and an abdominal x-ray, 0.485 rem.
   b. **Toxicity**
      (1) **Acute high dosage** produces:
         (a) Fever, diarrhea, and electrolyte disorders
         (b) Leukopenia, purpura, and hemorrhage
         (c) Ataxia, lethargy, convulsions, and death
      (2) **Chronic low level exposure** produces cancer of many organs.

2. **Nonionizing radiation** includes radio frequency, infrared, microwaves, and visible frequencies.
   a. **Exposure** is ubiquitous.
   b. **Toxicity.** High-dose directed exposure to microwaves will produce cataracts. Long-term effects to a variety of organ systems have not been well documented.

I. Biologic hazards

1. **Bacterial diseases**
   a. **Brucellosis,** a bacterial disease that causes fever, sweats, malaise, and weight loss, is most apt to affect veterinarians, animal attendants, farmers, packinghouse workers, rendering plant workers, tanners, and laboratory workers.
   b. **Tularemia,** a bacillary disease associated with skin ulcerations and a systemic syndrome, affects outdoor workers, hunters, trappers, foresters, veterinarians, and laboratory workers.
   c. **Leptospirosis,** which is characterized by fever, headache, and meningeal inflammation, affects farmers, construction workers, sewer workers, veterinarians, and packinghouse workers.
   d. **Anthrax,** a bacillary infection that manifests as skin ulcerations but may cause hemorrhagic mediastinitis, is almost exclusively seen in handlers of imported hides, wool, and goat hair.
   e. **Erysipeloid,** which is caused by a gram-positive bacillus that produces a local cellulitis or meningitis, affects butchers, kitchen workers, fish handlers, and tanners. It is contracted by contact with infected swine, cattle, sheep, fish, dogs, and rabbits.
   f. **Tetanus,** which produces muscle spasms, affects agricultural workers in particular.
   g. **Plague,** which may cause adenitis or pneumonia, affects shepherding families, farmers, ranchers, hunters, and geologists in sparsely populated areas of the western United States.
   h. **Tuberculosis,** which frequently manifests as a pulmonary infection, affects physicians, nurses, and laboratory workers.
   i. **Cutaneous granulomas** from *Mycobacterium marinum* (also known as *Mycobacterium balnei*) is seen primarily in fish handlers.
   j. **Psittacosis,** an influenza-like illness, affects pet shop workers, bird fanciers, zoo attendants, and individuals who raise and process poultry.

2. **Rickettsial and chlamydial diseases**
   a. **Rocky Mountain spotted fever and Colorado tick fever,** which are transmitted by tick bites and cause malaise, irritability, fever, muscle aches, and anorexia that may be severe and fatal, affect hunters, hikers, foresters, rangers, ranchers, farmers, trappers, and construction workers.
   b. **Q fever,** a self-limiting influenza-like illness that may include pneumonia, affects dairy farmers, ranchers, stockyard workers, and slaughterhouse workers.

3. **Viral diseases**
   a. **Hepatitis, especially HBV,** which is often contracted by contaminated needle sticks, is seen most often in health care workers, including dentists, dialysis technicians, blood bank workers, and physicians.
   b. **Rabies,** which is produced by animal bites, affects outdoor workers, especially in rural areas.
   c. **Cat scratch disease,** a regional lymphadenitis followed by skin lesions, affects dog and cat handlers.
   d. **Orf,** which is characterized by skin ulcers and regional lymphadenopathy, affects sheep and goat handlers.
   e. **Milker's nodules,** subcutaneous nodules caused by a pox virus, are contracted by dairy farmers when they milk cows that have mastitis.
   f. **New Castle disease** is an influenza-like illness found in poultry handlers.
4. **Fungal diseases**
   a. **Coccidioidomycosis,** an infection usually limited to the lungs but that may affect all organs, affects migrant farmers and other agricultural workers, construction workers, military personnel in endemic areas, and laboratory workers.
   b. **Histoplasmosis,** a systemic infection that produces lung granulomas, affects chicken farmers, pigeon breeders, laboratory personnel, and workers who clear old silos or clean up bird and bat feces.
   c. **Candidiasis,** a common infection between the fingers and around the nails, is seen in workers whose hands are frequently wet and prone to maceration, such as dishwashers, homemakers, bakers, food servers, bartenders, goose pluckers, and poultry packers.
   d. **Aspergillosis,** a pneumonia occasionally presenting as a fungus ball, affects farmers, grain mill workers, and bird handlers who handle grain and other decaying and fermenting vegetation.
   e. **Sporotrichosis,** a systemic disease precipitated by a thorn scratch and local ulceration, affects horticulturists, florists, gardeners, and others who work with sphagnum moss.

V. ORGAN SYSTEM APPROACH TO OCCUPATIONAL DISEASES

A. Pulmonary diseases

1. **Pneumoconioses**
   a. **Asbestosis,** a pleural and parenchymal fibrotic disease, affects insulation workers, pipe fitters, and construction workers.
   b. **Coal workers' pneumoconiosis (CWP),** a nodular interstitial disease, is seen in coal miners.
   c. **Baritosis** (from barium) affects chemical workers.
   d. **Hard metal diseases** (from tungsten or cobalt) affect welders and toolmakers and are primarily characterized by nodules visible on chest x-ray.
   e. **Mixed dust fibrosis** (i.e., several fibrogenic dusts together) affects welders and foundry workers.
   f. **Siderosis,** an interstitial disease with little effect on pulmonary function, results from iron oxide exposure and is seen primarily in welders.
   g. **Silicosis,** a progressive interstitial disease, results from silicon dioxide exposure and is seen in sandblasters, tunnelers, and foundry workers.
   h. **Talcosis** (from talc) affects rubber workers, talc miners, and millers.
2. **Asthma, or reversible bronchospasm,** has been observed following exposure to:
   a. **Isocyanates** in polyurethane foam and paint workers
   b. **Enzymatic detergents** in detergent manufacturing workers
   c. **Flour dusts** in bakers
   d. **Platinum salts** in jewelers and dentists
   e. **Aluminum solder flux** in electronics workers
   f. **Nickel** in metallurgists and electroplaters
   g. **Chromium** in electroplaters and welders
   h. **Wood dusts** in furniture workers
   i. **Cotton dusts** in cotton mill workers and card room workers who straighten the cotton fibers
3. **Bronchitis,** which is characterized by a daily cough with sputum production, is prevalent in:
   a. Coal miners
   b. Welders
   c. Foundry workers

4. **Hypersensitivity pneumonitis** (extrinsic allergic alveolitis), which produces an acute, febrile, 48-hour pneumonia, occurs as a result of exposure to:
   a. Moldy hay
   b. Moldy bagasse
   c. Mushroom compost
   d. Cork dust
   e. Maple bark
   f. Redwood dust
   g. Wood pulp
   h. Moldy barley
   i. Isocyanates
   j. Pigeon droppings
   k. Wheat flour

5. **Lung cancer** has been associated epidemiologically with exposure to:
   a. **Arsenic** in ore smelters and pesticide manufacturers
   b. **Acrylonitrile** in acrylic fiber manufacturers
   c. **Asbestos** in insulators, pipe fitters, and construction workers
   d. **Cadmium** in metal refiners, electroplaters, and battery manufacturers
   e. **Beryllium** in aerospace and electronics workers
   f. **Chloromethyl ethers** in ion exchange resin workers
   g. **Chromates** in chrome smelters and refining workers
   h. **Coke oven emissions** in coke oven workers
   i. **Fluorspar** in fluorspar miners
   j. **Hematite** in iron and hematite miners
   k. **Mustard gas** in the manufacture of mustard gas
   l. **Nickel** in battery makers, welders, and chemists
   m. **Uranium** in uranium mining
   n. **Vinyl chloride** in polyvinyl chloride makers
   o. **Formaldehyde** in manufacturers

6. **Infectious diseases** may be related to occupational exposures in special situations.
   a. An increased rate of **tuberculosis** has occurred in patients with silicosis and in health care workers.
   b. **Q fever** can occur in farmers, veterinarians, and slaughterhouse workers.
   c. **Anthrax** can occur in tanners and animal hair workers.
   d. **Coccidioidomycosis** can occur in construction workers in endemic areas.
   e. **Histoplasmosis** has occurred in farmers.
   f. **Leptospirosis** has occurred in longshoremen.

B. Cardiovascular diseases

1. **Coronary artery disease** has been associated with exposure to:
   a. **Carbon disulfide** in viscose rayon workers
   b. **Nitroglycerin** in munitions and pharmaceutical workers
   c. **CO**

2. **Cardiac arrhythmias** can occur as a result of exposure to:
   a. **Fluorocarbons** in refrigeration workers
   b. **Halogenated hydrocarbons**

3. **Peripheral vascular disease** manifests as **vibration white finger syndrome** in air hammer users. Vibration-induced damage to the microvasculature of the hand results in cold-induced vasospasm of the fingers on a nonautoimmune basis.

C. Hepatic diseases

1. **Health care workers** are at risk for HBV, hepatitis C (HCV), and non-A, non-B hepatitis.

2. **Hepatic necrosis** can occur as a result of occupational exposure to:
   a. **Carbon tetrachloride and other chlorinated hydrocarbon solvents** (e.g., in chemical workers)
   b. **Yellow phosphorus** (e.g., in pesticide workers)
   c. **Trinitrotoluene** (TNT) [e.g., in munitions workers]

3. **Intrahepatic cholestasis** has been observed in plastic resin workers following exposure to methylene dianiline.

D. Musculoskeletal disorders

1. **Low back pain** is one of the leading causes of time lost from work, second only to the common cold. Causes include:
   a. Heavy lifting
   b. Poor body mechanics
   c. Poor design of working environment or tasks

2. **Acute trauma disorders**
   a. Fractures
   b. Dislocations
   c. Strains

3. **Cumulative trauma disorders**
   a. **Bursitis,** including:
      (1) Olecranon bursitis (miners' elbow)
      (2) Infrapatellar bursitis (housemaid's knee)
      (3) Subcalcaneal bursitis (policeman's heel)
   b. **Tenosynovitis,** including:
      (1) De Quervain's disease (trigger thumb), which is seen in typists and switchboard operators
      (2) Lateral epicondylitis (tennis elbow)
   c. **Carpal tunnel syndrome** (median neuropathy), which is seen in manual workers and mail sorters
   d. **Degenerative joint disease,** including:
      (1) Osteoarthritis of the elbow and shoulders, which is seen in pneumatic drill operators
      (2) Osteoarthritis of the feet, which is seen in construction workers and dancers

E. Reproductive disorders. Reproductive health hazards are agents that cause reproductive impairment in adults and developmental impairment or death in the embryo, fetus, or child.

1. **Scope of the problem of reproductive health hazards**
   a. **Birth defects,** the causes of which are unknown in 60%–70% of cases, affect 7% of liveborn infants in the United States.
   b. **Exposure.** Over 60% of married women over age 20 work at some time during the 12 months prior to the birth of their children; of these, over 17% work in industries in which they face potential exposure to a teratogen.
   c. **Infertility.** Approximately 8.4% of couples in the United States in which the wife is of childbearing age are infertile.

2. **Mechanisms of action of reproductive stressors**
   a. **Agents that adversely affect human reproduction** may be chemical, physical, or biologic.
   b. **Men.** Toxic agents may affect the male reproductive system by acting directly on spermatogenesis or by acting on accessory organs of reproduction.
   c. **Women.** Toxic agents may affect the female reproductive system by causing ovulatory dysfunction, acting directly on the early conceptus, or by disrupting the intrauterine environment.
   d. **Adverse effects on the fetus** include:
      (1) Mutagenic alteration of inherited DNA
      (2) Teratogenic or generative alteration of organogenesis
      (3) Embryotoxic or fetotoxic degenerative damage to the developing fetus
      (4) Carcinogenic effect resulting in cancer in the child
   e. **The effect on the embryo or fetus** is determined by the:
      (1) Timing of exposure (the fetus, for example, is susceptible to the effects of various teratogens only during "critical windows" of organogenesis)
      (2) Dosage of the toxin
      (3) Ability of the mother and fetus to metabolize the toxin
      (4) Ability of the toxin to cross the placenta

3. **Examples of occupational reproductive hazards**
   a. **Lead exposure** in women has been associated with menstrual disorders, infertility, spontaneous abortion, stillbirths, and neonatal deaths. Lead exposure in men has been associated with abnormalities in sperm.

b. **Maternal ingestion of fish contaminated with methylmercury** has resulted in congenital Minamata disease in children.
c. **Maternal ingestion of rice oil contaminated with polychlorinated biphenyl** has resulted in congenital Yusho disease in children.
d. **Dibromochloropropane production workers** complaining of infertility were found to have dose-related reductions in sperm counts.
e. **Health care workers exposed to waste anesthetic gases** in operating rooms have been found to have increased rates of spontaneous abortion.

F. Cancer (Tables 12-2 and 12-3)

VI. MEDICAL SCREENING AND BIOLOGIC MONITORING

A. Medical screening for occupational disease is the application of routine or special tests to detect diseases in early stages (and before medical care has been sought) in workers exposed to known hazards.

1. **Uses.** Early detection of occupational disease in a worker or workers may result in the following:
   a. Removal of the workers from continued exposure
   b. Treatment and follow-up of illness
   c. Efforts to reduce exposure in the workplace

2. **Methods.** Occupational disease screening may employ any of the following evaluations, depending on the hazard and the subsequent illness:
   a. History
   b. Physical examination
   c. Laboratory analysis of blood, urine, or breath
   d. Chest x-ray
   e. Physiologic measurements (e.g., spirometry, full pulmonary function testing)
   f. Cytology (urine or sputum)
   g. Audiometry
   h. Biologic monitoring (see VI B)

3. **Timing** of tests depends on the natural course of the disease in question, including:
   a. Latency from exposure to development of illness
   b. Rate of disease progression
   c. Level and duration of the exposure

B. Biologic monitoring may be defined as the analysis of body tissues for toxins or toxin-metabolites.

1. **Uses** of biologic monitoring may include:
   a. Medical screening
   b. Confirmation of toxic exposure
   c. Assessing degree of toxicity

2. **Limitations** of biologic monitoring include the following.
   a. A relatively small fraction of the known hazardous agents can be assayed easily in the appropriate body tissues.
   b. In the case of many hazardous agents, there is a lack of well-established normal levels in unexposed populations with which to compare results.
   c. For most substances, there is insufficient data on dose-effect relationships, making interpretation of levels difficult.

3. **Timing** of samples and choice of tissue to be analyzed depend on:
   a. Rate of toxin absorption
   b. Pattern of toxin distribution into the tissues
   c. Elimination half-life in the tissue (e.g., blood, urine) that is being analyzed

4. **Selected hazards** (i.e., exposures to specific agents) for which biologic monitoring or medical screening is generally recommended can be found in Table 12-4.

Table 12-2. Cancer Sites for which Relationships with Occupational Exposures Are Well Established

Cancer Sites	Carcinogens or Industrial Process

Bladder	Benzidine
	β-Naphthylamine
	4-Aminobiphenyl
	Dyes
	  Auramine
	  Magenta

Blood (leukemia)	Benzene Radiation (x-rays)
Bone	Radium Mesothorium
Larynx	Ethanol (ethyl alcohol) manufacture* Isopropyl alcohol manufacture* Mustard gas Asbestos
Liver (angiosarcoma)	Arsenic† Vinyl chloride
Lung and bronchus	Arsenic Asbestos Bis (chloromethyl) ether Chromium compounds Coal carbonization Coal tar pitch volatiles Iron ore mining Mustard gas Nickel refining Radiation
Nasal cavity and sinuses	Isopropyl alcohol* Mustard gas Nickel refining Radium Mesothorium Woodworking
Peritoneum (mesothelioma)	Asbestos
Pharynx	Mustard gas
Pleura (mesothelioma)	Asbestos

Skin (epithelioma)	Arsenic†
	Coal tar products
	  Coal tar
	  Creosote
	  Pitch
	  Soot
	Mineral oils
	  Shale
	  Coal
	  Petroleum
	Radiation (x-rays)

Adapted from Decoufle P: Occupation. In *Cancer Epidemiology and Prevention.* Edited by Schottenfeld D, Fraumeni JF. Philadelphia, Saunders, 1982.

*By strong acid process.
†Inorganic compounds.

Table 12-3. Occupational Groups Associated with High Risks for Cancer

Groups	Types of Cancer
Benzoyl chloride manufacturers	Lung
Chemists	Brain Lymphatic tissues Hematopoietic tissues Pancreas
Coal miners	Stomach
Coke by-product plant workers	Colon Pancreas
Foundry workers	Lung
Leather workers	Bladder Larynx Mouth Pharynx
Metal miners	Lung
Petrochemical workers	Brain Multiple myeloma Stomach Leukemia Esophagus Lung
Painters	Leukemia
Printing workers	Lung Mouth Pharynx
Rubber industry workers	Bladder Leukemia Brain Lung Prostate Stomach
Textile workers	Nasal cavity Sinuses
Woodworkers	Lymphatic tissue (Hodgkin's disease)

Adapted from Decoufle P: Occupation. In *Cancer Epidemiology and Prevention*. Edited by Schottenfeld D, Fraumeni JF. Philadelphia, Saunders, 1982.

VII. OCCUPATIONAL MEDICAL SERVICES

A. Independent university or hospital services include:

1. **Clinical evaluations** of patients thought to be suffering from occupational disease (patients may be self-referred, or referred from physicians, lawyers, labor unions, companies by whom they are employed, or governmental agencies)
2. **Epidemiologic and laboratory evaluations** (supported by grants from the government or private industry) of newly suspected toxins
3. **Epidemiologic studies on worker cohorts** with various occupational exposures
4. **Preventive advice** to unions or industries on occupational health
5. **Communicating an understanding of the workplace environment** to practicing physicians, other health care professionals, and community groups

Table 12-4. Selected Hazards for which Medical Screening or Biologic Monitoring Is Useful and Readily Available*

Agent	Tests	Timing
Metals		
Arsenic†	Arsenic levels (in hair, nails, urine) Chest radiograph Sputum cytology	Periodic for chronic exposure or immediate for acute exposure
Cadmium	Cadmium levels (in urine) Low-molecular-weight proteins (in urine)	Periodic during exposure
Lead†	Lead levels (in blood) Zinc protoporphyrin (in blood) Complete blood count (CBC) Urinalysis (UA) Blood urea nitrogen (BUN) Creatinine clearance	Following acute exposure or periodic during chronic exposure
Mercury	Mercury levels (in blood, 24-hour urine)	Following acute exposure or periodic during chronic exposure
Organic solvents		
Benzene†	Total phenols (in urine) CBC	Periodic during chronic exposure
Methanol	Methanol levels (in serum) Arterial blood gas	Immediate following acute ingestion
Ethylene glycol	Ethylene glycol levels (in serum) Oxalate crystals (in urine) Arterial blood gas	Immediate following acute ingestion
Dusts		
Asbestos†	Chest radiograph Pulmonary function testing (PFT) Stool for occult blood	Periodic during and following chronic exposure
Silica	Chest x-ray PFT	Periodic during and following chronic exposure
Coal	Chest x-ray PFT	Periodic during and following chronic exposure
Cotton†	PFT	Periodic during exposure
Pesticides		
Organophosphates	Plasma cholinesterase Red blood cell (RBC) cholinesterase	Immediate following acute or periodic exposure or periodic during chronic exposure
Carbamates	Plasma cholinesterase RBC cholinesterase	Immediate following acute or periodic exposure or periodic during chronic exposure
Warfarin	Prothrombin time	Following acute ingestion
Asphyxiant gases		
Carbon monoxide	Carboxyhemoglobin	Immediate after acute or chronic exposure
Noise†	Audiometry in 500–8000 Hz range	Periodic during and following chronic exposure

*History and physical exam should be done in all cases.

†Occupational Safety and Health Administration (OSHA) standards require medical screening for exposure to these agents.

6. **Expert testimony** in toxic injury litigation or workers' compensation cases

B. **Government services** include:

1. **Laboratory, clinical, and epidemiologic research** to expand the knowledge of occupational medicine and toxins
2. **Advice to local, state, and federal government policymakers** concerning safety standards to protect the health of workers
3. **Epidemiologic and laboratory evaluation** of new chemicals
4. **Consultation to health professionals** concerning occupational health problems
5. **Publication of scientific reports** on occupational toxins
6. **Reviewing university research** for the purposes of funding and training in all disciplines of occupational health

C. **Labor union services** include:

1. Advice concerning **design and content of health and safety educational programs** for the membership
2. **Hazard evaluation and literature review** concerning local union plant health and safety problems
3. **Health and safety policy development,** both for collective bargaining and legislation
4. Aiding the membership in **epidemiologic or toxicologic study** of problems

D. **Corporate services** either in plants or on a contractual basis with community hospitals or outpatient facilities include:

1. **Pre-employment physical examinations** to assess the ability of employees to perform required tasks
2. **Periodic medical examinations and biologic testing** to monitor the adverse effects of toxins to which workers are exposed (e.g., pulmonary function testing for workers exposed to silica dust)
3. **Recommendations concerning preventive programs** to control toxins in the plant environment
4. **Acute medical therapy** for injuries and illnesses and in some programs, case management
5. **Advice to personnel departments regarding work restrictions** for partially incapacitated employees and an employee's ability to return to work following an illness
6. **Disability evaluations**
7. **Identification of, and communication with, medical consultants** concerning workers suffering illness or injury on the job
8. **Policy development** for collective bargaining and legislation

E. **Hospital, group practice, or primary care services** provide many of the services outlined in VII D on a contract basis.

VIII. ETHICAL ISSUES. The primary responsibility of the occupational medicine physician is to ensure the health and safety of the patient (i.e., the employee). This goal may conflict with economic or other interests of the employer, the employee, or the health care institution in which the physician practices. Thus, the physician may face frequent ethical dilemmas requiring careful consideration.

A. **Perspectives of various parties may differ** and present sources of conflict or pressure on the occupational health practitioner. These perspectives include:

1. **Employer's perspective.** The employer's financial interest will generally dictate that employee health be balanced against corporate finances. Against the costs of reducing workplace exposures and safety hazards via re-engineering, protective equipment, and other job modifications, the employer must consider the following costs:

a. Workers' compensation insurance
b. Liability for employee exposure (e.g., asbestos lawsuits)
c. Treatment and rehabilitation of injured patients

2. **Employee's perspective.** The physician may encounter potential dilemmas arising from social, financial, or other aspects of the diagnosis of a work-related illness. These include:
   a. **Threatened loss of job** following notification of employer of occupational disease
   b. **Employee desire for confidentiality** when reporting of exposure violation to public health authority is warranted
   c. **Employee resistance to undesirable job modification** (e.g., uncomfortable protective equipment) recommended by physician
   d. **Employee resistance to early return to work** following job-related injury

3. **Hospital's perspective.** Physicians employed by hospitals providing occupational health services may come into conflict with the hospital's economic concerns, which include:
   a. Benefits derived from high injury rates, leading to increased utilization of treatment and rehabilitation services
   b. Increased benefits associated with increasingly invasive therapy (e.g., back surgery versus conservative back therapy)
   c. Expectation of patient referral to hospital medical staff when other physicians at another hospital are known to be more competent

B. **Resolving ethical conflicts.** In an effort to assist physicians in resolving these conflicts, the **American College of Occupational Medicine (ACOM) Code of Ethical Conduct** offers the following principles for physicians providing occupational medical services:

1. To accord the highest priority to the health and safety for the individual in the workplace
2. To make or endorse only statements that reflect the physician's observations or honest opinion
3. To avoid allowing the physician's medical judgment to be influenced by any conflict of interest
4. To treat as confidential whatever is learned about individuals served, releasing information only when required by law or overriding public health considerations or when requested by the individual to confer with other physicians
5. To communicate understandably to those the physicians serve any significant observations about the individual's health, recommending further study, counsel, or treatment, where indicated

BIBLIOGRAPHY

American Conference of Governmental Industrial Hygienists (ACGIH): *1991–1992 Threshold Limit Values for Chemical Substances in Physical Agents and Biological Exposure Indices,* 2nd printing. Cincinnati, ACGIH, 1991.

Levy BS, Wegman DH: *Occupational Health.* Boston, Little, Brown, 1983.

National Institute for Occupational Safety and Health (NIOSH): *NIOSH Pocket Guide to Chemical Hazards.* Washington, DC, US Department of Health and Human Services, Centers for Disease Control, NIOSH, June 1990.

Parmeggiani L: *Encyclopaedia of Occupational Health and Safety,* 3rd edition. Geneva, International Labour Office, 1981.

Rom WN: *Environmental and Occupational Medicine.* Boston, Little, Brown, 1983.

LaDue J (ed): *Occupational Medicine.* Norwalk, CT, Appleton & Lange, 1990.

STUDY QUESTIONS

Directions: Each of the numbered items or incomplete statements in this section is followed by answers or by completions of the statement. Select the **one** lettered answer or completion that is **best** in each case.

1. Occupational asthma is typically caused by all of the following EXCEPT

(A) isocyanates
(B) cotton dust
(C) nickel
(D) flour dust
(E) zinc oxide

2. Hazardous exposures inherent to welding include all of the following EXCEPT

(A) metal fumes
(B) ultraviolet light
(C) irritant gases
(D) metal dusts
(E) heat

3. All of the following cancers have been associated with occupational exposure EXCEPT

(A) bladder cancer
(B) lung cancer
(C) hematopoietic cancer
(D) breast cancer
(E) liver cancer

Directions: Each item below contains four suggested answers of which **one or more** is correct. Choose the answer

A if **1, 2, and 3** are correct
B if **1 and 3** are correct
C if **2 and 4** are correct
D if **4** is correct
E if **1, 2, 3, and 4** are correct

4. Which of the following inorganic dusts can cause lung disease with possible significant clinical impairment?

(1) Coal dust
(2) Silica dust
(3) Asbestos
(4) Iron dust

5. Occupational cancer has been associated with which of the following substances?

(1) Talc
(2) Arsenic
(3) Hydrogen sulfide
(4) Benzene

6. Exposure to which of the following is suspected to cause reproductive system dysfunction in health care workers?

(1) Ethylene oxide
(2) HBV
(3) Waste anesthetic gases
(4) Tuberculosis

1-E	4-A
2-D	5-C
3-D	6-B

SUMMARY OF DIRECTIONS

A	B	C	D	E
1,2,3 only	1,3 only	2,4 only	4 only	All are correct

7. Which of the following information in an individual's occupational history would be important when that person is being evaluated for a possible occupational disease?

(1) Complete history of all jobs ever held by the patient
(2) Known hazards in the workplace
(3) Presence or absence of illness in the patient's coworkers
(4) Temporal relationship between exposure and onset of illness

8. Repetitive motions may cause which of the following musculoskeletal conditions?

(1) Carpal tunnel syndrome
(2) Degenerative joint disease
(3) Tenosynovitis
(4) Fractures

Directions: Each group of items in this section consists of lettered options followed by a set of numbered items. For each item, select the **one** lettered option that is most closely associated with it. Each lettered option may be selected once, more than once, or not at all.

Questions 9–13

Match each of the following characteristic clinical effects with the appropriate pesticide.

(A) Organophosphates
(B) Methyl mercury
(C) Dibromochloropropane (DBCP)
(D) Warfarin
(E) Chlorphenoxy compounds

9. Hypoprothrombinemia
10. Decreased sperm production
11. Cholinergic syndrome
12. Chloracne
13. Ataxia

Questions 14–16

For each metal listed below, select the condition that is most likely to result from chronic exposure to it.

(A) Cancer
(B) CNS dysfunction
(C) Both
(D) Neither

14. Lead
15. Mercury
16. Arsenic

7-E	10-C	13-B	16-C
8-A	11-A	14-B	
9-D	12-E	15-B	

ANSWERS AND EXPLANATIONS

1. The answer is E *[V A 2].*
Occupational asthma is caused by a variety of classes of compounds, by both immunologic and direct irritant mechanisms. Occupational asthma has not been described among workers exposed to zinc oxide. Asthma is seen among spray painters and polyurethane foam workers exposed to isocyanate, in cotton mill workers exposed to cotton dust, in electroplaters exposed to nickel, and from flour dust exposure ("baker's asthma").

2. The answer is D *[III C 1–5].*
Welding produces exposure to ultraviolet light created by the electric arc or flame. Irritant gases may include ozone and the oxides of nitrogen. Dusts are solid particles created by such activities as grinding, while fumes are solids created by condensation from a gaseous state such as that produced by superheating metal in welding. Although welders may be exposed to ambient metal dust from nearby sources, it is not a hazard inherent to welding itself.

3. The answer is D *[Table 12-2].*
Breast cancer has yet to be connected to any occupational exposure. Bladder cancer is associated with exposure to leather dyes, β-naphthylamine, benzidine, and 4-aminobiphenyl. Lung cancer is associated with exposure to asbestos, arsenic, chromium compounds, iron ore, mustard gas, nickel, and radiation. Leukemia is associated with exposure to benzene and radiation. Liver cancer is associated with exposure to arsenic and vinyl chloride.

4. The answer is A (1, 2, 3) *[IV C 1 a, b, d, e].*
Coal dust, silica dust, and asbestos each primarily cause interstitial lung disease, resulting in a pneumoconiosis, which may result in significant reduction of lung function and clinical impairment. Coal worker's pneumoconiosis (CWP) is characterized clinically by small rounded opacities on chest x-ray, obstructive or restrictive lung function abnormalities, and shortness of breath or chronic bronchitis. Silicosis is characterized by small rounded opacities on chest x-ray, impairment on lung function tests, and slowly or rapidly progressive dyspnea on exertion. Asbestosis is characterized by irregular densities on chest x-ray, impaired lung function, and slowly progressive shortness of breath. Siderosis, the pneumoconiosis caused by iron dust or iron oxide fumes, may cause significant radiographic abnormalities (rounded opacities) with little or no functional or clinical impairment.

5. The answer is C (2, 4) *[Table 12-2; IV C 1 f, F 3].*
Occupational cancer is caused by numerous compounds in a variety of sites. Arsenic has been associated with lung cancer in copper smelter workers. Benzene has caused leukemia in shoe manufacturers and others using benzene-containing glues. Pure talc is not associated with cancer, although it may be contaminated with asbestos, which is carcinogenic. Hydrogen sulfide is an asphyxiant gas and is not known to produce cancer.

6. The answer is B (1, 3) *[III F 2, 3].*
Ethylene oxide is mutagenic in animals and is a suspected teratogen. Operating room personnel exposed to waste anesthetic gases have been found to have increased rates of spontaneous abortion. Although hepatitis B virus (HBV) and tuberculosis may be serious infections that potentially could cause adverse effects during pregnancy, they do not affect the reproductive system per se.

7. The answer is E (all) *[II].*
The occupational history should look for a temporal relationship between the patient's exposures and the disease in question. Because of the long latency period between exposure and onset in some diseases (e.g., decades for pneumoconioses, cancer), a complete history of all jobs held in the past is necessary. The history should include a listing of the known hazards, the general conditions of the workplace, the nature of the exposure, and whether protective equipment is used. The presence of disease in coworkers may provide an important clue in identifying potential toxins and should not be overlooked in the occupational history.

8. The answer is A (1, 2, 3) *[IV G 5; V D 2 a, 3 b, c, d].*
Carpal tunnel syndrome results from entrapment of the median nerve by the tunnel formed by the carpal bones and the transverse carpal ligament. It is associated with repetitive motion requiring active finger flexion with the wrist flexed. Degenerative joint disease, or osteoarthritis, may develop from, or be ex-

acerbated by, occupations requiring frequent use of joints, especially with impact. Tenosynovitis also results from repetitive movements, especially when related to new activities. Fractures are acute trauma disorders.

9–13. The answers are: 9-D *[IV D 4 a (2)]*, **10-C** *[IV D 5 a (2)]*, **11-A** *[IV D 1 a (2)]*, **12-E** *[IV D 3 a (2)]*, **13-B** *[IV D 2 a (2)]*.
The rodenticide warfarin and similar compounds produce a depletion of vitamin K–dependent clotting factors, resulting in hypoprothrombinemia and bleeding.

Dibromochloropropane (DBCP), a nematocide, causes decreased sperm production and infertility among the workers who handled it. Agricultural use of DBCP was banned in the United States (except Hawaii) in 1979, and in Hawaii in 1985.

The cholinergic syndrome, including salivation, lacrimation, urinary and fecal incontinence, abdominal cramping, and increased respiratory secretions, is due to inhibition of acetylcholinesterase by the organophosphate insecticides. Carbamates have a similar effect.

The chlorphenoxy herbicides have been associated with chloracne and soft-tissue sarcoma.

The organic mercury compounds, including methyl mercury, cause central nervous system (CNS) dysfunction consisting of ataxia, dysarthria, and emotional disturbances.

14–16. The answers are: 14-B *[IV A 5 c]*, **15-B** *[IV A 6 c]*, **16-C** *[IV A 1 c; Table 12-2]*.
Lead poisoning causes diffuse central nervous system (CNS) dysfunction, which may manifest as an encephalopathy. Cancer is not associated with lead exposure. Mercury may cause neurologic disturbances, renal abnormalities, and skin and mucous membrane irritation. Inhalation of mercury vapors may lead to pulmonary difficulties (e.g., pneumonitis, bronchitis). Arsenic is also a neurotoxin and a lung carcinogen. In addition, exposure to arsenic fumes or dust may produce skin disorders (e.g., hyperpigmentation, hyperkeratosis, gangrene of the fingers and toes, nasal septal ulceration and perforation).

13 Environmental Health Issues

Samuel L. Rotenberg

I. INTRODUCTION. This chapter highlights the toxic effects of chemicals, environmental exposures, the relationship between exposure and effect, and the regulation and management of environmental risks.

A. Toxicity. All chemicals are toxic under some conditions of exposure. Because exposure to chemicals within the environment occurs all the time, it is important to understand the toxic effects that chemicals can cause and the doses at which these toxic effects are observed. The following are examples of chemicals normally assumed to be nontoxic or safe that produce toxic effects in humans under certain exposure conditions.

1. **Oxygen** is present in the atmosphere at a concentration of about 20% and is essential for respiration in higher organisms. However, oxygen causes vasoconstriction of the retinal vascular system of premature infants and can lead to permanent damage if exposure levels remain higher than atmospheric levels.
2. **Nitrogen** is a chemically inert substance that makes up about 78% of the atmosphere. However, at higher than atmospheric concentrations, nitrogen acts as a simple asphyxiant by excluding oxygen from the lungs. Nitrogen also is toxic when released into the bloodstream of divers who surface too rapidly.
3. **Water,** a major component of the environment, is essential to life; it is generally considered that humans can survive only a few days without water. However, water in the lungs blocks oxygen uptake and results in drowning, the cause of hundreds of deaths each year.

B. Exposure. Toxicity cannot occur without exposure to a chemical. An **exposure pathway,** or **route of exposure,** describes the processes and portals of entry required for a chemical in an environmental medium to become hazardous to humans or animals (see also IV B 1). Understanding an exposure pathway can be helpful in controlling and managing chemicals that enter the environment and may result in human or animal exposure.

C. Risk assessment is the process by which risks to humans are estimated from known toxicologic data. Although some chemicals in the environment pose very significant risks to the environment or to other species, most action to restrict chemical exposure occurs because of the potential effects on human health.

D. Managing and preventing risks to humans from chemicals present in the environment are two very difficult challenges facing modern society.

II. TOXIC EFFECTS OF CHEMICALS

A. Classification. Toxic effects of chemicals can be classified as threshold and nonthreshold effects, as well as according to the effects' duration and route of exposure, reversibility, and toxic endpoints.

Note.—This chapter was written by Samuel L. Rotenberg, Ph.D., in his private capacity. No official support or endorsement by the Environmental Protection Agency or any other agency of the federal government is intended or should be inferred.

1. **Nonthreshold and threshold effects**
   a. **Nonthreshold effects.** A chemical or insult is said to produce a nonthreshold effect if any exposure could result in the effect; that is, no safe dose or exposure can be established, and any exposure is associated with some risk. This does not imply, however, that any exposure *will* result in the effect. Only toxic effects that interact with genetic material, such as the following examples, currently are considered nonthreshold effects.
      (1) **Carcinogenesis** is the most important nonthreshold effect for humans. The causes of cancer and the changes in cancer incidence are important public health concerns. Cancer is a severe disease associated with pain, suffering, and death. One-sixth of the annual deaths in the United States are attributed to cancer.
      (2) **Mutagenesis** is an effect for which no threshold can be assumed. At present, it is not possible to estimate the significance of mutagenic effects of chemicals in humans.
   b. **Threshold effects.** A chemical or insult is said to produce a threshold effect if the effect occurs only at a certain level of exposure. Below the threshold exposure, the effect does not occur. **Teratogenesis** and **reproductive disorders as a result of chemical exposures** are considered threshold effects, because it is assumed that the chemicals involved act by a nongenetic interaction (i.e., an interaction that does not involve DNA) to alter fetal development or reproductive function.
   c. **General principles**
      (1) It is important to determine if the toxic effects of a chemical exposure (or other insult) demonstrate a threshold, because risk is estimated differently for threshold and nonthreshold effects.
      (2) The existence or absence of a threshold cannot be proven scientifically.
         (a) For data showing no apparent threshold, it could be argued that data at lower doses must be analyzed to show no effect at such doses.
         (b) For data showing an apparent threshold, it could be argued that a larger number of animals (or humans) in the low-dose group must be examined to show an effect at that dose.
      (3) Assumption of a nonthreshold is the most protective public health position. Less harm would occur if that assumption were wrong than if the converse assumption were made.

2. **Duration of exposure**
   a. **Acute effects** is a term describing the initial effects of exposure to very high doses or the effects that result from a single exposure, not the severity of the effects.
   b. **Chronic effects** is a term referring either to lifetime exposures or to the longest period of exposure time needed to produce an effect. Chronic does not reflect the persistence or reversibility of the effect but simply the length of exposure.
   c. **Subchronic effects** is a term referring to all lengths of exposures between acute and chronic.

3. **Reversibility of effects** refers to the inherent ability of the biologic system to return to normal function upon recovery; it does not refer to the ultimate toxic effect of an unlimited exposure. Many, if not most, toxic effects in humans are fully reversible.
   a. **Reversible effects** occur when no permanent change is made in the biologic system. The mechanism of reversibility depends on the chemical and its toxic effect. For example, cyanide acts by complexing with cytochrome a_3 in the respiratory chain to prevent utilization of oxygen as an electron receptor.
      (1) If sufficient cyanide binds to the cytochrome, completely blocking oxygen use, then death results.
      (2) However, if only a portion of the cytochrome a_3 is affected, the cyanide complexed to cytochrome gradually decreases over time, and the organism will survive. After complete recovery from cyanide poisoning, the organism will respond as if no past exposure had occurred.
   b. **Irreversible effects** occur when the biologic system does not return to its former state after removal of the toxic insult; some permanent change has occurred as a result of the chemical interaction.
   c. **Cumulative effects** occur when the chemical is sequestered (usually in a target organ) and does not affect the organ system until a critical body burden is present.

4. **Toxic endpoints.** The threshold, or safe dose, related to a particular toxic endpoint (i.e., eventual outcome of toxic effects) can be estimated by several methods, depending on the available

data base (i.e., information available about the chemical and its effects). Because a chemical has many toxic effects, a safe dose or acceptable daily intake level must be based on the most sensitive toxic endpoint and the most sensitive human population at risk. An unlimited number of toxic endpoints have been the subject of toxicity testing, ranging from toxic effects (e.g., death) to subtle effects (e.g., neurotoxicity).

a. Examples of toxic endpoints include:

(1) Teratogenesis
(2) Carcinogenesis
(3) Mutagenesis
(4) Reproductive effects
(5) Immune system effects
(6) Central nervous system (CNS) effects
(7) Irritation effects
(8) Organ system effects
(9) Mortality

b. Examples of tests or measurements used to confirm or identify toxic endpoints include:

(1) Physical observation
(2) Pathologic tests
(3) Neurologic tests
(4) Specific enzyme level measurements
(5) Body weight and organ measurements
(6) Analytic tests for specific chemicals (or metabolites)
(7) Behavioral tests

B. Evaluation of carcinogenic potential

1. Human epidemiologic studies. Most human epidemiologic studies involving cancer-causing chemicals are workplace exposure studies (see III B 2 b). Occupational exposures have two important factors necessary for a successful study in humans: relatively high exposure as compared to the general public and an exposed population that can be followed for long time periods.

a. Positive studies. Occupational exposure studies that correlate increased cancer incidence with exposure are directly applicable to human populations other than those in the studies. However, positive epidemiologic studies usually are limited to chemicals that are very potent carcinogens or that cause rare or unusual cancers. Table 13-1 lists some chemicals known to cause human cancer.

b. Negative studies. Studies that show no correlation between exposure and cancer incidence may reveal that the chemical is not a carcinogen. However, many confounding factors can prevent even a well-conducted study from demonstrating that a given chemical exposure increases cancer risks. The following are examples of such factors.

(1) Long latency periods. Latency period is defined as the time between the beginning of exposure and the appearance of cancer. Typical latency periods for human carcinogens are measured in years and decades, as shown in Table 13-1. If a chemical has a 20-year latency period, an epidemiologic study must follow workers for more than 20 years after the exposure before measurable increases in cancer incidence are seen.

(2) Small exposed populations limit the ability to detect carcinogens other than those that are potent or cause rare tumors. Because cancer incidences in nonexposed populations are appreciable, it is difficult to show a statistically significant increase in cancer in a small exposed population.

Table 13-1. Approximate Latency Periods for Human Carcinogens

Chemical	Cancer Site	Latency Period (years)
Arsenic	Skin and lung	20
Asbestos	Pleura and peritoneum	15–20
Benzene	Blood	10–20
Benzidine	Bladder	16
Chromium (VI)	Lung	10–20
Bis(2-chloromethyl)ether	Lung	8
Nickel	Lung and nose	20
Vinyl chloride	Liver angiosarcoma	15

(3) **Lack of lifetime study follow-up** for an exposed group compounds the problem of having a small exposed group and, thus, limits a study's ability to detect chemical carcinogens. When animals exposed to carcinogens are killed before reaching their usual life span and then examined for tumors, the cancer incidence is markedly decreased. Thus, negative human studies in which most participants are still alive may not detect an increased cancer incidence. Instead, the studies might erroneously conclude that the observed exposure does not increase cancer risk.

(4) **Other factors** also contribute to the incidence of cancer and complicate the analysis of human studies.

(a) In most workplace situations, workers are not exposed to a single chemical or agent. Also, workers often change occupations and, thus, are exposed to chemicals other than the one being studied.

(b) Genetic factors, smoking, diet, medication, and other lifestyle factors confound the analysis of human cancer rates.

c. **Suggestive studies.** Some epidemiologic studies show a correlation between chemical exposure and increased human cancer incidence but are not statistically significant. While suggestive studies can contain the same confounding factors present in negative studies, suggestive studies provide some indication that the chemical exposure increases cancer risk.

2. **Animal bioassay tests** for animal carcinogens are typically 2 years in length, which is the life span of the rats or mice used in the test. Exposure is by ingestion or inhalation, and all tissues are examined at the conclusion of the study.

a. **Dosage.** High doses used in animal bioassay tests are constantly criticized. It has been argued that the high dose itself is the reason that an animal bioassay is positive and that the chemical would not be carcinogenic at a low dose. This argument ignores the fact that most chemicals are not carcinogens, no matter how large the dose. Large doses of chemicals may be toxic, but they do not necessarily cause cancer.

(1) **Test-dose guidelines adopted by the Environmental Protection Agency (EPA)** for carcinogenic testing require that the highest dose used does not shorten the life span of the test species. Scientific justification for the use of high doses is both logical and practical.

(a) It has been demonstrated that the latency period is reduced at high doses. Since the life span of rats and mice is about 2 years, it is important that the cancer-causing effect show up within the 2-year life span.

(b) Experiments using animal species with a longer life span (e.g., dogs, cats, monkeys) would take decades to complete, thus lengthening the time needed to determine if a chemical is a carcinogen. Such experiments would also be costly because of the extra care needed for animals that are larger and live longer than mice and rats.

(c) There is no significant scientific advantage to knowing that a chemical causes cancer in animals of a higher order of species than the rodent.

(2) **A high-dose response might not indicate cancer-causing potential.** In a very small percentage of positive animal bioassay results, a high dose of a chemical could possibly alter the response at the target site and lead to cancer that would not occur at a low dose. This could be due to:

(a) **Metabolism of the chemical to the active carcinogenic metabolite.** If a chemical is metabolized by a different pathway at high doses and one of the metabolites along the high-dose pathway is the actual carcinogen, then low doses would not be expected to cause cancer because the cancer-initiating metabolite would not be produced.

(b) **Nonspecific or physical carcinogenesis.** If a physical irritant such as bladder stones were produced by high doses but not by low doses, then the presence of the stones may be directly responsible for bladder cancer.

b. **Route of exposure** for many animal bioassays is by ingestion. However, because exposure to chemicals in the environment (and workplace) usually is by inhalation, the validity of ingestion experiments has been questioned. Some chemicals have been proven to be animal carcinogens by both inhalation and ingestion experiments. Because the predominant difference between ingestion and inhalation exposure is the degree of absorption, both inhalation and ingestion animal bioassay experiments are valid for use in determining carcinogenic potential.

(1) **Inhalation.** A chemical absorbed into the bloodstream from the lungs passes directly to the heart and then into the systemic circulation.

(2) **Ingestion.** Chemicals absorbed from the stomach and intestines pass through the liver before entering the heart. Ingestion experiments are easier to control than inhalation experiments; many of the early experiments in the 1970s were performed by gavage tube.

(a) Since the liver is the predominant organ of metabolism for most chemicals, ingested chemicals are metabolized faster than inhaled chemicals.

(b) For some chemicals, the metabolized form is more toxic than the original chemical, while for other chemicals the converse is true.

(c) Unless all of an ingested chemical is metabolized by the liver after absorption, some will be carried back to the heart and into the systemic circulation.

c. **Advantages of animal studies**

(1) The exposure can be limited to a single chemical being tested.

(2) Several doses of a chemical can be used.

(3) Negative results from well-conducted studies in several species increase the likelihood that the chemical does not present a carcinogenic risk.

(4) Animal tests are relatively easy to conduct.

(5) Positive tests are relevant for humans.

d. **Disadvantages of animal studies**

(1) Positive results do not prove that the chemical is a human carcinogen. It is possible that the chemical is not metabolized by the same metabolite as it is in animals. Although this possibility exists in theory, it is most likely not true for most animal carcinogens.

(2) Estimating human cancer risks from animal cancer data requires converting animal exposure information and extrapolating and modeling dose-response information (see III A 3).

3. **Genotoxic tests.** Short-term tests have been developed to measure the ability of a chemical to interact with or alter DNA. Positive genotoxic test results are not considered sufficient to classify a chemical as a known carcinogen; however, positive results are suggestive and, thus, are often used to select chemicals for animal bioassays.

a. **Point mutations** are measured as an endpoint designed to test the ability of a chemical to cause a mutational event.

(1) The **Ames test,** the most well known and widely used of all short-term tests, measures the ability of a chemical to mutate a specific gene in *Salmonella typhimurium*. Because *S. typhimurium* is a bacterium, a chemical is tested in the presence and absence of a mammalian enzyme fraction to determine if a metabolic event (activation) is required for mutagenesis.

(a) **Advantages of the Ames test**

(i) About 90% of chemicals that test positive in the Ames test also are carcinogenic in animal bioassay tests.

(ii) It is a short-term, low-cost test that is easy to perform.

(b) **Disadvantages of the Ames test**

(i) Negative test results are common for metals and some chlorinated organics.

(ii) It is difficult to test volatile compounds.

(iii) Mutagenesis is not directly equated with carcinogenesis.

(2) **Other point mutation tests** use bacteria, yeast, or animal cell systems.

b. **Chromosome effects** are measured as changes in the structure or number of chromosomes or in the production of chromosome fragments. Many cell types are used, and exposure to the chemical can occur in vivo or in vitro.

c. **DNA damage** is measured as either direct breaks in DNA or the inability of a cell system to repair such breaks. Both bacterial and mammalian cell systems are used for DNA damage tests.

d. **Mammalian cell transformations** are changes in cells exposed to a chemical that cause the cell to induce tumors in recipient animals. Transformation often is accompanied by characteristic morphologic changes in the transformed mammalian cell.

4. **Evaluation for structural similarities to known carcinogens.** In the absence of animal or human data, structural similarities can be important in determining the likelihood that a chemical is a carcinogen, as shown in the following examples.

		Animal Evidence Needed				
		Sufficient	Limited	Inadequate	No data	No evidence
Human Evidence Needed	Sufficient	A	A	A	A	A
	Limited	B1	B1	B1	B1	B1
	Inadequate	B2	C	D	D	D
	No data	B2	C	D	D	E
	No evidence	B2	C	D	D	E

Figure 13-1. Human and animal evidence required to determine an Environmental Protection Agency (EPA) weight of evidence classification. *A* = human carcinogen; *B1* = probable human carcinogen; *B2* = probable human carcinogen; *C* = possible human carcinogen; *D* = not classified; *E* = no evidence of carcinogenesis for humans (see Table 13-2).

- **a.** An untested nitrosamine or benzidine derivative would be expected to be carcinogenic since so many different nitrosamines and benzidines have tested positive in animal bioassay tests.
- **b.** The three dichlorobenzene isomers would be expected to be carcinogens because the most highly chlorinated benzene, hexachlorobenzene, is an animal carcinogen, and benzene itself is a human carcinogen. Thus, it is logical, but not proven, that the dichlorobenzenes are carcinogens.

5. **Weight of evidence classification** describes the probability that the chemical is a human carcinogen. Figure 13-1 shows how available human and animal data for a chemical are integrated in a weight of evidence classification. The system used by the EPA to classify chemical carcinogens is summarized in Table 13-2. Table 13-3 lists examples of chemicals that show some evidence of carcinogenicity in humans; Table 13-4 lists examples of chemicals that show evidence of carcinogenicity only in animal tests; and Table 13-5 lists examples of chemicals that show no evidence of carcinogenicity in animal or human tests.
   - **a. The qualitative conclusion that a chemical is a possible, probable, or definite human carcinogen** is simply a determination of whether a chemical is a likely cause of cancer in humans. Only after a chemical is known to be carcinogenic can the potency of that carcinogen be determined. The **quantitative estimate of potency** for a carcinogen is separate from the qualitative weight of evidence conclusion concerning its carcinogenicity (see III A 2 a).
   - **b. Negative animal or human studies** often are cited as **reasons to modify** a qualitative weight of evidence conclusion or quantitative potency determination. As a rule, negative studies are not factored into the weight of evidence conclusion unless all studies are negative.

Table 13-2. Environmental Protection Agency (EPA) Weight of Evidence Classification for Carcinogens

Group	Description	Comment
A	Human carcinogen	Sufficient evidence in epidemiologic studies to support causal association
B1	Probable human carcinogen	Limited evidence of carcinogenicity in humans
B2	Probable human carcinogen	Sufficient evidence of carcinogenicity in animals
C	Possible human carcinogen	Limited evidence of carcinogenicity in animals
D	Not classified	Inadequate evidence of carcinogenicity in animals
E	No evidence of carcinogenesis for humans	No evidence of carcinogenicity in animals or humans

Table 13-3. Weight of Evidence Classification of Selected Chemicals Showing Evidence of Carcinogenicity in Human Epidemiologic Studies

Chemical (by class)	Human Epidemiologic Evidence	Animal Bioassay Evidence*	Weight of Evidence Classification
Metals			
Arsenic	Sufficient		A
Cadmium	Limited	Sufficient	B1
Chromium (VI)	Sufficient		A
Nickel	Sufficient		A
Inorganics			
Asbestos	Sufficient		A
Benzenes			
Benzene	Sufficient		A
Chlorinated volatiles			
Bis(2-chloromethyl)ether	Sufficient		A
Vinyl chloride	Sufficient		A
Miscellaneous organics			
Acrylonitrile	Limited	Sufficient	B1
Benzidine	Sufficient		A
Cyclophosphamide	Limited	Sufficient	B1
Diethylstilbestrol	Sufficient		A
1,2-Diphenylhydrazine	Limited	Sufficient	B1
Ethylene oxide	Limited	Sufficient	B1
Melphalan	Limited	Sufficient	B1
2-Naphthylamine	Sufficient		A

*Animal bioassay results are not shown for a chemical if sufficient human evidence exists.

(1) Some reasons that human studies could be negative even when the chemical is a carcinogen are given in II B 1 b. There are many experimental design problems that can result in a negative animal study.

(2) It is more difficult to make errors in an experimental protocol that shows a chemical to be carcinogenic when it is not than vice versa.

(3) In determining potency, a well-done negative epidemiologic study can establish **an upper limit of risk** in humans for a chemical that is a known animal carcinogen. However, to date, no human study has been able to establish such an upper limit.

III. DOSE-RESPONSE EVALUATION

A. Carcinogens

1. Carcinogenesis

a. Asbestos-induced cancer mortality is shown in Figure 13-2 for a group of asbestos workers. The relative risk of cancer death is plotted against the cumulative exposure to asbestos.

(1) These data are consistent with no threshold for asbestos-induced cancer deaths, or no safe dose of asbestos exposure. If a threshold existed, the plot would be expected to show a relative risk of 1 for some exposures greater than 0.

(2) Since these data show relative risk, the actual shape of the curves may not be meaningful.

b. Cancer resulting from 2-acetylaminofluorene (2-AAF). Table 13-6 shows the incidence of bladder and kidney cancer in mice fed various amounts of 2-AAF. The cancer incidence rates measured in this experiment are plotted in Figure 13-3. The experiment was performed to see whether a threshold would emerge for an animal carcinogen by lowering the dose and using larger numbers of animals in each exposure group.

(1) The data for bladder cancer may or may not be consistent with a threshold model of carcinogenesis.

(2) The liver tumor data clearly are not consistent with a threshold model.

Table 13-4. Weight of Evidence Classification for Chemicals Showing Some Evidence of Carcinogenicity in Animal Bioassay Tests

Chemical (by class)	**Animal Bioassay Evidence**	**Weight of Evidence Classification**
Metals		
Beryllium	Sufficient	B2
Lead (Pb)	Sufficient	B2
Pesticides		
Chlordane	Sufficient	B2
Dicofol	Limited	C
Toxaphene	Sufficient	B2
Inorganics		
Hydrazine	Sufficient	B2
Polyaromatic hydrocarbons		
Benzo[a]pyrene	Sufficient	B2
1-Naphthylamine	Limited	C
2-Naphthylamine	Sufficient	A*
Benzenes		
2,6-Dinitrotoluene	Limited	C
Hexachlorobenzene	Sufficient	B2
Phenols		
2,4,6-Trichlorophenol	Sufficient	B2
Chlorinated volatiles		
Chloroform	Sufficient	B2
1,1-Dichloroethylene	Limited	C
Trichloroethylene (TCE)	Sufficient	B2
Chlorinated nonvolatiles		
Polychlorinated biphenyls (PCBs)	Sufficient	B2
2,3,7,8-TCDD (dioxin)	Sufficient	B2
Miscellaneous organics		
Aflatoxin B_1	Sufficient	B2
Dimethylnitrosamine	Sufficient	B2
Ethylene oxide	Sufficient	B2
β-Hexachlorocyclohexane	Limited	C

2,3,7,8-TCDD = 2,3,7,8-tetrachlorodibenzo-*p*-dioxin.

*2-Naphthylamine is a known human carcinogen; thus, the weight of evidence classification is A.

c. **Cancer resulting from radiation** shows dose-response curves that are consistent with no threshold.
   (1) Radiation exposure is not identical to chemical exposure. However, radiation acts at the level of DNA, as do chemical carcinogens, and radiation-induced cancers show latency periods in humans as do chemical carcinogens.
   (2) Lack of an apparent threshold for radiation-induced cancers in humans is circumstantial evidence for lack of a threshold for chemical carcinogens.

2. **Human carcinogens** are chemicals or other insults that are thought to cause human cancer. There are about 30 known human carcinogens; for most of these, an animal model also exists. Table 13-7 lists examples of human and animal carcinogens and their associated tumor sites.
   a. **Potency** is the quantitative description of the ability of a chemical to cause cancer.
      (1) **Units.** Potency usually is expressed as a cancer risk in units of risk per mg/kg/day of exposure, or $(mg/kg/day)^{-1}$. Quantitatively, potency is the slope of the dose-response curve, where exposure is expressed in units of mg/kg/day and response is expressed as risk of cancer. The higher the numerical value of the cancer potency factor, the more potent the carcinogen.

Table 13-5. Chemicals Showing No Evidence of Carcinogenicity in Either Animal Bioassay Tests or Human Epidemiologic Studies (Weight of Evidence Classification D)

Chemical (by class)	Animal Bioassay Evidence	Chemical (by class)	Animal Bioassay Evidence
Metals		Pesticides	
Copper	Inadequate	Aldicarb	Inadequate
Manganese	Inadequate	Methoxychlor	Inadequate
Mercury	Inadequate	Miscellaneous organics	
Silver	Inadequate	Diethyl arsine	Inadequate
Benzenes		Glyphosate	Inadequate
Benzoic acid	Inadequate	Methyl ethyl ketone	Inadequate
Ethyl benzene	Inadequate	Inorganics	
Toluene	Inadequate	Cyanide	Inadequate
Xylenes	Inadequate		

(2) **Calculation.** Using the cancer potency factor for a chemical, risks associated with specific exposure situations can be calculated, or other units of interest can be derived, as shown here for benzene, which has a cancer potency factor of 0.052 (mg/kg/day)$^{-1}$.
   (a) **Assumptions.** For the purposes of this calculation, a body weight of 70 kg is assumed. Absorption into the body from air or water exposure is assumed to be 100%. Daily water intake is 2 L, and air intake is 20 m^3.
   (b) **Quantity.** The amount of chemical exposure associated with a given risk can be calculated. Exposure to 25 g of benzene over a lifetime corresponds to an excess cancer risk of 1 in 1000. Likewise, exposure to 25 mg of benzene corresponds to a risk of 1 in 1 million.
   (c) **Concentration.** The risk associated with unit concentration of a chemical in air or water can be calculated.
      (i) **Water.** The risk associated with drinking water containing benzene at 1.0 ppb (part per billion) [μg/L] over a lifetime is 20 in 100,000, or 2 in 1 million.
      (ii) **Air.** The risk associated with inhaling air containing benzene at 1.0 μg/m^3 over a lifetime is 34 in 100,000 or 3 in 1 million.

(3) **Examples.** Table 13-8 lists cancer potency factors of some known human carcinogens, as well as the concentration in drinking water and in ambient air that corresponds to a lifetime cancer risk of 10^{-6}, or 1 in 1 million. The body weight assumed in this calculation is 70 kg, and the exposure assumptions used are:
   (a) Lifetime exposure (70 years)
   (b) Breathing 20 m^3/day of ambient air
   (c) Drinking 2 L/day of water

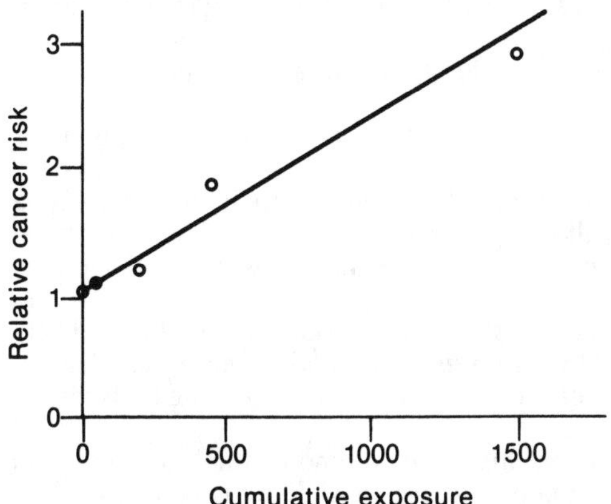

Figure 13-2. The dose-response curve for respiratory cancer mortality in a group of asbestos workers.

Table 13-6. Incidence of Bladder and Liver Tumors in Mice Fed 2-Acetylaminofluorene (2-AAF)

	Tumor Response*			
Dose (ppm)	**Bladder**	**Percentage**	**Liver**	**Percentage**
0	2/759	0.26%	20/762	2.62%
30	9/2105	0.43%	164/2109	7.78%
35	5/1357	0.37%	128/1361	9.40%
45	4/881	0.45%	98/888	11.0%
60	6/756	0.79%	118/758	15.6%
75	13/586	2.22%	118/587	20.1%
100	51/297	17.2%	76/297	25.6%
150	236/313	75.4%	126/314	40.1%

ppm = parts per million.

*Response is reported as the number of animals with the tumor compared with the total number of animals in the dose group and then calculated as a percentage.

b. **Extrapolation of cancer risk.** Human cancer risks from known human carcinogens are relatively easy to extrapolate. For simplification, it is assumed that the observed increase in cancer rate is directly proportional to the total exposure to the cancer-causing chemical.

3. **Animal carcinogens** are chemicals that test positive in a well-conducted animal bioassay test for carcinogenesis. Although several hundred chemicals are known animal carcinogens, most chemicals tested are not carcinogenic. Very few animal carcinogens are proven human carcinogens. There is a very high correlation of animal carcinogenicity with mutagenicity in short-term test systems.
   a. **Potency** is as defined for human carcinogens, but extrapolations to low-dose exposure and the shape of the dose-response curve at low doses have been assumed.
      (1) **Units** describing potency and expressions of cancer risks are as described for human carcinogens.
      (2) **Examples.** Table 13-9 lists cancer potency factors for some known animal carcinogens, as well as the concentration in drinking water and in ambient air that corresponds to a lifetime cancer risk of 10^{-6}, or 1 in 1 million. The exposure assumptions used to calculate this risk are the same as noted in III A 2 a (3).
   b. **Extrapolation of cancer risk.** Because data used to determine that a chemical is an animal carcinogen are obtained in animals and not in humans and under experimental rather than natural exposure conditions, extrapolations to human exposure must be made. These extrapolations can be made in several ways, as described below. In the absence of data to the contrary, the EPA assumes a surface area equivalency for conversion of doses in animal species to doses in humans.
      (1) **Body weight equivalency.** This method assumes that a given dose in mg/kg yields identical toxicologic effects in all species.
      (2) **Air exposure equivalency.** This method assumes that an air level in $\mu g/m^3$ yields identical toxicologic effects in all species.
      (3) **Food equivalency.** This method assumes that a food concentration in ppb yields identical effects.
      (4) **Water equivalency.** This method assumes that a water concentration in ppb yields identical effects.
      (5) **Surface area equivalency.** This method assumes that a given dose in mg/surface area yields identical toxicologic effects in all species. The pharmacologic basis for this assumption is that the metabolic rate of different species is more closely associated with surface area than with body weight.
   c. **Low-dose models.** Exposure of animals in a bioassay test is at doses higher than a likely environmental exposure. The absence of low-dose exposure and response data has resulted in many models and hypotheses of cancer mechanism and many methods for extrapolating to low-dose ranges.
      (1) Risks predicted at low doses from some of the more common models are shown in Table 13-10, and graphs of the dose-response curves are shown in Figure 13-4.
      (2) As a protective public health assumption, the EPA currently uses a multistage model that essentially assumes a linear dose response from the lowest observable data point.

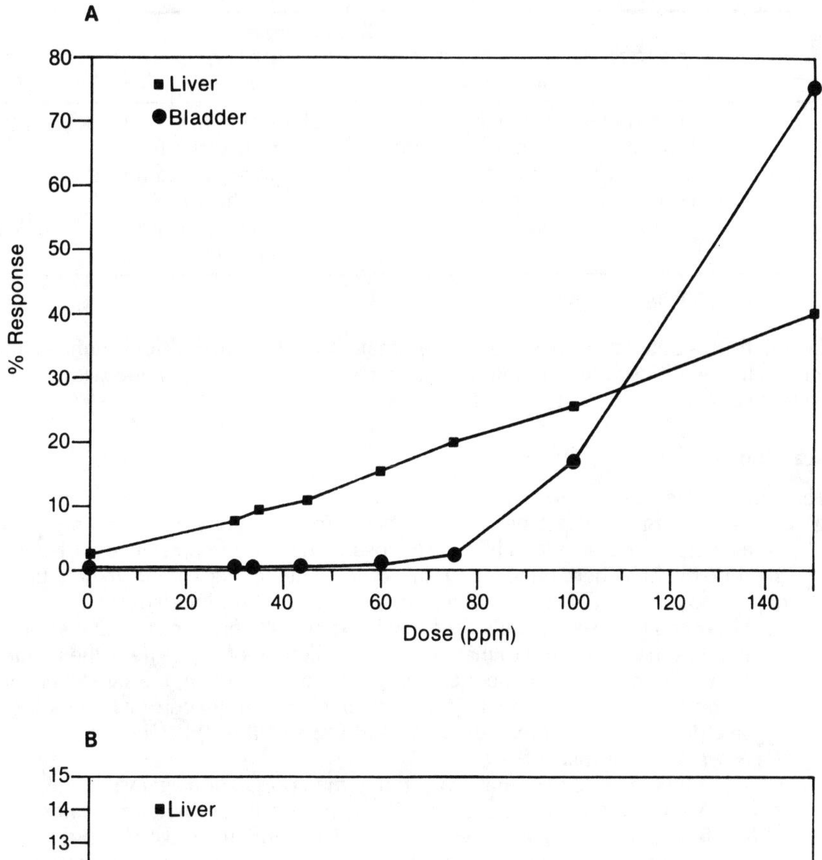

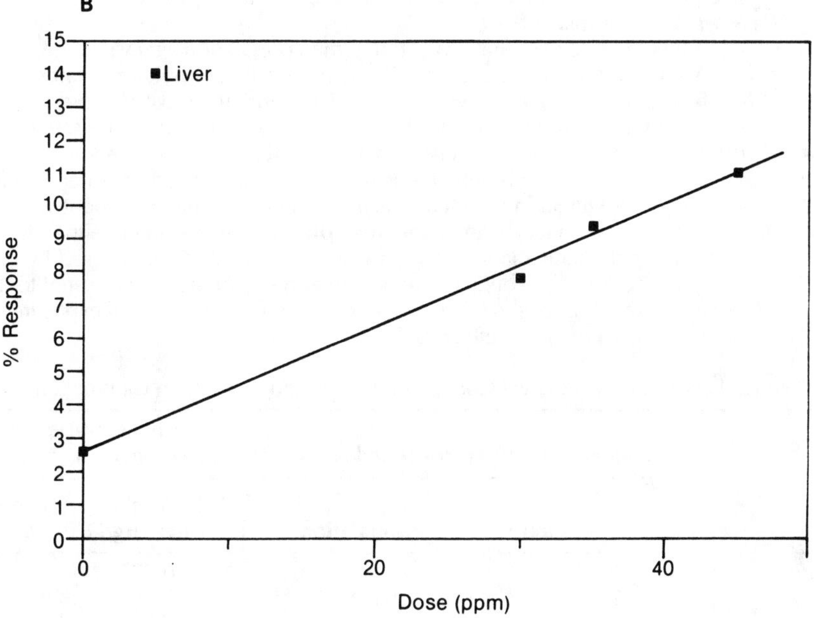

Figure 13-3. Liver and bladder tumor response in mice fed 2-acetylaminofluorene (2-AAF). (*A*) Dose-response curves. (*B*) Low-dose range of dose-response curve for liver tumors.

Table 13-7. Tumor Sites of Chemical Carcinogens in Humans and Animals

	Target Organ*	
Chemical	**Humans**	**Animals**
Aflatoxins	Liver (ingestion, inhalation)	Liver, stomach, colon, kidney (ingestion)
Benzidine	Bladder (ingestion, inhalation)	Liver (ingestion)
Diethylstilbestrol	Uterus, vagina (ingestion)	Mammary gland (ingestion)
Mustard gas	Lung, larynx (inhalation)	Lung (inhalation)
Vinyl chloride	Liver, brain, lung (inhalation)	Lung, liver, mammary gland, kidney (inhalation)

*Route of exposure is given in parentheses.

4. **Correlation of potency.** Cancer potency estimates from human data and animal data correlate remarkably well, usually differing by less than one order of magnitude with no discernible pattern.

B. Noncarcinogens

1. **Thresholds (safe doses)**
   a. **Determining thresholds.** Safe doses can be estimated for any period of time, but the usual estimate of a safe dose is for a lifetime exposure. In some circumstances, a 1-day or 10-day safe dose might be determined for a state or local health department to help them respond to an exposed population resulting from a contamination incident.
      (1) **Lifetime safe dose** is a daily dose that is expected to produce no adverse health effects in all humans exposed to that dose over a lifetime of exposure. When a lifetime safe dose is estimated for a chemical that also is a carcinogen, the safe level applies only to the noncarcinogenic toxic effects of that chemical. [In current terminology, lifetime safe doses are called reference doses (RfDs; see III B 4).]
      (2) **Most sensitive toxic effect**
         (a) A lifetime safe dose that protects a human population against the toxic effects that occur at the lowest exposure will also protect that population against the toxic effects that occur at a higher exposure. Therefore, the most sensitive toxic effect, or endpoint, should be used for the threshold determination of a safe dose.
         (b) The most sensitive toxic effect may not be easily determined—in part, because toxic effects are constantly being redefined. However, there often is reference to an adverse effect in the literature. This implies a judgment about what observed changes are, in fact, significant. Regardless of the integrity of either the observers or the judgments made in the past, any observed change caused by a chemical may decrease the ability of the person to respond to changes usual to their environment. Thus, observed changes that result from a chemical exposure should be considered the toxic effect itself.

Table 13-8. Potency Factors and Risk-Level Concentrations of Known Human Carcinogens

	Cancer Potency Factor [(mg/kg/day)$^{-1}$]		Concentration Needed to Produce 10^{-6} Lifetime Risk	
Chemical*	**Ingestion**	**Inhalation**	**In Drinking Water (μg/L)†**	**In Ambient Air (μg/m^3)‡**
Vinyl chloride	1.9	2.9×10^{-1}	0.025	0.029
Benzene	2.9×10^{-2}	2.9×10^{-2}	0.49	0.29
Nickel		8.4×10^{-1}		0.01
Arsenic	1.8	1.5×10^{1}	0.049	0.00057
Chromium (VI)		4.2×10^{1}		0.0002
Benzidine		2.3×10^{2}		0.000037
Bis(2-chloromethyl)ether		2.2×10^{2}		0.000039

*Chemicals appear in approximate order of inhalation potency.
†Exposure is by ingestion.
‡Exposure is by inhalation.

Table 13-9. Potency Factors and Risk-Level Concentrations of Known Animal Carcinogens

Chemical*	Cancer Potency Factor [(mg/kg/day)$^{-1}$]	Concentration Needed to Produce 10^{-6} Lifetime Risk
	Ingestion	**In Drinking Water (μg/L)†**
Dichloromethane (methylene chloride)	7.5×10^{-3}	4.7
Trichloroethylene (TCE)	1.1×10^{-2}	3.2
Tetrachloroethylene	5.1×10^{-2}	0.69
Chloroform	8.1×10^{-2}	0.43
Chlorophenothane (DDT)	3.4×10^{-1}	0.10
Chlordane	1.6	0.022
Hexachlorobenzene	1.7	0.021
Heptachlor	3.4	0.010
Polychlorinated biphenyls (PCBs)	4.3	0.0081
Aldrin	1.1×10^{1}	0.0032
Benzo[a]pyrene	1.2×10^{1}	0.0029
Dimethylnitrosamine	2.6×10^{1}	0.0013
Ethylene dibromide (EDB)	4.1×10^{1}	0.00085
Aflatoxin B_1	2.9×10^{3}	0.000012
2,3,7,8-TCDD (dioxin)	1.6×10^{5}	0.0000002
	Inhalation	**In Ambient Air (μg/m³)‡**
Tetrachloroethylene	1.8×10^{-3}	4.7
Trichloroethylene (TCE)	1.7×10^{-2}	0.5
Dichloromethane (methylene chloride)	1.4×10^{-2}	0.25
Ethylene oxide	3.5×10^{-1}	0.01
Benzo[a]pyrene	6.1	0.00057

2,3,7,8-TCDD = 2,3,7,8-tetrachlorodibenzo-*p*-dioxin.

*Chemicals in each list appear in approximate order of potency.
†Exposure is by ingestion.
‡Exposure is by inhalation.

(3) **Acute or emergency exposures.** A safe exposure level may be estimated for a contamination incident; that safe level will likely be much greater than the safe lifetime threshold level.

b. **Uncertainty factors** are used to reduce a safe human dose to reflect a condition other than the original exposure conditions.

(1) **Sensitive population.** If the sensitive population for a given chemical is unknown or if data on the chemical have been collected in a population that is not the most sensitive, an uncertainty factor of 10 is used to convert the observed exposure to a sensitive population exposure. This uncertainty factor typically is required when occupational exposure information or human experimental information is evaluated, since neither usually represents the most sensitive population.

(2) **Animal population.** An uncertainty factor of 10 is used to convert the results of animal studies to results in humans. A portion of this factor is the surface area–to–body weight dose issue discussed in III A 3 b (5); another consideration is that humans may be more sensitive than the animal species used for the tests.

(3) **Short-term results.** An uncertainty factor of 10 is used to convert short-term toxicologic test results to long-term results.

(4) **No-effect level.** An uncertainty factor of 10 is used to decrease the exposure when a no-effect level has not been established. This occurs when each of the exposure levels produced the same toxic effect.

(5) **Data base.** An uncertainty factor of 10 is used to decrease the exposure if the toxicologic data base is limited.

c. **Example.** Table 13-11 shows estimates of safe doses of toluene, using the available data base. These safe-dose estimates are for the noncarcinogenic effects of toluene. Additionally, toluene has been tested for carcinogenicity in an animal bioassay study and has not been determined to be carcinogenic. A conclusion drawn from this information would

Table 13-10. Dose-Response Relationships Extrapolated to Low-Dose Levels for Selected Models

	Proportion Responding within Each Model				
Dose	**Multihit***	**Weibull**	**Multistage**	**Single Hit**	**Log Logistic**
16	. . .	. . .	. . .	0.999	0.998
8	. . .	1.00	1.00	0.977	0.992
4	0.99	0.995	0.998	0.848	0.963
2	0.850	0.850	0.850	0.610	0.850
1	0.500	0.488	0.468	0.376	0.551
0.5	0.210	0.210	0.210	0.210	0.210
0.25	0.07	0.0798	0.0933	0.110	0.0544
0.125	. . .	0.0289	0.0431	0.0572	0.0123
0.0625	. . .	0.0103	0.0206	0.029	0.00269
0.01	0.00050	0.000657	0.00315	0.00470	0.0000473
0.001	0.0000035	0.0000206	0.000313	0.000470	0.000000294
0.0001	0.000000001	0.000000645	0.0000312	0.0000470	0.000000002

Parameters for models were chosen to produce identical responses at a dose of 0.5 and, if possible, at 2.0.

*Proportion responding was not calculated for all doses for this model.

state that the daily safe dose of toluene is not likely to be below 2020 μg/day and that this limit would be expected to be protective of children or other sensitive members of the population.

2. **Human exposure data.** In evaluating human exposure, many factors must be considered.
   a. **Route of exposure.** Many chemicals are not absorbed equally efficiently by all routes. When data using human studies are evaluated, the actual amount of chemical is most important for systemic toxicity. For irritation effects, the concentration in the environment is needed.
   b. **Workplace exposure recommendations** from the National Institute for Occupational Safety and Health (NIOSH) or the Occupational Safety and Health Administration (OSHA) may be used to estimate safe doses. NIOSH recommendations are health-based, whereas those from OSHA may be based on other factors (e.g., cost, available technology, politics).
      (1) Workplace exposures are for only 40 hours per week, so exposure limits must be reduced by the factor of 40/168, or 0.24, to correct for constant exposure (24 hr/day × 7 days = 168 hr).
      (2) One uncertainty factor of 10 is used to convert the exposure (of a presumed healthy population) to a sensitive population exposure, and another uncertainty factor of 10 is used to convert a "no adverse effect" exposure to a "no observed effect" exposure.
      (3) Thus, a dose that probably is safe for the general population would necessitate division of the recommended level by 420. Conservative toxicologists would probably reduce this further by a factor of 2, while industrialists would probably increase it by a factor of 5.
      (4) Air exposure limits in the workplace [i.e., threshold limit values (TLVs)] have been reduced over time, as the toxicologic data base has expanded and as understanding of toxicologic principles has become more sophisticated.
   c. **Experimental human exposure.** Short-term human exposure data are available for some chemicals. Such data are useful starting places for estimating safe doses where the toxicologic endpoints are observable and not life-threatening.
      (1) Advantages
         (a) The effects that are observed are relevant to humans.
         (b) Observations of toxic effects in humans at high doses can be used to direct animal toxicity experiments.
      (2) Disadvantages
         (a) Lack of long-term controlled exposure for experiments conducted with human volunteers limits the usefulness of some human exposure data.
         (b) Inability to control confounding factors and other chemical exposures complicates analysis of cause and effect.
3. **Animal exposure data.** As with human data, many factors must be considered for animal exposure information.
   a. **Route of exposure.** The actual dose to the animal depends on the route of exposure and the percent of chemical that is absorbed.

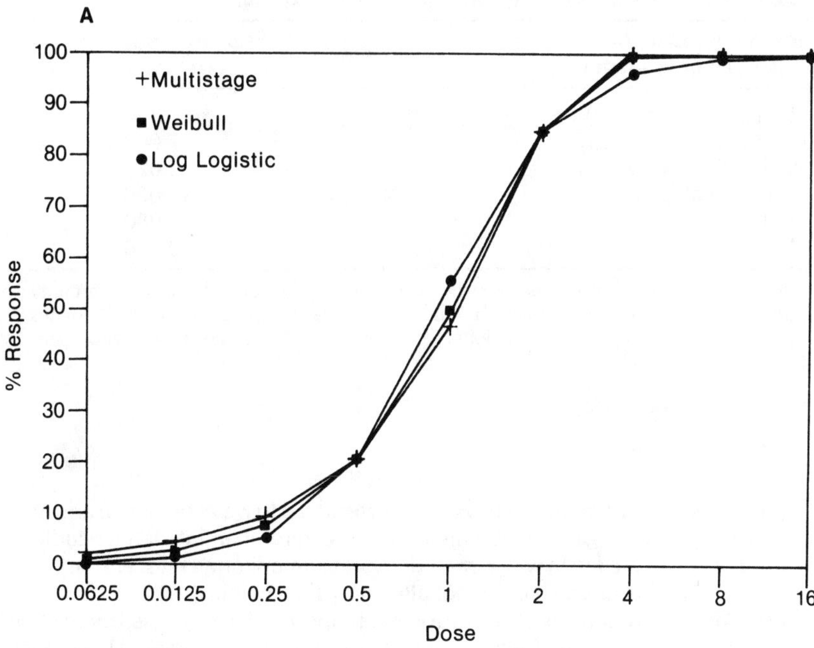

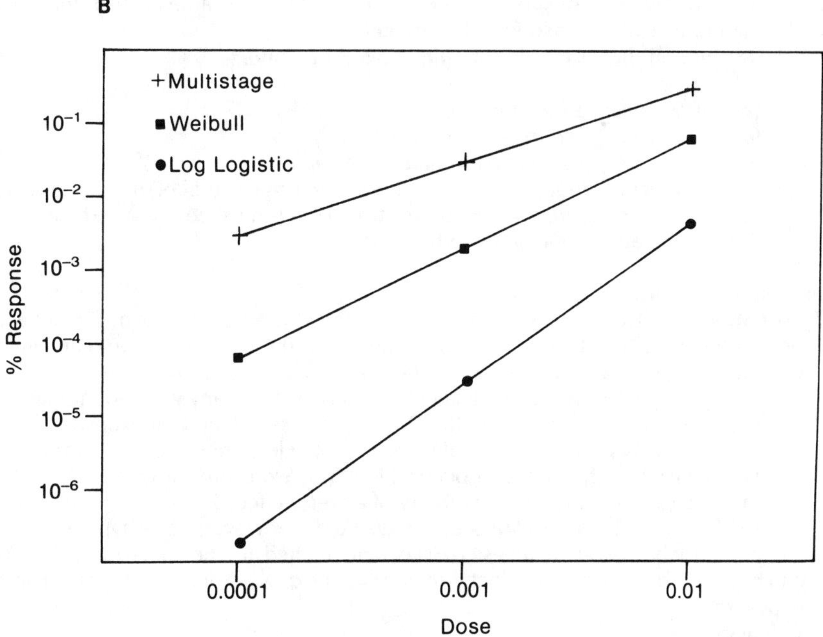

Figure 13-4. Dose-response curves for selected models. (*A*) Dose response at high doses. (*B*) Predicted dose response at low doses.

Table 13-11. Estimates of Safe Doses of Toluene Exposure

Toxicologic Data Base or Source of Estimate	Estimated Safe Dose (μg/day)*
Human (CNS/chronic)	2750
Rat (CNS/subchronic)	147,000
Rat (CNS/chronic)	2020
Mouse (teratogenic)	30,000
NIOSH	8980
EPA	20,200

Estimates of safe doses of toluene exposure were made by the author by using uncertainty and exposure factors to the human or animal toxicity data or to the safe exposure estimates of the National Institute for Occupational Safety and Health (NIOSH) or the Environmental Protection Agency (EPA).

CNS = central nervous system.

*Estimated for a 70-kg adult.

(1) **Ingestion studies** in which chemicals are added to water or food or are introduced into the animal by gavage tube are easier to control than **inhalation studies**. If ingested chemicals are fed in water or food, exposure monitoring must ensure that normal eating and drinking habits are not altered by the chemical.

(2) **Skin painting and injection** are routes of exposure that were used more often in the past than they are today. Each has some benefits for special types of toxicologic research, but neither is as useful for cancer bioassays as inhalation, ingestion, or feeding by gavage.

b. Metabolism. Although metabolic patterns are generally the same in all animal species, including humans, it is not so for all chemicals.

c. Advantages and disadvantages of animal exposure studies

(1) **Advantages**

(a) Exposure to a single chemical is controlled.

(b) Exposure is given in several doses.

(c) A wide range of toxic effects are observable.

(2) **Disadvantage.** Although similar to humans in many biochemical and physiologic functions, animals are not humans, so toxic effects must be evaluated with care to determine the actual relevance to humans.

4. Reference doses (RfDs)

a. Definition. The RfD for a chemical is a lifetime or chronic dose or exposure level that will protect the most sensitive human population from the most sensitive toxic effect of that chemical.

(1) Most likely, no adverse effects will be experienced by any group of humans exposed to levels equal to or less than the RfD, regardless of length of exposure.

(2) Conversely, exposure at or greater than the RfD level does not necessarily mean that an adverse health effect will occur. However, exposures at greater than RfD levels must be evaluated for the possibility of adverse effects.

b. Units. RfDs typically are expressed in mg/kg/day. However, using typical exposure assumptions for body weight, ingested water, and inhaled air, the numerical value of the RfD can be expressed in μg/L to reflect drinking water exposure or $\mu g/m^3$ to reflect ambient air exposure.

c. Calculation

(1) RfD is calculated by dividing a "no observed" or "lowest observed" effect value by a factor of 10 for each of the uncertainties that are valid for a given set of toxicologic data.

(2) Pertinent modifying factors may further reduce the final calculated RfD. Modifying factors are meant to reflect some professional judgment about the quality of available toxicologic data. They typically range from 1 to 10, with 1 being the default value.

d. Examples. Table 13-12 shows the RfD and chemical class of selected chemicals.

Table 13-12. Reference Doses (RfDs) for Selected Chemicals

Chemical (by class)	RfD	
	Ingestion (mg/kg/day)	Inhalation (mg/kg/day)
Metals		
Chromium (III)	1.4†	5.7×10^{-7}
Lead (Pb)	(3.0×10^{-3})*	
Pesticides		
Chlordane	(5.5×10^{-5})†	
Inorganics		
Cyanides	(2.2×10^{-2})†	
Nitrate	1.6†	
Nitrite	(1.0×10^{-1})†	
Phosphine	(3.0×10^{-4})†	
Polyaromatic hydrocarbons		
Anthracene	(3.0×10^{-1})*	
Naphthalene	4.0×10^{-3}	
Benzenes		
Toluene	(3.0×10^{-1})†	5.7×10^{-1}
Trinitrotoluene (TNT)	(5.0×10^{-4})†	
Xylenes	1.8†	(8.6×10^{-2})†
Phenols		
Phenol	(6.0×10^{-1})†	
Chlorinated volatiles		
1,1-Dichloroethane	1.0×10^{-1}	1.0×10^{-1}
Trichloroethylene (TCE)	(7.4×10^{-3})*	(3.1×10^{-3})*
Chlorinated nonvolatiles		
Polychlorinated biphenyls (PCBs)	(1.5×10^{-3})*	
Miscellaneous organics		
Acetone	(1.0×10^{-1})†	3.0
Methyl ethyl ketone	5.0×10^{-2}	2.2×10^{-1}
Strychnine	(3.0×10^{-4})†	
Tetraethyl lead	(1.0×10^{-7})†	

*RfD was estimated by the author.
†Oral RfD is currently verified by the Environmental Protection Agency's (EPA's) RfD work group.

IV. ROUTES OF EXPOSURE

A. General principles

1. **Environmental fate** of a chemical is a description of how and to what extent a chemical is removed from one medium or transferred from one medium to another.
   a. **Mediums,** or environmental compartments, include air, water (both surface water and groundwater), sediment, soil, aquatic organisms, plant organisms, and particulates.
   b. **Movement between mediums** is dependent mainly on the physical and chemical properties of the chemical, the concentration of the chemical, metabolism, and chemical transformation.
      (1) **Physical and chemical properties** control the affinity of a chemical for one environment compared to another.
      (2) **Concentration of a given chemical** in each medium is a factor controlling the rate of transfer from one medium to another. In most environmental situations, one medium normally exists without any of the chemical.
      (3) **Metabolism** (usually by microorganisms) is important for some chemicals in some mediums.

(4) **Chemical transformation** may play a major role in removal of a chemical from a medium. The transformation product may also be a toxic chemical. Photo-oxidation is an example of a chemical transformation that takes place in air. Some of the parameters that could affect the rate are:
   (a) Light intensity
   (b) Wavelength of light
   (c) Humidity
   (d) Temperature
   (e) Particles

(5) **The rate of transfer between mediums** can be modified by the following factors.
   (a) **Mixing or aeration** increases the volatile organic transfer rate from water to air.
   (b) **Fish with a high fat content** accumulate higher concentrations of nonpolar organics than fish with a low fat content.
   (c) **Insoluble metal precipitate** slows down metal transfer from water to sediment.
   (d) In **sandy soils,** water-soluble organics have a groundwater migration rate similar to that of other organics (as opposed to clay soils, in which the water-soluble organics migrate much faster than the others).

(6) **Principles governing chemical movement between mediums** [Characteristics of polarity are discussed in IV A 2 a (2).]
   (a) **Volatile chemicals** tend to move toward air.
   (b) **Nonpolar chemicals** tend to transfer to sediment and fish.
   (c) **Water-soluble organics** tend to move with water through soil.
   (d) **Water-insoluble (nonpolar) organics** tend to move slowly through soil.

(7) **Examples** (see Table 13-13)
   (a) Trichloroethylene (TCE; a volatile organic chemical) is significantly removed from contaminated groundwater by aeration or air stripping.
   (b) Polychlorinated biphenyls (PCBs; nonpolar organics) are found at much greater concentrations in fish and sediment samples than in the surrounding water.
   (c) Methyl ethyl ketone (a water-soluble organic) tends to move in soil with the groundwater.
   (d) Dioxins and dibenzofuranes (nonpolar organics) rarely migrate with groundwater flow.

c. **Physical parameters that help to predict the environmental fate of chemicals**

(1) **The octanol water partition coefficient (K_{ow})** describes the partitioning of a chemical between octanol and water.

Table 13-13. Physical Properties of Selected Chemicals

Chemical (by class)	S_w (mg/L)	P_v (mm Hg)	H (atm – m^3/mol)	K_{ow} (ml/g)	BCF (L/kg)
Volatile organics					
Benzene	1.8×10^3	9.5×10^1	5.6×10^{-3}	8.3×10^1	5.2
Chloroform	8.2×10^3	1.5×10^2	2.9×10^{-3}	3.1×10^1	3.8
1,1-Dichloroethylene	2.3×10^3	6.0×10^2	3.4×10^{-2}	6.5×10^1	5.6
Toluene	5.4×10^2	2.8×10^1	6.4×10^{-3}	3.0×10^2	1.1×10^1
Vinyl chloride	2.7×10^3	2.7×10^1	8.2×10^{-2}	5.7×10^1	1.2
Nonvolatile organics					
Chlordane	5.6×10^{-1}	1.0×10^{-5}	9.6×10^{-6}	1.4×10^5	1.4×10^4
Polychlorinated biphenyls (PCBs)	3.1×10^{-2}	7.8×10^{-5}	1.1×10^{-3}	5.3×10^5	1.0×10^5
Metals					
Arsenic	Very dependent on specific compound				4.4×10^1
Cadmium					8.1×10^1
Chromium					1.6×10^1
Lead (Pb)					4.9×10^1
Other					
Asbestos	1.0×10^{-11}	Very low		Unknown	8.0×10^{-2}
Cyanides	5.0×10^5	Species dependent		Very low	1.0

S_w = water solubility; P_v = vapor pressure; H = Henry's law constant; atm = atmospheres; K_{ow} = octanol water partition coefficient; BCF = bioconcentration factor.

(2) **Henry's law constant (H)** describes the ratio of the concentration of a chemical in the atmosphere with that in solution.
(3) **Vapor pressure (P_v)** describes the contribution to pressure that a chemical would produce in the gas phase at a given temperature. The higher the vapor pressure, the greater the tendency to volatilize.
(4) **Bioconcentration factor (BCF)** describes the affinity of the chemical for aquatic organisms. High BCF values indicate an accumulation of the chemical in fish compared to the water in which they swim.
(5) **Water solubility (S_w)** describes the maximum amount of a chemical that could be dissolved in water at a given temperature.

2. **Absorption.** Physical and chemical properties and concentration determine the extent of absorption.
   a. **Inhalation of chemicals**
      (1) **Chemicals adsorbed onto particulates** are absorbed slowly relative to gas phase chemicals.
         (a) Water solubility increases the absorption rate of chemicals on particulates.
         (b) Water-insoluble chemicals are absorbed by being engulfed by macrophages.
         (c) Because particles must penetrate to the alveoli before the chemicals adsorbed onto them can be available for absorption, the size and shape of the particle itself is important [see IV C 1 a (2)].
      (2) **Gas phase chemicals** are absorbed into the bloodstream at rates that increase with an increase of the polarity of the molecule.
         (a) **Characteristics of polar chemicals**
            (i) Water-like
            (ii) High dielectric constants
            (iii) Soluble in water
            (iv) Insoluble in oil
         (b) **Characteristics of nonpolar chemicals**
            (i) Fat-like
            (ii) Low dielectric constants
            (iii) Insoluble in water
            (iv) Soluble in oil
   b. **Absorption of ingested chemicals**
      (1) Inhaled particles greater than 6–10 μm in diameter are trapped by the cilia in the nasal passages and upper bronchial tree and enter the body by ingestion.
      (2) Particles and metal compounds in general are absorbed to a lesser extent after ingestion than after inhalation.
   c. **Absorption through the skin or mucous membranes** is possible, but environmental exposure by direct contact is usually insignificant compared to exposure by inhalation or ingestion.
      (1) Nonpolar chemicals are absorbed to a much greater degree than polar chemicals because of the properties of skin.
      (2) Dilute concentrations of chemicals in air or water are absorbed to a lesser degree through skin than when ingested or inhaled.
      (3) Abraded skin or mucous membranes are more likely to absorb chemicals than intact skin.
      (4) Absorption of chemicals is not a prerequisite for local or irritative effects. Irritants act directly by damaging the skin or exposed mucous membrane.

3. **Metabolism.** Alteration in the metabolic pathway or rate of metabolism can change a toxic response by affecting the amount of toxic metabolite delivered to the systemic circulation. Almost all of the metabolic transformations that occur in living systems are enzyme-catalyzed reactions.
   a. **Metabolic pathway** describes the chemical intermediates to which a chemical is converted during metabolism. In general, the metabolic pathways of a chemical are similar for most organisms. However, there are often differences in pathways among microorganisms, plants, and animals. There are sometimes differences in metabolic pathways within animal or bacterial species and even within strains of the same species.
   b. **Rate of metabolism** describes the time course of the metabolism and is usually a quantitative statement of the disappearance of a toxic chemical or the appearance of a given metabolite (see II B 2 b).

4. **Target organ dose** is the amount or concentration of chemical to which the systemic target is exposed; this dose can be measured if there is sufficient knowledge about the toxic mechanism and the actual target site. Such doses are measured in different units from doses describing exposures.
   a. Target organ doses might use units such as mg/L (of blood supplied to organ) or mg/kg (of target organ weight) rather than an exposure dose in units such as mg/kg (of body weight).
   b. Blood levels of chemicals after exposure are useful for systemic toxicants, but many samples are needed to determine the accurate time course of blood levels of a chemical after a given exposure.
   c. Without detailed knowledge of how a chemical interacts at a sensitive target organ to cause a toxic effect, blood level measurements contribute little to the understanding of the toxic effect.

B. Mediums and routes of exposure

1. **Routes of exposure** refer to the points of entry into the body for local effects and to the points of absorption into the bloodstream for systemic effects.
2. **Mediums** are the materials that contain the chemical that causes the toxic effect.
   a. Air as a medium contains chemicals in the vapor or gas phase and chemicals adsorbed onto particles entrained in air.
   b. Water as a medium refers to drinking water, surface water, groundwater, or rain.
   c. Soil refers to materials mixed with or adsorbed to soil particles.
   d. Food refers to fish, plants, and animals.
3. **Relationships.** The medium of chemical exposure is sometimes associated with a given route of exposure. However, multiple routes of exposure should be considered.
   a. Water is associated with ingestion, but other exposures result from direct contact (e.g., bathing) and inhalation (e.g., showering).
   b. Soil is associated with direct contact, but other exposures result from inhalation (due to entrainment of particles) and ingestion.

C. Specific exposures listed by medium and route of exposure

1. **Air exposures** can be classified by both space and activity.
   a. **Ambient air** is the outdoor air surrounding everything, in the absence of any activity that might change its composition. For convenience, ambient air can be divided further into the following categories.
      (1) **Gas phase components or gases** are chemicals in the vapor phase.
      (2) **Particulates** are solid materials suspended in air. The shape and size of particle is the most important factor in determining how much of the particulate material will be inhaled into the lungs.
         (a) In general, particles larger than 1 μm and smaller than 10 μm in diameter will reach the alveoli.
         (b) Particles smaller than 1 μm in diameter are usually exhaled.
         (c) Particles larger than 10 μm are deposited in the upper lungs (and ultimately ingested).
   b. **Indoor air** is the air present in buildings where people live or work, in the absence of any industrial activity that might change the air.
      (1) **Lifestyles** affect exposure to toxic chemicals. For example, smoking leads to direct exposure of the smoker and indirect exposure of others in the indoor area. Exposure to the carbon monoxide (CO) in smoke reduces the ability to use oxygen for metabolism. Exposure to the polynuclear aromatic hydrocarbons (many of which are known animal carcinogens) adsorbed onto particulates is probably responsible for the increased lung cancer rates of both smokers and exposed nonsmokers.
      (2) **Home maintenance activities** can contribute to chemical exposure.
         (a) **Formaldehyde** offgassing, or release from improperly cured urea foam formaldehyde insulation, can result in exposure to high levels of formaldehyde that can be detected by a characteristic odor and that can cause a chronic response in humans. If the insulation is properly applied, no formaldehyde is released, and no exposure occurs.
         (b) **Radon** accumulation occurs when homes are insulated or otherwise modified to reduce air exchange with the outside.

(i) Although less air exchange results in energy savings, the "air-tight" home prevents dissipation of the radon that enters through the basement slab or crawl space into the lower levels of the home.

(ii) Naturally occurring radioactive radon results from decay of radium in the soil. Radium is present in all soils, but it is more concentrated in granite and black shale.

(iii) Because radiation is a nonthreshold insult, increased lung cancer incidence is expected as a result of increased radon exposure.

(c) **Solvent exposure** from paint removal or painting activity occurs through indoor use of materials containing solvents.

(d) **Termiticide** (e.g., aldrin and chlordane) exposure can occur from the improper application of the pesticide for home termite control.

(3) **Water containing volatile organic compounds (VOCs)** can contribute to indoor air levels of those chemicals. Chloroform, an animal carcinogen, is one of the important halomethanes produced by the process of chlorinating surface waters. Several of the other halomethanes produced are also animal carcinogens. Thus, VOCs are present in much of the drinking water supplied to cities. The regulatory limit for total halomethanes in drinking water is 100 ppb. This limit is a technology-based limit (chemical chlorination process and tvpical equipment used) rather than a health-based limit. Despite the fact that chlorinauon of surface water supplies leads to the presence of carcinogens in the finished drinking water, the chlorination does perform the needed function of removing bacterial contamination from drinking water. However, there may be alternative technologies that accomplish the disinfection without introducing carcinogenic chemicals into the finished drinking water.

(a) Activities such as showering, bathing, clothes washing, cooking, and cleaning can release VOCs contained in the water.

(b) The amount of chemical released from water depends on a number of factors, such as physical and chemical properties of the VOC, concentration, temperature, and agitation of the water.

(c) Air exposure to VOCs affects both individuals involved in the activity releasing the chemical (e.g., the individual taking a shower) and the other occupants of the house as the chemical is dispersed in the indoor air.

(d) VOCs are removed from indoor air by the exchange with outside air.

(e) Both monitoring and modeling of VOCs in indoor air (see V B 2, D) indicate that total individual indoor air exposure to VOCs from drinking water is about the same as the exposure from drinking 2 L of the same water each day.

(4) **Deterioration of asbestos insulation** in office buildings, schools, and homes can lead to exposure to asbestos fibers. Although damage by contact with water is the most common cause of asbestos exposure, removal activities can lead to very high air exposures if appropriate precautions are not taken. Asbestos is a known human carcinogen, and exposure to any concentration is associated with an increase in cancer risk.

(5) **Hobbies,** such as building model airplanes, can contribute to indoor air exposure to solvents found in glue and paint.

c. **Recreational air exposure** can lead to chemical exposure as VOCs are released from water used to fill swimming pools and from streams used by fishermen.

d. **Occupational air exposure** is important because exposure to chemicals often occurs at high concentrations and for an appreciable fraction of an individual's lifetime.

2. **Water exposure** can be categorized by the source of the water or by the activity resulting in exposure to a chemical in water.

a. **Drinking water.** Most of the drinking water in the United States comes from **public water supplies,** which are regulated under the **Safe Water Drinking Act**. Some drinking water comes from **private wells, which are not regulated**. Public water is obtained from:

(1) Surface water (e.g., rivers)

(2) Groundwater (e.g., wells)

b. **Fish and other aquatic organisms** accumulate chemicals in their edible flesh; thus, ingestion of fish results in human exposure to these chemicals.

(1) The ratio of concentration of chemical in edible flesh to the concentration of chemical in the water in which the fish lives is the BCF. BCFs refer to the concentration ratio at equilibrium or after enough time has passed so that no change in the ratio is observed.

(2) Typically, inorganic metals do not bioaccumulate, while organic chemicals accumulate, depending on their polarity and the extent of metabolism. Table 13-13 lists the BCFs for some chemicals.

c. **Direct exposure**

(1) Activities that involve contact of water with skin or mucous membranes can result in absorption directly through skin. Examples of such activities are bathing and swimming.

(2) Mucous membranes and abraded skin allow more rapid transport of chemicals in water than does intact skin.

(3) Chemicals adsorbed to particulates are absorbed very slowly through the skin as compared to the same chemical dissolved in water.

(4) Quantities of chemicals absorbed through the skin are usually small relative to amounts absorbed through other routes of exposure.

3. **Land disposal.** Waste piles, dumps, spills, releases onto land, road oiling, and land treatment are all units or activities that are classified as land disposal. Landfills should only be used to dispose of nonliquid wastes, while surface impoundments are designed for liquid waste storage.

a. **Direct contact.** Exposures from direct contact with a solid or semisolid material containing a chemical can occur, but, in general, this contact is not appreciable except in special circumstances, such as high concentrations, long exposure times, or by chemicals that can damage skin.

b. **Food.** Uptake of chemicals by vegetables from the soil can occur.

(1) Rates of uptake, or the amount of chemical accumulated in the plant, depend on the:

(a) Physical and chemical properties of the chemical

(b) Species of vegetable

(c) Soil conditions

(2) Different parts of the vegetable accumulate chemicals from soil differently; thus, human exposure depends on what portion of the plant is normally eaten.

c. **Particulates.** Entrainment of particles into air from soils can be a significant route of exposure.

(1) The physical properties of the chemical in soil determine to what extent the chemical will be adsorbed to particulates that are small enough to be entrained.

(2) The factors that affect entrainment are:

(a) Particle size

(b) Water content

(c) Meteorology

(d) Site topography

(e) Vegetation

(f) Physical activity (e.g., dirt biking)

d. **Ingestion.** Direct ingestion of soil, and therefore of the chemicals found in soil, is considered significant only in young children (see V C 2 e).

(1) The actual amount of soil ingested by small children is a matter of vigorous current debate, with extremes of ingestion ranging from 0.1 to 10 g/day.

(2) Ingestion is likely to occur for only a small portion of a lifetime.

(3) Dirt also could be ingested by population groups other than small children if those groups worked with soil and then consumed food in the same area.

e. **Groundwater contamination.** Leaching of toxic chemicals from landfills has been the cause of chemical contamination of many public and private wells. Landfills and surface impoundments leak. Chemicals from materials and wastes placed in land disposal units eventually leak out into the soil and groundwater beneath the disposal site.

(1) **Double liners** that are now required for hazardous waste landfills and surface impoundments can delay the migration of hazardous constituents from the unit, but cannot prevent leaching. Typically, liners and double liners retard migration for periods ranging from decades to centuries.

(2) **Past disposal practices** are responsible for much of the groundwater contamination throughout the United States. Two examples of the worst kinds of poor management and lack of environmental controls follow.

(a) Placing liquid wastes into unlined surface impoundments has caused significant leakage.

(b) Disposing of bulk liquid spent solvent wastes in municipal or sanitary landfills (which are specifically designed for garbage and trash) has also led to leakage. When properly designed and operated, sanitary landfills do not endanger public health or the environment.

(3) The **concentration of chemicals** in groundwater underneath the site is dependent on many factors, including:

(a) Waste composition
(b) Liner integrity
(c) Physical and chemical properties
(d) Groundwater flow rate
(e) Rainfall
(f) Soil type
(g) Other wastes present
(h) Geology

4. **Other exposures** to toxic chemicals can occur as by-products of everyday activities, such as use of food, drugs, medications, and cosmetics.

a. **Food.** Toxic effects of exposure to foodstuffs or additives in food are commonly known.

(1) **Ethanol** (i.e., alcohol) is consumed as a beverage, providing calories as well as enhancing the pleasures of eating; it is also a toxic chemical affecting nearly all who consume it.

(a) Ethanol exposure can lead to liver damage as a chronic toxic effect.
(b) Traffic fatalities caused by drunk drivers can also be considered toxic effects of ethanol.

(2) **Peanut butter** contains the chemical aflatoxin, which is released by a mold that grows on the peanuts. Processed peanut butter contains trace amounts of aflatoxin.

(a) Aflatoxin is an animal carcinogen and, therefore, a probable human carcinogen.
(b) Consuming peanut butter is associated with some excess cancer risk when compared with not eating peanut butter.

(3) **Food additives** have known toxic effects, although many are safe to almost all individuals at the levels used in food.

(a) **Monosodium glutamate (MSG)** is used as a flavor enhancer in some types of Asian cooking and causes a characteristic headache in some individuals who consume food prepared with MSG.
(b) **Sulfite** used to preserve fruit and wine can result in a severe allergic reaction in a small group of people.

b. **Drugs, medicines, and cosmetics** are other examples of materials that, because of their chemical makeup, can cause some toxic effects in humans.

V. EXPOSURE EVALUATION

A. **General principles.** Physical presence and exposure are not synonymous. A chemical may be present at very high concentrations in a medium yet pose no health hazard because exposure cannot occur from the medium due to the physical or chemical state of the chemical.

1. **The chemical state of an element** refers to its oxidation state, or valence. Because physical properties of an element or compound depend on the oxidation state, release of the chemical into a medium may be affected by its oxidation state.

a. **Inorganic elements** often have many oxidation states in the environment, while **organic chemicals** generally have a single oxidation state.

b. **Changes in the oxidation state** of a chemical may affect availability of that chemical to a given medium.

(1) **Chromium** in the hexavalent state, Cr(VI), is a human carcinogen, while trivalent chromium, Cr(III), is not. Many industries use Cr(III) in manufacturing processes, and wastes from these processes contain chromium. If the chromium is in the Cr(III) form and oxidation to Cr(VI) is prevented, exposure presents no cancer risks.

(2) **Lead** in the ionic state (Pb^{2+}) is extremely toxic to small children, impairing nervous system development. Elemental lead (Pb) is the lead used in automobile batteries and in lead bullets.

(a) Lead from battery-crushing operations (reclamation) can migrate to groundwater because the concentrated sulfuric acid used in batteries oxidizes lead from Pb to Pb^{2+}, which can then leach to groundwater; therefore, drinking water may contain lead.

(b) In the absence of a source of concentrated acid, lead from bullets used at a practice range is very unlikely to migrate into groundwater and pose a health problem. Lead bullets are not oxidized to ionic lead to any appreciable degree.

(c) Acid from acid rainfall is more than 100-fold less acidic than the acid used in car batteries.

2. **The physical form of a chemical** refers to its physical association with other materials or to some property of the chemical.
   a. **Binding and trapping** of a chemical can prevent its release. Asbestos insulation used to insulate pipes or to protect structural steel against collapse during a fire contains 30%–60% asbestos. If the insulation is intact, no asbestos fibers are released into the air, thus preventing exposure and consequent increased cancer risk. Contact with water from leaking roofs and pipes results in the release of asbestos into the air, resulting in exposure and an increased cancer risk. If there is no damage to the insulation, no exposure occurs, even though asbestos is present in large quantities.
   b. **Lack of water solubility** can retard the release of a chemical. Many of the common salts of lead are relatively insoluble in water. For example, the concentration of $Pb(SO_4)_2$ (lead sulfate) in water of pH = 9 is 1 mg/L. However, as the pH drops and the medium becomes more acidic, the solubility increases; at pH = 5.5, the solubility is 10 g/L. Thus, solid lead sulfate spilled into water dissolves very slowly at a pH above 9 but dissolves rapidly at a pH less than 6.
   c. **Containment** is another method that makes a chemical unavailable to a medium.
      (1) Transformers most often contain a mixture of PCBs and chlorobenzenes. Exposure to these substances cannot occur unless the transformer ruptures in use or the insulating fluid leaks or spills during normal operation and maintenance.
      (2) Solvents stored in 55-gallon drums are not an exposure source if the drums are always closed during management.

B. Chemical analysis

1. **Analytic methodology** determines concentrations of contaminants in all mediums and materials. Analyses of air, water, soil, and sediment are routine while analysis of fish tissue is less common.
   a. **Priority pollutants.** There are 129 chemicals or classes of chemicals that are designated as priority pollutants. These chemicals either are commonly used in commercial processes or are unusually toxic. Chemicals most relevant to the environment are listed in Table 13-14. This list was developed to settle the 1976 lawsuit against the EPA by the Natural Resources Defense Council (NRDC).
   b. **Analysis of organic and inorganic compounds** is by methods that are highly specific to the organic or inorganic compound measured.
      (1) Gas chromatography is the basic method for analyzing organic compounds.
      (2) Atomic absorption is the basic method for analyzing inorganic heavy metals.
   c. **The detection limit** is the minimum amount of a chemical that can be positively identified by an analytic method.
      (1) In aqueous samples, the detection limit is about 1 ppb for most chemicals.

Table 13-14. Priority Pollutants

Category	Number	Examples
Metals	13	Arsenic, lead, and silver
Pesticides	7	Chlordane, chlorophenothane (DDT), and toxaphene
Inorganics (other)	2	Asbestos and cyanides
Polyaromatic hydrocarbons	5	Naphthalene
Benzenes	7	Benzene, dichlorobenzene, and dinitrotoluene
Phenols	7	Phenol and pentachlorophenol
Chlorinated volatiles	14	Haloethers, trichloroethylene (TCE), and vinyl chloride
Chlorinated nonvolatiles	3	Dioxins and polychlorinated biphenyls (PCBs)
Miscellaneous organics	7	Acrylonitrile, benzidine, and nitrosamines

(2) In air and soil, detection limits are higher.

(3) In special situations, detection limits are lower than routinely obtained (e.g., stack sampling for determining hazardous waste incinerator permit conditions or soil testing for PCBs, dibenzodioxins, and dibenzofuranes). Low detection limits raise analytic costs.

d. **The units of measurement** for determining the concentration of chemicals in various mediums are as follows.

(1) **Air levels** are generally stated as:

(a) Parts per million or billion (ppm or ppb) on a volume per volume basis

(b) Milligrams or micrograms per cubic meter (mg/m^3 or μg/m^3) on a weight per volume basis

(2) **Water concentrations** are generally given as ppm or ppb on a weight per weight basis. Because 1 ml of water weighs about 1 g at temperatures found in the environment, ppm is equivalent to mg/L and ppb to μg/L.

(3) **Soil concentrations** are usually given as ppm or ppb, and these are equivalent to mg/kg soil or μg/kg soil, respectively. Note that the soil is not dried to remove water before analysis.

(4) **Particulate concentrations** in air are measured as mg/m^3 or μg/m^3, which represent the amount of particulate material contained in 1 m^3 of air.

2. **Environmental monitoring** involves sampling and analysis.

a. **Monitoring environmental mediums,** such as water, air, fish, or soil, for chemicals has direct implications for humans exposed to those mediums.

b. **Monitoring materials** (e.g., spent solvent, used oil, asbestos insulation, waste streams, chemical ingredients) for chemicals usually has an indirect relationship to exposure and represents only a *potential* for a chemical to be released into a medium.

3. **Monitoring individuals** for parameters of exposure is divided into three areas. For each area, appropriate sampling and analytic methods are important.

a. **Sampling the air** around an individual for chemicals and using a radiation-sensitive badge are ways to measure individual exposure.

b. **Measurement of tissue or body fluid levels** of a chemical or metabolite can verify exposure.

(1) **Blood and urine** are the most common body fluids analyzed. Fat biopsy for chemicals is occasionally used; however, fat samples are much more difficult to obtain than blood or urine.

(2) **A metabolite** may need to be measured rather than the original chemical because chemicals are often metabolized by the body.

(3) The **relationship** of body fluid levels to exposure is known for relatively few chemicals. Usually the relationship is known only if the chemical is of low acute toxicity and the chemical is used industrially, where medical surveillance, including body fluid analysis, occurs.

c. **Body functions can also be measured.** For example, blood cholinesterase measurements are used to determine pesticide exposure. However, usually blood cholinesterase levels are used only to indicate a need for therapy or to stop a known exposure. Rarely can functional tests measure the amount of exposure.

C. **Models** are a set of assumptions used to estimate exposures. As such, models estimate exposures for individuals to the extent that the assumptions made are accurate. Models are useful because of the ability to determine the change in exposure when one of the assumptions is changed. Thus, individual variation in exposure can be obtained.

1. **Assumptions** that are used to estimate exposures must be as accurate and reasonable as possible since they directly affect the exposure estimate. Assumptions are sometimes deliberately made to protect public health. Common assumptions used for the models are listed below.

a. **Body weight** is 70 kg for adults and 10 kg for children.

b. **Life span** is 70 years for humans.

c. **Water consumption** is 2 L/day for adults and 1 L/day for children.

d. **Air inhalation** is 20 m^3/day for adults.

e. **Particles** larger than 10 μm in diameter are ingested, particles less than 1 μm in diameter are exhaled, and particles of intermediate size are retained in the lungs.

f. **Fish consumption** is 6.5 g/day of edible flesh. [This amount is a national average and may not be the correct amount for individuals who eat fish frequently. An alternative amount of 50 g/day (i.e., about two 6-ounce servings of fish flesh per week) can be used.]

g. **Soil ingestion** is 0.1 g/day for adults and 0.2 g/day for children under 6 years of age.

2. **Models in mediums**
   a. **Models for air exposure** to a chemical are determined by using air levels of the chemicals obtained by modeling or monitoring, combined with exposure assumptions.
      (1) **Inhaled volume** of 20 m^3/day is a total volume per day and is summed over all daily activities. The inhaled volume of air per individual varies with:
         (a) Age
         (b) Health status
         (c) Body weight
         (d) Work output or physical activity
      (2) **Absorption** of a chemical in air into the bloodstream is measured in inhalation exposure. Absorption is determined from existing experiments, estimated from structurally similar chemicals, or assumed to be complete. Absorption of chemicals adsorbed to particles deposited in the lungs is assumed to be 100%.
   b. **Models for drinking water exposure** use a daily volume of water consumed and an absorption factor determined by experiment or assumption.
   c. **Models for fish ingestion** depend on the amount and species of fish ingested.
      (1) The average amount of fish consumed in the United States in 1980 was 6.5 g/day of edible flesh. This value is useful only as an average and cannot be used to estimate the actual risks to individuals who include fish in their diet on a regular basis (see V C 1 f).
      (2) The fat content of the edible flesh is directly related to the amount of chemical that has accumulated. BCFs are standardized to a weighted fat content of 3.0%. Table 13-15 shows the fat content of some selected fish species.
   d. **Models for direct exposure** from contaminated water or soil are not commonly used because absorption usually contributes much less to the total exposure than do inhalation and ingestion. However, an estimate of dermal exposure from chemical contaminants in soil can be made using factors such as 1.5 mg of soil per cm^2 of exposed surface area for dust adherence, 1% absorption, and surface areas of 2000 cm^2 and 1000 cm^2 for the exposed areas of adults and children, respectively.
   e. **Models for soil ingestion** use an estimate of soil consumed and an absorption factor determined by experiment or assumption.
      (1) The assumed amount of dirt ingested is 0.1 g/day. However, young children are known to ingest a significant amount of dirt. More representative estimates for children are 0.2 g/day; however, some observers have estimated up to 10 g/day.
      (2) Children are assumed to be exposed for only a portion of their 70-year life span; it is commonly estimated that exposure takes place for 10 years.
      (3) Exposure may not occur every day, and sometimes exposure for a certain number of days per year is assumed.

Table 13-15. Fat Content of Edible Flesh of Some Fish Species

Ocean		Freshwater		Shellfish	
Species	**Percent Fat**	**Species**	**Percent Fat**	**Species**	**Percent Fat**
Bluefish	3.3	White perch	4.0	Soft clam	1.9
Cod	0.3	Yellow perch	0.9	Crab	1.9
Eel	18.3	Brook trout	2.1	Crayfish	0.5
Tuna	4.1	Lake trout	10.0	Lobster	1.9
Atlantic		Rainbow trout	11.4	Mussel	2.2
Herring	11.3	Lake whitefish	8.2	Octopus	0.8
Mackerel	12.2			Eastern oyster	7.8
Ocean perch	1.2			Western oyster	2.2
Salmon	13.4			Scallop	0.2
Pacific				Shrimp	0.8
Herring	2.6			Squid	0.9
Mackerel	7.3				
Ocean perch	1.5				

D. Modeling is a procedure by which concentrations of a chemical released into air, water, or land are estimated from knowledge of emission, or release rates, and assumptions about the movement and fate of the chemical in the environment.

1. **Air dispersion modeling** can be used to estimate concentrations of a chemical at various locations around a point of emission. A variety of modeling approaches are reasonable, and choice depends on the characteristics of the emission source, terrain, and meteorology. Air modeling can be used for particulates as well as gas phase chemicals.
   a. **Factors affecting the concentration of a chemical** include:
      (1) Emission rate
      (2) Temperature
      (3) Chemical and physical properties
      (4) Meteorology
      (5) Stack height (i.e., of smokestacks)
      (6) Terrain
      (7) Environmental fate
   b. **Examples of environmental releases.** Air modeling has successfully approximated actual measured concentrations of:
      (1) VOCs released from sewage treatment plants
      (2) Solvent releases from vented storage tanks
      (3) Particulate releases from smelters
      (4) Chemical releases from industrial processes
   c. **Outputs of air modeling** are typically concentration isopleths of the chemical averaged over some time period. Modeling can also identify the location, or point, of maximum air concentration of the chemical.

2. **Surface water modeling** is used to estimate concentration of a chemical in surface water after releases into the water.
   a. **The three most common releases** are by:
      (1) Direct discharge into the water
      (2) Groundwater discharge into the surface water
      (3) Sediment or soil release of adsorbed chemicals
   b. **Factors affecting the concentration of a chemical** at a given location in surface water include:
      (1) Emission rate
      (2) Chemical and physical properties
      (3) Environmental fate
      (4) Velocity of water flow
      (5) Temperature
      (6) Dilution
      (7) Treatment
   c. **Examples of environmental releases.** Surface water modeling approximates the actual water concentrations measured in:
      (1) Solvent released into a stream as a spill
      (2) Acid waste discharge allowed by an environmental permit
      (3) PCBs released from sediments in a river
   d. **Surface water modeling results** are a chemical's water concentration and the variation of that concentration over time at a given physical location, usually a public drinking water supply intake.

3. **Groundwater modeling** is used to estimate concentrations in groundwater from chemical releases onto or into soil. The groundwater could be used for private or public drinking water wells, or it could become surface water as it is discharged into streams.
   a. **Factors affecting the concentration of a chemical** in groundwater include:
      (1) Emission rate
      (2) Physical and chemical properties
      (3) Groundwater flow rate
      (4) Soil type
      (5) Environmental fate
      (6) Geology
   b. **Examples of releases to soil.** Groundwater modeling successfully approximates concentrations of chemicals in groundwater monitoring wells in:

(1) Solvent tanks leaking directly into soil
(2) PCBs released into a river by groundwater flow from material spilled onto and buried in soil

c. **Groundwater modeling results** are expressed as:
(1) Concentration of a chemical at various locations
(2) A variation of concentrations with time

VI. REGULATION OF CHEMICALS IN THE ENVIRONMENT.

Chemicals in the environment are regulated on a programmatic basis that includes environmental mediums and end uses.

A. Air. The **Clean Air Act of 1970 (CAA)** and subsequent amendments is the most important federal law protecting the air that people in the United States breathe. It establishes ambient air standards for six pollutants and emission standards for those six and other chemicals. The CAA does not have jurisdiction over workplace exposure.

1. Concentration standards

a. **Criteria pollutants.** Six pollutants have been labeled "criteria" pollutants. Because none of the six were believed to be carcinogens, threshold, or safe, levels were established. (Recent data have shown Pb to be carcinogenic, although it is still not regulated as such.) The criteria pollutants are:
(1) CO
(2) Pb
(3) NO_2
(4) Ozone
(5) Particulates
(6) Sulfur dioxide

b. **Sources.** Both mobile and stationary sources of emission are regulated under the CAA. Exemptions from regulations exist for some sources based on the industrial process and on the amount of the pollutant emitted.
(1) **Emissions from automobiles** contribute significant amounts of all criteria pollutants except sulfur dioxide.
(2) **Stationary sources,** including utility boilers, manufacturing processes, and chemical storage, emit many chemicals.

c. **"Right to know" laws.** Some states or local jurisdictions have "right to know" laws or similar types of legislation that establish local ambient air standards.

2. Emission controls

a. **Hazardous air pollutants** are chemicals that may result in an increase in mortality or an increase in a serious reversible illness.
(1) **Criteria pollutants.** The hazardous air pollutants identified by the EPA, most of which are animal or human carcinogens, include:
(a) Asbestos
(b) Benzene
(c) Beryllium
(d) Mercury
(e) Radionuclides
(f) Vinyl chloride
(2) **Sources.** The CAA requires the EPA to identify sources and set emission standards with an "ample margin of safety to protect the public health."
(a) The EPA has identified the industrial processes that emit large quantities or result in high ambient concentrations of each hazardous air polllutant.
(b) Since any exposure to a carcinogen is associated with some risk of cancer, risk assessments have been conducted for each source of a hazardous air pollutant.
(c) Risk management decisions are made for each emission from each source. The decision is based on the risk to the individual and the total population and on the possible potential reduction of risk with available technology.

b. **Unregulated chemicals.** The EPA has virtually no authority to regulate releases of chemicals other than criteria and hazardous air pollutants.
(1) **Toxic chemical releases** are currently unregulated except for a small number of sources of hazardous air pollutant releases. Both "normal" process releases, or losses, and emergency, or accidental, releases require tight environmental controls.

(2) **Indoor air quality** is currently unregulated. Radon accumulation, VOCs from drinking water, formaldehyde, and CO are examples of chemicals that are not controlled in indoor air.

(3) **Air releases from environmental cleanup activities,** such as sewage treatment plants, hazardous waste incinerators using solvents as fuels, or air stripping of VOC contaminants from groundwater, are usually not controlled.

B. Water. The **Clean Water Act of 1972 (CWA)** and the **Safe Drinking Water Act** (**SDWA**; 1974) are the two federal laws responsible for protecting water as an environmental medium.

1. **Drinking water standards.** Public drinking water is regulated by establishment of standards. Private wells used by single families are not regulated. Public drinking water can be pumped from either groundwater or surface water. Only the finished water is regulated, not the water source prior to treatment.

   a. **Maximum contaminant levels (MCLs)**

      (1) **Definition.** The MCL is a concentration maximum for a chemical or constituent that may not be exceeded in drinking water regulated under the SDWA.

      (2) **Applicability.** MCLs are enforceable water standards for public water supplies only, not for private drinking water wells.

      (3) **Limits.** MCLs have been finalized for the following **regulated contaminants,** the majority of which are listed in Table 13-16, along with the MCL value in units of μg/L:

         (a) Microorganisms
         (b) Radioactivity
         (c) A group of seven metals, listed in Table 13-16
         (d) A group of organic pesticides, listed in Table 13-16
         (e) Some inorganic anions
         (f) Total haloforms
         (g) A group of organic chemicals, listed in Table 13-16

Table 13-16. Selected Chemicals Regulated by the Safe Drinking Water Act (SDWA)

Chemical (by class)	MCL	Chemical (by class)	MCL
Inorganic metals		Organics	
Arsenic	50	Benzene	5
Barium	2000	Carbon tetrachloride	5
Cadmium	5	Chlorobenzene	100
Chromium	100	Dibromochloropropane	0.2
Lead (Pb)	5	*o*-Dichlorobenzene	600
Mercury	2	*m*-Dichlorobenzene	600
Selenium	50	*p*-Dichlorobenzene	75
		1,2-Dichloroethane	5
Pesticides		1,1-Dichloroethylene	7
Alachlor	2	*cis*-1,2-Dichloroethylene	70
Aldicarb	3*	*trans*-1,2-Dichloroethylene	100
Aldicarb sulfone	2*	1,2-Dichloropropane	5
Aldicarb sulfoxide	4*	Ethylbenzene	700
Altrazine	3	Ethylene dibromide	0.05
Carbofuran	40	Pentachlorophenol	1*
Chlordane	2	Polychlorinated biphenyls (PCBs)	0.5
2,4-D	70	Styrene	0.1
Endrin	2*	Tetrachloroethylene	5
Heptachlor	0.4	1,1,1-Trichloroethane	200
Heptachlor epoxide	0.2	Trichloroethylene (TCE)	5
Lindane	0.2	Toluene	1000
Methoxychlor	400	Vinyl chloride	2
Toxaphene	5	Xylenes	10,000
2,4,5-TP silvex	50		

MCL = maximum containment [all MCL values are in units of μg/L, which is equivalent to parts per billion (ppb)]; 2,4-D = 2,4-dichlorophenoxy acetic acid; 2,4,5-TP silvex = 2, 4, 5-trichlorophenoxy propionic acid.

*This is a proposed MCL value.

b. **Unregulated toxic organic chemicals.** Regulatory concentration limits (i.e., MCLs) for more VOCs and other organic chemicals have been proposed, and those chemicals are shown as asterisked values in Table 13-16. These are only *proposed* concentration limits; they are not legally enforceable. A discussion of allowable concentrations of chemicals in drinking water can be found in VI B 1 a.

(1) **For noncarcinogens,** the proposed MCLs are protective of the most sensitive human population.

(2) **For carcinogens,** the levels proposed would result in a lifetime risk no greater than 10^{-5}, or 1 in 100,000.

2. **Effluent standards** are limits for discharge into waters of the United States; they regulate many industries that discharge priority pollutants and other chemicals.

a. **Sources.** Most discharge sources are regulated, for example:

(1) Industrial manufacturing process discharges
(2) Cooling water tower discharges
(3) Storm water runoff
(4) Chemical industry discharges
(5) Groundwater treatment discharges
(6) Municipal sewage treatment plant effluents

b. **Effluent limitations**

(1) The first set of effluent standards were developed in the early 1970s and were based on controlling the following conventional pollutants:

(a) Suspended solids
(b) Oil and grease
(c) Extremes of pH
(d) Fecal coliform
(e) Biologic oxygen demand

(2) Discharge permits usually do not govern individual chemical contaminants but instead limit only conventional pollutants.

(3) Effluent permits currently being issued by the EPA and the states limit amounts of priority pollutants discharged and require that dischargers use the best available treatment technology. Thus, regulation of effluent discharges is technology-based, not health-based.

c. **Unregulated chemicals**

(1) There are no concentration limitations for chemical constituents for current or future use of:

(a) Groundwater
(b) Recreational water
(c) Streams
(d) Lakes and ponds

(2) Underground injection wells, which are a potential source of groundwater contamination, are also unregulated.

(3) Health-based standards rather than technology-based standards are needed for drinking water.

C. **Land.** The **Resource Conservation and Recovery Act** (**RCRA;** 1976) and the **Comprehensive Environmental Response, Compensation, and Liability Act** (**CERCLA,** or **Superfund;** 1980) are the two federal laws governing regulation of present and future land disposal practices and cleanup.

1. **Land disposal units and activities** include:

a. **Landfills** for:

(1) Municipal wastes
(2) Hazardous wastes
(3) Industrial residues
(4) Infectious or pathologic materials

b. **Surface impoundments or lagoons** for:

(1) Wastewater treatment
(2) Hazardous waste treatment or storage
(3) Equalization basins
(4) Storm water runoff

c. **Waste piles** used for accumulating any noncontainerized solid nonflowing materials

d. **Land treatment** for waste application onto, or incorporation into, the soil surface

2. **Waste management practices**
   a. **Liners** used for any land disposal units eventually fail.
      (1) Recent regulations require two liners and a leachate collection system between the double liners. However, many of the existing surface impoundments and landfills do not have any liners.
      (2) Originally, liners were compacted from clay available near the site; however, synthetic plastic liners are the liners of choice for almost all waste materials.
   b. **Liquids** are not suitable for landfill disposal.
   c. **Inorganic wastes** are generally more suitable for landfill disposal than organic wastes.
      (1) **Organic compounds** can cause synthetic liners to fail because they are sometimes incompatible with the liner.
      (2) **Inorganic materials** that have been removed (e.g., mined) from the earth cause minimal problems of containment when placed back into the earth.
   d. **Treatment by encapsulation** or similar processes can retard the mobilization of soluble constituents for many years, thus delaying and diluting the appearance of a chemical in groundwater beneath the land disposal unit.

3. **Standards**
   a. **Prohibitions.** Hazardous wastes that may not be discarded in landfills include:
      (1) Liquid hazardous wastes
      (2) Solvents
      (3) Some dioxin-containing wastes
      (4) Other selected organic wastes
   b. **Emissions.** Releases from land disposal units are controlled.
      (1) Groundwater monitoring is required for all land disposal units.
      (2) Indicator parameters are used to determine if a unit is leaking.
      (3) Remedial activity is required for releases.
   c. **Closure.** Requirements for clean closure are part of all land disposal permits issued.
      (1) Removal of all wastes and contaminated residues is required for storage or treatment surface impoundments.
      (2) Capping and groundwater monitoring is required for 30 years for all landfills.

4. **RCRA and CERCLA cleanup activities.** Both RCRA and CERCLA have regulatory and enforcement provisions for cleaning up land disposal sites. Activities range from emergency removal of waste materials when an imminent and substantial danger exists to remedial activity planned and executed over a several-year period when cleanup is needed but no emergency exists.
   a. **CERCLA versus RCRA**
      (1) **CERCLA** usually is implemented when a responsible party chooses not to cooperate or when no responsible party exists (e.g., in a case of bankruptcy).
      (2) **RCRA** is used when responsible parties have an existing RCRA permit; it was used prior to the existence of CERCLA.
   b. **Determining a cleanup strategy**
      (1) **The extent of contamination** at the site, including the identity of the chemical contaminants and their distribution space, must be known.
      (2) **Acceptable levels** of the contaminant for the site are then determined, using the following procedures for both Acts. (Numerical values are discussed in VI C 4 c.)
         (a) **For groundwater,** the concentration of the chemical in the groundwater is compared to the cleanup standard. For each chemical contaminant of groundwater, typically, no further cleanup is required if the concentration is less than the cleanup standard.
         (b) **For contaminated soils,** the concentration of the chemical in the soil is compared directly to the cleanup standard. Again, typically, no further cleanup is required if the leachate concentration is less than the cleanup standard.
      (3) **Technologies** that can achieve the desired cleanup levels, as well as the cost of those technologies, must be identified.
      (4) **The least costly remedial activity** that can reduce the risk from the site to an acceptable level typically is implemented.
   c. **Numerical values for RCRA and CERCLA cleanup**
      (1) **If an MCL is available,** it is usually used to determine the final cleanup level required in groundwater for a given chemical. However, MCLs are sometimes neither protective at the 10^{-6} level for carcinogens nor fully protective for noncarcinogens.

(2) **When no MCL exists** for a chemical, the following criteria are used.
(a) **For carcinogens,** the concentration in drinking water (or soil) that corresponds to an excess cancer risk of 10^{-6} is used as the maximum concentration allowed after cleanup.
(b) **For systemic toxicants,** the concentration in drinking water (or soil) that is safe to ingest daily over a lifetime is used as the maximum concentration allowed after cleanup.

5. **Unresolved land disposal issues**
a. **Lack of adequate enforcement** of existing standards and regulations is the most significant land disposal problem.
b. **Developing new treatment techniques** to treat waste materials to reduce the reliance of societies on land disposal is a significant technologic challenge.
c. **Lack of public confidence** in the government's commitment to protect public health is one of the obstacles in siting hazardous waste management facilities.
d. **Lack of adequate capacity** for hazardous and nonhazardous wastes is also a serious concern.

D. **Food.** The **Food and Drug Administration (FDA)** regulates levels of chemicals in food through the authority of the **Food, Drug, and Cosmetics Act**. Several thousand substances are regulated.

1. **Food additives** may serve any of the following purposes in foods:
a. To flavor
b. To color
c. To preserve
d. To sweeten
e. To emulsify
f. To prevent caking
g. To stabilize
h. To bleach
i. To enhance flavor

2. **Classifications**
a. Substances can be classified according to **how the additive gets into food.**
(1) **Intentional** food additives are added during some part of the commerical or home preparation of the food. Examples of intentional food additives are:
(a) Sodium benzoate, which is used as a food preservative
(b) MSG, which is used as a flavor enhancer
(c) Agar-agar, which is used as a stabilizer
(d) Vanillin, which is used as a flavor
(e) Caramel, which is used to add color
(2) **Unintentional** food additives are substances that are not deliberately added but are in the food as a result of the growth process or from harvesting or storage. Examples of unintentional food additives are:
(a) Antibiotics, which are used to control diseases
(b) Residues of pesticides, which are used to control insects
(c) Chemicals that are used for storage or packaging purposes
(d) Radioactivity from fallout after nuclear weapons testing
b. Substances can also be classified according to **the degree of regulation**.
(1) Hundreds of additives are **generally recognized as safe (GRAS)** because of historic use in food and the lack of reports of adverse health effects. This group is the least regulated of all substances added to food.
(2) Substances in the GRAS group have been evaluated for toxicity using modern toxicologic methods, resulting in the removal of some chemicals from the GRAS group.
(3) All remaining food additives are stringently regulated.

3. **Carcinogens** are banned as intentional food additives because of the Delaney Amendment to the Food Additive Amendment of 1958. This farsighted amendment prohibits the FDA from considering as "safe" any chemical that has caused cancer in humans or animals.
a. **Cyclamate** was banned as an artificial sweetener in 1970 because it caused bladder cancer in animals. However, it is likely that the bladder tumors resulted because exposure was by pellet implantation. Other lifetime studies, in which exposure was by ingestion, have failed to demonstrate a tumorigenic response. Thus, it is likely that cyclamate should not be considered an animal carcinogen.

b. Saccharin was banned as an artificial sweetener in 1977 because it caused tumors in laboratory animals; however, the U.S. Congress stayed the ban.

(1) In 1977, when the saccharin ban was proposed, no other artificial sweetener was considered safe, making saccharin the only low-calorie sweetener used by the general public. Opponents of the ban argued that the risk of adverse health effects from obesity and diabetes outweighed the risk of cancer.

(2) Further testing of saccharin confirmed that it is an animal carcinogen. This contrasts with further testing of cyclamates, which did not confirm cyclamates as an animal carcinogen. Thus, potential health risks from the two food additives are not comparable.

c. A number of dyes used as food colors have been banned because of their carcinogenicity in animal bioassays.

4. Action levels are chemical concentrations at which the FDA will take action to remove a food containing that chemical from the market. The FDA has set action levels for more than 20 chemicals in various foodstuffs. Over half of these chemicals are pesticides. Action levels function as follows.

a. They are not permissible levels of contamination if the contamination is avoidable. They represent **the maximum concentration of unavoidable contamination,** resulting from growth, harvest, storage, and preparation.

b. They apply to selected foods. For a given chemical, separate action levels are set in each food or foodstuff, as is shown in the following examples.

(1) Endrin has an action level of 0.05 ppm in asparagus and 0.3 ppm in fish and shellfish.

(2) Chlordane has an action level of 0.8 ppm in rendered animal fat and 0.3 ppm in fish.

E. Consumer products. The **Consumer Product Safety Commission (CPSC)** administers several laws developed to protect consumers from unsafe products that are otherwise unregulated.

1. Tris(2,3-dibromopropyl)phosphate (TRIS) was used to make children's sleepwear fire-resistant. The requirement for fire-resistant sleepwear is part of the Flammable Fabrics Act. After TRIS was determined to be a potent animal carcinogen, the CPSC banned its use and required that treated garments be removed from the market.

2. Formaldehyde is a gas that is produced when urea foam formaldehyde insulation is improperly formulated. Formaldehyde is an animal carcinogen that produces nasal cancer in rats.

a. Proper preparation at the site of installation prevents offgassing of formaldehyde. In a small percentage of installations, the insulation is not mixed properly, and the insulation does not produce the desired polymer; thus, formaldehyde is released into the interior of the home.

b. The CPSC banned the use of urea foam formaldehyde insulation because of the potential for improper formulation. However, the ban was rescinded by court order after an industrial lawsuit.

(1) The use of urea foam formaldehyde insulation has declined dramatically because of the publicity accompanying the CPSC ban.

(2) Existing urea foam formaldehyde insulation that was properly formulated and has "set up," or polymerized, does not produce formaldehyde (nor does it do so when first installed).

F. Toxic chemicals. The **Toxic Substances Control Act (TSCA;** 1976) is the federal law that regulates production and use of new chemicals and previously unregulated chemicals.

1. Application. TSCA applies to all chemicals except foods, drugs, cosmetics, and pesticides.

2. Regulation. Before a new chemical can be produced for industrial or commercial use, the EPA must review the available toxicologic data base. The EPA has the power to regulate any chemical judged to pose an unreasonable risk of injury to human health or to the environment. **Regulatory options** that have been used under TSCA include:

a. Banning
b. Labeling requirements
c. Disposal requirements
d. Exposure precautions
e. Informational requirements

3. Specific chemicals regulated under TSCA are:

a. Asbestos. TSCA requires notification of the public if friable (i.e., crumbly) asbestos is found in public schools and establishes removal and disposal requirements.

b. **PCBs.** TSCA regulates the use, treatment, and disposal of PCBs.
c. **Dioxins.** TSCA regulates the disposal of dioxin-containing waste.

G. **Radiation and radioactive materials.** The **Atomic Energy Act** is the most important federal law regulating radioactive substances. This Act is administered by the Nuclear Regulatory Commission for nonmilitary purposes, while the Department of Defense is responsible for military controls. Also, some radioactivity in environmental mediums is controlled by various laws administered by the EPA.

1. **Sources**
   a. **Ionizing radiation** occurs naturally or is synthetic and includes:
      (1) Cosmetic irradiation incident to the earth's surface
      (2) Naturally occurring radionuclides in the earth's crust
      (3) Radiation from medical diagnostic or treatment machines
      (4) Radionuclides prepared for medical, technical, or scientific uses
      (5) Nuclear power reactors
      (6) Nuclear weapons
   b. **Nonionizing radiation** that occurs naturally is ultraviolet light, a component of sunlight.

2. **Effects.** Both ionizing and nonionizing radiation can cause cancer. Since cancer is a nonthreshold effect, cancer incidence is directly proportional to exposure.

3. **Controls**
   a. **Concentration standards** exist for radioactivity in some mediums, such as:
      (1) Drinking water
      (2) Milk
   b. **Emission standards** or controls exist for releases into:
      (1) Air
      (2) Groundwater
      (3) Surface water
   c. **Radiation exposure** is controlled for:
      (1) Workplaces
      (2) Medical x-rays
   d. **Radioactive material exposure** is controlled for:
      (1) Nuclear power generation
      (2) Nuclear weapons production and storage
      (3) Scientific and medical research

H. **Workplace.** The **Occupational Safety and Health Act (1970)** is the most important federal law regulating workplace exposure. Because occupational exposure to chemicals is discussed in Chapter 12, only a few areas of concern are noted here.

1. The Act includes significant exemptions for some occupational groups of workers and for workplaces employing small numbers of workers.

2. Other laws also control some workplace exposures, and these regulate:
   a. **Air.** The EPA may act if a pollution source is presenting an imminent and substantial danger to anyone.
   b. **Hazardous waste management.** The EPA may act to protect workers' health.
   c. **State or local jurisdictions**
   d. **Chemicals in commerce.** The EPA may act to protect workers.

3. Occupational standards are intended to assure that an employee shall suffer no material impairment of health or functional capacity even if exposed throughout his or her working life. However, occupational standard-setting is as much a political process as a scientific or medical process. Historically, workplace standards have been made more stringent as our scientific and medical data bases increase.

I. **Drugs and cosmetics.** The Food, Drug, and Cosmetics Act administered by the FDA is the major federal law regulating drugs and cosmetics. Although exposure to drugs and cosmetics is voluntary, the routes of exposure differ. Cosmetic exposure is by direct contact, the absorption of chemicals by this route is much slower than drug absorption via ingestion or inhalation.

1. **Drugs** are chemicals that are used because of specific effects that they cause in humans.
   a. **Doses** of drugs must be high enough to produce the desired effect, and such high doses often cause other effects that are considered toxic. Side effects are not unusual because chemicals can interact at many sites in humans.
   b. Use of a drug is an example of a **risk management decision**. The benefits of the drug therapy must be considered in conjunction with:
      (1) The risks of not using the drug
      (2) The risks of side effects
      (3) The risks and benefits of alternate available therapies
   c. The classification of drug use as licit or illicit is not relevant in considering toxic effects.
   d. **Drug abuse** is the excessive use of a drug because of nonmedicinal effects of the drugs. Chemicals that are not drugs can also be abused, and such abuse differs only in that the chemical is not regulated as a drug (e.g., glue sniffing, where the chemical is the solvent toluene). Although drug abuse occurs with licit and illicit drugs, most of the public focus on drug abuse is on the illegal use of narcotics, barbiturates, amphetamines, cocaine, and psychedelic drugs (see Chapter 11). However, the most abused drugs in our society are the legal drugs alcohol and tobacco.
2. **Cosmetics.** Because exposure to chemicals in cosmetics is by direct application to skin or mucous membranes, only small amounts of chemicals are expected to pass through the skin into the systemic circulation. Thus, toxic effects from cosmetic application are usually confined to effects on the skin or mucous membranes.

VII. MANAGEMENT OF ENVIRONMENTAL RISKS

A. Risks

1. **Definitions**
   a. **Risk** is the likelihood of a given toxicologic endpoint resulting from a specified exposure situation. Environmental risks are often associated with exposure to chemicals but are also the result of exposure to other insults, such as microorganisms or radiation.
   b. **Safety** is the opposite of risk and is the probability that a given toxicologic endpoint will not occur as a consequence of a specified exposure.
2. **Voluntary and involuntary risks**
   a. **Voluntary risks** are those accepted by individuals or society with some knowledge that the activity involved has risks; however, the extent or severity of the risks may not be accurately or fully understood. Causes, consequences, and probabilities for some voluntary risks are listed in Table 13-17.
   b. **Involuntary risks** are those risks about which individuals or society have no knowledge or control and are usually imposed on the individual or groups. Examples of involuntary risks are listed in Table 13-17.
3. **Risk assessment** is the scientific determination of the identity and probability of adverse human health effects from exposure to a chemical or insult.
   a. **Components.** Information from scientific and technical disciplines are integrated into a complete risk assessment.
      (1) **Hazard identification** is the identification of the health effects or toxicologic endpoints that result from exposure to a chemical or insult.
      (2) **Dose-response evaluation** is the quantitative relationship between exposure and toxic effect.
      (3) **Exposure evaluation** is the quantitative estimate of population and individual exposure to the chemical or insult.
      (4) **Risk characterization** is the integration of all of the toxic effects, dose-response, and exposure evaluation information.
   b. **Results** of risk assessments for carcinogens and noncarcinogens are expressed differently.
      (1) **Noncarcinogens.** A risk assessment for a noncarcinogen results in an estimate of the exposure to the noncarcinogen compared to a threshold or safe exposure. If the ratio of exposure to threshold is less than 1, then a toxic effect is unlikely to occur. Conversely, if the ratio is greater than 1, a toxic effect may occur in the exposed individual.
      (2) **Carcinogens.** A risk assessment for a chemical carcinogen results in an estimate of the maximum excess cancer risk from exposure to the carcinogen. Because of the uncertainties and protective public health assumptions, the cancer risk derived is the upper

Table 13-17. Voluntary and Involuntary Risks

Cause and Activity	Consequence	Individual Lifetime Risk*	Lifetime Risk* per 1 Million Population
Involuntary			
Home accidents	Death	1/1190	840
Traffic accidents (using seat belts)†	Death	1/114	8750
Being struck by lightning	Death	1/28,500	35
Pneumonia	Death	1/45	22,300
Outdoor exposure to radon	Lung cancer	1/2000	500
Voluntary			
Coal mining accidents‡	Death	1/17	58,500
Coal mining black lung disease‡	Death	1/3	369,000
Traffic accidents (without seat belts)†	Death	1/114	8750
Truck driving accidents‡	Death	1/220	4500
Smoking one cigarette per week	Lung cancer	1/3500	285
Smoking one cigarette per day	Lung cancer	1/500	2,000
Smoking one pack of cigarettes per day	Lung cancer	1/25	40,000

*Lifetime risks are shown in two equivalent ways: the lifetime risk of death for an individual and the lifetime risk per 1 million population.

†Risk is the excess risk of death in a traffic accident when not using seat belts. The seat-belt use and the non–seat-belt excess risk were determined from the total traffic accident risk using the assumption that half of the deaths would be prevented by the use of seat belts. The total risk of death from traffic accidents is the sum of the seat-belt use risk and the non–seat-belt use excess risk; this total is 1/57 or 17,500 per 1 million.

‡Lifetime risk assumes a 70-year lifetime exposure; however, the occupational exposure of coal miners and truck drivers is 45 years.

limit of the true risk. This means that the actual risk is not likely to be greater than the estimated risk and may in fact be much less.

4. **Scientific policy.** Risk assessment for most chemicals or insults is not an exact quantitative science because the scientific data base is rarely sufficient. In the absence of sufficient data to determine a relationship, scientific policy decisions are made. These decisions combine the available data with protective public health assumptions. The following scientific policy decisions have been made.
   - **a.** Animal studies are valid indications of human carcinogenic potential.
   - **b.** Animal bioassay tests using high doses are valid predictors of human response.
   - **c.** Benign tumor formation in animal bioassays is considered a cancer-producing response.
   - **d.** Both inhalation and ingestion routes of exposure are valid methods for animal bioassays.
   - **e.** The most sensitive animal bioassay response is valid to estimate human cancer potency.
   - **f.** No threshold is a valid assumption for carcinogenesis.
   - **g.** Dose conversions between species use surface-area equivalence.
   - **h.** High- to low-dose extrapolation models predicting linearity at low doses are valid.

5. **Uncertainties.** Because some of the components of a quantitative risk assessment include assumptions that are protective of public health, there are some uncertainties associated with the resulting risk assessment. These uncertainties can be classified into two groups:
   - **a.** Those that are the result of scientific policy decisions
   - **b.** Those that are the result of assumptions about human exposure (in general, the area with the greatest uncertainty for risk assessment)

6. **Risks of living.** Life is not risk-free. Individual and societal decisions involving risk affect the cause and time of death but not the fact of death.
   - **a. Daily life.** The lifetime risk of death from "normal" activities is shown for a few examples in Tables 13-17 and 13-18.
   - **b. Chemical exposure.** Exposure and associated cancer risks for a few selected chemicals are shown in Table 13-18. Note that the chemical concentrations used are those actually measured in an ambient environmental medium.
   - **c. Radiation exposure.** Exposure and associated cancer risks from radiation are also shown in Table 13-18.

Table 13-18. Cancer Risks from Chemical or Radiation Exposure

Chemical or Radiation	Exposure Conditions (concentration)	Individual Lifetime Risk*	Lifetime Risk per 1 Million Population*
Benzene	Rural ambient air (4.5 μg/m³)	1/64,400	16
	Urban ambient air (8.9 μg/m³)	1/32,600	31
	Self-service gasoline station (780 μg/m³)†	1/750,000	1
Chloroform	Rural ambient air (0.20 μg/m³)	1/215,000	5
	Urban ambient air (0.49 μg/m³)	1/87,800	11
	Chlorinated surface drinking water supply (10 μg/L)‡	1/570,000	2
	Chlorinated surface drinking water supply (75 μg/L)‡	1/76,000	13
	Daily shower using surface water supply (75 μg/L)§	1/87,700	11
Asbestos	Office building with friable asbestos (58 ng/m³)‖	1/22,900	41
Radon	Indoor exposure (1 pCi/L)#	1/514	1940
Radiation	Yearly chest x-ray	1/20,000	50
Arsenic	Remote ambient air (0.0004 μg/m³)	1/575,000	2
	Urban ambient air (0.003 μg/m³)	1/76,700	13
	Ambient air near smelters (0.03 μg/m³)	1/7670	130
	Occupational exposure at smelter (1 μg/m³)‖	1/1220	823
	Occupational exposure at smelter (10 μg/m³)‖	1/122	8230
PCBs	Eating bluefish (2.0 ppm)**	1/4000	249
Chlordane	Private home air levels after misapplication (2.1 μg/m³)#	1/2200	454
Saccharin	Drinking two 12-ounce cans of diet soda per day	1/3330	300

pCi = picocuries; PCBs = polychlorinated biphenyls.

*Lifetime risks are shown in two equivalent ways: the lifetime risk of death for an individual and the lifetime risk per 1 million population. Exposure is assumed to be 70 years.

†Assumes a 5-minute exposure per week.

‡Environmental Protection Agency (EPA) limits for total haloforms in drinking water are 100 μg/L.

§Exposure was modeled by the author, assuming one 15-minute shower per day.

‖Occupational exposure is based on a 40-hour work week, 46 weeks per year for 45 years.

#Assumes a 14-hour exposure per day.

**Assumes an ingestion of one 6-ounce portion of bluefish per month.

B. Risk management is the process of choosing between regulatory or risk reduction options. Risk assessments are important to risk management decisions. Without some human health risk, there would be little need for a risk management decision. Almost all risk management decisions fall into at least one of the following categories:

1. **Legal or regulatory.** Regulations and laws often require or prohibit certain actions.
2. **Health.** Public or individual health consequences of a risk management action is the "pure" risk assessment contribution to risk management.
3. **Ethical.** Individuals (e.g., physicians or toxicologists) and social institutions (e.g., hospitals or government agencies) often have ethical considerations that affect risk management decisions.
4. **Practical.** Good management is usually the most important consideration for activities that are unregulated but pose some risk.
5. **Other.** In addition to human health considerations, other concerns are integrated into risk management decisions, including:
   - **a.** Economics
   - **b.** Politics
   - **c.** Public expectations

d. Social considerations
e. Technical feasibility

C. Health professional risk management. Health professionals and government officials most often respond to environmental exposures involving chemicals that are carcinogens or that pose other serious health consequences.

1. Strategy for present exposure
a. Symptoms, if present, should be treated.
b. Exposure should be verified.
(1) If analytic results show the presence of the chemical in a medium and if exposure is likely, it is reasonable to assume that exposure has occurred.
(2) If analytic results are not available or not likely to be available, and a simple and inexpensive blood or urine test can yield an unequivocal result, then body fluid samples should be analyzed. If the results of a test will not alter treatment or reduce exposure, no tests should be performed; the existence of exposure should be assumed.
c. Presumed exposure should be reduced by whatever means necessary.

2. Strategy for past exposure
a. Symptoms, if present, should be treated.
b. It should be assumed that exposure has occurred for purposes of determining potential health effects.
c. A test of environmental medium of body fluids should be recommended only if a test result would alter some action to be taken.

3. Toxic endpoints of special concern are carcinogenesis, teratogenesis, and reproductive effects. Uncertainties exist in estimating risks or effects from carcinogens and teratogens. It is important that these risks and uncertainties be communicated to patients.
a. Carcinogenesis. Exposure to a cancer-causing chemical will at most increase the lifetime cancer risk of the individual. For many chemical exposures, estimates (risk assessments) show that the excess cancer risk is quite small, on the order of 10^{-6}, or 1 in 1 million lifetime risk. For other chemical exposures, the risks estimated may be appreciable, such as 10^{-4}, or 1 in 10,000 lifetime risk. Whatever the actual number, it is reassuring to know what the risk is rather than worrying about what it might be. Since risk assessments estimate the maximum likely risk and represent an upper bound or limit, the actual risk may be much smaller.
b. Teratogenesis and reproductive effects. Exposure to chemicals that cause teratogenic or reproductive effects are not likely to result in those effects unless the exposure is massive. Society places a special value on protecting the developing fetus and the process of reproduction. However, these toxic effects are likely threshold responses (i.e., safe doses, or thresholds, exist). Generalization cannot substitute for data, but as a rule, when teratogenic or reproductive effects are found, other toxic endpoints are also observed. Therefore, if exposure to a chemical is far below the level needed for any other toxic effect to occur, that exposure is unlikely to cause reproductive or teratogenic effects.

D. Risk communication. How health workers and other professionals communicate health risk information is important. Often a person's acceptance of both the scientific risk assessment and the risk management recommendations depends on the ability of the personnel involved to communicate. The following guidelines are recommended for physicians.

1. Preparation. The basis of the risk assessment process, including the health effects and exposure data, assumptions, and uncertainties, should be known by the physician.

2. Honesty. The physician's recommendations are more likely to be believed and followed by the patient if the physician communicates honestly. Known information should be communicated directly and accurately. The physician should also mention anything that is not known, or cannot be known, about the situation.

3. Concern. The physician should listen carefully to the patient's concerns and feelings and respond with care and sympathy.

STUDY QUESTIONS

Directions: Each item below contains four suggested answers of which **one or more** is correct. Choose the answer

A if **1, 2, and 3** are correct
B if **1 and 3** are correct
C if **2 and 4** are correct
D if **4** is correct
E if **1, 2, 3, and 4** are correct

1. Safe doses for threshold responses of chemicals are determined

(1) by applying uncertainty factors
(2) by the technical ability to control the chemical in a medium
(3) to be protective of the most sensitive human population
(4) from controlled laboratory experiments with human volunteers

2. Examples of nonthreshold effects include which of the following?

(1) Respiratory failure
(2) Cancer formation
(3) CNS depression
(4) Mutagenesis

3. Environmental scientists have been called in to analyze a trichloroethylene (TCE) spill that occurred alongside a highway. The scientists plan to use modeling and monitoring to assess the health dangers presented by TCE in the groundwater. In both modeling and monitoring,

(1) the maximum potential concentration of TCE in the medium would be estimated
(2) the release rate and environmental fate of TCE would be measured
(3) the movement of TCE in the medium would be a concern
(4) the results would be reported in the same concentration units

4. PCBs appear in appreciable concentrations in

(1) groundwater
(2) sediment
(3) air
(4) edible fish tissue

5. Trichloroethylene (TCE) is a known animal carcinogen. Which of the following are potential shortcomings of a negative epidemiologic study describing TCE production workers?

(1) Small group size
(2) Lack of quantitative TCE exposure information
(3) Lack of lifetime follow-up of workers
(4) Workers' exposure to other chemicals

1-B
2-C
3-D
4-C
5-B

ANSWERS AND EXPLANATIONS

1. The answer is B (1, 3) *[III B 1–3].*
Thresholds, or safe doses, are determined for the most sensitive toxic endpoint (i.e., the toxic effect that is observed at the lowest dose or exposure) and in the most sensitive human population. If the safe dose was not determined for the most sensitive human population, then it could not protect that population from potential toxic effects. Uncertainty factors estimate threshold doses by adjusting available toxicologic data to ensure that the most sensitive toxic endpoint is considered and that the most sensitive human population is protected. Controlled laboratory experiments with humans rarely provide the basis for the most sensitive toxic endpoint for a variety of reasons. The most sensitive endpoints are often chronic effects, and human studies are usually not carried out over extended time periods. The ability to control a chemical is determined by both the available technology and management decisions. In the past, the chemical industry may have determined safe exposures based on the cost of controls. In contrast, safe doses are explicitly determined based on health.

2. The answer is C (2, 4) *[II A 1, 2].*
Only toxic effects that are the result of the interaction of a chemical with genetic material are currently considered nonthreshold effects. All other interactions of a chemical result in threshold toxic effects. Both mutagenesis and carcinogenesis are believed to result from permanent alterations in genetic material. Mutational events may be either in germ cells, in which case they are heritable, or in somatic cells, in which case they only affect the organism in which the event occurs. Although mechanisms of carcinogenesis are complex and not well understood, some alteration of genetic material is regarded as an early requirement. Each of the other two toxic endpoints, respiratory failure and central nervous system (CNS) depression, are toxic effects that may be caused by a variety of chemicals acting systemically but not at the level of DNA.

3. The answer is D (4) *[V B 2, C, D].*
The essential difference between modeling and monitoring is that modeling makes use of reasonable assumptions about environmental fate and movement of chemicals while monitoring simply measures the chemical concentration in a medium. Both yield estimates of the concentration of the given chemical species [in this case, trichloroethylene (TCE)] in an environmental medium (here, groundwater). However, monitoring results are not necessarily estimates of the maximum concentration because the results are obtained at the time of measurement and not at the time of likely maximum concentration. Wind speed and direction can alter measured air levels, increased flow and agitation can alter surface water measurements, and soil type and rate and direction of groundwater flow can alter groundwater levels. Monitoring results are not dependent on factors such as emission or release rates or environmental fate because monitoring results express only what is present and measurable, no matter how the chemical got there. However, results from modeling are very dependent on any assumptions made about the emission or release rate or the environmental fate of a chemical. For example, an increased amount of TCE released to the soil will result in an increased concentration of TCE in groundwater. Similarly, TCE is not likely to be degraded appreciably by soil bacteria (or chemically transformed otherwise in soil). Thus, the concentration modeled in groundwater would not be reduced by a biotransformation factor.

4. The answer is C (2, 4) *[IV A 1 b (1)–(7), c; Table 13-13].*
Polychlorinated biphenyls (PCBs) have high octanol water partition coefficients (K_{ow}) and high bioconcentration factors (BCFs) relative to other classes of organic chemicals and metals. The K_{ow} describes the partition of a chemical between oil-like and water-like mediums, while the BCF describes the uptake of chemicals into fish tissue from the surrounding water. PCBs tend to move from water into sediment because of the organic content of sediment and the high value of K_{ow} (5×10^5). PCBs tend to move from water to edible fish tissue because of their high BCF value (10^5). Neither groundwater nor air should contain appreciable concentrations of PCBs because of low water solubility (about 30 ppb) and low vapor pressure.

5. The answer is B (1, 3) *[II B 1 b (1)–(4)].*
Negative human epidemiologic studies are quite common for many known animal carcinogens. Assuming that the study is well designed, a study is usually negative because of small group size. The chemical carcinogen is often not sufficiently potent to produce an excess of cancer incidence that can be observed in small groups of exposed workers. Another common reason that a study is negative is the lack of a lifetime follow-up of the exposed group. Thus, some cancers are not given sufficient time to appear in the human population. Exposure to other chemicals may be a reason for high cancer incidence in controls or for cancer responses that are not dose-related to trichloroethylene (TCE), but it is not a reason for negative studies. Also, while a lack of quantitative exposure information can make quantitative estimation of the potency of a carcinogen difficult, this difficulty is not related to negative studies in humans.

14 Legal Aspects of Medical Practice and Community Medicine

Arnold J. Rosoff

I. INTRODUCTION. Health care practice is more regulated today than ever before. Therefore, it is important that health care providers have a basic knowledge of the law and its applications to assure their own legal safety and that of their institutions, to control their practice environment, and to take an active role in shaping future legal developments through the political process. Health care regulation takes many forms.

A. Medical malpractice litigation brought by private parties is a form of regulation that focuses on the quality of care. The incidence of such litigation, which reached crisis levels in the early 1970s, runs in cycles, declining for a few years and then rising precipitously.

B. State regulation of practitioners, facilities, practice organizations [e.g., health maintenance organizations (HMOs)], and health financing programs is widespread, even in states where pressures to limit government intervention in the private sector are strong.

C. Federal regulation through publicly funded programs (e.g., Medicare, Medicaid) is a potent control factor. Although the conditions required for participation in these federally funded programs are rigorous, few health care institutions or providers can survive without the service revenues generated by such participation.

II. THE U.S. LEGAL SYSTEM

A. Precedent. The common law system is based on case precedent. The principle of adhering to precedent is referred to as *stare decisis,* Latin for "let the decision stand."

1. Except in special circumstances (and to some extent in Louisiana, where the legal system is based on French civil law), **legal principles established in one case are followed in similar cases in the same jurisdiction**. Cases do not have to follow precedent if they can be distinguished as significantly different from the precedent-setting case.
2. **Case precedents are not binding upon courts in other jurisdictions (i.e., in other states) or upon higher courts in the same jurisdiction.** However, even if a precedent is not binding, it may be persuasive—that is, it may influence the development of the law.

B. Civil versus criminal suits. The same act may constitute grounds for both a civil suit and a criminal prosecution. However, these two legal actions are independent, and the outcome of one has little or no impact on the outcome of the other.

1. **Civil suits** are those involving individuals, groups, or other parties acting in a nonpublic capacity.
   a. **Plaintiffs** (i.e., individuals who begin the suit) in civil suits generally seek to obtain compensation for injuries suffered through the wrongful acts of **defendants** (i.e., individuals who are being sued). A suit may have multiple plaintiffs and defendants. A decision pertaining to one plaintiff or defendant does not necessarily pertain to other plaintiffs or defendants in the same suit.
   b. A defendant who loses a civil suit is said to be **liable for damages**. The term **guilty** is not technically applicable to a civil suit.

2. **Criminal suits** are those brought by the federal, state, or local government to enforce laws that exist for the protection of society at large.
   a. **Criminal actions** are brought to punish the wrongdoer with a fine, imprisonment, or both.
   b. The principal purpose of punishing convicted criminals is **deterrence**.
   c. A defendant who loses a criminal suit is said to be **guilty**.

C. **Burden of proof.** The standard of proof required in criminal prosecutions is higher than the standard required in civil litigation.

1. Plaintiffs in a **civil suit** must prove their case by a **preponderance of evidence**—that is, the court must be persuaded that the material elements of the case more likely than not are in favor of the plaintiff.

2. The prosecution in a **criminal case** must prove its case **beyond a reasonable doubt**. This is consistent with the presumption by our legal system that the accused is **innocent until proven guilty**.

3. The party bringing the suit, the plaintiff or the prosecutor, generally bears the burden of proving all material elements in the case. Special circumstances may shift the burden of proof of certain elements to the defendant; however, this is an infrequent occurrence.

D. **Jury versus nonjury trials**

1. A **right to trial by jury** exists for most civil and criminal claims under federal and state constitutions, but a jury trial is not automatic. Unless one of the parties makes a request, the case is **docketed** (i.e., scheduled) for a nonjury trial. In fact, most cases are tried before a judge alone.

2. **Issues in equity,** a special subset of the law, must be heard by a judge alone (e.g., cases of mental incompetence or guardianship).

E. **Functions of judge and jury**

1. **Jury.** The function of the jury is to decide disputed issues of fact, where such issues exist. A **summary judgment** (i.e., a quick disposition of a case without a trial or resort to jury) will be entered when the judge determines that there are no material factual issues to be decided.

2. **Judge.** The function of the judge is to control the procedural aspects of the trial, to supply the applicable law, and to decide disputed issues of law. If a jury is used, it may announce the verdict, but it is bound to apply the law as instructed by the trial judge.

F. **Statute of limitations**

1. **Definition.** A statute of limitations is a procedural rule that establishes a maximum period of time during which a legal suit may be initiated. After the statutory period is over, a suit cannot be initiated regardless of how strong the case may be.

2. **Purpose**
   a. A statute of limitations requires parties to bring their suits to court while evidence is still fresh so that factual issues can be determined accurately.
   b. It also provides a cutoff date after which parties can be confident that no suit can be brought.

3. **Length of the statutory period.** The period allowed for initiating suit may vary from jurisdiction to jurisdiction for suits concerning similar legal matters. It also may vary within a given jurisdiction for suits concerning different legal matters. For example, the statute of limitations is commonly 4–6 years for contract actions and 1–3 years for personal injury actions. The statute of limitations can be **tolled** (i.e., stopped from running) in special circumstances—for example, if the defendant is absent from the state or is mentally incompetent and, therefore, unable to be sued. The beginning of the statutory period for medical malpractice is defined variously as:
   a. The date the alleged malpractice took place
   b. The date the physician-patient relationship was terminated
   c. The date the patient discovered the alleged malpractice
   d. The date the patient discovered, or by exercise of due care, should have discovered, the alleged malpractice (this is the most commonly used definition)

G. Measure of damages

1. **Determining the appropriate measure of damages** is as important, and sometimes just as difficult, as determining whether the defendant is liable. A number of different measures may be used, either separately or in combination.
   a. **Compensatory damages** compensate the plaintiff financially for the harm caused by the defendant. Tangible economic losses, such as expenses for remedial care, loss of wages, and future loss of earnings due to physical impairment, are the principal elements of compensatory damages.
   b. **Pain and suffering, mental anguish, and loss of consortium** (i.e., loss of marital companionship, especially of a sexual nature) attempt to provide dollar compensation for losses that are real and discernible but that cannot be measured readily in financial terms.
   c. **Punitive damages**—that is, damages in excess of normal compensation—may be awarded against a defendant who acted in a grossly negligent manner or with deliberate wrongful intent. Their purpose is to punish wrongdoers and to deter them and others from acting similarly in the future. The defendant must pay punitive damages to the plaintiff along with any other damages awarded. The amount is generally computed with regard for the degree of culpability of the defendant's actions and the defendant's ability to pay.
   d. **Nominal damages** are awarded when the plaintiff has been able to establish the defendant's wrongdoing and, thus, the defendant's liability but has not been able to prove that the plaintiff suffered any monetary loss. A small sum, such as one dollar, is awarded as a symbolic acknowledgment that the plaintiff won the suit.
2. **Legal expenses.** Under the American legal system, each party bears its own legal expenses, regardless of who won the litigation. However, court costs are assessed against one or the other or both parties at the discretion of the court. By contrast, in Britain, the winning party can recover reasonable attorneys' fees from the losing party.

III. TORT LAW

A. Definition. Torts are civil wrongs—that is, injuries to an individual's person, property, or reputation. Torts can be **deliberate** or **negligent**. Under absolute, or strict, liability, certain undesirable acts may be considered torts even when the **tortfeasor**—that is, the individual who committed the tort—acted neither deliberately nor negligently. **Remedies** in tort suits generally are meant to compensate the aggrieved party to restore as nearly as possible the position the victim would have enjoyed had the tort not been committed. When a tortfeasor's conduct is particularly culpable, punitive damages may be awarded.

B. Negligent torts. Most of the litigation relating to failures of medical care involves alleged negligence by health care providers.

1. **Negligence liability.** An individual who has been the victim of tortious conduct can sue for damages. However, unless the following four conditions (the "four Ds") are satisfied, there can be no recovery for the negligent tort.
   a. **Duty.** A duty is an obligation recognized by the law, the breaching of which is subject to legal sanctions.
      (1) To recover damages, the plaintiff must establish that she was owed a duty and the nature and extent of that duty.
      (2) The duty, or **standard of care,** generally must be established by **expert testimony** as to common practice within the relevant professional community.
   b. **Dereliction.** The plaintiff must prove that the defendant performed significantly below the legally required standard of care.
   c. **Damage.** The plaintiff must prove that he was harmed and establish the nature and extent of that harm.
      (1) In medical malpractice litigation, damages may be based on **physical injury, psychological harm,** and **reputational loss**.
      (2) **Economic losses** suffered by the plaintiff generally are not recoverable unless they are coupled with some other harm suffered. For example, the costs incurred by the patient for tests or hospitalization that were determined to be unnecessary cannot be recovered from the physician who prescribed the care unless the patient suffered harm other than economic waste.

d. **Direct causation.** There can be no liability unless the defendant's negligence was the proximate cause of the plaintiff's injuries.
   (1) A **proximate cause** is a factor without which the harm would not have occurred. It must be the predominant factor causing the harm. In medical malpractice cases, proximate cause is often difficult to establish since bad outcomes can occur even in the absence of negligence.
   (2) Under the **"loss of a chance" theory,** some courts have begun to award damages if the plaintiff can establish that the defendant's acts significantly reduced the patient's chances of survival or recovery. This liberal definition of causation makes it easier to recover damages in cases of medical malpractice.

2. **Standard of care**
   a. **Reasonable care.** The care usually required is that degree of care that a reasonably prudent individual would exercise in similar circumstances. The standard of care generally is fixed by reference to the customary practice of a given profession. Because the judge and jury cannot possibly know the customary practice of all professions, this must be established in court by expert testimony.
      (1) Participation as an **expert witness,** which must be voluntary, is secured through negotiation of a **witness fee**. In contrast, testimony as to one's factual observations can be compelled through use of a **subpoena** (i.e., a court order to appear and testify).
      (2) It is widely claimed, especially by plaintiffs' attorneys, that a **conspiracy of silence** among physicians makes it difficult to obtain expert testimony on behalf of plaintiffs in medical malpractice cases.
   b. **Locality rule,** still followed in a few jurisdictions, has largely been replaced by a new approach—**national standards** for health care practice.
      (1) **"Strict locality" rule** requires that expert testimony on the standard of care be drawn from the geographic community in which the alleged malpractice occurred. In the late 1800s, courts recognized that customary medical and surgical practices in isolated areas were not on par with those in progressive urban areas, and a differential standard of care was allowed.
      (2) **"Same or similar community" standard** measures the defendant's performance by reference to closely comparable medical communities. This liberalization of the locality rule makes it easier for plaintiffs to obtain expert testimony in support of their cases.
      (3) **National standards** have been adopted by some jurisdictions, especially in cases where specialty care is rendered by board-certified practitioners. Some states also apply national standards set by the Joint Commission on Accreditation of Hospitals to measure hospital care (*Hall v. Hilbun,* Mississippi, 1985).
   c. **Generalist versus specialist standards**
      (1) When a physician claims the ability to provide the type of care that normally is rendered by a specialist, the standard of care applied is that of the appropriately trained specialist.
      (2) Under emergency circumstances in which specialty care is not available, a general practitioner may provide care that normally is rendered by a specialist. In such cases, a generalist standard should be applied to measure the adequacy of the care rendered.
      (3) Failure to refer a patient to a specialist when specialty care is indicated subjects the attending physician to liability, a case known as **negligent nonreferral**.
   d. **Court-imposed standards of care.** The legally required standard of care may be fixed by a court at a level higher than that of prevailing professional practice.
      (1) In *Helling v. Carey* (Washington, 1974), the state's highest court held that customary professional practice is not absolutely determinative of reasonably prudent care. In this case, two ophthalmologists were held liable for not using a tonometer test for glaucoma even though it was not customary to use this test on patients of the plaintiff's age unless there was an indication of a visual field disorder.
      (2) Although Washington's legislature enacted a reform measure intended to overrule the *Helling* precedent, the state supreme court has resisted application of the new law (*Gates v. Jensen,* Washington, 1979).
      (3) The *Helling* precedent has not been widely followed, but it is generally thought to be sound. Under clear-cut circumstances—that is, where it is obvious what lay opinion would think good care requires—other courts can be expected to use a similar approach.

3. **Proof of dereliction**
   a. Whether or not the defendant performed up to the required standard of care is a factual matter, generally requiring proof.
      (1) Although expert witnesses cannot be compelled to testify as to matters of opinion, they can be required (subpoenaed) to testify as to factual matters that they directly observed in the care of the patient (plaintiff).
      (2) Care may have been so deficient that a judge or lay jury may infer negligence even in the absence of expert testimony under the doctrine of ***res ipsa loquitur,*** Latin for "the thing speaks for itself." Thus, the plaintiff is spared the burden of producing further evidence of negligence.
   b. Today, some jurisdictions allow the plaintiff to introduce recognized medical texts as proof of accepted professional practice. However, some jurisdictions exclude such evidence as **hearsay** because the author of the text is not present in court, under oath, and subject to cross-examination.

C. **Deliberate torts.** Although most medical suits involve negligent torts, there is significant opportunity for suits charging deliberate torts. To establish the required **intent** to support such a charge, it is not necessary to show that the defendant specifically meant to harm the plaintiff but only that the defendant deliberately performed the wrongful act. Of the possible types of deliberate torts, the following are the most significant in the medical area.

1. **Battery,** which is defined as touching an individual without permission, often leads to health care suits.
   a. The wrongful act to be avoided under battery is the invasion of a person's **right of bodily inviolability**.
   b. A valid ground for complaint exists even if the defendant intended no harm and the patient suffered no physical damage. Monetary awards generally are small unless there is physical damage or the defendant meant to cause harm.
   c. Cases of alleged **sexual assault** by physicians are considered battery actions.

2. **Fraud and deceit** are important grounds for deliberate tort suits. Cases in which a physician deliberately misrepresents facts to obtain a patient's consent for a procedure are treated as matters of fraud and deceit. These cases can be distinguished from the more common cases of **informed consent** (see V).

3. **Breach of confidentiality** involves a disclosure of information about a patient's case without his permission. This theory can support a suit based on a number of specific theories, including:
   a. **Breach of an implied contract duty** to keep patient information confidential
   b. **Invasion of privacy**
   c. **Defamation,** in cases where the disclosure of information might have negative consequences for the patient's personal, social, or business life
   d. **Unprofessional conduct**

4. **Bad faith breach of contract** is an innovative approach to convert a tort action into a contract action, which has had some success to date (see IV F).

D. **Institutional liability.** Increasingly, courts are holding health care institutions liable for malpractice committed by individuals in some relationship with the institution.

1. **Vicarious liability** occurs when one party is held responsible for something that another does or fails to do.
   a. Under the vicarious liability principle of ***respondeat superior,*** Latin for "let the master answer," the employer (institution) is responsible (liable) for torts committed by its employees (e.g., nurses, house staff) within the scope of their employment.
   b. Under the **apparent agency,** or **ostensible agency,** doctrine, the institution may also be liable for torts of people not employed by it (i.e., **independent contractors**), if the circumstances reasonably made it appear to the patient that the person in question was an employee or agent of the institution.
      (1) Institutional liability is less likely, but still possible, if the patient and the person in question had a relationship outside the institutional context (e.g., as physician and patient).
      (2) To avoid liability, the institution must take steps to assure that patients understand the independent contractor status of the person in question.

2. **Corporate negligence** is an evolving legal theory by which an institution may be held directly (not vicariously) liable for a tort committed by an independent contractor, such as a staff physician, practicing in or through the institution.
   a. The institution has a duty to all patients treated in its facilities to take reasonable steps to assure the competence of all who are allowed to practice there.
   b. Liability can result from failing to check credentials adequately before granting staff privileges to an unqualified practitioner or from allowing privileges to be retained when the institution knows, or should know, that the practitioner poses a risk to patients.
   c. Many states have adopted variants of this theory since the landmark case, *Darling v. Charleston Community Memorial Hospital* (Illinois, 1965).

3. **Charitable immunity,** an outmoded doctrine barring tort suits against nonprofit hospitals, has been abandoned in most states.

4. **Governmental immunity** still prevails in several jurisdictions, preventing or limiting suits against institutions run by governmental units.
   a. In states where the doctrine exists, the facts and circumstances of the individual case may determine whether the doctrine applies.
   b. Immunity for the institution may not extend to all health professionals practicing there. The key question is whether the individual was acting as an agent of the institution in the particular instance.

5. **Peer review and professional discipline** are being strengthened in response to increased institutional liability pressures.
   a. The federal **Health Care Quality Improvement Act of 1986** requires hospitals and other health care entities, state licensure agencies, and malpractice liability insurers to report to a national registry **(National Practitioner Data Bank)** incidents raising substantial question about a physician's ability to practice medicine safely.
      (1) Institutions must consult this registry when granting staff privileges and periodically thereafter.
      (2) Civil immunity is granted to health care entities that engage in peer review if prescribed due process safeguards for the practitioner are observed.
      (3) Suits challenging peer review and related staff privilege denials as a violation of federal antitrust law are also blocked (*Patrick v. Burget,* US Supreme Court, 1988).
   b. States also are improving medical licensure and discipline mechanisms, providing various services and supports for "impaired physicians" (i.e., generally those suffering from substance abuse and other personality disorders), and demanding mandatory reporting by professionals of those known to pose a threat to patient safety.

IV. CONTRACT LAW

A. **Definition.** A contract is a **consensual agreement** between two (or more) parties whereby each undertakes defined obligations to the other. The law recognizes a contract, when properly entered into, as legally binding and provides sanctions for its breach. Two elements are essential for the creation of a contract.

1. **Consideration** is an item, act, or forbearance that one party gives to the other to bind a contract. The contract is not binding unless each party gives, or promises to give, consideration to the other.
   a. **Example.** Bill promises to wash Al's car, in return for which Al gives Bill $5.00. A binding contract has been made. The consideration passing from Al to Bill is the $5.00 (an item); Bill's undertaking to wash Al's car is the consideration passing from Bill to Al. As alternative forms of consideration, Al could have agreed to mow Bill's lawn (an act) or could have agreed not to ask Bill's girlfriend out on a date (a forbearance).
   b. Something that a party already has a preexisting obligation to do cannot serve as consideration for a new contract. Thus, if Al was already under contract to mow Bill's lawn whenever it needed mowing, a redundant promise by Al to do that same thing could not serve as consideration for Bill's undertaking to wash Al's car.

2. **Offer and acceptance.** An **offer by one party** and an **acceptance by the other,** which may occur formally or informally, are essential to the establishment of a consensual relationship and, thus, to the formation of a contract.

a. The offer and acceptance constitute a **bargained-for-exchange,** through which the consideration given by one party is recognized as the agreed-upon price for the undertaking by the other party. This aspect of giving up something in return for action or forbearance by the other party is described by the term ***quid pro quo,*** Latin for "this for that."

b. The law provides complex guidelines by which to determine whether an offer and acceptance have taken place, an issue that often is not clear-cut.

B. Express versus implied contracts

1. **Express contracts** are those that are stated in words, whether spoken or written.

2. **Implied contracts** are those in which the agreement of a party is not expressly stated but may be inferred from the party's conduct. It is possible for the consent of both parties to be given by implication. For example, in the health care context, most contracts for care are implied. Patients register their willingness to enter into a contract by presenting themselves to health care providers for care. Providers register their willingness to enter into a contract by providing that care.

   a. When the parties agree upon a price, that price becomes a part of the contract, whether or not others would consider it reasonable.

   b. When the parties do not agree on a price, the law presumes that a reasonable price was intended. What constitutes a reasonable price is a factual matter, which may be determined by the court.

C. Measure of damages. The purpose of damages in a contract action is to place the aggrieved party (i.e., the one against whom a breach has been committed) as nearly as possible in the position she would have enjoyed had the contract been performed as agreed. This approach to compensatory damages attempts to give an aggrieved party the **benefit of the bargain** that was embodied in the contract.

1. In general, **only economic losses are considered** in awarding damages for a contract breach. Emotional distress and other intangible harms are not compensable, except in rare circumstances.

2. Similarly, punitive damages generally are not awarded against a breaching party, even though the breach may be deliberate (see IV F for a possible exception).

D. Breach of warranty. An application of contract law to the health care setting can be seen in suits brought by patients against health care providers for failure to obtain the positive results that the providers allegedly contracted to deliver—that is, for breach of a warranty of cure.

1. This approach, where allowed, may permit recovery of damages even though the provider has not been negligent in the provision of care. The patient's complaint is not that the provider failed to perform according to professional standards but that the provider failed to deliver the promised result.

2. At least one court has held that the proper measure of damages in such a suit is the difference in value between the result promised by the provider and the result actually obtained—a **benefit of the bargain approach,** which is derived from classic contract actions outside the health care field (*Hawkins v. McGee,* New Hampshire, 1929).

3. Some courts have awarded damages following the rules for tort-based suits, allowing compensation only for deterioration of the patient's condition after care as compared to his condition before care was rendered (*Sullivan v. O'Connor,* Massachusetts, 1973).

4. Courts generally are reluctant to allow contract-based claims in medical malpractice cases. Some courts restrict the use of contract theories by imposing two important requirements.

   a. No breach of warranty is possible unless the provider makes a specific promise of cure.

      (1) Positive projections of the benefits of a planned treatment or promises that providers will "do their best" do not constitute a warranty upon which a suit can be based.

      (2) Providers should choose their words carefully to avoid crossing the line from a general reassurance to a specific promise of positive outcome.

   b. Some courts insist that the alleged promise may be expressly stated in a written document before it can serve as a basis for a breach of warranty suit.

E. Statute of limitations. One motivation for using a contract theory is that the statute of limitations for these actions may be longer than those for tort actions (see II F).

F. **Bad faith breach of contract.** This curious hybrid of contract and tort law is increasingly being applied in the health insurance context. Under the doctrine, a third party payer that deliberately breaches a contract to provide or pay for health services may be liable for the harm suffered as a result of the nontreatment as well as for punitive damages.

1. To recover damages, it must be shown that the payer knew or should have known that the services were appropriate and were covered by the plan.
2. Bad faith denial of coverage claims increasingly arise from attempts to contain health care cost by reducing testing and treatment services (*Sarchett v. Blue Shield,* California, 1987).
3. Such suits are increasingly being brought against HMOs and other organizations that link provision of and payment for services.

V. INFORMED CONSENT

A. **Basic concept.** The law requires that diagnostic, medical, and surgical procedures be authorized by a **voluntary, knowledgeable consent of the patient or the patient's legal representative**. This important aspect of patients' rights originates from the principles regarding battery.

1. Case law early in this century declared that "every human being of adult years and sound mind has a right to determine what shall be done with his own body" (*Schloendorff v. Society of New York Hospital,* New York, 1914). This is the root premise of the developing law of informed consent.
2. Since the late 1950s, courts increasingly have held that a patient's consent to treatment, even if formally obtained and documented in writing, is legally ineffective if the patient was not informed adequately about the treatment, including the inherent risks (*Salgo v. Stanford University Hospital,* California, 1957).

B. **Defining informed consent obligations.** Two approaches have evolved for defining the health care provider's informed consent obligations.

1. The older, **physician-based approach,** first adopted in the case of *Natanson v. Kline* (Kansas, 1960), requires that physicians disclose to patients all that is customary in the profession to disclose in similar situations. The law essentially adopts the **professional community standard**. Thus, in court, the patient (plaintiff) is required to produce expert testimony as to what physicians customarily tell their patients—obviously a difficult evidentiary burden. About half the states follow this approach.
2. The newer, **patient-based approach,** adopted in the landmark case of *Canterbury v. Spence* (US Court of Appeals for the District of Columbia Circuit, 1972), requires that physicians disclose all that a reasonably prudent patient would consider material to the decision to accept or reject the proposed treatment. A factor is material if, either alone or in combination with other factors, it significantly would affect the patient's decision. Because expert testimony as to a "standard disclosure" is not needed, it is generally easier for patients to sue on informed consent grounds in states using this approach.

C. **Required disclosure elements.** Under either the physician-based or the patient-based approach, the following elements must be disclosed in language that the patient reasonably can be expected to comprehend:

1. **Diagnosis,** including the disclosure of any reservations the physician has about the diagnosis
2. **Nature and purpose of the proposed treatment**
3. **Risks and consequences of the proposed treatment,** which includes only risks and consequences of which the physician has, or reasonably should have, knowledge
4. **Feasible treatment alternatives,** which includes other treatment modalities that the medical community would consider using in this particular case, regardless of the personal treatment preferences of the physician making the disclosure
5. **Prognosis without treatment** (i.e., if the patient elects not to have the recommended treatment, he must be informed of the implications of this choice)

D. Causation. To recover damages for a physician's failure to disclose information, a patient must convince the court that she would have made a different decision about the treatment had the information been known. Obviously, this is a difficult, speculative determination, which requires the court to determine, after a bad clinical result has occurred, what the patient would have chosen before the fact, not knowing the outcome.

1. Most courts base the causation analysis on an **objective standard**—that is, what an "average, reasonable patient" would have chosen.
2. A few courts use a **subjective standard**—that is, what "this particular patient" would have chosen.

E. Therapeutic privilege. Many courts have recognized that a physician may be justified under certain limited circumstances to withhold information in the patient's best interest.

1. This privilege applies *only* when a patient is unusually sensitive, anxious, or emotional. A general policy of not disclosing information because of the presumed hypersensitivity of patients is not an acceptable basis for this privilege.
2. A physician relying on therapeutic privilege should document carefully why the information in question should be withheld from the particular patient.
3. When the physician's use of therapeutic privilege is challenged, it must be determined whether the physician followed sound medical judgment in withholding information.

F. Consent. When the patient is adult and competent, the authority to give or withhold consent to treatment rests exclusively with the patient, unless she makes a valid delegation to someone else.

1. A **power of attorney** executed in writing by a competent adult (the patient) can delegate the responsibility for health care decisions to another competent adult. The provider should take care to ascertain that the decision in question lies within the scope of the expressly authorized delegation, since the law interprets powers of attorney narrowly.
   - **a.** Many states hold that a power of attorney becomes ineffective when the individual giving it becomes incompetent. This is consistent with the general principle of agency law that an agent can have no greater capacity to act than his principal has.
   - **b.** A **durable power of attorney,** which remains effective even after the giver of the power becomes incompetent, is recognized in several states. This form of power is most useful in the health care setting.
2. The **legal age of majority** varies from state to state but is usually 18 or 19 years of age. Individuals who have not attained this age cannot give legally effective consent except in the following situations.
   - **a. Emancipated minors** (i.e., minors who are married, live away from their parents' home, or are financially independent) are regarded as having an adult capacity to consent to health care.
   - **b.** Some states, by statute, have fixed a **lower age of consent** for health care, especially regarding the diagnosis and treatment of sexual and reproductive problems (e.g., contraception, abortion, pregnancy, venereal disease) and drug or alcohol abuse.
   - **c.** Some states, by case law, recognize a **mature minor exception,** allowing minors to give consent to health care under certain circumstances, such as when there is a pressing need for care, when the consent of a parent or guardian cannot be obtained easily, and when the minor patient has sufficient mental ability to understand the implications of the treatment.
3. **Next of kin.** When a patient is incapable of giving consent because of age, incompetency, or incapacity, the law holds that the closest available relative can authorize care on the patient's behalf.
   - **a.** The President's Commission for the Study of Ethical Problems in Medicine and Biomedical and Behavioral Research (1983) defined **competency** as "the patient's capability to understand information relevant to the decision and to reason about relevant alternatives against a background of reasonably stable personal values and life goals."
   - **b.** A health care provider who acts on the belief that a person is the patient's next of kin is legally protected if this turns out not to be the case. To assure protection, the provider should document the basis for believing that a person is the patient's next of kin.
   - **c.** A difficult legal matter results when the next of kin refuses to authorize care that the provider believes is urgently needed. In such cases, a **court order** authorizing the treatment

must be obtained. Where time or other circumstances do not permit this, the provider is not liable for action taken on sound medical judgment. However, this is a very risky situation, turning, as it does, on a court's after-the-fact determination of what the exigent circumstances required. **Extreme caution is advised.**

4. **Emergency situations.** The law recognizes an exception to the requirement of consent in cases where the patient is unconscious or otherwise unable to give consent and the need for care is so urgent that it is not feasible to contact the patient's next of kin.
   a. The rationale for this emergency consent exception is that, unless the health care providers have information to the contrary, they are entitled to presume that the patient would have chosen the care others have chosen in similar circumstances.
   b. The exception does not extend beyond situations where immediate action must be taken to preserve life or, in some states, to prevent serious physical harm.
   c. The circumstances justifying the emergency consent exception should be documented, including all efforts to contact next of kin before treatment is rendered.
   d. **Administrative authorization**—that is, consent for treatment granted by the administration of a health care facility—helps merely to document the applicability of the emergency consent doctrine. Health care facility administrators have no inherent power to grant consent on behalf of patients.

VI. PATIENT'S RIGHTS

A. **Refusal of treatment.** A patient who is competent to give consent also is entitled legally to withhold it for whatever reasons he deems sufficient. This is true even if refusing treatment may result in serious harm or death.

1. When a patient refuses treatment, the provider should document all of the information given to the patient concerning the consequences of the refusal. Failure to provide such information or the inability to prove that it was provided could result in liability on informed consent grounds (*Truman v. Thomas,* California, 1980).

2. When the competence of the patient to make the treatment decision is questionable, the provider may rely on the principles of emergency consent and consent by the next of kin. Again, great care is advised, and a court order authorizing treatment should be obtained when feasible.

B. **Terminally ill and vegetative-state patients.** Numerous state court decisions over the last 15 years have held that terminally ill patients and those in a "persistent vegetative state" have a right to refuse life-supporting care that would serve only to prolong the process of dying or a meaningless existence.

1. Patients do not have an unrestricted "right to die." Courts and legislatures dealing with this matter have defined rather narrowly the cases in which patients can refuse life support.

2. Ending years of speculation on how it would rule on the issue, the U.S. Supreme Court held in 1990 that a patient does have the constitutional right to decline life-sustaining treatment (*Cruzan v. Director, Missouri Department of Health,* US Supreme Court, 1990). However, the Court also upheld the right of the state to require strong evidence of the patient's desires on the matter.

3. Some courts traditionally have distinguished between the use of ordinary and extraordinary life-support measures. **Ordinary measures** generally have been held to include the provision of nutrition and hydration via nasogastric or other types of feeding tubes; **extraordinary measures** encompass cardiopulmonary resuscitation and the use of a ventilator to maintain respiration.
   a. Calling the use of a respirator extraordinary treatment, the New Jersey Supreme Court allowed an irreversibly brain-damaged and comatose young woman to be removed from the respirator that was presumably sustaining her life (*In re Quinlan,* New Jersey, 1976).
   b. In 1985, the New Jersey Supreme Court held that it might be appropriate to discontinue nasogastric feeding and hydration for a senile, semiconscious 84-year-old nursing home patient who was in failing condition but whose death was not thought to be imminent (*In re Conroy*, New Jersey, 1985).
      (1) **Extraordinary care** was defined as care in which the expectable benefits to the patient cannot be justified when weighed against the burdens.

(2) Strict procedural safeguards were imposed to assure that the rights of nursing home patients are protected.

4. **"No code," or "do not resuscitate" (DNR),** orders entered by the attending physician generally are legally acceptable in appropriate cases involving terminally ill patients. If the patient is unconscious or incompetent, family members should be consulted about the DNR decision. Extreme care should be taken when it is known or suspected that a relative opposes the entry of a DNR order.
   a. The physician should document carefully the consent of the patient or the next of kin to the entry of a DNR order.
   b. Pain-killing drugs may be used even when this may accelerate the death of a terminally ill and failing patient. However, no jurisdiction has officially condoned active euthanasia.
   c. Although some providers have been reluctant to enter a DNR order overtly in the patient's chart, such a frank acknowledgment of the DNR decision is advisable, provided that the steps outlined above have been followed.

5. Numerous states sanction the use of a **living will** or **natural death directive** by which a patient can direct what care should be rendered in a terminal illness if the patient is not competent at that time to provide such direction. Even in states that have not yet officially recognized the legal validity of such devices, their use should help to protect those who act in response to sound medical judgment and the patient's documented wishes.

C. **Substituted judgment analysis.** Termination-of-treatment decisions for incompetent patients commonly are made by attempting to ascertain what the patients would choose for themselves if able.

1. The *Quinlan* case established this principle as flowing from the patient's right of self-determination.

2. The substituted judgment approach works best when the patient, before becoming incompetent, either expressed her wishes on the issue of termination-of-treatment or otherwise revealed enough about her beliefs so that her wishes on the issue reasonably can be inferred.
   a. *Superintendent of Belchertown State School v. Saikewicz* (Massachusetts, 1977) demonstrated the unique challenge of using substituted judgment analysis where the patient had never been competent. The court made its treatment decision for Joseph Saikewicz, a 67-year-old man who had been profoundly retarded since birth, based on speculation as to what a person who had never been competent would choose if he were competent long enough to exercise rational free will.
   b. In the "Brother Fox" case, the clergyman being maintained on a respirator had stated on several occasions that he would not wish to be kept alive that way (*In re Eichner,* New York, 1981).
   c. The New Jersey Supreme Court's *Conroy* decision established a three-tiered analytic framework for applying substituted judgment.
      (1) A **"subjective" test** is used when patients expressly have stated their wishes at some previous time (e.g., as in the "Brother Fox" case).
      (2) A **"limited objective" test** is used when the patients' wishes can be inferred from known religious, ethical, or lifestyle beliefs (e.g., *Brophy v. New England Sinai Hospital, Inc.,* Massachusetts, 1986).
      (3) A **"pure objective" test** is used when no information is available from which to infer what the particular patient would have wanted. Inferences must be drawn based upon what the "average" person would desire in such a situation.

VII. ACCESS TO CARE

A. **Duty to render care.** The law is struggling to balance the right of providers to choose whom they will serve against the pressing need of the community to have quality health care services readily available.

1. **Individual practitioners.** An individual health care practitioner has no common law duty to render care to anyone she has not accepted as a patient, even when a person is in need of immediate care. The physician who does not respond to such a call for aid has no liability for harm suffered by the patient.
   a. **Moral duty.** There is a clearly recognized moral and professional duty, however, to render care to the best of the practitioner's ability under the circumstances.

b. **Abandonment.** Once a physician accepts a patient for care, the obligation to provide care within the scope of the agreed relationship continues until either the patient terminates the relationship or the physician terminates it with the patient's consent or with sufficient advance notice to allow the patient to secure an alternative source of care.
(1) The principle of abandonment is the source of the physician's legal obligation to arrange adequate coverage for a patient's care when the physician is not going to be available.
(2) Because of the possibility of an abandonment charge, the practitioner should document when a physician-patient relationship has terminated and provide the patient with unequivocal notice that this has occurred.

2. **Statutory imposition of duty to render care.** Alone among U.S. jurisdictions, Vermont has adopted legislation requiring all citizens to do what they reasonably can to lend aid and assistance in emergency situations. The sanction for failing to obey the law's mandate is a minor criminal fine.
a. Although the law makes no specific mention of health care professionals, it applies to them as well.
b. Presumably, states could require health care professionals to aid in emergencies as a condition of licensure. No state has adopted such a requirement, however, and politically, if not constitutionally, it would be problematic.

3. **Good samaritan statutes.** These statutes have been passed in all states to encourage physicians to render care in emergencies.
a. Such statutes grant immunity from civil liability for injuries caused by a physician's good faith attempts to render care in emergency situations.
b. There is generally no immunity if the physician is grossly negligent—that is, if the physician acts with wanton or reckless disregard for the consequences of her actions—or if she is acting within the ordinary scope of her duties.
c. Some statutes cover health care professionals other than physicians, such as nurses, paramedics, and various emergency medical technicians. The immunity generally extends only to people who act within the scope of their properly certified abilities.
d. Even in the absence of good samaritan protection, persons attempting to assist in an emergency would run little risk of being held liable for harm suffered by the person they sought to aid. The standard for a good-faith volunteer's actions is any action that other persons similarly qualified would be expected to do under similar circumstances.

B. **Health care facilities.** Private hospitals are under no common law duty to accept patients or render care in emergencies. Public hospitals (i.e., those operated by federal, state, or local governments) have a broader obligation to provide care to the public. The law acts in various ways to encourage or require hospitals to expand access to their services.

1. **Common law principles** have been developed in case law to require privately owned and operated health care institutions to admit patients or at least to give them initial treatment, advice, and referral.
a. *Wilmington General Hospital v. Manlove* (Delaware, 1961) held that a private hospital that maintains an emergency department whose existence is known to the general public undertakes an obligation to provide emergency care to those presenting for treatment in an emergency situation. The rationale for the ruling was that the hospital led the public to rely on the availability of the emergency service and could not unilaterally frustrate this reliance.
b. The rendering of initial appraisal and advice may be held to constitute an acceptance of a patient for care. Failure to admit the patient after such initial steps have been taken could lead to a charge of abandonment (*O'Neill v. Montefiore Hospital,* New York, 1960).

2. **Hospital licensure statutes** in many states require general acute-care hospitals, even private institutions, to maintain emergency facilities and treat the general public in emergency situations (*Thompson v. Sun City Community Hospital, Inc.,* Arizona, 1984).
a. As in the *Thompson* case, some states provide public funds to pay for hospitals that render uncompensated emergency care.
b. A key issue in such cases is when the emergency status ends and the patient can be transferred safely to another institution.

3. Conditions for participation in the Medicare and Medicaid programs require that general acute-care hospitals must maintain emergency treatment facilities. In addition, these laws require hospitals to accept Medicare and Medicaid beneficiaries for treatment. Amendments to

the **Medicare and Medicaid laws** under the **Consolidated Omnibus Budget Reconciliation Act of 1985** (COBRA) require hospitals to render emergency care to all patients presenting with an "emergency medical condition" or in "active labor."

- **a.** These **"antidumping" provisions** apply to all hospitals that participate in Medicare and Medicaid, but the provision of care applies to *all* patients, not just the beneficiaries of these programs.
- **b.** Strict safeguards are imposed against medically inappropriate "economic transfers," with strong penalties for their violation.

4. Rules for tax-exempt status under the federal tax laws (Internal Revenue Code section 501-C-3) contemplate that hospitals will maintain emergency facilities open to the general public. They do not, however, require tax-exempt hospitals to admit all patients regardless of their ability to pay for care.

5. Federal hospital financing laws (Hill-Burton Act of 1945) require that hospitals constructed or improved with federal funds must provide a reasonable volume of free or reduced-cost care to the general public. The **Hill-Burton free-care obligation** helps to assure access to hospital care for persons who might not otherwise be admitted or treated (*American Hospital Association v. Schweiker,* US Court of Appeals, 7th Circuit, 1983).

6. The **Joint Commission on Accreditation of Healthcare Organizations** (JCAHO) requires general acute-care hospitals to maintain emergency facilities and staffing and to render initial appraisal and advice to individuals presenting for emergency treatment.

VIII. PUBLIC HEALTH, GOVERNMENTAL POWER, AND INDIVIDUAL RIGHTS

A. Bases of governmental power. Under the Constitution of the United States, the powers of the state (i.e., the government at the federal, state, and local levels) are limited. Much power and discretion are left to individuals to live as they wish and to control their own destinies. However, two intrinsic types of governmental power are implicitly allowed.

1. Police power is the inherent authority of the state to take necessary steps to protect public health, welfare, safety, and morals.

- **a.** Police power can be exercised when the state has a "legitimate interest" in an activity and undertakes action "reasonably related" to the protection of that interest.
- **b.** It must be balanced against the rights of the individual. When the individual right involved is a "fundamental right," the state cannot take action unless it can demonstrate a "compelling interest."

2. *Parens patriae* (Latin for "the state as parent"). When individuals cannot take adequate care of themselves, the state is both empowered and obliged to take protective action (i.e., to assume a "parent" role).

B. Prohibition of dangerous activities and other governmental interventions are justified under either police power or *parens patriae,* depending on who is at risk from the activity.

1. Activities that pose a threat to society, such as going to school with a communicable disease, are regulated under police power.

2. Activities that pose a threat only to the individual, such as riding a motorcycle without a helmet, are regulated under *parens patriae.*

3. Activities that pose a threat to both the individual and society, such as driving an automobile while intoxicated, can be regulated under both doctrines.

4. The nature and extent of the state intervention must be weighed against the seriousness of the harm to be avoided and the degree of interference with the rights of individuals. The following examples illustrate how such balancing may be done.

- **a. Mandatory quarantine** of individuals with contagious diseases like hepatitis A can be sustained legally because the disease is highly contagious through casual contact. Also, it has a finite, relatively brief period of contagion; thus, the quarantine would be for a limited time.
- **b.** As a general matter, public schools may not exclude a child with human immunodeficiency virus (HIV) infection or acquired immune deficiency syndrome (AIDS). The following factors support this policy decision.
  - **(1)** Present knowledge of the disease indicates that it cannot be spread by casual, nonsexual contact.

(2) The period of contagion is indefinite, potentially necessitating a lifelong quarantine.
(3) Education of children is highly valued.

C. **Police tests.** In certain cases, physical tests of individuals may be necessary to obtain evidence of criminal activity. Determining the ability of law enforcement officials to order these tests against the will of the person being tested requires knowledge of the constitutional rights of the individual. An **essential requirement for a test's constitutionality** is that it must be able to prove what it purports to prove. A test cannot be used unless it has demonstrable scientific basis; some debate as to its efficacy is tolerable, however. **Key factors in the law's allowance of compulsory tests** are the extent of the bodily invasion, the health risk to the subject, and the strength of the need to obtain evidence in this way.

1. **Blood tests** can be ordered by the police when there is reasonable cause to believe that a crime has been committed and necessary evidence can be obtained by a blood test.
   a. A **search warrant** must be obtained from a court if time and circumstances permit.
   b. If the time required to obtain a court order would result in the destruction of evidence, the need for a judicial warrant is obviated (*Schmerber v. California,* US Supreme Court, 1966).
   c. Blood tests are justifiable because the degree and duration of the bodily invasion are minor and the risk to the subject is minimal.

2. **Invasive tests** are less likely to be upheld as legal. In *Rochin v. California* (US Supreme Court, 1951), the forcible pumping of a suspect's stomach to retrieve drug capsules that he allegedly swallowed was held to be a violation of the suspect's rights to due process.

3. **Breath analysis (breathalyzer)** to determine intoxication is performed routinely and upheld by the courts. It is a simple, noninvasive, painless, and risk-free test.
   a. In some states, consent to such tests is made a condition of obtaining a driver's license; in others, the use of highways is taken as implied consent.
   b. Statutes treat a suspect's refusal to allow breath analysis as supporting the presumption that the suspect is guilty of intoxication.

4. **Urinalysis** is treated like breath analysis from the standpoint of individual rights and routinely is allowed because the test is noninvasive, harmless, and poses no risk to the subject.

5. **Skin and hair samples** may be removed for identification purposes.

6. **Semen samples** for rape and paternity identification pose a different and obvious problem. While removal of the samples poses no physical threat to the subject, the subject's cooperation obviously is needed. Thus, this test cannot be compelled without consideration of the subject's legal rights.

7. **Removal of bullets** cannot be compelled without a court order since the time required for this step would not result in the loss of evidence.
   a. The judge must consider medical testimony as to the possible danger to the subject. Removal of a bullet cannot be authorized if it would jeopardize the life or safety of the subject.
   b. Legal problems are often avoided by the subject's desire to have the bullet removed.

8. **Health care personnel** cannot be compelled to perform tests whether on police request or court order.
   a. Even if police have a legal right to order a particular test, private individuals have no obligation to assist them.
   b. Provided that the police appear to be within their rights in ordering a test, health care personnel are legally protected if they choose to participate.
   c. To guard against later challenges, health care personnel should insist on documentation of the police order before performing the test.
   d. If the subject consents to the test, a consent form signed by the subject should be obtained.

D. **Reporting requirements for diseases and incidents**

1. **Confidentiality of information** regarding patients' treatment must be scrupulously respected.
   a. Both professional and legal requirements exist to protect against unauthorized disclosure of information related to patient treatment.
   b. Health care personnel can be held liable for violation of the right of privacy, defamation, breach of trust, or breach of implied contract if improper disclosure of information results in harm to the patient.

2. **Disregard of confidentiality.** There are situations where revealing information about a patient's condition or treatment may be both ethically and legally required.
   a. The **Code of Medical Ethics of the American Medical Association** (AMA) recognizes and supports the disregard of patient confidentiality when there is a higher duty owed to the community or when the law requires the reporting of information. The following is an illustrative (not exhaustive) list of the types of information that must be reported in most states:
      (1) Gunshot, knife, and other wounds indicative of a crime or other breach of the peace
      (2) Communicable diseases, including most venereal diseases
      (3) Evidence of use or abuse of, or addiction to, drugs or other substances prohibited by law
      (4) Evidence of abuse or neglect of children, the elderly, animals, or other parties not capable of protecting themselves
      (5) Epilepsy or other neurologic, visual, or motor control disorders, which make it dangerous to operate a motor vehicle or other device, thereby posing a threat to the individual and society
   b. Health care personnel who reveal information without patients' knowledge or against their objection should observe the following cautions.
      (1) Disclosure of information should be made only to the proper authorities.
      (2) Disclosure should not go beyond what is required by the situation and the law. Confidences should be preserved as far as possible.
      (3) The reasons for and circumstances surrounding disclosure of confidential information should be documented carefully in a patient's record.
      (4) Professional and personal ethics, as well as practical considerations, may dictate telling the patient that disclosures will be made to the proper authorities. In the absence of specific statutes, however, there is no legal duty to make such a disclosure to the patient.
   c. **Civil immunity** (i.e., protection from a lawsuit charging defamation) is granted to health care providers who disclose patient confidences in good faith with reasonable justification. Disclosure is not protected if it is unnecessary or is motivated by malice or a desire to embarrass the patient.
   d. A growing number of states requires, pursuant to case law, that **mental health professionals** (and presumably other health care providers) report reliable indications that a mentally disturbed individual intends to do harm to an identifiable individual or group.
      (1) *Tarasoff v. Regents of the University of California* (California, 1976) held that a psychotherapist had a duty to warn the intended murder victim of one of his patients.
      (2) The *Tarasoff* decision, and others following its reasoning, is highly controversial because of the chilling effect it may have on counselor-patient communications and because of the burden it puts on counselors to distinguish between patients' idle talk and real threats of harm.

E. **Discrimination** in employment based on physical condition is strictly limited under the federal **Americans with Disabilities Act of 1990**.

1. This Act covers employment agencies, labor organizations, and employers, except for those with fewer than 15 employees, in industries affecting interstate commerce.

2. Covered entities cannot discriminate against a "qualified individual with a disability" because of that disability. A qualified individual is one who can "perform the essential functions of the employment position" or who can do so if the employer makes a "reasonable accommodation."

3. Asymptomatic HIV infection would not render an individual unqualified unless that individual would "pose a direct threat to the health or safety of other individuals in the workplace."

4. In addition to employment, the Act also prohibits discrimination in "public accommodations," defined to include hospitals and medical offices. Thus, although the Act helps to secure access to health care services for those with HIV, it includes no provision for financing such services.

BIBLIOGRAPHY

Bierig J, Portman R: The Health Care Quality Improvement Act of 1986. *St. Louis U Law J* 32:977, 1988.

Danner D, Sagall E: Medicolegal causation: a source of professional misunderstanding. *Am J Law Med* 3:303–308, 1977.

Eisenberg J, Rosoff A: Physician responsibility for the cost of unnecessary medical services. *N Engl J Med* 299:76, 1978.

Gosfield A: Navigating through JCAH's new quality assurance and medical staff standards. *Health Aff (Millwood)* 4:3, 1987.

Price S: The sinking of the "captain of the ship." *J Legal Med* 10:323–356, 1989.

Roth M, Levin L: The dilemma of *Tarasoff:* should psychotherapists protect their patients or society? *Law Med Health Care* 11:104, 1983.

Shoenberger A: Medical malpractice injury: causation and valuation of the loss of a chance to survive. *J Law Med* 6:51–84, 1985.

Symposium on AIDS and the rights and obligations of health care workers. *Md Law Rev* 48:1–245, 1989.

COURT CASES

American Hospital Association v Schweiker, 721 F 2d 170 (US Court of Appeals, 7th Circuit, 1983)

Brophy v New England Sinai Hospital, Inc, 497 NE 2d 626 (Massachusetts, 1986)

Canterbury v Spence, 464 F 2d 772 (US Court of Appeals, DC Circuit, 1972)

In re Conroy, 486 A 2d 1209 (New Jersey, 1985)

Cruzan v Director, Missouri Department of Health, 110 SCt 2841 (US Supreme Court, 1990), certiorari denied 383 US 946 (1966)

Darling v Charleston Community Memorial Hospital, 211 NE 2d 253 (Illinois, 1965)

In re Eichner, 420 NE 2d 64 (New York, 1981)

Gates v Jensen, 595 P 2d 919 (Washington, 1979)

Hall v Hilbun, 466 So 2d 856 (Mississippi, 1985)

Hawkins v McGee, 146 A 641 (New Hampshire, 1929)

Helling v Carey, 519 P 2d 981 (Washington, 1974)

Natanson v Kline, 350 P 2d 1093 (Kansas, 1960)

O'Neill v Montefiore Hospital, 202 NYS 2d 436 (New York, 1960)

Patrick v Burget, 106 SCt 1658 (US Supreme Court, 1988)

In re Quinlan, 355 A 2d 647 (New Jersey, 1976)

Rochin v California, 342 US 165 (US Supreme Court, 1951)

Salgo v Stanford University Hospital, 317 P 2d 170 (California, 1957)

Sarchett v Blue Shield, 729 P 2d 267 (California, 1987)

Schloendorff v Society of New York Hospital, 105 NE 92 (New York, 1914)

Schmerber v California, 348 US 757 (US Supreme Court, 1966)

School Board of Nassau County v Arline, 480 US 273 (US Supreme Court, 1987)

Sullivan v O'Connor, 296 NE 2d 183 (Massachusetts, 1973)

Superintendent of Belchertown State School v Saikewicz, 370 NE 2d 417 (Massachusetts, 1977)

Tarasoff v Regents of the University of California, 551 P 2d 334 (California, 1976)

Thompson v Sun City Community Hospital, Inc, 688 P 2d 605 (Arizona, 1984)

Truman v Thomas, 611 P 2d 902 (California, 1980)

Wilmington General Hospital v Manlove, 174 A 2d 135 (Delaware, 1961)

STATUTES

Americans with Disabilities Act of 1990, PL 101-336, 104 Stat 327
Health Care Quality Improvement Act of 1986, 42 USC §§11101–11152
Hill-Burton Act of 1945, 42 USC §291
Consolidated Omnibus Budget Reconciliation Act of 1985, 42 USC §1395 *et seq*

STUDY QUESTIONS

Directions: Each of the numbered items or incomplete statements in this section is followed by answers or by completions of the statement. Select the **one** lettered answer or completion that is **best** in each case.

1. The Anglo-American common law system places great emphasis on adherence to precedent. Which of the following Latin phrases is used to summarize this principle?

(A) *Res ipsa loquitur*
(B) *Stare decisis*
(C) *Parens patriae*
(D) *Quid pro quo*
(E) *Habeas corpus*

2. Which of the following statements regarding the plaintiff's burden of proof in a medical malpractice suit is true?

(A) The plaintiff is required to prove the material elements of his or her case beyond a reasonable doubt
(B) The plaintiff is allowed to present proof to a jury only if the defendant agrees; otherwise, the case is heard by a judge
(C) Once the plaintiff demonstrates injury in the course of receiving medical care, the burden of proof shifts to the defendant to show lack of negligence
(D) The plaintiff cannot recover damages, even though the defendant's negligence is clear, unless it is proved that the defendant's negligence was the proximate cause of the plaintiff's injury
(E) The plaintiff is relieved of the burden of proof if the court feels the defendant's acts are sufficiently offensive to deserve public censure

3. Which of the following legal doctrines may be used, in appropriate circumstances, to relieve the plaintiff of the burden of introducing expert testimony to prove the defendant's negligence?

(A) Burden of proof
(B) Hearsay
(C) *Res ipsa loquitur*
(D) Conspiracy of silence
(E) Contributory negligence

4. Which of the following is a provision of the Health Care Quality Improvement Act of 1986?

(A) Health care institutions are required to consult the National Practitioner Data Bank when granting staff privileges and periodically thereafter
(B) Emergency rooms must treat patients regardless of the patient's ability to pay
(C) Physicians are granted immunity from civil liberties for injuries caused by the physician's good faith attempts to render care in emergency situations
(D) Physicians must disclose all information that a reasonably prudent patient would consider material to the decision to accept or reject a proposed treatment
(E) Standards of reasonable care were established at the federal level

5. The "antidumping" provisions of the Consolidated Omnibus Budget Reconciliation Act of 1985 (COBRA) seek to assure access to hospital services for which of the following groups?

(A) Incompetent or unconscious patients
(B) Medicare beneficiaries
(C) Medicaid eligibles
(D) All emergency patients

6. All of the following are implied contracts EXCEPT

(A) dining in a restaurant
(B) taking a cab
(C) signing an apartment lease
(D) consulting with a physician as a patient

1-B	4-A
2-D	5-D
3-C	6-C

7. All of the following statements regarding the duty of health care providers to report to the authorities information learned in the course of treating patients are true EXCEPT

(A) the basic, *legal* principle is that patients' confidences must be respected unless there is compelling reason to divulge them
(B) the AMA's Code of Medical Ethics prohibits physicians from divulging patients' confidences
(C) most states require that providers report the treatment of conditions, such as gunshot or knife wounds, that are indicative of a crime or other breach of the peace
(D) some states require mental health professionals to report to the authorities indications that a mentally disturbed individual plans to harm an identifiable individual or group
(E) civil immunity protecting those who divulge patients' confidences is lost if the disclosure was not necessary and was prompted by the provider's desire to cause harm or embarrassment to the subject of the disclosure

Directions: Each item below contains four suggested answers of which **one or more** is correct. Choose the answer

A if **1, 2, and 3** are correct
B if **1 and 3** are correct
C if **2 and 4** are correct
D if **4** is correct
E if **1, 2, 3, and 4** are correct

8. The starting point for the statute of limitations applicable to medical malpractice suits in United States jurisdictions is the date that the

(1) alleged malpractice took place
(2) alleged malpractice was discovered by the patient
(3) alleged malpractice was discovered, or should have been discovered, by the patient
(4) the physician-patient relationship was terminated

9. In civil suits, punitive damages are sometimes awarded for which of the following reasons?

(1) To collect additional money to support the court system
(2) To punish the wrongdoer for an act that is particularly culpable
(3) To allow a token recovery in cases where the defendant's wrongdoing has been established, but the plaintiff has not been able to prove that he or she suffered any monetary loss
(4) To deter others from committing the same kind of socially undesirable act as committed by the defendant

---

7-B
8-E
9-C

SUMMARY OF DIRECTIONS

A	B	C	D	E
1,2,3 only	1,3 only	2,4 only	4 only	All are correct

10. Expert testimony is required to establish a defendant's negligence in medical malpractice cases unless the

(1) case involves specialty care rendered by a board-certified specialist
(2) court is able to locate a recognized medical text from which the relevant information can be obtained
(3) plaintiff is unable to obtain an expert witness willing to testify against the defendant
(4) care rendered by a defendant was so obviously negligent that a lay jury can discern it without expert testimony

11. A physician's duty to render care to a patient is described by which of the following statements?

(1) By accepting a license to practice medicine, physicians implicitly undertake that they will serve all patients in urgent need of care when none is procurable from another available source
(2) Physicians have no duty to accept someone as a patient, even in dire emergencies
(3) Good samaritan statutes in many states require physicians to come to the aid of persons threatened with serious and urgent medical problems
(4) Physicians can be held liable for abandonment if they accept a patient and later discontinue care without being discharged by the patient or giving the patient adequate notice

12. Privately owned and operated hospitals may be required to render care to all individuals, including those they might otherwise choose not to serve, by the

(1) reliance of the public on the hospital's custom of providing emergency services
(2) federal Hill-Burton program for financing of hospital capital expenditures
(3) Medicare and Medicaid amendments of 1985, which require participating hospitals to maintain emergency facilities and treat all individuals presenting with emergency medical conditions or in active labor
(4) federal tax laws governing the grant of tax-exempt status to nonprofit hospitals

13. Which of the following tests can the police order a criminal suspect to undergo without first obtaining a court order if the time required to get a warrant would cause information to be lost?

(1) Blood sample
(2) Urinalysis
(3) Breath analysis
(4) Removal of a bullet

10-D
11-C
12-A
13-A

Directions: Each group of items in this section consists of lettered options followed by a set of numbered items. For each item, select the **one** lettered option that is most closely associated with it. Each lettered option may be selected once, more than once, or not at all.

Questions 14–17

For each concept or doctrine listed below, select the legal term that most closely represents it.

(A) *Parens patriae*
(B) *Res ipsa loquitur*
(C) Substituted judgment
(D) Police power
(E) Therapeutic privilege

14. The government has the legal authority to take protective measures to safeguard individuals who are incompetent or otherwise unable to care for themselves

15. When decisions are made on behalf of unconscious or incompetent patients, care must be taken to assure that the decision is what the patients would have chosen for themselves

16. The plaintiff is relieved of the burden of introducing expert testimony to establish the defendant's negligence because a lay jury can discern the lack of care without expert guidance

17. While physicians are generally required to disclose information to their patients concerning the diagnosis, treatment, risks, alternatives, and prognosis, this obligation is waived if the physician feels it is in the patient's best interest to withhold information

Questions 18–20

Match the test definition with the appropriate test.

(A) Subjective test
(B) Documented test
(C) Relative test
(D) Limited objective test
(E) Pure objective test

18. Used when the patient has expressly stated his wishes at some previous time

19. Used when the patient's wishes can be inferred from known religious, ethical, or lifestyle beliefs

20. Used when no information is available from which to infer what the particular patient would have wanted

Questions 21–24

For each of the legal concepts or doctrines described below, select the term that most accurately describes it.

(A) Corporate negligence
(B) Ostensible agency
(C) *Respondeat superior*
(D) Vicarious liability
(E) Independent contractor

21. If an independent contractor reasonably appears to be working as an employee of a health care institution in a particular incident, the institution can be held liable for that person's improper actions

22. Under appropriate circumstances, one party can be held legally responsible for the wrongful acts of another

23. An employer is held liable for the torts of its employees committed within the scope of the employment

24. A hospital may be held responsible to take reasonable steps to assure that those who practice in or through the institution, even if they are independent contractors and not employees, are qualified to practice safely

---

14-A	17-E	20-E	23-C
15-C	18-A	21-B	24-A
16-B	19-D	22-D	

ANSWERS AND EXPLANATIONS

1. The answer is B *[II A 1, 2].*
Stare decisis means "let the decision stand." It is believed that justice is best served by equal treatment —that is, by having the law applied consistently in all similar cases. Existing precedents are generally followed by other courts at the same level or at lower levels in the same jurisdiction unless the case can be distinguished on its facts from the one that established the precedent or situations have changed in such a way as to make the precedent no longer appropriate.

2. The answer is D *[III B 1 a–d].*
An individual can sue for damages as a result of alleged failures in medical care. However, to recover damages, the plaintiff must prove by a preponderance of evidence that a duty of care (an obligation recognized by the law, the breaching of which is subject to legal sanctions) was breached, that dereliction (i.e., that the defendant performed significantly below the legally required standard of care) existed, that damage (i.e., that the plaintiff was harmed) resulted from a failure of medical care, and that the defendant's negligence was the proximate cause of the plaintiff's injuries. Proof "beyond a reasonable doubt" is required only in criminal cases. A given situation can be the basis for both a civil and criminal suit.

3. The answer is C *[III B 3 a].*
Res ipsa loquitur, Latin for "the thing speaks for itself," applies when an occurrence is so unusual that a court can infer negligence from the mere fact of its happening. All courts hold that, at the least, when this doctrine is applicable, the plaintiff does not have to produce expert testimony to establish that there was negligence. Some courts hold that a rebuttable presumption of the defendant's negligence is established, shifting the burden of proof to the defendant.

4. The answer is A *[III D 5 a].*
The federal Health Care Quality Improvement Act of 1986 requires hospitals and other health entities, state licensure agencies, and malpractice liability insurers to report to a national registry (the National Practitioner Data Bank) any incidents raising substantial questions about a physician's ability to practice medicine safely. Institutions must consult this registry when granting staff privileges and periodically thereafter. Civil immunity is granted to health care entities that engage in peer review if prescribed due process safeguards for the practitioner are observed. Suits challenging peer review and related staff privilege denials are also blocked (*Patrick v. Burget,* U.S. Supreme Court, 1988).

5. The answer is D *[VII B 3].*
The Consolidated Omnibus Budget Reconciliation Act of 1985 (COBRA) requires hospitals to serve all patients presenting with an emergency medical condition and those in active labor. These "antidumping" provisions apply to all hospitals that participate in Medicare and Medicaid, but the provision of care obligation applies to *all* patients, not just to the beneficiaries of these programs.

6. The answer is C *[IV B 1, 2].*
Signing an apartment lease is an express contract because it is stated in words, in this case written, but they could also be spoken. An implied contract is one in which the agreement of a party is not expressly stated but may be inferred by the party's conduct. When one enters a cab, goes to a restaurant, or sees a physician, it is assumed that certain services will be provided and that the recipient of these services will, in turn, provide remuneration for the services.

7. The answer is B *[VIII D 1, 2].*
The American Medical Association's (AMA's) Code of Medical Ethics places great importance on the maintenance of patients' confidences; however, the AMA does recognize situations in which revealing information about a patient's condition or treatment may be both ethically and legally required. A patient's confidentiality can be disregarded when there is a higher duty owed to the community or when the law requires the reporting. Disclosures should be made only to the proper authorities, and they should not go beyond what is required by the situation and by the law. Civil immunity is granted to health care providers who disclose patients' confidences in good faith and with reasonable justification; however, disclosures are not protected if they are unnecessary or are motivated by malice or a desire to embarrass the patient.

8. The answer is E (all) *[II F 3 a–d].*
The statute of limitations is a procedural rule that establishes a maximum period of time during which a legal suit may be initiated. The beginning of the statutory period for medical malpractice suits in the United States is generally defined as the date: (1) the alleged malpractice took place, (2) the alleged malpractice was discovered by the patient, (3) the alleged malpractice was discovered or should have been discovered by the patient, and (4) the physician-patient relationship was terminated. Definition (1) is the

simplest, but perhaps the most unfair to the plaintiff if the statutory period is running against him while he is unaware that there has been an act of malpractice. Definition (2) guards against the unfairness to the plaintiff but is arguably unfair to the potential defendant, since the plaintiff (patient) could be lax in investigating symptoms that would lead to the discovery of an error in treatment. Definition (3) is favored by most jurisdictions as the fairest, although it may be difficult to determine when a reasonably diligent patient should have discovered the malpractice. Definition (4), which is used in very few jurisdictions, assumes that while the patient is still under the care of the same physician, it is unfair for the statutory period to run because it is unlikely that the patient would discover that he has been the victim of malpractice.

9. The answer is C (2, 4) *[II G 1 c].*
Punitive damages, that is, damages in excess of normal compensation, may be awarded to punish a defendant for an act that is particularly culpable and to deter wrongdoers from acting similarly in the future. When punitive damages are awarded, the defendant must pay the plaintiff (not the state to support the court system), along with any other types of damages awarded. A token recovery in cases where the defendant's wrongdoing has been established but when the plaintiff is unable to prove a monetary loss as a result describes the situation in which *nominal* (not punitive) damages are awarded.

10. The answer is D (4) *[III B 1 a (1), (2), 2 a (1), (2), b, 3 a (1), (2)].*
In cases where the court can see that "the matter speaks for itself" (*res ipsa loquitur*), most jurisdictions will excuse the plaintiff from introducing expert testimony to establish the appropriate professional standard of care. Specialty care may have a bearing upon the standard of care to be applied—that is, a local versus a national standard—but does not address how the plaintiff goes about proving what that standard is. Some states allow the plaintiff to use medical texts in lieu of expert testimony to establish a point about the standard of care, but the burden of proof lies with the plaintiff. Under our adversary system, the court, with very rare exceptions, does not undertake independent research to answer questions upon which a subject piece of litigation turns. When the plaintiff is unable to secure an expert witness—perhaps because of the conspiracy of silence—it generally means that the plaintiff's suit will fail as a result of the plaintiff's inability to provide the burden of proof. The doctrine of *res ipsa loquitur* provides the only major exception to this unfortunate fact of life.

11. The answer is C (2, 4) *[VII A 1–3].*
Physicians have no inherent duty to take on any patients or render care except at their own choosing. Good samaritan statutes offer civil immunity to physicians who render care under difficult, emergency conditions, but they do not compel physicians to render such care. Once physicians have accepted a patient, they cannot unilaterally discontinue the relationship, unless the patient is given sufficient notice to allow the patient to secure needed assistance from another source.

12. The answer is A (1, 2, 3) *[VII B 1–6].*
Private hospitals, while under no inherent common law duty to accept patients or render care in emergencies, are encouraged under certain circumstances to render care to individuals they might otherwise choose not to serve. For example, a hospital that maintains an emergency department whose existence is known to the general public undertakes an obligation to provide emergency care to those individuals presenting for treatment in an emergency situation. Medicare and Medicaid programs have conditions for participation, including the requirement that general acute-care facilities maintain emergency treatment facilities and that these facilities treat *all* patients presenting with an emergency medical condition or in active labor, not just the beneficiaries of these programs. The Hill-Burton free-care obligation requires that hospitals constructed or improved with federal funds must provide a reasonable volume of free or reduced-cost care to those unable to pay. While rules governing tax-exempt status consider the maintenance by hospitals of emergency facilities open to the general public, they do not require tax-exempt hospitals to admit all patients regardless of their ability to pay for care.

13. The answer is A (1, 2, 3) *[VIII C 1–8].*
In certain cases, physical tests may be necessary to obtain evidence of criminal activity. However, if a test is painful, invasive, or poses a significant risk to the patient, it must be authorized by a court order. Both breath analysis and urinalysis are painless, noninvasive tests that pose no risk to the subject and, therefore, can be ordered by the police without a warrant. The police would be justified in proceeding without a warrant to get a blood sample if the information sought might be lost if the drawing of blood were delayed to obtain a court order. Removal of a bullet is subject to stringent safeguards to protect the health and inviolability of the suspect. A bullet may be removed without a court order only if the subject's life is in danger.

14–17. The answers are: 14-A *[VIII A 2],* **15-C** *[VI C],* **16-B** *[III B 3 a (2)],* **17-E** *[V E 1–3].*
Parens patriae ("the state as parent") is applied to individuals who are unable to care for themselves. Under these circumstances, the state is both empowered and obliged to take protective action—that is, to assume the role of parent.

The Supreme Court of New Jersey in the *Claire Conroy* case established elaborate criteria for determining the wishes of the patient. Thus, under the doctrine of substituted judgment, care must be taken to assure that any decisions that are made for unconscious or incompetent patients, particularly in regard to care, be as close as possible to those the patients would have chosen for themselves.

Under the doctrine of *res ipsa loquitur* ("the thing speaks for itself"), a judge or lay jury may infer the defendant's negligence even in the absence of expert testimony. Thus, the plaintiff is spared the burden of producing evidence of negligence, which can be difficult as a result of a conspiracy of silence among physicians.

The exercise of therapeutic privilege, the exception to the physician's duty to disclose information, must be related to properly documented concerns that the physician has about the mental or emotional status of the patient. A general policy of not disclosing information to patients because of a presumed hypersensitivity is not an acceptable basis for this privilege.

18–20. The answers are: 18-A, 19-D, 20-E *[VI C 2 c (1)–(3)].*
The substituted judgment doctrine attempts to respect patients' rights by choosing the treatment approach for unconscious or incompetent patients that they would choose if able to do so. Obviously, the best situation for applying substituted judgment is when one knows what the patient would have chosen. The "subjective test" applies when the patient has expressed an opinion at some time on the specific question. The "limited objective test" applies when the patient has not expressly stated any wishes on this point, but there are other known factors, such as the patient's religious, ethical, or lifestyle beliefs, from which the patient's wishes can reasonably be inferred. The "pure objective test" is used when no information is available from which to infer what the particular patient would have wanted. Inferences must be drawn based on what the "average" person would desire in such a situation.

21–24. The answers are: 21-B, 22-D, 23-C, 24-A *[III D 1, 2].*
Vicarious liability occurs when one party is held liable because another does something improper. Under the vicarious liability principle of *respondeat superior* (Latin for "let the master answer"), the employer or institution is responsible for torts committed by its employees within the scope of their employment. Under the "ostensible agency," or "apparent agency," doctrine of vicarious liability, an individual is treated legally as an employee of an institution if it reasonably appears to the patient that he is such. To avoid liability, the institution must make the patient understand the independent contractor status of the person in question.

Corporate negligence is an evolving legal theory by which an institution may be held directly (not vicariously) liable for a tort committed by an independent contractor (i.e., a staff physician) practicing in or through the institution.

15
Medical Ethics

Thomas K. McElhinney

I. DEFINITIONS

A. Ethics is a discipline that includes the study of ideals for human conduct and an understanding of the moral life, in which actions are judged as right or wrong and persons and institutions are judged as praiseworthy or blameworthy. Ethics may be seen as a subdivision of **philosophy** or of **theology**. Usually, one position is given dominance over the other, depending on the individual's own bias.

1. **Philosophical ethics** is concerned with the study of the moral life and with analysis of ethical judgments.
2. **Theological ethics** is the study of moral behavior, which provides judgments of proper conduct, drawing from specific religious sources.

B. Divisions of ethics. Like many disciplines, ethics has historical, theoretical, and practical dimensions (Figure 15-1).

1. **Descriptive ethics** is concerned with analyses of facts obtained from anthropological, historical, psychological, or sociological studies. Such comparative studies and cross-cultural inquiries are conducted without imposing judgments of the relative merits of the various systems.
2. **Normative ethics** concerns inquiry into actions and their worth.
   a. **General normative ethics** discusses principles of human conduct and how evaluations are to be effected. For example, arguments may be generated in favor of decisions by consequences or by the inherent rightness or wrongness of certain actions (see II).
   b. **Applied normative ethics** concerns the judgments of specific moral problems. It includes medical ethics, legal ethics, business ethics, and other professional ethics.
3. **Metaethics** is the study of the meaning and justification of ethical discourse and the nature of moral concepts. It is concerned with questions such as "Why should one be good?" or, even more basically, "What does good mean?"

C. Moral and nonmoral values or goods. Both moral and nonmoral values are used in ethical analysis.

1. **Moral values or goods** are judgments of conduct, character, or actions of individuals, groups, or institutions (e.g., a saintly person, a despicable act).
2. **Nonmoral values or goods** are distinctions applied to estimates of the common worth of objects (e.g., a valuable painting, a good computer).
3. **Value levels** (adapted from Jurrit Bergsma and Raymond S. Duff, 1980) include personal values, group values, and society's values. Ethical conflict arises when any one value conflicts with another.
   a. **Personal values** are the interpretations of worth that an individual holds.
      (1) Although people may share many views about the relative merits of specific actions, even identical twins express different values. Personal values appear to be formed early in life and often are strongly held.
      (2) When an individual acts differently from the other members of a group, it may be because her personal values cannot accommodate to the mood of the others. In a value sense, each person truly hears "a different drummer."

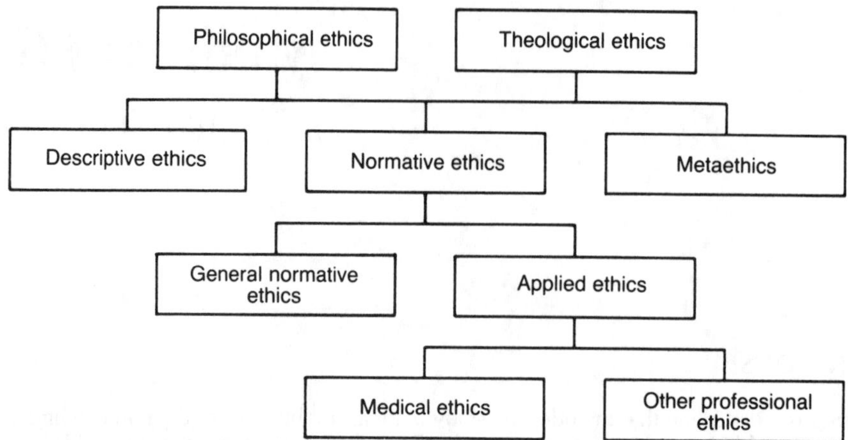

Figure 15-1. Divisions of ethics.

b. **Group values** are the norms of family, work, or organization that an individual adopts.
   (1) By association with others, an individual comes to accept shared values, perhaps the "good of the team," rather than his own personal desires. There is no conflict when the individual's own values correspond to those of the group, which is most often the case. An individual opposed to abortion would have least conflict in a hospital setting where the policy was not to do abortions.
   (2) Unfortunately, group values change. A new supervisor may create policies that lead to conflicts for employees who had enjoyed congruence between their personal and group values.

c. **Society's values** are general norms that are applicable to an individual or a group. The individual, or the group with which an individual is associated, may experience value conflict with a larger framework of values. In medicine, for example, government or other third-party payment plans may require financial loss unacceptable to a hospital (an individual's group) as well as treatment differences unacceptable to an individual physician's personal values. As value disruption increases, institutions are paralyzed, and individuals experience heightened stress.

D. Virtues and vices

1. **Virtues** are desirable character traits (i.e., they are a form of positive valuation about the moral worth of the agent).
   a. **Compassion** is a cardinal virtue of a health professional; it implies the ability to "suffer with" a patient.
   b. **Integrity** of a health professional is expected by a patient; it is a virtue that demands honesty and allows the communication of personal matters that ordinarily would not be shared with those closest to the patient.
   c. **Example.** However much a physician may deplore certain behaviors, either for their supposed moral deficiencies or for their association with physical and emotional debility, the virtuous physician does not condemn the individual nor rejoice in the pain and suffering that that individual's actions may have incurred.

2. **Vices** are undesirable character traits but not necessarily simply the opposite of virtues (a debated issue in moral philosophy). **Examples** include:
   a. **Greed** that might put a physician's financial interests before a patient's health through an unnecessary operation
   b. **Deceit** that would lead a medical student to prepare inaccurate reports to cover up a failure to provide care

E. Duties and rights

1. **Duties** are moral obligations owed by an individual, group, or institution to another individual, group, or institution.

2. **Rights** generally are correlative to duties and are claims by an individual, group, or institution on another individual, group, or institution.
   a. One consideration about rights is the strength of the claim; that is, is this particular right imposing enough to make others respond?
   b. It is also a problem to judge between competing rights, such as that of the woman to freedom with her body and the fetal claim to life. Even if both rights are believed to exist, their relative strengths are much debated.

F. **Sources of morality.** One or more sources may be drawn upon in any ethical situation. These sources operate as the basis for rights (and duties) and for the development of principles. The following are commonly used sources for moral opinion.

1. **Social contract** is the theory that specific rights may be drawn from implicit and explicit agreements by members of a society. This theory locates morality in **human custom**.

2. **Natural law** in morality may be regarded as the source of universal norms for human conduct. This theory holds that these norms can be discovered by **reason** and by an **understanding of human nature**.

3. **Divine command** is the belief that God **reveals** (directly or through inspired scripture) norms by which humans shall live.

4. **Individual insight** is the **direct perception** by the individual of what is right either through intuition or common sense.

II. NORMATIVE ETHICAL THEORIES.

Specific methods for ethical decision making center on either the consequences that are expected (**teleology**) or the nature of the actions themselves (**deontology**). Historically, many ethicists have argued that the two positions are exclusive (i.e., that dependence on either the results or the nature of what one does is, in the end, determinative).

A. **Deontological theories** involve **duty-based ethics,** in which right actions are determined independently of the moral goods or the consequences of those actions.

1. **Act deontology**
   a. **Definition.** Act deontology holds that no rules can apply to specific judgments, as each situation is unique.
      (1) Each act is evaluated as a particular event according to its rightness or wrongness. When emphasized as "decision," this position is an existentialist ethic, that is, one made from the individual perception of the situation without references that others may validate other than through their own experiences.
      (2) This ethical position is **subjective**.
   b. **Drawbacks**
      (1) Act deontology provides no ethical guidelines.
      (2) It is based on individual perception (it is more emotive than rational).
      (3) It ignores the usefulness of rules.

2. **Rule deontology** is the more popular deontological position.
   a. **Definition.** Rule deontology holds that a rule or rules may be applied to decide ethical problems.
      (1) **Monistic rule** deontology holds that one rule dominates all other rules. An example of such a rule would be Immanuel Kant's (1785) practical imperative "So act as to treat humanity, whether in thine own person or in that of any other, in every case as an end withal, never as a means only."
      (2) **Pluralistic rule** deontology holds that many moral rules exist (e.g., natural rules, the ten commandments) and that these rules must guide proper ethical decision making.
      (3) ***Prima facie* duties**—a modern modification of rule deontology—makes a distinction between those rules (duties) that seem appropriate for a certain situation and what may actually be best to do (the actual duty).
   b. **Drawbacks**
      (1) With rule deontology, there is no agreement on one primary rule.
      (2) Judging conflicts among rules is difficult.

B. **Teleological theories** are forms of **consequence-based ethics,** in which right actions are determined by the moral goods (results) produced without regard to the nature of the action.

1. **Egoism**
   a. **Definition.** Egoist theory holds that acts must be judged on the individual's best long-term interest. The good of the actor may be pleasure (hedonistic), but it also may be knowledge, power, or self-interest.
   b. **Drawbacks**
      (1) Egoist theory provides no guides or rules to settle conflicts. There are no means by which to decide what is best.
      (2) There are no general principles to validate individual interest as primary human conduct.

2. **Act utilitarianism** avoids the weaknesses of egoism by moving beyond self-interest.
   a. **Definition.** Act utilitarianism theory promotes moral conduct that produces the greatest balance of good over evil. A balance of good and evil is applied to every action.
   b. **Drawbacks**
      (1) With act utilitarianism, it is difficult to assess consequences. Further, when two acts have equal consequences, they may still differ according to rightness of some principle.
      (2) Act utilitarianism ignores the usefulness of rules.

3. **Rule utilitarianism**
   a. **Definition.** Rule utilitarianism theory uses rules to assess the balance of good and evil. Thus, there is conformity of actions to valuable rules.
   b. **Drawbacks**
      (1) With rule utilitarianism, there is no way to judge between contradictory rules with equal consequences.
      (2) The greatest good for the greatest number may be quite unjust to a minority.

C. **Mixed ethical theory.** Many modern writers attempt to mix the two extremes of ethical theory, attending to the "rightness" of an action in terms of its nature and the "goodness of the act" in terms of what will be accomplished (although right and good may be used in reverse fashion). Even the most extreme opponents of deontological or of teleological thinking often have great respect for the values of their opponent's views.

1. **Advantages of a mixed theory**
   a. The best moral act will attend to traditional norms and values and will also achieve agreeable results.
   b. It is especially true that persons seeking to do what appears to be a right action also hope for positive results. However convinced they may be of the correctness of their position, they are cognizant of unpleasant consequences and do not desire that suffering may ensue.
   c. A virtuous person, convinced of the rightness of a position, does not rejoice in the misery of others (see I D).

2. **Drawback.** A mixed view does not provide a final answer as to what will be the deciding factor to resolve a particular ethical problem.

III. **MEDICAL ETHICS** is a branch of applied normative ethics supported by philosophical and theological presuppositions. It involves the study of general problems relating to health care, health care institutions, and biomedical research. While many issues are difficult to resolve because of conflicting social, political, and economic pressures, there is considerable agreement about the general values that buttress the health profession. Moral disagreements often are amenable to rational discussion. The major ethical debates currently in medicine have arisen from new technologies, increased respect for patient's rights, and financial restraints. Interest in medical ethics will remain strong as long as significant value differences exist and as long as ethics addresses the concrete concerns of patients and practitioners.

A. **Background.** The teaching of modern medical ethics began in the early 1960s. At present, virtually every medical school and several medical specialty boards require courses in medical ethics, largely because:

1. **New medical technologies** (e.g., genetic screening, life-support equipment) challenge traditional patterns of care.

2. **Demands of public interest groups** create new responses from the health care professions to questions concerning patients' rights.

3. Physicians and other health care professionals are concerned about the **moral climate** of their own fields.

B. Moral questions in medicine. Virtually every contact between a patient and a health professional contains moral dimensions, especially those contacts that place demands on the health professional. Most often the values of the patient, the health care worker, and the sponsoring institution conform, and there is no moral conflict. However, when values conflict, there is a need for medical ethical reasoning. The anatomy of moral conflict is best observed in an analysis of value levels.

1. **Physician's values.** Each physician has personal values; values formed at the level of practice partnership, service, or hospital; and values shared with other members of professional organizations and other general medical groups. At times, demands from various levels may cause the physician internal conflict. When, for example, a physician who is opposed to abortion is a member of a medical group that is working for abortion rights, then the resultant pull of values between personal belief and professional loyalty is a subject for medical ethics.

2. **Patient's values.** Since patients also hold value claims at three levels similar to those of the physician, the possibilities for conflict are significantly increased. A physician opposed to abortion who practices at a hospital supporting abortion rights may argue for a woman's right to have an abortion against the wishes of the patient's spouse and parents. Although not agreeing with the hospital policy nor the woman's choice, the physician may feel a moral duty to represent both value levels (the physician's group values and the patient's personal values) to a spouse and parents whose values coincide with the physician's personal values.

C. Professional codes of conduct. Almost all health professions, including many of the various medical specialties, have their own codes of conduct. Many codes, including the principles of the American Medical Association (AMA), are interpreted through judicial reviews conducted by the sponsoring organization and published for the benefit of the members.

1. **The Hippocratic Oath,** once widely subscribed to by graduating medical students, has been revised in favor of new interpretations of desirable medical behavior. While outdated in many ways, the major principles of the oath, which are the key components of most medical moral codes, are to:
   a. Do no harm
   b. Keep confidential the information learned through one's work

2. **The AMA's Principles of Medical Ethics** is a statement of professional principles that is revised periodically. The articles of the most recent AMA code of ethics is shown in Figure 15-2. A major contrast between the AMA's Principles of Medical Ethics and the Hippocratic Oath is a **shift in the balance of rights** between physician and patient.
   a. **Physicians' rights** assumed in the Hippocratic Oath are now spelled out, especially in the

I. A physician shall be dedicated to providing competent medical service with compassion and respect for human dignity.

II. A physician shall deal honestly with patients and colleagues, and strive to expose those physicians deficient in character or competence, or who engage in fraud or deception.

III. A physician shall respect the law and also recognize a responsibility to seek changes in those requirements which are contrary to the best interests of the patient.

IV. A physician shall respect the rights of patients, of colleagues, and of other health professionals, and shall safeguard patient confidences within the constraints of the law.

V. A physician shall continue to study, apply and advance scientific knowledge, make relevant information available to patients, colleagues, and the public, obtain consultation, and use the talents of other health professionals when indicated.

VI. A physician shall, in the provision of appropriate patient care, except in emergencies, be free to choose whom to serve, with whom to associate, and the environment in which to provide medical services.

VII. A physician shall recognize a responsibility to participate in activities contributing to an improved community.

Figure 15-2. Articles of the American Medical Association's Principles of Medical Ethics. (Reprinted from American Medical Association: Principles of Medical Ethics. In *Current Opinions,* Prepared by the Council on Ethical and Judicial Affairs. Chicago, AMA, 1989, p ix.)

AMA's statement regarding "whom to serve, with whom to associate, and the environment in which to provide medical services" (Article VI).

b. **Patients' rights** to protection from sexual abuse and from gossip about their situation and to choose certain interventions considered wrong for the Hippocratic physician (e.g., surgery, abortion, use of "poisons") have been extended.

3. **Patient's bills of rights,** which appear in a variety of forms, bring the patient more fully into the decision-making process than was allowed within the philosophy of the Hippocratic Oath. For example, patients' rights enumerated in the List of Patient's Rights in California (Section 70707 of California Administrative Code, Revised November 1984) include:
   a. The right to participate actively in decisions regarding one's medical care
   b. The right to receive reasonable responses to requests for service
   c. The right to an explanation of the medical bill, regardless of the source of payment

IV. ETHICAL DECISION MAKING IN THE CLINICAL SETTING.

Applied medical ethics seeks to relate general normative ethical theory to concrete decisions that must be made about specific situations. Standard decision-making procedures can be used. The following is a useful method for considering clinical ethical problems.

A. Elements of the case method (Figure 15-3)

1. **Premise.** The premise is an action statement regarding conduct that should be initiated or discontinued because of a moral obligation of the physician to the patient or to an involved institution. Normally, the premise is stated as, "I (We) should (should not) do. . . ." When opposite choices appear attractive, a positive action statement should be used as the original premise.

2. **Ethical argument.** The ethical argument consists of reasons for the premise and justifications for the reasons. Objections to the premise should be held until later in the argument.

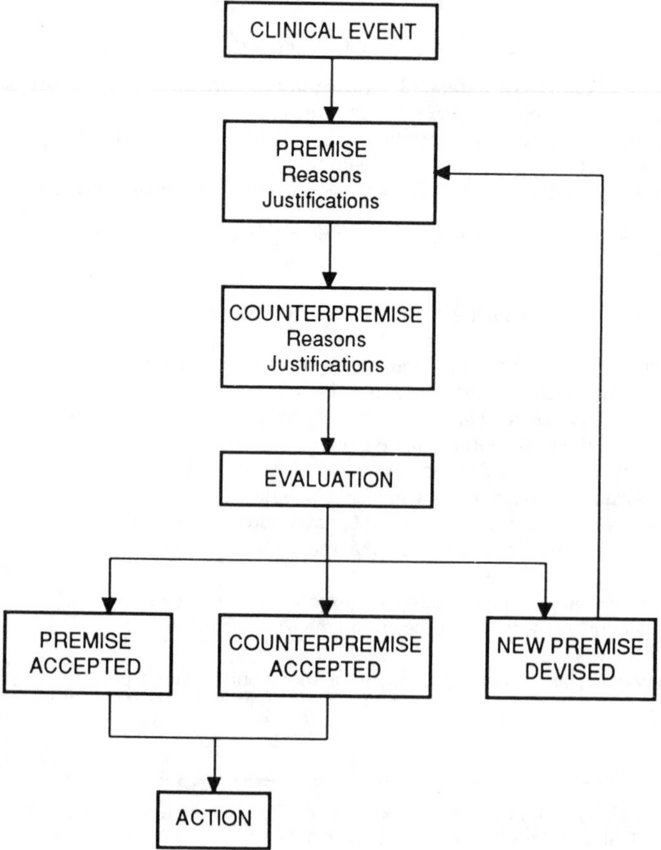

Figure 15-3. Ethical decision making in the clinical setting.

a. All **reasons** that support the premise should be listed, with medical, legal, social, and personal reasons separated from moral ones.
b. A **justification** should be provided for each moral reason listed. Justifications are "reasons for the reasons" and generally move to more abstract and general concepts.

3. **Counterpremises.** For each premise, there will be one or more counterpremises. This phase of hypothesis testing proceeds as follows.
   a. List the first counterpremise.
   b. List all reasons that support the counterpremise, including objections to the premise.
   c. Sort the moral reasons from the other reasons.
   d. Provide justifications for each moral reason.
   e. List other counterpremises, if any, and complete steps a through d.

4. **Evaluation** consists of weighing the several reasons to determine their relative importance and to select the most important elements. When conflict remains, outside input (e.g., from colleagues, other professionals, patients and their families, ethics committees, other counselors) may help to define the problems better.
   a. **General guidelines**
      (1) **Consistency.** The decision should be one that could be supported in all similar cases.
      (2) **Coherence.** The decision should have internal logic and conform to the general treatment plan for the patient unless there is an overriding reason for altering that plan.
   b. **Alternatives** include:
      (1) Accepting the original premise
      (2) Accepting a counterpremise
      (3) Developing a new premise as a modification of an earlier premise or counterpremise, in which case the reasoning process should be repeated.

5. **Action.** Medical ethical decision making is directed to an action or to a determination not to act. Eventually, one may need to proceed without the agreement of other interested parties.
   a. In such cases, the moral imperative includes continued dialogue with those whose positions were not supported.
   b. Moral choice should not be confused with the adversarial proceedings of legal action. Moral choice in difficult situations must preserve a sensitivity to the values of those whose choices are rejected.

B. Example of clinical ethical decision making. The following fictitious example is controversial. Therefore, it is possible to weight the arguments differently from this suggestion. It also is possible to promote different reasons or justifications.

1. **Case description.** An 85-year-old diabetic woman with associated renal problems lives in her own home and conducts a part-time telephone business. She recently developed gangrene in her left foot and refuses to give consent to operate, saying she is ready for death and wants to "go to heaven a whole person." Her two children want the operation done immediately. A psychiatric consult concludes that, although the patient is oriented and generally aware of her situation, she may be considered incompetent to assess fully the gravity of her situation. Repeated explanations by her physician, by the hospital staff, and by her children have failed to change the patient's mind.
   a. **Premise:** Seek a court order to obtain medical guardianship and then operate on the patient.
   b. **Ethical argument**
      (1) **Reason 1:** The situation is life threatening. **Justification 1:** There is a duty to save life.
      (2) **Reason 2:** If the patient does not understand, she should not decide. **Justification 2a:** Letting her decide is, in effect, doing harm by omission. **Justification 2b:** A physician should do no harm.
      (3) **Reason 3:** The psychiatrist has judged the patient incompetent to make a medical decision. **Justification 3:** The expert opinion of the consultant is respected in most cases.
      (4) **Reason 4:** The children desire this medical intervention. **Justification 4:** The children have a vested interest in the patient's well-being and, if she is incompetent, would ordinarily make medical decisions for her.
   c. **Counterpremise:** Accede to the patient's wishes.
   d. **Ethical argument**
      (1) **Reason 1:** The patient has a right to refuse treatment. **Justification 1a:** Permitting the

patient's decision respects her as an individual. **Justification 1b:** Accepting the patient's opinion is accepting her autonomy.

(2) **Reason 2:** If the patient understands other things, perhaps she does understand the situation. **Justification 2:** There is a need to appreciate that she may have a different value scheme, which should be respected.

(3) **Reason 3:** At her age, she will not live long anyway. **Justification 3:** Accept the fact that any intervention will have only a short-term benefit.

e. **Evaluation.** The weight of law hinges on the psychiatric testimony but does not compel action.

(1) The life-threatening aspect would lead many physicians to proceed with the operation, completely overriding the patient's wishes. The children's preference for intervention would help to influence this decision. It is assumed that the physicians would have the patient's well-being in mind.

(2) Had the children agreed with the patient, it would be much harder to override their decision, but, if the patient were a minor and agreed with the parents to refuse treatment (e.g., on religious grounds), then the health team might seek court approval for the medical intervention.

(3) The argument about age seems irrelevant, if not prejudicial, in this case.

f. **Action:** Go to court, and then proceed with the operation.

2. **Commentary.** This case might go either way, depending on the physicians and others who are involved and how they evaluate the different parameters. Consider, for example, how much clearer the decision might be if the patient came from a nursing home and did not have a business. Although there is a psychiatric consult, evidence suggests that the patient recognizes her problem but is choosing a way of resolving it that is based on a value system that is different from that of the hospital or her family. Her religious perspective is not recognized. Even if her clergy did not back her interpretation, she would have the right to hold her own interpretation.

V. GENERAL MEDICAL PRINCIPLES.

Medical ethics may be divided into a consideration of some persistent general principles and into specific moral problems (see VI). The general principles discussed in this section can be rated in different hierarchies. For example, the maxim, "first, do no harm," is not always the primary rule for a physician's conduct. Unless a monistic position is taken, the priority of principles must be established case by case.

A. **Fidelity.** By their professional standing, physicians and other health professionals make certain promises to society and, thus, to individual patients. Fidelity is the duty to observe the pledges made by the profession.

1. **Truthfulness.** One of the most troubling of the promises is that of telling patients the truth within the bounds of fidelity.

a. The general assumption that physicians should have the sole authority to decide how much to tell their patients (**directed paternalism**) has been challenged by the courts and by physicians' organizations.

b. A complete disregard for fidelity occurs when the physician adopts an attitude of "care less" truth-telling, that is, without sensitivity to the nature of what is communicated. Bluntness in truth-telling is not necessarily a virtue.

2. **Confidentiality.** Access to a patient's records may be obtained legally by health professionals, hospital personnel, and insurance or government representatives. General guidelines of confidentiality include:

a. Limiting access to those who have a legitimate need

b. Avoiding idle conversation about patients

c. Using pseudonyms and altering other identifying data when presenting cases in conferences and teaching situations

B. **Autonomy.** A basic understanding of the relations between individuals in a moral situation posits autonomy on the part of the moral decision maker. Increasingly, medical ethics has stressed the autonomy of the patient or recipient of health care.

1. **Truth-telling.** In a manner similar to fidelity, the recognition of autonomy requires that the patient have access to the truth about his condition.

2. **Decision making.** One mark of autonomy is the ability to make rational decisions, especially when considering one's own future. Truly moral decisions incorporate respect for the patient's own desires and needs.

3. **Respect for individuals.** A health professional must remember that illness often weakens a patient's independence; it is, therefore, necessary to help the patient according to his individual needs so that autonomy is practiced.

C. **Beneficence.** The medical profession has a responsibility to do good for patients and the general public. This responsibility may be exercised through the care of individual patients or through efforts directed to preventing or ameliorating health problems in a community. Beneficence includes all efforts to increase the health of a community.

D. **Nonmaleficence.** The duty to "do no harm" is one of the oldest guiding principles of the medical profession.

1. **Deliberate acts to harm.** Only under limited concepts of self-defense is it permissible to harm another person. The exception in medicine is a harm (hurt) needed to help, heal, or cure the patient (e.g., a surgical incision, breaking confidentiality by telling authorities of threats made by a patient against another person).

2. **Calculated risk**
   a. When possible harm may occur, there must be a compensating and compelling possibility of benefits to justify the action. The side effects of medications are calculated risks, with moral permissibility to increase risks when the benefits are most important (e.g., to use almost toxic concentrations with certain tumors).
   b. For health care professionals, standards of "due care" include knowledge, craft (skill), and perseverance.

E. **Justice.** Equitable distribution of benefits and burdens constitute the subject matter of the principle of justice.

1. **Procedural justice.** One means of just distribution is the establishment of rules. To be fair, exceptions to rules should be clearly built into the procedures. The distribution of services on the basis of "first come, first served" is an example of a procedural rule.

2. **Distributive justice.** Equal sharing may not always be the most just way to distribute benefits or burdens; additional claims may be involved. Claims requiring decisions based on distributive justice arise when resources are limited; thus, reductions on spending for health care generate the questions of who shall have health care and who shall not (see VI B).

3. **Compensatory justice.** Punishment as retribution is one form of compensatory justice. The more positive aspect is the attempt to reward victims for losses that are not the consequences of their own action (e.g., quotas to combat discrimination).

4. **Individual and society.** Often issues of justice rest on claims of the rights of individuals against claims of the society in which the individual lives. Decisions made for the "good of society" are particularly painful when they discriminate against an individual patient. The physician is often caught between primary duty to the patient and obligations to society.

VI. **SELECTED MORAL PROBLEMS.** Each problem discussed in this section represents a question of limits and of the moral conflict at the boundaries.

A. **Limiting technology.** New pharmacologic agents and sophisticated diagnostic and therapeutic techniques allow physicians access to procedures that alter the traditional relations between physician and patient. Problems associated with technology include the following.

1. **Initiating life-support treatment.** Legal and moral uncertainties surrounding the removal of life-support systems have, in turn, raised issues about initiating treatment at the onset of a medical crisis.
   a. To not initiate treatment means the loss of a life that might be saved.
   b. To begin treatment means the possibility of sustaining individuals who have no prospect for recovery, which can be costly in terms of patient, staff, and family suffering as well as in the use of resources that might be applied to other health problems.

2. **Withdrawing life-support techniques** has been better accepted than not initiating treatment, yet both decisions are difficult.
   a. General philosophical and social agreement with the Roman Catholic distinction of ordinary and extraordinary treatment has facilitated the development of procedures for withdrawing **ventilation support**.
   b. More problematic, and often subject to judicial review, are the cases where conscious persons ask that treatments be discontinued and those where the change involves withholding **nutritional support**. One troubling group of problems centers in the patients classified as **persistent vegetative state (PVS),** who may survive for decades as long as care is given. Deciding how much support shall be given and when, if ever, certain support may be withdrawn is widely debated, and the regulations are constantly shifting.

3. **Terminating life.** In the Netherlands, laws have been passed to permit physicians to assist terminally ill patients to die by active means (e.g., injection of a lethal drug). Physicians in the United States are debating this precedent.

4. **Control and autonomy.** Many of the new technologies promise methods of mind and behavior control, which have beneficial effects for some patients but which could also be used by repressive governments, or even by well-meaning but paternalistic health professionals. It is difficult to establish limits between the beneficial applications of technology and uses that may debase individuals and populations.

B. **Limiting resources.** The availability and types of medical care are restricted by the choices of individual physicians about their practices and through the process of congressional budget setting. Choices of **microallocation** (decisions affecting individuals) and **macroallocation** (decisions about which goods are available) produce many ethical questions.

1. **The right to treatment.** Ideal moral consensus expects that individuals be treated equally with respect to health care. However, the complexity of treatment systems and the diversity of illnesses make such an ideal impossible to maintain. Decisions by society determine which diseases and patients receive support, resources, and access to treatment. For example, the decision to fund renal dialysis changed a limited resource to a more readily available therapy but at significant economic expenditure. The right to treatment as decided by society determines:
   a. What diseases get funded
   b. Which patients receive support for catastrophic illnesses
   c. Which treatments shall be limited because of the patient's age (too young or too old)
   d. Which theory of justice can best serve the decisions about the right to treatment

2. **Individual physician's decisions.** Although some government intervention has attempted to redistribute physicians by requiring certain locations for practice to repay educational assistance, physicians remain relatively free to choose where they practice and in what specialty. They also choose whom they will serve and, to a great extent, how much time they will spend with each patient. Those physicians working within prepaid plans report pressures to meet quotas. Physicians as a group, with some intervention by society, still determine:
   a. How many physicians will be trained
   b. The eligibility of physicians to pursue certain medical specialties and subspecialties
   c. The time that physicians should spend with patients
   d. The fees for their services

3. **Medicine and other social needs.** The total expenditure on health care by society is balanced against other needs of that society—for example, defense, education, and measures against crime.
   a. If it is determined that American expenditures on health care need to be changed, responsible parties must be assigned to decide how the money should be reallocated.
   b. It is also important to determine how much money and resources would be allocated to prevention, maintenance of good health habits, and treatment of existing illnesses, especially those affecting small numbers of people or those having high individual cost.

C. **Limiting research.** The new technologies are the result of the burgeoning research that occurred during and after World War II. The problems associated with research, although generally present throughout history, were highlighted by the medical experiments performed on humans in Nazi concentration camps. Articles written in the past 20 years continue to direct attention to unethical behavior by experimenters.

1. **Deception.** It should be determined when, if ever, deception is necessary in research. The investigator must ask if an altered design or a different protocol could obtain the necessary information; if not, under limited and controlled circumstances where the risk of harm seems minimal, it may be possible ethically to use deception.

2. **Informed consent.** The rights of individuals to choose risks has led to the move for informed consent in research. At one end of the spectrum, this doctrine means freedom to reject participation; at the other end, it requires a thorough evaluation of the individual's role in the experiment.
   a. **Children** cannot grant informed consent because of their limited capacity to assess risks and benefits. Nontherapeutic research in children generally is proscribed even where limited risk exists.
   b. **Prisoners** once served as a major source of research subjects. As the doctrine of informed consent was strengthened, it became apparent to some that consent by those held in special restraint may be impossible to obtain. Critics of prisoner research argue that consent that offers good financial rewards to generally poorly paid convicts, that allows relaxation from otherwise strenuous and tedious duties, or that promises consideration for early parole or favorable attention when parole comes up is not comparable to the consent of nonprisoners. Additionally, since the concept of consent includes the right to refuse, prisoners who may be judged "uncooperative" for not volunteering to be research subjects do not have the same right of nonparticipation as do other potential subjects. Those advocating prisoner research refer to elevated prisoner morale from a sense of contributing to society, the chance to earn extra money, and relief from the monotony of prison life, as positive factors that promote freely informed consent from prisoners.
   c. **Proxy consent.** For small children, the mentally retarded, and comatose patients, consent must be obtained from a legal guardian. Great restraints have been placed on proxy consent except in cases of possible therapeutic benefit for the patient or, in fatal illnesses, for others with the same disease.

3. **Privacy.** One constraint on researchers is the need to maintain patient confidentiality. However, with the general use of computerized records the problem of access to private information has increased.

4. **Reporting unethical research.** Journal editors have disagreed about the editorial responsibility for ensuring that published papers adhere both to high standards of research and to ethical means of obtaining data. The pressure of the news media for information as well as the fame and fortune to be gained by being "first" exacerbate this problem.

D. **Limiting risk of disease.** The continuing problem of the health profession to weigh the risks of the increased incidence of a disease against other public and private goods, such as the invasion of privacy, the rise of unnecessary panic, and confidence in health care has been illuminated by the health problems generated by acquired immune deficiency syndrome (AIDS).

1. **General ethical concerns** involving infectious diseases, such as AIDS, venereal disease, and the common cold, raise some very interesting questions. For example, attempts to limit the spread of a disease may place unnecessary restrictions on individuals not affected by the illness. General ethical concerns include:
   a. Caring for infected individuals
   b. Reducing the spread of the disease
   c. Finding treatments and eventually cures
   d. Accepting AIDS as a professional risk

2. **AIDS** is a new human experience, yet it parallels the diseases (e.g., leprosy) and plagues (e.g., Black Death) of the past. Physicians need to be alert to the rapidly changing knowledge of AIDS. In addition to the questions raised generally by infectious diseases, the following concerns are related to the AIDS epidemic:
   a. Locating funding for the growing number of infected individuals
   b. Bypassing experimental protocols for compassionate use
   c. Maintaining confidentiality for those individuals for whom fear of their illness may be coupled with prejudice about their suspected lifestyles
   d. Determining an equitable commitment of health care and research resources to AIDS as compared with other medical and social problems.

3. **Public health issues,** such as smoking, the use of alcohol or other drugs, or the possession of firearms, also raise issues of control and judgment concerning who shall be limited and in what ways. These items also balance the cost of measures to reduce ill effects while still permitting freedom to choose lifestyles.

BIBLIOGRAPHY

American Medical Association: Principles of Medical Ethics. In *Current Opinions.* Prepared by the Council on Ethical and Judicial Affairs. Chicago, AMA, 1989, p ix.

Beauchamp TL, Childress JF: *Principles of Biomedical Ethics,* 3rd edition. New York, Oxford University Press, 1989.

Bergsma J, Duff RS: A model for examining values and decision-making in the patient-doctor relationship. *The Pharos,* 1980, pp 7–12.

Edelstein L: The Hippocratic Oath: text, translation and interpretation. In *Ancient Medicine.* Edited by Temkin O, Temkin CL. Baltimore, Johns Hopkins Press, 1967, pp 3–63.

Institute of Science, Ethics, and the Life Sciences: *Hastings Center Report,* Hastings, NY.

Kant I: *Fundamentals of Principles of the Metaphysics of Morals,* Buffalo, NY, Prometheus Books, 1987 (translation; originally published in 1785 in German).

Kennedy Institute of Ethics: *Bioethicsline,* National Library of Medicine, Washington, DC.

Kennedy Institute of Ethics: *Encyclopedia of Bioethics,* 4 vols. New York, Free Press, 1978.

Kennedy Institute of Ethics: *Kennedy Institute of Ethics Journal,* Baltimore, Johns Hopkins University Press.

Society for Health and Human Values: *Newsletter,* McLean, VA.

STUDY QUESTIONS

Directions: Each of the numbered items or incomplete statements in this section is followed by answers or by completions of the statement. Select the **one** lettered answer or completion that is **best** in each case.

1. The study of ethics is generally divided into all of the following areas EXCEPT

(A) descriptive ethics, in which comparative and cross-cultural analyses are done
(B) normative ethics, in which there is an inquiry into actions and their worth
(C) metaethics, in which ethics itself is studied to determine questions about moral concepts
(D) evaluation, in which the best answers are determined

2. A physician is told by her colleagues in a group practice that the reason she is seeing fewer patients is because she spends too much time with each one. She argues, however, that her view of the physician's role demands the time she spends. This example represents which of the following conflict-of-value levels?

(A) Physician's personal–physician's group
(B) Physician's personal–physician's society
(C) Physician's group–physician's society
(D) Physician's group–patient's rights
(E) Physician's personal–patient's rights

3. Which of the following statements is most clearly about nonmoral values?

(A) My mother is a good woman
(B) Anyone who curses God is bad
(C) He was wrong to lie
(D) Her car was a good buy
(E) The doctor did an excellent job of telling the patient that she had cancer

4. Factors that can be expected to continue the importance of medical ethics include all of the following EXCEPT

(A) the rise of new technologies
(B) the demands of the public
(C) new moral discoveries
(D) physician concern

5. All of the following are general guidelines for observing the principle of confidentiality EXCEPT

(A) limiting access to patient information
(B) avoiding idle conversation about patients
(C) using false names and altering data when teaching
(D) not lying to patients

6. The onset of the AIDS epidemic poses the usual ethical challenges of dealing with infectious diseases along with special concerns for all of the following EXCEPT

(A) locating funding for the rapidly growing number of affected individuals
(B) bypassing experimental protocols for compassionate use
(C) senility that often accompanies later stages of the disease
(D) maintaining confidentiality for those individuals for whom fear of their illness may be coupled with prejudice about their suspected lifestyles

---

1-D	4-C
2-A	5-D
3-D	6-C

Directions: The item below contains four suggested answers of which **one or more** is correct. Choose the answer

A if **1, 2, and 3** are correct
B if **1 and 3** are correct
C if **2 and 4** are correct
D if **4** is correct
E if **1, 2, 3, and 4** are correct

7. Moral limits on research include the

(1) need for informed consent
(2) high cost of equipment
(3) need for ethical means of conducting research
(4) scarcity of researchers

7-B

ANSWERS AND EXPLANATIONS

1. The answer is D *[I B 1–3].*
Evaluation is part of the process of decision making but is not an area into which the study of ethics is generally divided. The standard divisions of ethical inquiry are descriptive ethics; normative ethics, which is the most common area for medical and other applied questions; and metaethics.

2. The answer is A *[I C 3 a–c].*
The physician's view of her role is conflicting with the physician's group. While it might be argued that the conflict is with patient's rights, the structure of the patient encounter is largely the responsibility of physicians.

3. The answer is D *[I C 2].*
A statement about nonmoral values is a judgment of the worth of an object—in this case, someone's car. Statements about a person's character or conduct are moral values.

4. The answer is C *[III A 1–3].*
Basic moral theory has changed little since Socrates, Plato, and Aristotle made contributions that formally established the field 2500 years ago; it is, therefore, unlikely that medical ethics will be important because of new moral discoveries. However, changing technology, public demand, and physician concern have prompted the current interest in medical ethics and will be significant in the future of medicine and of medical ethics.

5. The answer is D *[V A 1, 2 a–c, B 1].*
While truthfulness is a desirable moral behavior, it is related to the principles of fidelity and autonomy rather than to confidentiality. Limiting access to information, avoiding idle conversation about patients, and using simple means to change patient information when teaching are general guidelines for observing the principle of confidentiality. It is important to note, however, that access to a patient's record may be obtained *legally* in certain situations.

6. The answer is C *[VI D 2].*
While senility may accompany later stages of the acquired immune deficiency syndrome (AIDS) complex, dealing with the incompetent patient is no different in AIDS patients than in any other terminal illness.

7. The answer is B (1, 3) *[VI C 2, 4].*
Informed consent is one doctrine that has arisen in response to a concern about unethical practices. Informed consent not only means freedom to reject participation but also requires a thorough evaluation of an individual's role in an experiment. For example, prisoners once served as a major source of research subjects, but it has been argued that perhaps incarcerated populations can never really be "free" to give their consent. Unethical research practices may lead to publishing restrictions and general rejection by the scientific community. The high cost of equipment and the scarcity of researchers may limit the ability to conduct research, but they are not *moral* limits. It may be a moral problem of the *allocation of resources* not to fund expensive equipment or the training of researchers.

16 Health Care Professionals

Brett J. Cassens

I. STAFFING ISSUES.

I. STAFFING ISSUES. Five percent of the work force is employed in medically related occupations. Because of the large number of health care professionals and the costs of their education, training, wages, and salaries, staffing issues are a major priority.

A. General staffing concerns

1. Attracting **adequate numbers of health care personnel** has always been a concern of society. This is especially true of physicians, whose costly training takes 7 years or more.
2. **Wages and salaries.** Medical care is labor intensive, and wages and salaries constitute a major percentage of the costs.
   - **a.** An average of 407 people were employed in community hospitals for every 100 patients in 1988, compared with 226 employees for every 100 patients in 1960.
   - **b.** Labor costs for these personnel in 1989 constituted 54% of the adjusted average cost per patient per day ($637).

B. Physician staffing concerns

1. **Shortages.** A perceived shortage of physicians received widespread publicity in the 1960s as society struggled to improve access to medical care through Medicare and Medicaid.
2. **Expansion of facilities.** During the 1960s and early 1970s, federal funding supported the construction of new health professional schools and expansion of classes through the **Health Professions Education Assistance Act of 1963**. Between 1964 and 1975, the following occurred.
   - **a.** The **number of medical schools** rose from 88 to 114, a 30% increase.
   - **b.** The **total enrollment of medical students** rose from 32,428 to 54,074, a 67% increase (Table 16-1).
3. **Maldistribution.** Despite this astounding increase in physicians, **underserved areas persist** as a result of maldistribution. Physicians tend to cluster near urban areas, avoiding rural and economically depressed communities. Even in physician-dense cities, physicians' services are not accessible to everyone. Table 16-2 demonstrates the variations in the geographic density of physicians.
   - **a.** Early evaluation of physician shortages assumed that expanding the total number of physicians would lead to more physicians in underserved areas. This diffusion of physicians has not occurred.
   - **b.** Relatively poor physician reimbursement in rural areas may contribute to this maldistribution. Medicare reimbursement reforms are seeking to reduce this disparity and make rural practice more economically attractive.
4. **Predicting physician supply (surpluses or shortages)** is a highly controversial issue. Various studies have been commissioned to address this vital issue.
   - **a. The Graduate Medical Education National Advisory Committee (GMENAC)** was chartered in 1976 by the Department of Health Education and Welfare [now the Department of Health and Human Services (DHHS)] to project physician staffing requirements for the year 1990 and for each specialty.
     - **(1) Findings.** The report predicted an excess of 70,000 physicians by 1990, particularly in the areas of general surgery, obstetrics and gynecology, radiology, and general internal medicine. A physician surplus would mean unnecessary educational costs absorbed by the medical care system or the taxpayer (see II C 1, 2) and increased competition among physicians for available revenues.

Table 16-1. Graduates of Health Professional Schools and Number of Schools, According to Profession, in the United States: Selected 1950–1991 Estimates and Projections for 2000

Year	Medicine	Osteopathy	Nursing*	Dentistry
		Graduates		
1950	5553	373	25,790	2565
1960	7081	427	29,895	3253
1970	8367	432	43,103	3749
1975	12,714	702	73,915	4969
1978	14,393	963	77,874	5324
1979	14,966	1004	77,132	5424
1980	15,135	1059	75,523	5256
1981	15,667	1151	73,985	5550
1982	15,985	1017	74,052	5371
1983	15,824	1317	77,408	5756
1986	16,100	1667	77,000	5200
1988	15,947	1601	64,800	4618
1990	16,240	1480	68,400	4390
2000	16,080	1460	57,800	4080
		Schools		
1950	79	6	1304	42
1960	86	6	1128	47
1970	103	7	1340	53
1975	114	9	1362	59
1978	122	12	1358	59
1979	125	14	1374	60
1980	126	14	1385	60
1981	126	15	1401	60
1982	127	15	1432	60
1983	127	15	1466	60
1988	127	15	1442	55
1991	126	15	1460	55

Data are based on reporting by health professional schools. (Adapted from Bureau of Health Professions: *Report to the President and Congress on the Status of Health Personnel in the United States.* Health Resources and Services Administration. DHHS Pub No HRS-P-OD 84-4, Rockville, MD, 1984; unpublished data; and American Chiropractic Association: unpublished data.)

*Some nursing schools offer more than one type of program. Numbers shown for nursing are the number of nursing programs.

(2) **Recommendations** included reduced medical school enrollment, a 20% reduction in residency programs in areas of projected surpluses, and financial incentives to attract residents to primary care and away from oversubscribed specialties.

b. **The Council on Graduate Medical Education (COGME),** which was convened by the federal government to reassess physician staffing issues, issued its report in 1988.

(1) **Findings.** The report predicted a surplus but provided no estimate as to its magnitude.

(2) **Recommendations.** Alluding to substantial uncertainties in the projection, the council made no recommendations.

c. **Surpluses in the early 1990s are not evident; in fact, growing shortages have been predicted** (Schwartz, 1988).

(1) **Findings.** Factors contributing to possible shortages include:

(a) Increased demand for services caused by escalating numbers of people with the acquired immune deficiency syndrome (AIDS)

(b) The aging of the population as the baby-boom generation of the 1940s and 1950s reaches middle age

(c) The demands of newer technology

(2) **Recommendations**

(a) Shortages of 7000 physicians by the year 2000, and perhaps 50,000 by 2010, could result if current policies constrain the number of medical graduates.

Table 16-2. Nonfederal Physicians, Civilian Population, and Physician-Population Ratios by Census Division for 1990

Census Division	Nonfederal Physicians	Civilian* Population (thousands)	Physician-Population Ratio
Total†	584,921	246,553	237:1
New England	41,578	12,998	320:1
Middle Atlantic	112,147	37,660	298:1
East North Central	88,069	42,231	209:1
West North Central	36,049	17,777	203:1
South Atlantic	102,277	42,541	240:1
East South Central	27,752	15,314	181:1
West South Central	49,397	26,798	184:1
Mountain	27,894	13,397	208:1
Pacific	99,758	37,837	264:1

Reprinted from Roback G, Randolph L, Seidman B: *Physician Characteristics and Distribution in the US*. Chicago, American Medical Association, 1992.

*Population estimates as of July 1, 1989.

†Includes the 50 states and Washington, DC, but excludes Possessions.

(b) Determining what constitutes the optimum demand for services is the key to determining the optimum number and location (supply) of physicians. As long as major segments of the population are underserved because of limited geographic and financial access to care, needs appear to exceed availability.

C. Nurse staffing concerns. In the 1960s, many geographic areas reported shortages of nurses despite the large number of registered nurses (RNs) in the United States. In 1983, there were 1,404,000 RNs and 549,000 licensed practical nurses (LPNs) in the United States. By 1988, RNs numbered 2,033,000. Eighty percent, or 1,627,000, of RNs filled 780,000 full-time equivalent positions. Despite this apparent surplus, 15% of available positions were vacant in major cities.

1. Shortages. In contrast to the controversy over physician supply, a clear and profound shortage of RNs has existed for several years. The Commonwealth Fund published a report (1989) analyzing nursing shortages and proposed solutions. Six major metropolitan areas were studied, and 15% of budgeted RN positions were vacant in four of these six areas.

a. Decreased supply

(1) Low salaries. In the early 1980s, nursing wages compared poorly with those in occupations traditionally held by men. Consequently, women increasingly shifted to better paying professions.

(2) Shrinking pool of nursing applicants. Until recently, the overwhelming majority of nursing students were 18- to 24-year-old single, white females. This segment of the population has shrunk as the baby-boom generation of the 1940s and 1950s ages. From 1983 to 1987, nursing enrollment dropped from 250,000 to 185,000 students, a 26% decrease.

(3) Changing demographics of nursing. In the last 20 years, the population of RNs has changed from single young women to predominantly married women with children. These women are, on average, 35–40 years old. Demands of family life make full-time hospital nursing unattractive because of the night and weekend work. Thus, these older nurses often leave hospital work. By the time they are 12 years beyond graduation, only 15% are hospital staff nurses compared to 63% of new graduates.

b. Increased demand. The number of full-time RNs working in hospitals increased 21% from 1980 to 1987. Employment increased from 622,000 to 758,000 full-time equivalents. Causes include:

(1) Increased complexity of medical care. Technologically complex surgery and intensive care units require more staff. While the number of general hospital beds has decreased, intensive care units have expanded, employing 40% of hospital staff nurses.

(2) Aging population. By the year 2000, 5 million Americans will be 85 years and older as a result of more sophisticated care and technology. By comparison, only 2 million Americans were that old in 1980.

(3) **Increased educational demands for nursing.** From 1980 to 1987, demand for RNs increased greatly, while hospital use of LPNs decreased from 228,000 to 170,000 full-time equivalents. This shift reflects the belief of the nursing profession that a better educated nurse is needed to meet the demands of the more technological care setting. It has, in fact, been suggested that all RNs should have a Bachelor of Science in Nursing (BSN) degree.

(4) **Poor physician-nurse relations.** The relationship between physicians and nurses has been a topic of discussion and concern within both professions. The authoritarian and sexist nature of some physician-nurse interactions remains a concern, but conditions appear to be improving.

2. **Remedies for nursing shortages.** Proposals for ameliorating the shortage include:
   a. Recruiting nursing students from nontraditional groups (e.g., the poor, minorities, men)
   b. Developing programs to retrain unemployed workers from other occupations
   c. Providing educational programs to train current health care workers (e.g., LPNs) to become RNs
   d. Offering more flexible schedules and increased pay for night and weekend work
   e. Increasing nursing efficiency by using nurses' aids, "nurse extenders," and patient care assistants
   f. Attracting part-time workers by creating in-house agencies and encouraging them to work more hours by raising pay and benefits as they work more hours per week
   g. Reducing nursing workload by investing in labor-efficient equipment and nursing units

II. PHYSICIANS

II. PHYSICIANS control most medical care expenditures and are, with rare exception, the only practitioners licensed to diagnose and treat medical problems. Two philosophies of medicine dominate today: **allopathic** and **osteopathic** medicine. The terms allopathic and homeopathic were coined by Samuel Hahnemann, the 18th century German physician who was the founder of the homeopathic philosophy of medicine. He believed that illnesses could be treated best by dilute solutions of elements thought to be related etiologically to a given symptom—thus, the term homeopathy, which refers to employing treatments "like the disease." In retrospect, Hahnemann's therapeutic conservatism doubtlessly saved many who would have died from the heroic methods of the day.

A. **Allopathic physicians,** who graduate with a Doctor of Medicine (MD) degree, constituted 95% of the 615,421 physicians practicing in the United States in 1990. **Allopathic, or conventional, medicine** originated in the heroic therapies of bloodletting and purging. The term allopathic refers to the concept that heroic medical treatments bore little relationship to the diseases to which they were applied.

1. **Medical education.** Medical degrees are granted by colleges and universities after 3 or 4 years of study beyond the baccalaureate degree.
   a. **Enrollment.** In 1990–1991, 64,986 students were enrolled in 127 accredited medical schools in the United States. This is 90 fewer students than in 1989–1990. Table 16-3 shows the peak enrollment in 1983–1984, with a gradual decline in each recent year.
      (1) Enrollment in medical schools has declined for the last 5 years but is projected to increase gradually in the next decade (Table 16-4).
      (2) A total of 29,243 students applied for first-year positions in medical schools in 1990, and 17,206 were accepted, making the ratio of applicants to positions 1.7:1. This second year of moderate increases in applicants reverses a 15-year downward trend.
      (3) In the last 50 years, the ratio of applicants to positions has never fallen below 1.6:1. This low ratio is thought to be encouraging to students, who see a stronger likelihood of acceptance into medical school. Figure 16-1 demonstrates the relationship of applications to acceptances.
   b. **Women** constitute 37% of all medical students, though fewer than 20% of practicing physicians are women.
      (1) Thirty-nine percent of the 1990–1991 entering class were women, with eight medical schools having a majority of women in the first year. In 1990–1991, 24,100 women were enrolled.
      (2) The rapid increase in female applicants in the early 1980s offset the decline in male applicants. From 1985 to 1989, however, the number of female applicants declined by 12% (Figure 16-2). In 1990, female applicants surprisingly increased by 12%.

Table 16-3. Medical School Students and Graduates over 20-Year Period

Academic Year	Number of Schools	Enrollments: Total	Enrollments: First Year*	Enrollments: Intermediate Years†	Graduates
1970–1971	103	40,487	11,348	20,165	8974
1980–1981‡	126	65,497	17,204	32,626	15,667
1981–1982	126	66,485	17,320	33,180	15,985
1982–1983	127	66,886	17,230	33,832	15,824
1983–1984	127	67,443	17,175	33,941	16,327
1984–1985	127	67,090	16,992	33,779	16,319
1985–1986	127	66,604	16,929	33,484	16,125
1986–1987	127	66,142	16,779	33,527	15,836
1987–1988§	127	65,742	16,686	33,109	15,887
1988–1989	127	65,150	16,781	32,749	15,620
1989–1990	127	65,081	16,749	32,996	15,336
1990–1991‖	126	64,986	16,803	32,684	15,499#

Reprinted from Jonas HS, Etzel SI, Barzansky B: Educational programs in US medical schools. *JAMA* 266(7):913, 1991.

*First-year enrollment includes students repeating the year.

†Intermediate years include final-year students who did not graduate.

‡Ponce (Puerto Rico) School of Medicine and the University of South Dakota, Sioux Falls, did not provide information; 1979–1980 enrollment was used for these schools.

§Howard University, Washington, DC, did not provide information; 1986–1987 data were used for this school.

‖Hahnemann University, Philadelphia, PA, and the University of Texas, Galveston, did not provide information; 1989–1990 data were used for these schools.

#Estimated in April 1991.

c. **Minorities.** Approximately 28% of new enrollees were categorized as minority group members (Table 16-5).
   - **(1)** With one exception (i.e., the Asian or Pacific Islander category), there has been essentially no change in the percentages of black, Hispanic, or Native American medical students in the last 10 years (Figure 16-3).
   - **(2)** In absolute numbers, both male and female black enrollees increased in 1990, to 567 and 701, respectively. This demonstrates a sustained increase for black women.
   - **(3)** By contrast, applications from Asian Americans and Pacific Islanders have increased by 57% since 1983. These groups constituted 15% of first-year enrollees in 1990–1991. In the 1980 census, 1.6% of Americans were Asian or Pacific Islanders. This is by far the most rapidly growing segment of medical school entrants.

d. **International medical school graduates.** The number of Americans studying in foreign medical schools is unknown but appears to be declining.
   - **(1)** In 1984, 247 Americans studying abroad transferred to U.S. medical schools, while 340 did so in 1985.
   - **(2)** Since then, however, there has been a steady decline to 117 in 1990–1991.

Table 16-4. Number of New First-Year Students and Graduates Projected by Medical Schools*

Academic Year	First-Year Class	Graduates
1991–1992	15,946	16,002
1992–1993	15,946	16,142
1993–1994	15,950	16,247
1994–1995	15,953	16,169
1995–1996	15,956	16,162

Reprinted from Jonas HS, Etzel SI, Barzansky B: Educational programs in US medical schools. *JAMA* 226(7):913, 1991.

*Hahnemann University, Philadelphia, PA, and the University of Texas, Galveston, did not provide information.

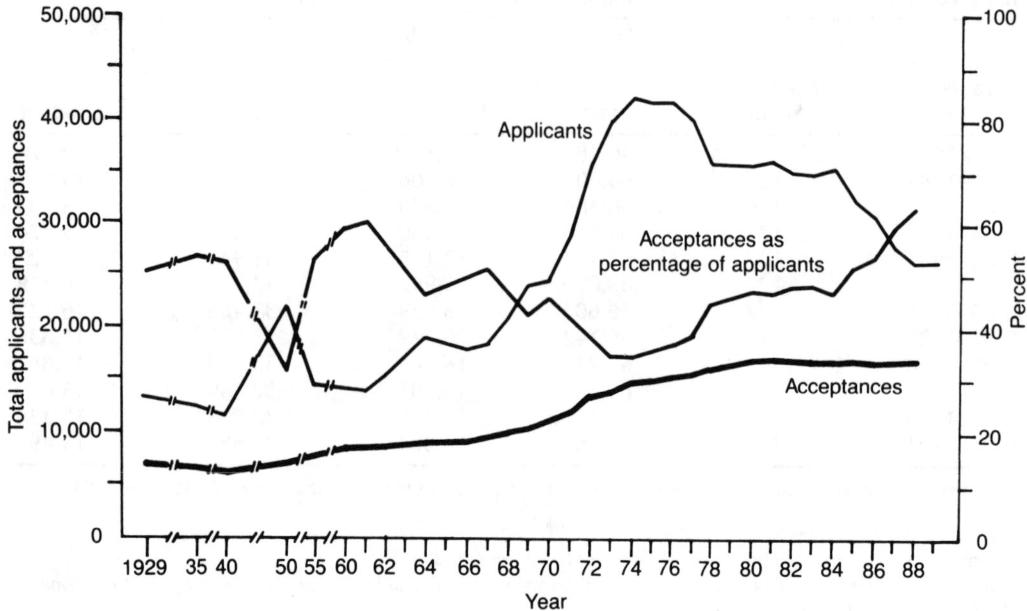

Figure 16-1. Applications and acceptances to U.S. medical schools and acceptances as a percentage of applications. (Reprinted from Relman AS: The changing demographics of the medical profession. *N Engl J Med* 321:1541, 1989.)

(3) Considering the current high percentage of U.S. applicants being accepted into medical school, it is unlikely that Americans will study abroad in large numbers.

(4) **Fifth Pathway programs** usually provide lectures and clinical rotations for Americans who have graduated from foreign medical schools to prepare them for residency programs in the United States.

(a) Since 1988, only seven U.S. medical schools offered Fifth Pathway clinical experiences, compared to 25 such programs in 1983.

(b) Of 290 applicants in 1990–1991, 67 students were admitted. This is down from 1,969 applicants and 374 admitted in 1984–1985.

2. **Graduate medical education** (i.e., training programs beyond medical school) is accredited by the Accreditation Council for Graduate Medical Education (ACGME) of the American Medical Association (AMA).

a. **Residency programs** for most specialties entail 3 postgraduate years (PGY-I, PGY-II, PGY-III).

(1) In 1991, 22,468 PGY-I positions (formerly known as internships) were estimated to be available for the 15,499 graduates of U.S. medical schools.

(2) The total number of residents on duty in 1988 declined compared to 1987—that is, there were 81,410 residents in 1987 and 81,093 residents in 1988. However, this number has increased substantially from the low of 74,500 residents in 1985. This temporary decline has been followed by increases to 82,902 in 1990.

(3) While the primary care specialties of family medicine, pediatrics, and internal medicine have been promoted in recent years, only 39% of students enter such programs.

(4) Surgery, which is generally overrepresented, showed a decrease in PGY-I positions, as did internal medicine and pediatrics.

(5) The number of graduates of foreign medical schools in American residency programs, referred to as international medical graduates (IMGs), is steadily declining. IMGs decreased from 25% of all residents in the mid-1970s to 16.8% of all residents in 1985. However, between 1989 and 1990, there was a 22% increase, resulting in IMGs accounting for 18% of all residents. A total of 2817 Americans graduating from foreign medical schools worked in residency programs in the United States, down from 5100 in 1988.

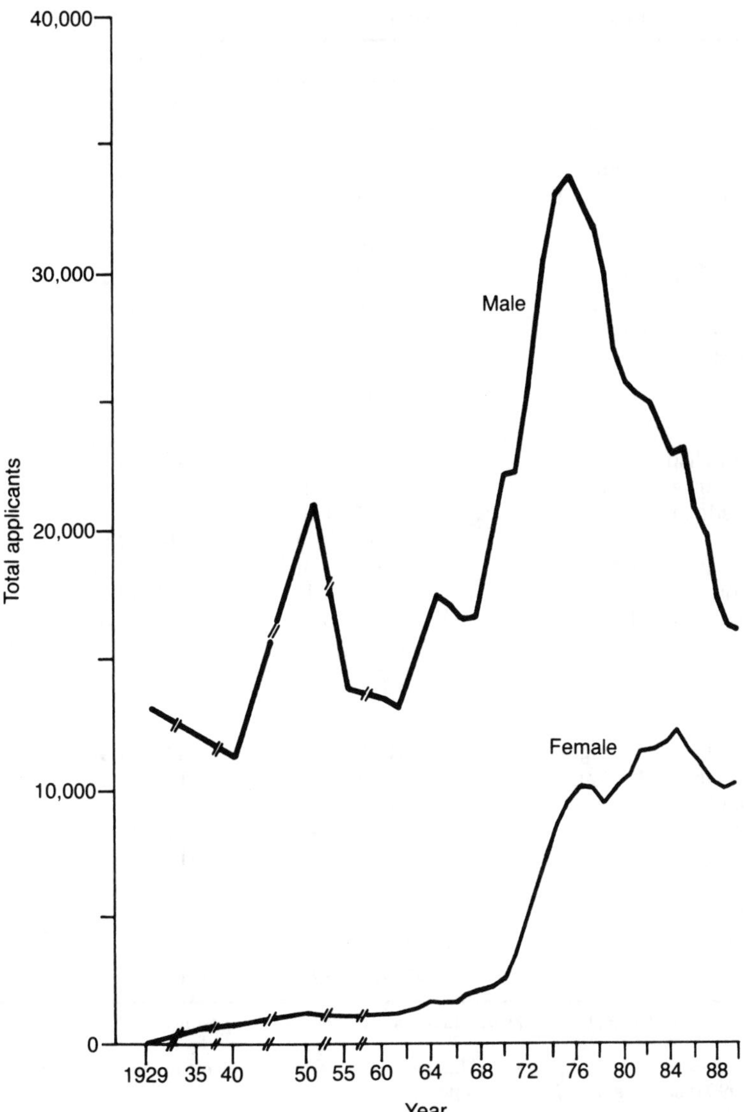

Figure 16-2. Applications to U.S. medical schools from 1929 to 1989. (Reprinted from Relman AS: The changing demographics of the medical profession. *N Engl J Med* 321:1540, 1989.)

b. **Fellowship programs** entail subspecialty training following residency programs in a general specialty (e.g., residents complete 3 years of general internal medicine before entering a 2-year fellowship program in infectious diseases).

c. **Board certification or board eligibility** is the endpoint of specialty training. Each of the 24 specialties has its own board or, in two cases, a conjoint board formed by representatives of two or more other boards. While board certification has no legal significance like licensure, it does establish a practitioner as a specialist. Some forms of insurance compensate specialists at higher rates.

3. **Licensure.** Regulation of medical practice is a function of the states and territories. Texas passed the first modern licensure and medical practice act 100 years ago. While medical graduates are licensed as "physicians and surgeons" and, thus, are not legally restricted to practice in a specialty, liability coverage and hospital privileges act to limit the scope of practice.

   a. **Eligibility for licensure** requires:

      (1) Graduation from a medical school accredited by the Association of American Medical Colleges (AAMC)

Table 16-5. Race and Ethnic Background of Medical School Enrollees, 1990–1991*

	Number (%)		
	Men	Women	Total
First-year enrollment†			
Blacks (not of Hispanic origin)	567 (3.4)	701 (4.2)	1268 (7.6)
Native Americans or Alaskan Natives	45 (0.3)	30 (0.2)	75 (0.5)
Mexican Americans	172 (1.0)	102 (0.6)	274 (1.6)
Puerto Ricans	132 (0.8)	93 (0.5)	225 (1.3)
Puerto Ricans (mainland)	60 (0.4)	43 (0.2)	103 (0.6)
Other Hispanics	177 (1.0)	135 (0.8)	312 (1.8)
Asians or Pacific Islanders	1552 (9.2)	974 (5.8)	2526 (15.0)
All other students‡	7599 (45.2)	4421 (26.3)	12,020 (71.5)
Total	10,304 (61.3)	6499 (38.7)	16,803 (100.0)
Graduates			
Blacks (not of Hispanic origin)	401 (2.6)	510 (3.3)	911 (5.9)
Native Americans or Alaskan Natives	29 (0.2)	14 (0.1)	43 (0.3)
Mexican Americans	167 (1.0)	87 (0.6)	254 (1.6)
Puerto Ricans	134 (0.9)	81 (0.5)	215 (1.4)
Puerto Ricans (mainland)	43 (0.3)	18 (0.1)	61 (0.4)
Other Hispanics	177 (1.1)	100 (0.6)	277 (1.7)
Asians or Pacific Islanders	1035 (6.7)	597 (3.8)	1632 (10.5)
All other students‡	7929 (51.2)	4177 (26.9)	12,106 (78.1)
Total	9915 (64.0)	5584 (36.0)	15,499 (100.0)
Total enrollment			
Blacks (not of Hispanic origin)	1878 (2.9)	2337 (3.6)	4215 (6.5)
Native Americans or Alaskan Natives	152 (0.2)	120 (0.2)	272 (0.4)
Mexican Americans	688 (1.1)	420 (0.6)	1108 (1.7)
Puerto Ricans	534 (0.8)	334 (0.5)	868 (1.3)
Puerto Ricans (mainland)	215 (0.3)	154 (0.2)	369 (0.5)
Other Hispanics	715 (1.1)	456 (0.7)	1171 (1.8)
Asians or Pacific Islanders	5313 (8.2)	3212 (4.9)	8525 (13.1)
All other students‡	31,327 (48.2)	17,131 (26.4)	48,458 (74.6)
Total	40,822 (62.8)	24,164 (37.2)	64,986 (100.0)

Reprinted from Jonas HS, Etzel SI, Barzansky B: Educational programs in US medical schools. *JAMA* 266(7):913, 1991.

*Hahnemann University, Philadelphia, PA, and the University of Texas, Galveston, did not provide enrollment information; 1989–1990 data were used for these schools.

†First-year enrollment data include students repeating the year.

‡All other students include whites (not of Hispanic origin) and non–U.S. citizen foreign students of various race and ethnic backgrounds.

(2) Successful completion of an objective examination—either Steps I, II, and III of the U.S. Medical Licensing Examination (USMLE) or the Federal Licensing Examination (FLEX)

(3) Completion of 1 year of postgraduate medical training

b. Reciprocity of licensure permits a physician licensed in one state to seek similar privileges elsewhere in the United States. Licensure is usually limited to a fixed number of years after completion of the USMLE examinations or FLEX. Thereafter, an applicant may be required to take a state licensing examination.

c. Maintenance of licensure. Although states currently do not require reexamination to maintain licensure, many seek evidence of 50 credit hours of continuing medical education (CME) per year.

B. Osteopathic physicians graduate with the Doctor of Osteopathy (DO) degree. In 1991, 31,000 osteopathic physicians were in practice, comprising 5% of practicing physicians in the United

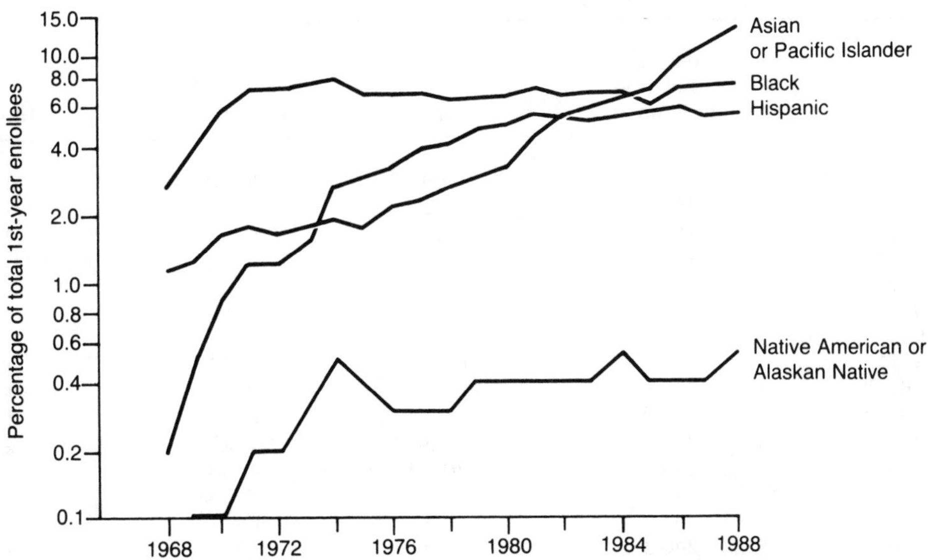

Figure 16-3. First-year enrollment of minority students in U.S. medical schools, 1968–1988, expressed as a percentage of total first-year enrollment. Schools of osteopathic medicine are not included. [Reprinted from Department of Health and Human Services: *United States: 1990.* Pub No (PHS) 91-1232. Hyattsville, MD, DHHS, 1991, p 36.]

States (Table 16-6). **Osteopathic medicine** (literally "bone treatment") was developed by Andrew Taylor Still in the 1870s. Still was educated informally in allopathic medicine but was wary of the poisonous compounds used in the therapies of the day. Through a chance discovery, he learned to alleviate his own headaches by applying tension to the cervical spine. Based on his theories of musculoskeletal manipulation, he abandoned medications for this new osteopathic therapy, which he felt could enhance the body's natural healing ability.

1. **Osteopathic education.** Study leading to the DO degree requires 4 years of education beyond the baccalaureate degree. Curriculum content closely parallels that required for allopathic physicians, with the addition of training in manipulation therapy. Manipulation is now largely used as an adjunct to more traditional medical treatments.
   a. **Enrollment**
      (1) In 1990, a total of 6800 students were enrolled in osteopathic schools.
      (2) Approximately 1530 students graduated in 1990, which is a decline from a peak of 1600 in 1988.
      (3) There are currently 15 schools of osteopathy (Michigan and New Jersey have both allopathic and osteopathic medical schools).
   b. **Women and minorities.** Although Still's original school pioneered the admission of both blacks and women, ironically the percentages of blacks and women in osteopathy schools in the 1983–1984 school year were smaller than those in allopathic medical programs; however, in 1991, 6% of entering osteopathic students were black, and 33% were women, numbers similar to allopathic schools.

2. **Graduate osteopathic education** for osteopathic physicians has been limited until recently. Traditionally, osteopathic physicians have followed a primary care path. Currently, 91% of all DOs are in general practice, pediatrics, or internal medicine.
   a. **Seventy-five percent of osteopathic students** complete a rotating internship, labeled Year I, in an osteopathic hospital in order to become a member of the American Osteopathic Association. Following Year I, osteopathic physicians may elect general practice or select a training program in 46 accredited osteopathic specialties. These residency years are numbered R1, R2, and R3. Osteopathic physicians are increasingly seeking specialty training.
   b. **Twenty-five percent of osteopathic students** enter a national resident matching program in their fourth year of school and go directly into allopathic residencies. These numbers

Table 16-6. Estimates and Projections of Physicians, 1950–2000 (thousands)

Year	Total U.S. Population (millions)	Physicians		
		Total	Medical Physicians	Osteopaths
Actual				
1950	152.3	219.9	209.0	10.9
1955	165.9	240.2	228.6	11.6
1960	180.7	259.5	247.3	12.2
1965	194.3	288.7	277.6	11.1
1970	205.1	326.2	314.2	12.0
1975	215.9	384.4	370.4	14.0
1980	227.8	457.5	440.4	17.1
1981	230.1	466.7	448.7	18.0
1982	232.5	483.7	465.0	18.7
1983	234.8	501.2	481.5	19.7
1984	237.0	506.5	485.7	20.8
1985	239.3	520.7	498.8	21.9
1986	241.7	534.8	511.6	23.2
1987	243.9	548.5	524.1	24.4
1988	246.3	562.0	536.3	25.7
Projections				
1990	248.7	587.7	559.5	28.2
1995	255.2	645.5	611.1	34.4
2000	259.6	696.5	656.1	40.0

Reprinted from Health Insurance Association of America: *Source Book of Health Insurance Data—1991*. Washington, DC, Health Insurance Association of America, 1991.

have increased rapidly. Between 1986 and 1990, osteopathic residents in allopathic programs increased from 1543 to 2872, an 86% increase. This substantial increase is attributed to the shortage of osteopathic residency positions and a 300% increase in osteopathic graduates in the past 20 years.

C. Costs of medical education. The costs of medical education and salaries for health care personnel, especially physicians, are major components of medical care costs today. For example, medical school costs $40,000 or more per year.

1. **Expenditures by medical schools.** Medical school and graduate medical education expenses are increasing by 10% per year, with medical school expenditures for 1989–1990 exceeding $18.6 billion.
   - **a.** Approximately 40% of revenues come from patient care.
   - **b.** Approximately 23% of revenues come from federal funds. Recently, federal support through grants and contracts has stabilized after many years of declining.
2. **Medical student debt.** Rising medical school costs are reflected in increased medical student debt.
   - **a.** In 1985, the average graduating student owed $30,256, and 10% of graduates owed over $50,000.
   - **b.** By 1988, the average graduating student owed $38,500, and 24% of graduates had a debt in excess of $50,000.
   - **c.** For 1990 graduates, the mean debt was $46,200, but the percentage of graduates with debt declined from 81.3% to 78.8%.

III. NURSES. A key component of the health care system, nurses have been in critically short supply for the last decade. Despite the high demand for nurses, enrollment in nursing schools has declined since 1983, when enrollment peaked at 250,000 students. However, in 1988 and again in 1989, there were modest increases, and enrollment grew to 201,000 students. While cause for optimism, these increases are still inadequate to meet growing needs for RNs.

A. Registered nurses (RNs) constitute 80% of nurses in the United States.

1. **Qualifications and training.** Three types of educational programs qualify a student to become an RN. (Table 16-7).
   a. **Diploma programs** are the oldest form of nursing education and are typically sponsored by hospitals. Living adjacent to the sponsoring hospital, student nurses participate in a 3-year program of didactic work and firsthand experience working in the hospital. Diploma programs are being replaced by associate and bachelor degree programs. In 1989, graduates of diploma programs numbered 4826, down from 20,000 15 years earlier (Figure 16-4).
   b. **Associate degrees** in nursing are granted after 2 years of study, usually at a junior college. Associate degree students acquire limited practical experience. Students with associate degrees comprise the largest number of graduates. As with the other types of RN programs, graduates with associate degrees have declined sharply from a high of 45,000 in 1985 to a low of only 37,400 in 1988. Interestingly, 1989 showed a 1.2% increase in associate degree graduates. By comparison, graduates of bachelor degree and diploma programs declined by 12% and 19%, respectively.
   c. **Bachelor of Science degrees** in nursing (BSNs) are granted by 4-year colleges or universities and require more extensive class work. As medicine has become increasingly technologically sophisticated, nursing leadership has advocated an emphasis on advanced nursing degrees. It has been proposed that nursing staffs be composed entirely of RNs with baccalaureate degrees, but the realities of the nursing shortage preclude this [see I C 1 b (3)]. As general interest in nursing has declined, so have the number of graduates of BSN programs. In 1989, 30% (18,997) of RNs who graduated that year earned a BSN.

2. **Specialization**
   a. **Hospital-based nurses** often elect to practice in one specialty, such as pediatrics, operating room, medical and surgical, or intensive care nursing, for prolonged periods. The technical complexity of care, including more complex monitoring and drug regimens, is the principle force behind this specialization.
   b. **Nurses working outside the hospital**
      (1) Community health nurses are nurses who work outside of hospitals. Community

Table 16-7. Educational Requirements for Nurses

Educational Level	Training Required beyond High School	Curriculum	Training Site
Registered nurse			
PhD and DNS (Doctor of Nursing Science)	3–5 years post-baccalaureate	Academic program integrated with practical work throughout the years	University
Master's degree	5–6 academic years	1- to 2-year academic program integrated with practical work	University, hospital, and community health agencies
Baccalaureate degree	4 years and summer sessions	4-year academic program integrated with practical experience	University, hospital, and community health agencies
Diploma	27–36 months	1-year academic program and 2 years of practical experience with clinical courses	Hospital
Associate degree	2 years	2-year academic program integrated with practical experience	Junior college
Licensed practical nurse	1 year	1-year academic program integrated with practical experience	Vocational technical school and hospital

Reprinted from Snook DI: *Hospitals: What They Are and How They Work.* Rockville, MD, Aspen Publishers, 1981, p 81.

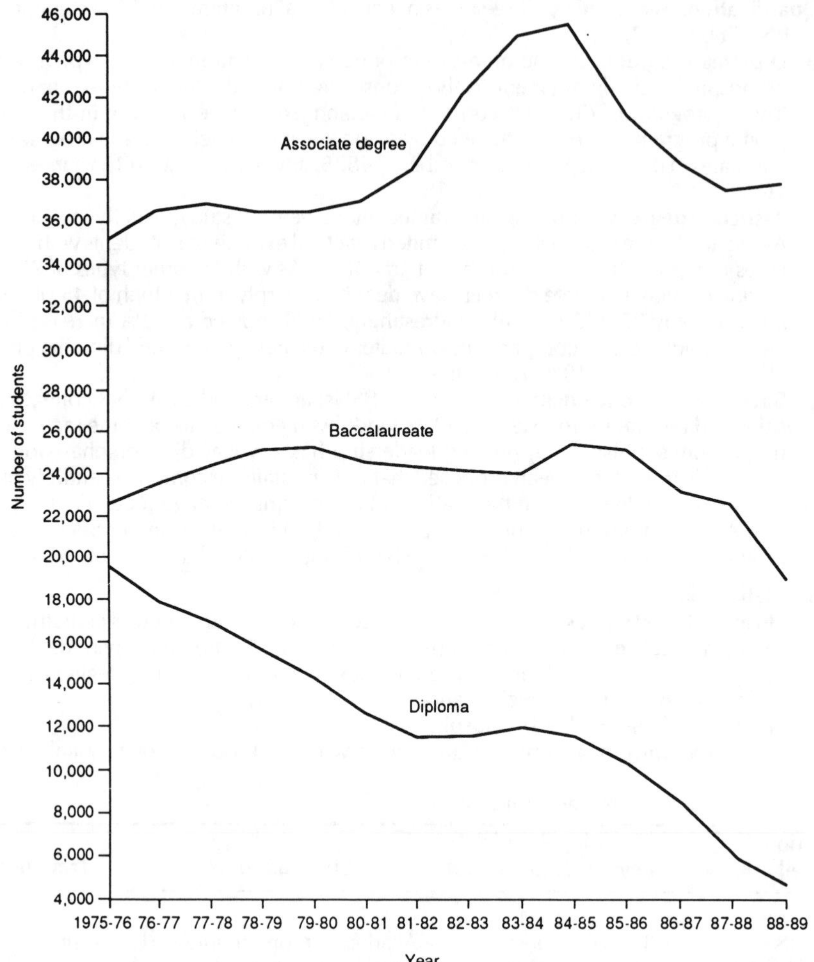

Figure 16-4. Number of students graduating from initial programs leading to an RN degree in the United States and outlying areas from 1975–1976 to 1988–1989, by type of program. (Adapted from Smith H: *Facts about Nursing, 1986–1987.* Kansas City, MO, American Nurses' Association, 1989, p 29.)

health nurses are increasingly in demand to provide **home health care services**. Because their practices are independent of direct physician review, they traditionally have been required to have a BSN.

(2) Public health nurses are community nurses employed by local, state, or federal government.

(a) Public health nurses develop and implement programs in immunization, maternal and infant health, and control of infectious diseases.

(b) In 1988, it was estimated that 94,500 full-time equivalent positions were available in public health nursing, or 38 per 100,000 population.

(c) In California and Minnesota, a nurse is licensed as a public health nurse (LPHN). While a licensure fee is required, there are minimal additional educational requirements beyond the BSN.

3. Licensure. RN licensure is handled by state boards of nursing. Each state administers a licensing examination. All nurses must be licensed to provide patient care. Additional licenses must be obtained for each state in which a nurse wishes to practice.

B. Licensed practical nurses (LPNs) numbered 608,000 in 1991.

1. Qualifications and training

a. LPNs, or licensed vocational nurses (LVNs), are certified health workers trained in basic manual skills and techniques for assisting RNs in patient care. A major limitation of LPNs is that they are not permitted to dispense medication, although they can hand it to a patient once an RN has dispensed it.

b. LPNs must train for 1 year. There were 30,400 graduates in 1990 from 1048 LPN and LVN programs. Both numbers of programs and graduates plummeted in the mid-1980s. Yearly graduates fell from a high of 47,000 to a low of 28,000 in 1988. Enrollment has rebounded in the 1987–1989 period, however, and suggests a healthy renewal of interest in LPN and LVN jobs.

2. **Salaries** for LPNs are lower than those for RNs; thus, a hospital ward usually is staffed with one or two RNs who are assisted by several LPNs.

3. **Licensure** for LPNs is similar to that for RNs (see III A 3).

IV. DENTISTS.

Dentistry generally is confined to care of the teeth and oral cavity.

A. Education

1. **Schools.** In 1991, there were 55 dental schools in the United States granting Doctor of Dental Surgery (DDS) or Doctor of Medical Dentistry (DMD) degrees (equivalent degrees) to students after 4 years of study.

2. **Areas of study.** Dental and medical students study similar subjects (e.g., pharmacology, anatomy, physiology), but dental students focus on the clinical and technical aspects of oral and tooth diseases.

3. **Enrollment.** In 1990, 4400 students graduated from dental school.

B. Licensure. Each state has a board of dentistry and laws regulating the practice of dental medicine. Licensing examinations are required, and practitioners must obtain a license for each state in which they wish to work.

C. Types of practice. In 1990, an estimated 150,800 dentists were in active practice in the United States. A surplus of dentists exists, with an average of 60 dentists per 100,000 civilian population.

1. **General dentistry,** the most common type of practice, involves oral diagnosis, repair of dental structures, and preventive dentistry. Preventive dental care is becoming more common with the advent of dental insurance, which is held by over 60 million Americans.

2. **Specialty practice** may be in one of eight specialties recognized by the American Dental Association (ADA). Specialty training requires 1–4 years of additional training. There are 17,000 dental specialists listed in the United States. The eight dental specialties are:
   - **a.** Dental public health
   - **b.** Endodontics (treatment of diseases of the pulp)
   - **c.** Oral pathology
   - **d.** Oral surgery
   - **e.** Orthodontics (treatment of tooth and oral structural problems)
   - **f.** Pediatric dentistry
   - **g.** Periodontics (treatment of diseases of the oral mucosa and gums)
   - **h.** Prosthodontics (replacement of teeth and dental structures by substitutes)

V. MIDLEVEL PRACTITIONERS

include nurse midwives, nurse practitioners, and physician's assistants. These professionals usually work with, and are supervised by, physicians. They are seen as physician extenders (i.e., they increase a physician's productivity), although their skills in areas such as health education and prevention may exceed those of a physician. In a few states, midlevel practitioners are licensed to practice independently. Most midlevel practitioners are either licensed or regulated by state nursing or medical boards. The quality of care provided by midlevel practitioners compares favorably with that provided by physicians treating similar problems.

A. Nurse practitioners are RNs who have completed additional study in a specific area (e.g., pediatrics). There are approximately 26,000 active nurse practitioners.

1. **Education.** Most programs, which grant a Master of Nursing (MSN) degree, last 1 or 2 years and prepare candidates for diagnosing and treating patients within their areas of expertise.

2. **Certification.** Candidates must pass a certifying examination and then are registered or licensed through state nursing boards.

B. **Nurse midwives** are RNs with special training in managing uncomplicated pregnancies, childbirth, postpartum, gynecologic phases of the reproductive cycle, and normal newborns. There are an estimated 2500 certified midwives currently living in the United States, 70% of whom are practicing.

1. **Education.** University programs for nurses with bachelor's degrees grant master's degrees after 1 or 2 years of midwifery study and experience. Additional 9- to 12-month programs are available to RNs with diplomas and associate degrees.

2. **Certification.** The American College of Nurse Midwives (ACNM), a professional organization of midwives founded in 1955, administers a national certifying examination. Successful completion of this examination plus evidence of sufficient clinical experience leads to certification and the title certified nurse midwife (CNM).

3. **Licensure.** Most states require licensure that is specific to nurse midwives and require close cooperation with, and supervision by, an obstetrician.

C. **Physician's assistants (PAs)** are specially trained health care workers who function under the supervision of licensed physicians. PAs working in surgical practices are known as surgeon's assistants. In 1990, over 21,000 PAs were in practice, and about one-third of them were women.

1. **Education.** The first educational program for PAs was based on former military corpsmen—that is, military medics returning to civilian life were given additional medical education to provide them with an official status in civilian medical care. Since 1965, over 50 programs have been accredited by the Committee on Allied Health Education and Accreditation (CAHEA), a voluntary organization established by the AMA in 1976 that is made up of 14 members, representing government, the public, and numerous health organizations. Programs last 18–24 months and cover the basic medical sciences and clinical skills. Certificates or degrees are awarded upon completion of the program.

2. **Certification** is achieved on examination by the National Commission on Certification of Physician's Assistants. A certified PA must pass an examination every 6 years.

3. **Licensure or registration** varies by state, but a state's Board of Medical Examiners usually oversees licensure.

4. **Practice patterns.** Generally, PAs, who numbered over 21,000 in the United States in 1990, take medical histories, perform physicals, order diagnostic studies, and initiate treatment. PAs are viewed as economically attractive alternatives to physicians' services.
   a. Ten years ago, most PAs worked in a physician's office.
   b. Today, 64% of PAs are based in institutions and are replacing house staff on some services.

VI. **ALLIED HEALTH PERSONNEL** include professionals and workers in the fields of patient care, public health, and health research who assist independent practitioners in providing health services. They are defined as individuals working under the general supervision of a physician in providing medical services to members of the public while exercising independent judgment within their areas of competence. Over 8 million allied health personnel were active in 1990, and 33,942 allied health professionals graduated in 1990. Table 16-8 lists 26 CAHEA-accredited allied health occupations.

A. **Education.** A high school diploma or equivalent is necessary for admission to all programs. The programs may also require college level work or a baccalaureate degree. The program itself may be as short as 6 months for an electroencephalogram technician to 4 years for a radiographic technologist.

B. **Certification** of allied health professionals is carried out by individual professional organizations. For example, a respiratory therapist must take the test administered by the National Board of Respiratory Therapy. Upon successful completion, the candidate would be a registered respiratory therapist (RRT). Some allied health professions do not have certification processes, but some states may require registration or licensure.

Table 16-8. Enrollments and Graduates by Occupation, 1989–1990

Occupation	Enrollments*			Graduates*
	Full-Time	Part-Time	Total	Total
Anesthesiologist's assistant	40	7	47	20
Cardiovascular technologist	155	0	155	61
Cytotechnologist	247	13	260	210
Diagnostic medical sonographer	597	38	635	338
Electroneurodiagnostic technologist	172	4	176	63
Emergency medical technician-paramedic	2089	1260	3349	1817
Histologic technician/technologist	168	15	183	104
Medical assistant	8751	2056	10,807	4516
Medical illustrator	75	27	102	36
Medical laboratory technician (associate degree)	4216	920	5136	1444
Medical laboratory technician (certificate)	1476	56	1532	848
Medical record administrator	1577	715	2292	671
Medical record technician	2538	1612	4150	1165
Medical technologist	5259	475	5734	3024
Nuclear medicine technologist	1200	53	1253	611
Occupational therapist	7322	664	7986	2424
Ophthalmic medical technician/technologist	110	19	129	72
Perfusionist	338	7	345	206
Physician's assistant	2897	120	3017	1120
Radiation therapy technologist	949	13	962	542
Radiographer	18,061	632	18,693	7402
Respiratory therapist	6983	929	7912	2830
Respiratory therapy technician	5451	581	6032	2886
Specialist in blood bank technology	64	15	79	49
Surgeon's assistant	95	0	95	48
Surgical technologist	2325	187	2512	1435
Total	73,155	10,418	83,573	33,942

Reprinted from American Medical Association: *Allied Health Education Directory.* Chicago, AMA, 1991.

*Enrollment and graduate data were provided by the 2827 programs accredited as of July 1990 and 80 programs that were discontinued in 1989–1990. Data reflect the 1989–1990 academic year.

C. Licensure of allied health personnel is not uniform and, because of the cumbersome task of establishing individual state examinations for the many allied professions, certification by a national organization has been proposed. By contrast, physical therapists are not nationally certified but must apply for registration or licensure in each state in which they wish to practice. Diagnostic radiographic technicians may be required to pass a state licensing examination, even though they might be registered or certified.

VII. PHARMACISTS, OPTOMETRISTS, AND PODIATRISTS

A. Pharmacists. There were 164,000 pharmacists in the United States in 1989. They provide a range of services from retail pharmacy to clinical pharmacology. Pharmacy education usually requires 5 years of a combination of undergraduate work and pharmacy experience. Registered pharmacists have completed the required educational program and passed appropriate examinations. All states register or license pharmacists.

B. Optometrists are trained to diagnose eye disorders and fit corrective lenses. The educational program leads to a Doctor of Optometry (OD). In 1989, there were 4600 students of optometry and approximately 1100 graduates. Over 26,000 optometrists are practicing today.

C. Podiatry. According to the American Association of Colleges of Podiatric Medicine, podiatry involves examining, diagnosing, treating, and preventing diseases or conditions affecting the foot and its related structures. In 1990, over 12,000 podiatrists were in practice (i.e., 4.8 podiatrists per 100,000 population).

1. **Education.** There are currently seven colleges of podiatric medicine. The oldest was founded in 1912. These colleges offer 4-year programs leading to the Doctor of Podiatric Medicine (DPM) degree. In 1990, 2600 podiatric students were enrolled, and 600 graduates received the DPM.
2. **Postgraduate training.** Ninety percent of graduates pursue advanced training in one of the 180 programs in the United States. These programs may be rotations, residencies, podiatric orthopedic residencies, or podiatric surgical residencies.
3. **Licensure.** Licensure of podiatric physicians is required in all states. Twelve states, however, require podiatric medical residency training before licensure.

BIBLIOGRAPHY

American Medical Association: *Allied Health Education Directory.* Chicago, AMA, 1991.

American Medical Association: *Physician Characteristics and Distribution in the US.* Chicago, AMA, 1992.

Commonwealth Fund: What to do about the nursing shortage. Unpublished paper, New York, Commonwealth Fund, 1989.

Department of Health and Human Services: *Health United States, 1990.* Hyattsville, MD, DHHS, 1991.

Department of Health and Human Services: *Sixth Report to the President and Congress on the Status of Health Personnel in the United States.* Washington, DC, US Printing Office, 1988.

Eisenberg C: Medicine is no longer a man's profession: or, when the men's club goes coed, it's time to change the regs. *N Engl J Med* 321:1542–1544, 1989.

Gonzales ML (ed): *Socioeconomic Characteristics of Medical Practice, 1990/91.* Chicago, American Medical Association, 1991.

Health Insurance Association of America: *Source Book of Health Insurance Data—1991.* Washington, DC, Health Insurance Association of America, 1991.

Marder WD, Kletke PR, Silberger AB, et al: *Physician Supply and Utilization by Specialty: Trends and Projections.* Chicago, American Medical Association, 1988.

National League of Nursing: *Nursing Data Review, 1991.* New York, National League of Nursing Press, 1991.

Relman AS: The changing demographics of the medical profession. *N Engl J Med* 321:1540–1541, 1989.

Schwarz WB, Sloan FA, Mendelson DN: Why there will be little or no physician surplus between now and the year 2000. *N Engl J Med* 318:892–897, 1988.

STUDY QUESTIONS

Directions: Each of the numbered items or incomplete statements in this section is followed by answers or by completions of the statement. Select the **one** lettered answer or completion that is **best** in each case.

1. Which of the following statements about the cost of medical education is correct?

(A) The rise in the cost of medical education generally has been lower than the overall rate of inflation
(B) Nearly 40% of medical school revenues come from direct patient care
(C) Nearly 60% of the revenues that support medical education come from federal funding
(D) Federal support of medical education remains strong and continues to grow as a percentage of all revenue
(E) The average medical student with debt owes twice as much now as compared with 5 years ago

2. True statements about the report issued by the GMENAC in 1976 include all of the following EXCEPT

(A) it predicted an excess of surgeons by the year 1990
(B) it predicted an excess of internists by the year 1990
(C) it projected physician staffing requirements for different geographic areas of the United States
(D) it recommended reducing medical school enrollment
(E) it recommended financial incentives to attract residents to primary care

3. Which of the following is a true statement regarding female medical school applicants?

(A) Women comprise 20% of all medical students
(B) The increase in female applicants in the 1980s paralleled the increase in male applicants
(C) Since 1985, the number of female applicants has consistently increased
(D) Some medical schools have a majority of women in the first-year class

4. All of the following statements accurately describe osteopaths EXCEPT

(A) students of osteopathy complete the same number of years of medical school as allopathic students
(B) there are approximately one-sixth as many osteopathic students as allopathic students
(C) osteopaths are licensed in all 50 states
(D) osteopaths have a high specialization rate
(E) osteopathic medicine differs from allopathic medicine because osteopathic physicians use manipulative therapy

---

1-B
2-C
3-D
4-D

Directions: Each item below contains four suggested answers of which **one or more** is correct. Choose the answer

A if **1, 2, and 3** are correct
B if **1 and 3** are correct
C if **2 and 4** are correct
D if **4** is correct
E if **1, 2, 3, and 4** are correct

5. There were approximately 608,000 LPNs in the United States in 1991. Accurate statements about LPNs include which of the following?

(1) Their salaries are lower than those of RNs
(2) They assist patients with personal care
(3) They are referred to as LVNs in some states
(4) They usually dispense routine medications

6. All of the following are requirements for eligibility for licensure as an allopathic physician EXCEPT

(1) graduation from an AAMC accredited medical school
(2) successful completion of Steps I, II, and III of the USMLE or of FLEX
(3) completion of 1 year of postgraduate medical training
(4) declaration of a specialty

7. Statements that accurately describe nursing in the United States include

(1) LPNs outnumber RNs 2 to 1
(2) nursing educators encourage the BSN degree
(3) diploma nursing programs are university based
(4) a high level of specialization has evolved in nursing practice

Directions: The group of items in this section consists of lettered options followed by a set of numbered items. For each item, select the **one** lettered option that is most closely associated with it. Each lettered option may be selected once, more than once, or not at all.

Questions 8–11

Match each of the following descriptions with the appropriate type of medical practitioner.

(A) Allopathic physicians
(B) Osteopathic physicians
(C) Certified nurse practitioners
(D) Physician's assistants
(E) Pharmacists

8. The first educational program for these practitioners was based on the training given to military medics returning to civilian life who were given additional medical education to provide them with an official status in civilian medical care.

9. The original basis for the educational program for these practitioners is in the theories of musculoskeletal manipulation.

10. The educational program for these practitioners usually requires 5 years of a combination of undergraduate and on-the-job experience.

11. These practitioners must have a master's degree to practice.

5-A
6-D
7-C
8-D
9-B
10-E
11-C

ANSWERS AND EXPLANATIONS

1. The answer is B *[II C 1, 2].*
Nearly 40% of medical school revenues come from direct patient care. The funding for undergraduate medical education has changed radically as federal support has diminished. Now constituting less than 24% of all revenues, federal funds have only recently stabilized instead of declined. The shortfall must be offset by patient billings and increased tuition. From 1985 to 1990, the debt owed by the average student with debt rose 54%, from $30,000 to $46,200. Additionally, the cost of medical education has risen by more than 10% a year, which is over twice the rise in inflation.

2. The answer is C *[I B 4 a].*
The Graduate Medical Education National Advisory Committee (GMENAC) produced a report projecting physician staffing requirements for the year 1990 and for each specialty, but geographic maldistributions in the United States were not addressed. The report predicted an excess of 70,000 physicians in the year 1990, particularly in the areas of general surgery, obstetrics and gynecology, radiology, and general internal medicine. Recommendations included reduced medical school enrollment, a 20% reduction in residency programs in areas of projected surpluses, and financial incentives to attract residents to primary care and away from oversubscribed specialties.

3. The answer is D *[II A 1 b].*
In 1990–1991, women formed a majority of the first-year class in eight medical schools in the United States. Women comprise 37% of all medical students, although fewer than 20% of practicing physicians are women. The rapid increase in female applicants in the early 1980s offset the decline in male applicants. From 1985 to 1989, however, the number of female applicants gradually declined. In 1990, female applicants increased by 12%, or 1250 applicants, a remarkable increase.

4. The answer is D *[II B].*
Developed in the 1870s by Andrew Taylor Still, osteopathy was founded on the concept that musculoskeletal therapy could speed the body's natural healing ability. Upon completing 4 years of osteopathic school, which is very similar to the medical curriculum of their allopathic colleagues, osteopathic physicians complete an internship and are eligible for licensure anywhere in the United States. A total of 6600 osteopathic students attend any of 15 schools compared to a total of 65,000 students in 102 allopathic medical schools. Traditionally, osteopathic physicians have followed a primary care path. Currently, 91% of all osteopathic physicians are in general practice, pediatrics, or internal medicine.

5. The answer is A (1, 2, 3) *[III B 1, 2].*
Licensed practical nurses (LPNs) provide much of the hands-on care of patients, but they are prohibited from dispensing drugs. Because LPNs earn lower salaries than registered nurses (RNs), it is common for a hospital to employ fewer RNs but several LPNs to assist them. LPNs are known as licensed vocational nurses (LVNs) in some states.

6. The answer is D (4) *[II A 3].*
Medical graduates are licensed as "physicians and surgeons" and, thus, are not legally restricted to practice in a specialty. However, liability coverage and hospital privileges limit the scope of practice. Eligibility for licensure requires graduation from a medical school accredited by the Association of American Medical Colleges (AAMC), successful completion of an objective examination [either Steps I, II, and III of the U.S. Medical Licensing Examination (USMLE) or the Federal Licensing Examination (FLEX)], and completion of 1 year of postgraduate medical training.

7. The answer is C (2, 4) *[III A 1 a–c, 2].*
As nursing has become increasingly specialized and technical, the education of nurses has become more demanding, emphasizing the 4-year program required for a Bachelor of Science degree in nursing (BSN). Diploma nursing programs are primarily those established by hospitals and lack the university or college affiliation to grant a BSN degree. There are more than twice as many registered nurses (RNs) as licensed practical nurses (LPNs).

8–11. The answers are: 8-D *[V C]*, **9-B** *[II B]*, **10-E** *[VII A]*, **11-C** *[V A 1].*
The first educational program for physician's assistants (PAs) was based on the training given to military medics returning to civilian life who were given additional medical education to provide them with an

official status in civilian medical care. Generally, PAs take medical histories, perform physical examinations, order diagnostic studies, and initiate treatment.

Osteopathic physicians' training is based on Andrew Taylor Still's theories of musculoskeletal manipulation. Study leading to the Doctor of Osteopathy (DO) degree requires 4 years of education beyond the baccalaureate degree. Curriculum content closely parallels that required for allopathic physicians, with the addition of training in manipulation. In 1989, osteopathic physicians comprised 10% of practicing physicians in the United States.

Pharmacy education usually requires 5 years of a combination of undergraduate work and pharmacy experience. Registered pharmacists have completed the required educational program and passed appropriate examinations.

Certified nurse practitioners are registered nurses (RNs) who have completed additional study in a specific area, such as pediatrics. Most programs, which grant a Master of Nursing degree, last 1 or 2 years and prepare candidates for diagnosing and treating patients within their areas of expertise.

17
Health Care Services

Brett J. Cassens

I. OVERVIEW OF THE HEALTH CARE SYSTEM. In the 1990s, the United States has been confronted with having, simultaneously, limited access to care for 37 million Americans and the most expensive health care system in the world (e.g., over $700 billion was spent on health care by 250 million Americans in 1991). This chapter discusses the current approach to care in the United States and presents promising improvements for this system in the 21st century. The success of health services is measured in longevity, prevalence of disease in a given population, and the functional status of the population. Both individuals and institutions constitute the system that provides personal and public health.

A. Personal health care is the service provided to an individual by a health professional to preserve or restore health. There are several categories of personal health care.

1. **Ambulatory care,** or **outpatient services,** refers to services provided for nonhospitalized patients in medical offices, clinics, emergency departments, urgent care centers, and physical therapy offices.
2. **Hospital care,** or **inpatient services,** refers to institutional services that include bed and board. Physicians, nurses, and ancillary personnel work together to provide intensive, sophisticated care in the hospital environment.
3. **Long-term care** refers to health care services provided in nursing homes or by home health care specialists who provide personal medical care for patients who have not completely recovered but are not sick enough to remain hospitalized.

B. Public health is defined as the combination of sciences, skills, and beliefs that are directed to the maintenance and improvement of the health of an entire population. Public health typically is in the domain of government. According to the World Health Organization (WHO), governments should demonstrate a responsibility for their peoples' health by providing adequate health and social services. In the United States, federal, state, and local governments provide health services.

1. **Federal government involvement in health care** is a function of the **Department of Health and Human Services (DHHS),** established in 1953 as the Department of Health, Education, and Welfare (DHEW) and renamed DHHS in 1979.
   a. Figure 17-1 shows the organization of DHHS. The Secretary, a cabinet level position, makes recommendations to the President regarding the health, welfare, income security, policies, and programs of the United States.
   b. **The Public Health Service (PHS)** is the division of DHHS that is responsible for public health services, research, and, to a limited extent, personal health care (e.g., Indian Health Service). The Assistant Secretary for Health and the Surgeon General head the PHS, which has its origins in the Marine Hospital Act of 1798. The seven major divisions of the PHS are listed in Figure 17-2.
2. **State and local governments** fund 85% of all public health activities, usually through cooperative programs. Control of infectious diseases; medical laboratory services; environmental health, including air, food, and water quality; maternal and children's health; health education; immunizations; and vital statistics are major responsibilities of state and local health departments. Federal agencies, especially the Centers for Disease Control (CDC), regularly provide funding, technical assistance, and personnel to support local health departments on unusual or complex public health problems [e.g., rubella outbreaks, acquired immune deficiency syndrome (AIDS)].

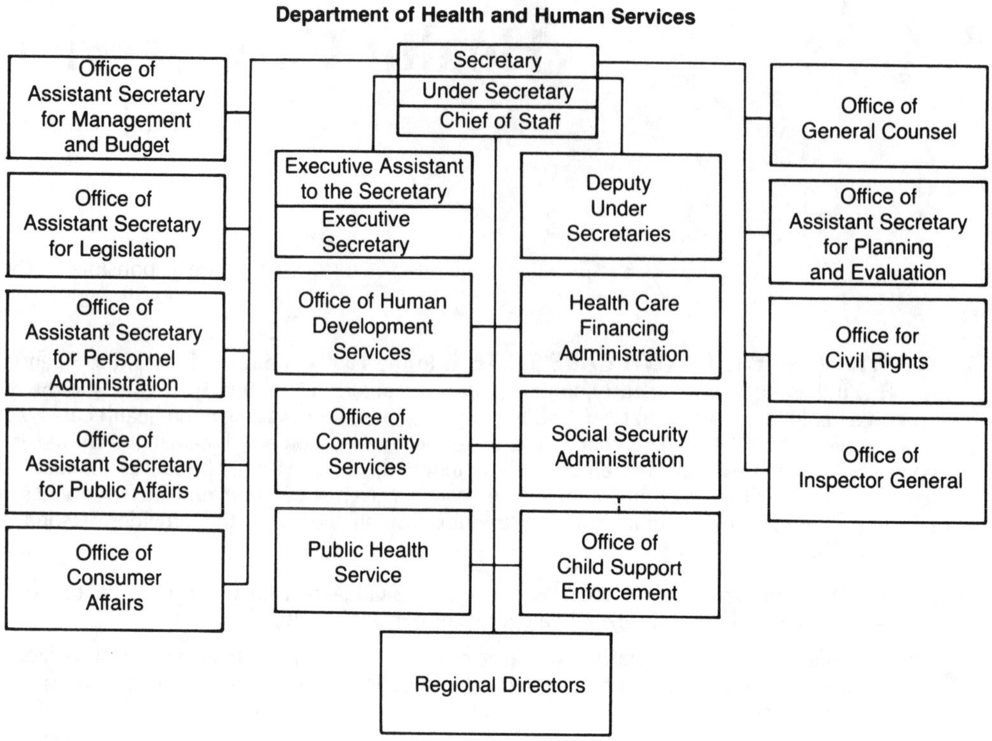

Department of Health and Human Services

Secretary
Under Secretary
Chief of Staff
Office of Assistant Secretary for Management and Budget
Office of Assistant Secretary for Legislation
Office of Assistant Secretary for Personnel Administration
Office of Assistant Secretary for Public Affairs
Office of Consumer Affairs
Executive Assistant to the Secretary
Executive Secretary
Office of Human Development Services
Office of Community Services
Public Health Service
Deputy Under Secretaries
Health Care Financing Administration
Social Security Administration
Office of Child Support Enforcement
Office of General Counsel
Office of Assistant Secretary for Planning and Evaluation
Office for Civil Rights
Office of Inspector General
Regional Directors

Figure 17-1. Organization of the Department of Health and Human Services (DHHS).

a. **State health departments** are headed by boards of health or by a secretary or commissioner of health. In the latter case, governors appoint their health officers and exercise significant political control over the appointees. The state department of health sets minimum standards for hospitals, nursing homes, and laboratories and licenses institutions and many health professionals. In rural and unincorporated areas, the state has responsibilities for immunizations, rabies control, and water and air quality.

b. **Local health departments.** Cities, large municipalities, and counties also may have boards

Divisions of the Public Health Service

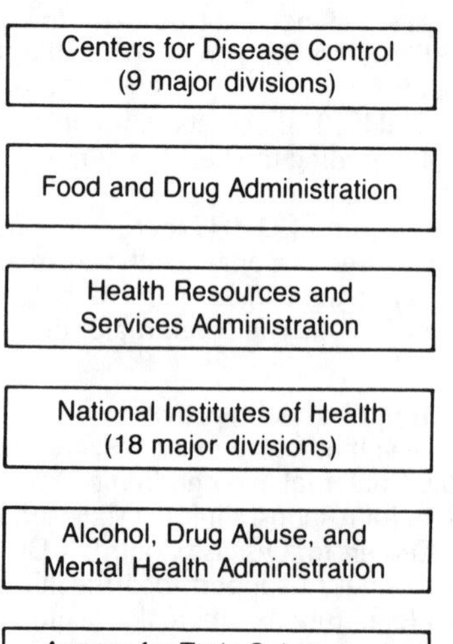

Figure 17-2. Organization of the U.S. Public Health Service (PHS)—a division of the Department of Health and Human Services (DHHS).

of health, health commissioners, or directors of public health. While the local responsibilities parallel those of the state, local services may exceed those of the state. Most local health departments operate with boards of health composed of community members. Such boards advise on health matters and formulate codes of health that govern the community. Many cities provide free community health centers, but few still support large municipal hospitals, such as Cook County Hospital in Chicago and Bellevue Hospital in New York City.

II. CHARACTERISTICS OF MEDICAL PRACTICES.

The 650,000 physicians [Doctors of Medicine (MDs) and Doctors of Osteopathy (DOs)] in the United States direct and are responsible for the activities of the 8 million other health care workers. In the past, physicians were either general practitioners or specialists, depending on whether or not they completed a residency program beyond the obligatory internship. However, virtually all medical students today enter residency programs in a particular specialty.

A. Primary care providers are central to the medical system because they are the first contacts of patients seeking care. Efforts to streamline and economize medical practice have placed increasing importance on the role of the primary care physician.

1. **Primary care physician.** According to the American Medical Association (AMA), the primary care physician generally is contacted by the public directly and provides a range of services, including the treatment of chronic illnesses, preventive and emergency care, and patient counseling.
2. **Primary care specialties** include family medicine, internal medicine, and pediatrics. All other specialties are not primary care. During the last 5 years, the number of resident physicians trained in primary care has declined; only 33% of practicing physicians are in these primary specialties. The number of primary care physicians is expected to continue to decline in the forseeable future.
3. **The primary care physician's role** is alternately described as a keystone or a gatekeeper. The difference is significant.
   a. The **keystone role** of the primary care physician holds that primary care physicians coordinate the care provided by an increasing number of disparate specialists and technicians, each of whom is concerned with only a single aspect of an individual's overall medical condition. As a keystone, the primary care physician oversees these interactions and ties them together as effectively as possible, just as a keystone unites and caps the sides of an arch.
   b. The **gatekeeper role** of the primary care physician, by contrast, also coordinates care but additionally controls and limits access to other specialists. For example, primary care physicians in health maintenance organizations (HMOs) [see II D 2 a] provide a broad scope of medical services, thus avoiding expensive, unnecessary referrals to specialists. Family practitioners, for example, competently treat acne, usually without dermatologic consultation.
   c. **Pros and cons of these two conceptual models**
      (1) **Advocates of the keystone concept** argue that patients should be free to select whomever they wish for a service, and the specialist, though potentially more expensive, may actually be more efficient by virtue of his expertise and superior level of care. Non–primary care specialists, in particular, favor patient freedom to exercise preference for one specialist over another.
      (2) **Advocates of the gatekeeper function** accept the restrictions of patient choice but believe that this loss of freedom is justified because better care results when it is provided by one physician rather than numerous consultants. Recent research has shown a 6% decrease in physician charges in a randomized trial of gatekeeper versus open access to consultants. Critics charge that HMOs reward primary care providers for not referring, thus providing incentives for not making referrals, even when they are medically indicated. The expanding influence of managed care delivery systems, like HMOs and preferred provider organizations (PPOs) [see II D 2 c], predicts a greater role for primary care gatekeepers.
      (3) **From the patient standpoint,** freedom of choice remains an important option. An increasingly popular form of health insurance is an **open-ended HMO**. Subscribers are enrolled in a managed-care setting and may receive services at little cost from their

designated provider. However, they may opt to see physicians outside of the plan but are responsible for a percentage of the cost, usually 30%–40%.

B. Organization of physician practice. The choice between solo and group practice and between self-employment and employee status are important issues that confront physicians today. Office visits continue to be a major portion of physician-patient contact each year; over two-thirds of all encounters with physicians are office visits, with the remaining one-third consisting of hospital rounds, emergency room, and outpatient department visits.

1. **Solo practice.** Two-thirds of physicians practice alone. As entrepreneurs, they are at risk for all aspects of the business. They tend to work longer hours (i.e., 59 versus 57.7 hours per week for physicians in nonsolo practice). They see 9% fewer patients per week (i.e., 115 versus 125 for physicians in nonsolo practice), and they earn somewhat lower net incomes (i.e., $140,000 versus $147,000 per year for physicians in practice with one or more other physicians).

2. **Group practice** originated with the advent of the Mayo Clinic in the 1880s. It was viewed with suspicion, and members of groups were sometimes sanctioned by local medical societies in the belief that groups foster an impersonal, "corporate" medical practice.
   a. **Definition.** The AMA considers a medical group practice to be three or more physicians organized to provide medical care, such as consultation, diagnosis, and treatment, who share equipment, records, and personnel and who distribute income from the medical practice according to some prearranged plan.
   b. **The disadvantage of group practice** is essentially the perceived loss of independence attendant upon working in a group setting. Decisions require consensus and compromise. The group culture establishes norms for professional and sometimes personal behavior.
   c. **The advantage of group practice** is that groups, on average, provide better care because the patients' problems are discussed among the various members of the group. The group fosters a sharing of expertise and, in multispecialty groups, ease of referral without fear of losing the patient to the consultant.
   d. **Positions in group practices.** In 1988, 156,000 positions were offered in the 16,579 groups registered in the AMA census. In 1984, by contrast, 15,500 groups were counted with 140,000 positions. In 1988, 30% of all physicians not employed by the federal government were members of medical groups.
   e. **Growth in the numbers of medical groups** has slowed. The annual increase in numbers of groups formed between 1984 and 1988 was less than 2% per year, whereas in the prior 4 years (1980–1984), the rate of increase had been 11% per year. Explanations for this change include the following.
      (1) Physicians may find the current medical economic climate unfavorable to the formation of new groups and may prefer the relative security of joining an established group practice.
      (2) Increased overhead expenses and diminished Medicare reimbursement may be driving groups out of business or into mergers.
   f. **Medical group size** typically is small, numbering only three or four practitioners, usually in a single specialty. Fifty percent of single specialty medical groups are of this size and are the fastest growing type of group. Single specialty groups increased in number by 442% in the last 23 years. However, the average size of all groups has increased to nine physicians per group. The largest group contains more than 2000 physicians, while 118 groups report 100 or more physicians, according to the 1990 AMA report.

3. **Self-employed and salaried physicians.** The traditional solo entrepreneur is becoming a thing of the past, as young physicians opt for more limited time commitments and early guarantees of a stable income. As recently as 10 years ago, salaried positions for physicians were limited. Now, as hospitals and large health care corporations provide patient care through clinics, HMOs, and urgent care centers (see V B), the number of salaried positions is growing. Fully 45% of physicians under the age of 35 are now working as employees. However, over the first 11 years of experience, the percentage drops to 24% and remains in this range. Women are twice as likely to be employed over all age ranges compared to their male counterparts.
   a. **Work patterns** of self-employed and salaried physicians differ significantly. Although both groups work an average of 47 weeks per year, AMA statistics reveal a shorter work week for salaried physicians (i.e., 49 versus 55 hours for self-employed physicians). Similarly, salaried physicians have fewer patient visits but longer patient hospital stays (i.e., 7.5 days versus 4.5 days per hospitalization for patients of self-employed physicians).

b. **Income.** For the self-employed physician, **annual net income before taxes** is the total amount of money earned in the practice (gross income) per year less expenses (**overhead**). Rent, insurance of several types, office staff salaries, and supplies are all paid by the employer/physician and deducted from the gross earnings of the practice. This net income is **taxable income**. For salaried physicians, salary is net income. Average net income for self-employed physicians is $160,000 versus $113,000 for salaried physicians. The greater financial risk and longer hours of self-employed physicians translates into 27% higher earnings.

4. **Midlevel practitioners** include physician's assistants, nurse midwives, and nurse practitioners. There are approximately 48,000 of these health professionals, providing many of the services of physicians. Although most midlevel practitioners work under the supervision of physicians, a small number practice independently in some states. With salaries in the range of $40,000–$50,000 annually, they are attractive alternatives to more expensive physician personnel. Although the scope of practice of midlevel practitioners is more limited than physicians, they have replaced house physicians in some hospitals and some nursing homes and physicians in rural and city clinics. These providers increasingly compete with physicians for the growing number of salaried positions in health care organizations.

C. **Practice economics** is an unfamiliar area for the physician first entering the job market. Yet, the ability of physicians to earn adequate salaries is essential to their ability to retire the substantial debts accumulated during the course of their education and for job satisfaction.

1. **Physician numbers** are large, contributing to a more competitive job market. A ratio of 150 physicians per 100,000 population is thought to be ideal. In 1989, 234 physicians were available per 100,000 population in the United States. This is a 20% increase over 1980. Physician extenders (e.g., physician's assistants, nurse practitioners) are also more numerous each year, and increasing numbers are accepting salaried positions in institutions rather than in physicians' practices. Efforts to contain health care expenditures by reducing physicians' fees combined with rapidly rising office overhead are making medical practice less financially attractive than previously.

2. **Average annual net income of physicians** in 1988 was $144,700, including pensions and retirement plan contributions. As a 9% increase over 1987, this represented a net gain of 5% over inflation. While a similar increase was seen in 1987, a much smaller gain was seen before that. Indeed, in 1984 and 1985, physicians' income increases failed to match the rate of inflation. Smaller increases in physicians' salaries are likely in the future.
   a. **Specialty differences.** Physicians are among the highest paid professionals in the United States, although this is not the case for physicians elsewhere in the world. In the United States, 50% of physicians earned less than $120,000, when the mean income among physicians was $145,000. This is partially attributable to variations in earnings among specialties. The highest earnings were among surgeons and the lowest among pediatricians and family physicians. Table 17-1 shows the low of $94,600 for family medicine and the high of $207,500 for surgeons. This disparity of 116% demonstrates the difference in compensations for procedure-oriented care such as surgery, compared to the cognitive services of pediatricians, internists, and family physicians.
   b. **Regional differences in net income** are shown in Table 17-2. Physicians in the mountain states of Arizona, Colorado, Idaho, Montana, Nevada, New Mexico, Utah, and Wyoming experienced the lowest net income of $132,100, while those in Alabama, Mississippi, and Kentucky earned $165,000. Income in Alabama, Mississippi, and Kentucky increased 17%, twice the national average. The reasons for these differences are not clear and vary from year to year.

D. **Managed care** refers to a system that integrates financing and delivery of appropriate health care services to subscribers of the health plan. Also referred to as **alternative delivery systems,** they include HMOs, PPOs, and independent practice associations (IPAs).

1. **Common elements of managed-care systems** include:
   a. Contracts with a selected panel of providers
   b. Explicit standards for selection of providers
   c. Formal quality assurance and utilization review programs
   d. Significant financial incentives for members to use providers and procedures covered by the plan

Table 17-1. Mean Physician Net Income (in thousands of dollars) after Expenses and before Taxes, by Specialty (1981, 1984, 1988)

	1981	1984	1988
All physicians	89.9	108.4	144.7
Specialty			
General/family practice	71.5	71.6	94.6
Internal medicine	83.4	104.2	130.9
Surgery	114.5	151.0	207.5
Pediatrics	63.5	73.7	94.9
Obstetrics/gynecology	111.0	118.8	180.7
Radiology	108.0	139.7	184.6
Psychiatry	70.5	85.1	111.4
Anesthesiology	115.2	143.9	194.5

Adapted from American Medical Association (AMA) Center for Health Policy Research: *Socioeconomic Characteristics of Medical Practice 1989.* Chicago, AMA, 1989, p 124.

2. Definitions

a. **Health maintenance organizations (HMOs)** [see Ch 18 V B] provide prepaid comprehensive health care for a fixed periodic payment. Preventive, diagnostic, and therapeutic services are provided to **enrollees** (i.e., individuals who are on the membership roster). The financial risk of excessive use of services is born by the HMO.

b. **Independent practice associations (IPAs)** are a form of managed care, where physicians are in private practice but agree to accept either a reduced fee or a capitation fee (see II D 2 f) for services rendered to all plan patients. Unlike an HMO, the IPA physician is also likely to see patients who are not IPA members. A provider may also belong to more than one IPA.

c. **Preferred provider organizations (PPOs)** are fee-for-service plans, where insured individuals are given financial incentives to use "preferred providers." Other than the agreed discount from their charges, physicians are not at financial risk, and patients may use any physician, though nonmember physicians' services require copayments or deductibles.

d. **Exclusive provider organizations (EPOs)** are a rare form of fee-for-service plan, where an employer selects hospitals and physicians with favorable charges. Patients within such plans are required to use the physicians and hospitals felt to be most cost-effective. Providers are at no financial risk.

e. **Health insuring organizations (HIOs)** are similar to HMOs, except that enrollees are placed in the HMO without choice. This type of plan is rare but is used by a few states to control costs of Medicaid programs; in these states, Medicaid coverage is offered to indigent patients only through the HIO.

f. **Capitation** is the typical form of reimbursement in prepaid plans. A provider receives a fixed payment per month per enrollee to provide a specified set of services to that individual. Capitation fees usually take age and sex into consideration. The physician does not bill the patient or the plan.

Table 17-2. Mean Physician Net Income (in thousands of dollars) after Expenses and before Taxes, by Census Division (1981, 1984, 1988)

	1981	1984	1988
New England	83.0	87.8	133.0
Middle Atlantic	82.4	99.3	134.9
East North Central	96.4	109.8	147.0
West North Central	85.6	109.1	138.2
South Atlantic	91.4	113.6	156.0
East South Central	94.8	121.8	165.0
West South Central	97.9	122.2	160.9
Mountain	87.9	101.5	132.1
Pacific	88.8	109.2	136.2

Adapted from American Medical Association (AMA) Center for Health Policy Research: *Socioeconomic Characteristics of Medical Practice 1989.* Chicago, AMA, 1989, p 124.

g. **Coinsurance** is a fixed percentage of the bill for medical services paid by the patient. **Copayment** is either the amount paid for a service according to coinsurance or a fixed amount paid per service. All forms of health insurance require that employees copay to reduce premiums and to constrain the use of services. For example, if an insurance policy or HMO has a 20% coinsurance plan, a complete physical costing $150 would cost the patient $30 and the insurance company $120. An HMO requiring $3 copayments collects this amount whenever the patient sees a provider.

h. **Deductible** is the amount an enrollee must pay each year before the insurance plan begins to pay. A typical deductible is $250–$500. If a patient incurred $800 of medical expenses in 1992, and the patient's plan has a $300 deductible, then the patient pays the first $300, and the plan would pay the remaining $500, less the copay. Insurance plans and HMOs may employ deductibles and copayments together.

3. **Prepaid medical care,** or **prospective reimbursement,** refers to the concept that hospitals or providers are paid a predetermined amount in advance for services that enrollees are entitled to receive. Implicit in prepayment is risk. A skillful provider with healthy patients might earn a handsome sum, whereas a less efficient physician or one with sick patients might earn a meager reimbursement relative to services rendered—that is, payment is independent of the health status of the patient or the efficiency of the provider.

   a. **History of prepaid health care**

      (1) The earliest prepaid health plans date back to the Great Depression. In 1929, the Ross-Loss Clinic contracted with the city of Los Angeles to provide prepaid health care to city employees. In 1934, consumers in Elk City, Oklahoma, organized a health cooperative, hired physicians, and provided services on a prepaid basis.

      (2) Despite the staunch resistance of medical societies to the concept of "contract" medicine, prepaid health care slowly spread in the 1940s and 1950s. It was during this period that the **Kaiser Health Plans** gained a strong foothold on the West Coast.

      (3) The **Medicare** and **Medicaid** programs established in 1964 have had a decisive effect on prepayment. These two programs rapidly inflated federal health care expenditures to such an extent that reform desperately was sought by 1969.

      (4) The concept of prepaid care that emphasizes health maintenance over expensive hospital care was the proposal of Paul Elwood, the Executive Director of the American Rehabilitation Foundation. He coined the term "health maintenance organization." His proposals eagerly were adopted by the Nixon administration, but strong resistance from organized medicine and liberals alike postponed passage of the **HMO Act** (Public Law 93-222) until 1973. This law funded only limited demonstration projects and overrode state laws that might prohibit HMOs. Amendments to the HMO Act in 1976 and 1978 finally spurred a true federal commitment to prepaid health care.

   b. **Prepaid health care today**

      (1) **Growth.** Although the 1971 projection of 1700 HMOs by 1977 proved wildly optimistic, recent growth has been impressive. Since 1984, the number of enrollees in HMOs has more than doubled, with over 35 million enrollees nationwide. By contrast, the number of HMOs peaked in 1988 at 633 and has declined slowly, but significantly, since. There are currently 575 HMOs in the United States. The decline in number of HMOs is largely due to plan terminations and mergers or consolidations. These factors account for approximately half of the plans no longer listed. The years 1985–1990 were a volatile period for HMOs, with rising costs forcing closures and consolidations.

      (2) Ironically, though prepayment was hailed as the means to reduce federal health care expenditures under **Medicare** and **Medicaid,** it was not until 1984, a decade later, that these programs were promoted within HMOs. Even then, the politics of prepayment was controversial. Opponents either feared that the poor and elderly might be underserved to the financial benefit of the plans or that calculations of cost of care would lead to windfall profits for the HMOs. By 1989, 2 million Medicare and 2.5 million Medicaid beneficiaries were enrolled in prepaid plans. Half of all Medicaid enrollees are in HIOs.

      (3) The **basic form of an HMO,** variations of which are illustrated in Figure 17-3, consists of the plan, a group of physicians, and a hospital. Enclosures in the circles indicate ownership by the plan. Straight-line linkages are contractual relationships.

         (a) **Staff-model HMOs.** In these HMOs, physicians are employed by the plan, while the hospitals may be plan-owned or independent.

         (b) **Group-model HMOs.** In these HMOs, physician groups contract with the plan, but the physicians remain employees of the group.

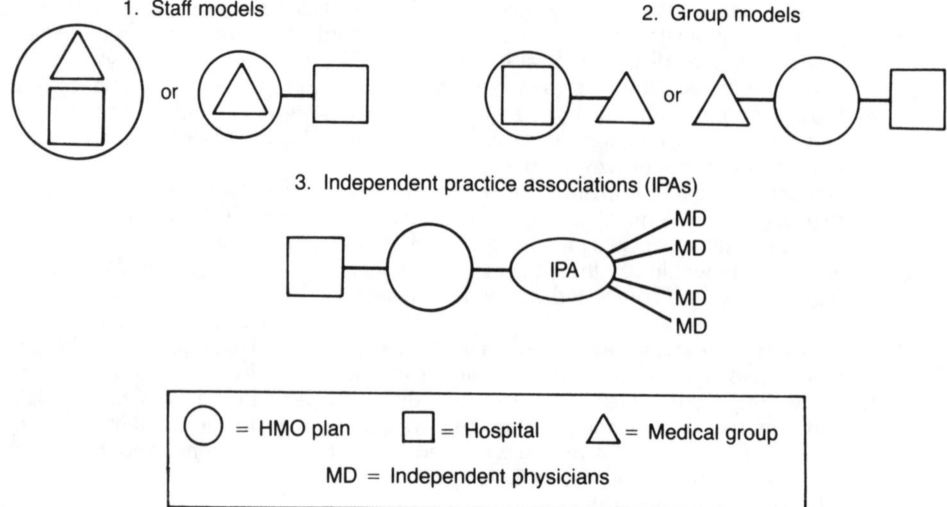

Figure 17-3. Health maintenance organization (HMO) models.

- **(c) IPAs** differ from staff- and group-model HMOs because the physicians are private practitioners who agree to see prepaid enrollees. Physicians band together on an IPA, and, then, this entity contracts with the HMO. Because of the independent position of the practitioner, IPAs are more palatable to organized medicine.

(4) Operation of an HMO

- **(a)** A group of investors, usually physicians and hospitals, formulate a plan for an HMO.
- **(b)** After licensure by the state insurance authority, the plan, which is actually an insurance company, formalizes contracts with hospitals and either hires physicians or contracts with a group.
- **(c)** The plan then attempts to convince employers in the area to offer the HMO health insurance to their employees for a premium, depending on whether the employee is single, married, or has a family.
- **(d)** The plan collects premiums, and the new enrollee selects a physician.
- **(e)** The plan begins providing services.
- **(f)** All routine and emergency care is provided at little, if any, charge to the enrollee.
- **(g)** If the HMO has an average number of sick patients, it will break even or perhaps make a small profit. If patients are quite ill, a debt is incurred. The distribution of financial risk is ideally dispersed among providers, hospitals, and the plan. The appropriate sharing of risk is fundamental to HMO management.

(5) Continued HMO development is inevitable as insurance companies start HMOs of their own to compete with independent prepaid plans. Triple option plans, under which an insurance company offers its own indemnity (traditional) plan, an HMO, and preferred provider options, are the wave of the future. Thus, one insurance company can offer these three different products to an employer.

E. Veterans Administration (VA) services. The VA provides extensive health services to eligible veterans. Medical care is provided without charge for any military service–related illness or disability. Veterans with non–service-related problems may receive care based on financial need. Hospital care, nursing home care, and outpatient medical and dental care are offered.

1. **Facilities.** VA facilities include 171 medical centers, 16 domiciliary facilities (see IV C 3), 225 clinics, 105 nursing homes, and 194 Vietnam veterans outreach facilities.

2. **Costs.** Health care expenditures within the VA totaled $11 billion or 2% of all health care dollars in the United States. Approximately 61% was spent for inpatient services, while 19% went to outpatient care.

3. **Eligibility.** Prior to 1989, eligibility requirements were minimal. Any American veteran could receive care, although priority was toward those with service-related injuries or disabilities.

Approximately 15% of the 30 million American veterans use VA services. In 1989, regulations were changed permitting only those with service-related disabilities or those with incomes under $18,000 to use the services.

4. **Educational programs.** In 1946, VA hospitals increased their affiliations with educational programs. Now, over 1000 different professional schools are affiliated with VA hospitals. It is estimated that 33% of medical students in clinical rotations and about 40% of house officers pass through the VA system each year.

III. HOSPITALS.

III. HOSPITALS. According to the **American Hospital Association (AHA),** a hospital is a licensed institution that is designed to provide medical diagnosis and treatment to patients and that has at least six beds, an organized physician staff, and continuous nursing services. In recent years, substantial changes in the roles and operations of hospitals have occurred. The patient length of stay has decreased dramatically, and financially pressed hospitals have consolidated or closed, as seen by the marked decline in hospitals in the last decade. In 1983, there were 6700 hospitals in this country; today there are only 5500.

A. History

1. In the 12th century, hospitals were established to provide shelter for the growing number of homeless individuals moving from the countryside to the cities. No medical treatment was provided, as little existed at the time. Incurables were not admitted.
2. American hospitals trace their ancestry to the Pennsylvania Hospital founded in Philadelphia in 1751. Only patients with curable illnesses (and, interestingly, psychiatric cases) who could not care for themselves or be cared for at home were admitted. Most care was simply room and board with nursing assistance. Physicians periodically attended the hospitalized ill, but most medical care of that time was delivered in the home.
3. By the beginning of the 20th century, the concepts of sepsis, surgery with anesthesia, and radiography heralded new technology, which was essentially institutionally based. As care became more sophisticated, home care was precluded. The hospital had become the doctor's workplace.

B. Definitions.

1. **Admissions** include the total number of patients, excluding newborns, accepted for care.
2. **Average length of stay** is the total number of patient days per year counting the day of admission but not the day of discharge, divided by the total number of patients discharged per year.
3. **Hospital discharge** is the completion of any continuous period of 1 night or more in a hospital as an inpatient. Deaths, transfers to other hospitals or nursing homes, and patients returning home are all considered discharges. The stay of a well newborn is excluded. The number of discharges does not equal the number of admissions because of the minimum length of stay requirement and the inclusion of sick newborns.

C. Types of hospitals.

C. Types of hospitals. Hospitals are classified according to the average length of stay, the type of ownership, and the focus of care.

1. **Short-stay and long-term hospitals.** Short-stay hospitals have an average length of stay less than 30 days. Long-term hospitals include psychiatric, rehabilitation, or chronic illness, such as tuberculosis and drug dependency. In 1989, there were 6185 short-stay and 535 long-term hospitals in the United States.
2. **Community and noncommunity hospitals.** Community hospitals are defined as nonfederal short-stay general hospitals whose facilities are open to the public. Noncommunity hospitals include federal hospitals, such as military, VA medical centers, and the Indian Health Service hospitals, as well as long-term hospitals.
3. **Voluntary, proprietary, and government hospitals**
   a. **Voluntary hospitals** are established by community members rather than by the government. They are not-for-profit organizations operated by churches, fraternal groups, and other community or charitable institutions. Voluntary hospitals can, of course, have revenue in excess of expenses, but it would be termed a "surplus." Not-for-profit organizations do not pay income or property tax.

b. **Proprietary hospitals** are operated for profit by individuals or corporations explicitly to make a profit, which is then returned to the investors.

c. **Government hospitals** may be federally funded (e.g., the VA system), state funded (e.g., state university hospitals, facilities for the mentally retarded), or supported by city and county funds (e.g., Cook County Hospital, Boston City Hospital for indigent individuals). Government hospitals are often large institutions with over 1000 beds. These numbered 1850 in 1989.

4. **General and specialty hospitals.** General hospitals provide both diagnostic and treatment services for patients with a variety of medical conditions, both surgical and nonsurgical. Specialty hospitals provide a particular type of service. Common specialty hospitals include, for example, children's, maternity, eye, and rehabilitation.

D. Hospital operations

1. **Hospital governance** consists of an appointed hospital board of community members, physicians, or members of the sponsoring organization, such as a religious order. The board delegates the day-to-day responsibilities of running the hospital to a hospital director, who is the chief executive officer. This person then manages other administrators and personnel who operate the various departments of the hospital.

2. The **medical staff** is a formal organization of practitioners who have been accepted by the board to practice in the hospital. These physicians elect officers and representatives who meet with the board to advise on medical matters.

3. **Hospital services** include medicine, surgery, obstetrics and gynecology, and pediatrics. Hospitals also may have rehabilitation and psychiatric units. As hospitals have become more sophisticated, highly specialized units have been established. Thus, oncology, stroke, and AIDS units are now common. In addition, most hospitals have a constellation of intensive care units, such as neonatal intensive care, surgical and medical intensive care, coronary care, respiratory care, and neurologic intensive care.

4. **Ancillary services** encompass all of the departments that assist physicians in diagnosing and treating patients. The principal ancillary service departments, which are staffed by various allied health professionals, include anesthesia, clinical laboratories, radiology, respiratory care, pharmacy, and physical medicine.

5. **Hospital licensure and accreditation**

   a. **Hospital licensure** is a legal function carried out by individual states. All states license hospitals and have standards for the construction and operation of hospitals. All nonfederal hospitals must be licensed to operate.

   b. **Hospital accreditation** is, in theory, voluntary, although over 95% of allopathic hospitals are accredited. The Joint Commission on Accreditation of Health Care Organizations (JCAHO), formerly the Joint Commission on Accreditation of Hospitals, is comprised of representatives of the AMA, the American Dental Association (ADA), the AHA, the American College of Physicians (ACP), and the American College of Surgeons (ACS). Detailed hospital standards are established and updated by the JCAHO, which does on-site surveys every 3 years if a hospital is fully accredited.

      (1) Hospitals must be accredited to receive federal funds for patient care under Medicare.

      (2) Osteopathic hospitals are accredited by the American Osteopathic Association (AOA).

E. Statistical measures. A number of statistics reflect hospital activity.

1. **Admissions.** Both admissions and discharges (see III B) are used to tabulate the number of patients who have received care. Steadily increasing until 1983, total admissions to community hospitals dropped 11% in the last decade to 31.1 million in 1989. Large decreases in admissions affected both rural and urban hospitals in 1988–1989. Admissions to rural hospitals dropped 2.7%, while admissions to urban hospitals declined 0.7%. Considering that both the general population and, particularly, the population over the age of 65 have increased by more than 10% in this time, these declines are a dramatic evidence of the shift to outpatient care.

2. **Average length of stay** of 7.6 days per admission has remained stable for years. The implementation of **diagnosis-related groups (DRGs)** in 1984 steadily has decreased length of stays

(see Ch 18 IV C 1). A half-day reduction was effected by this emphasis on alternatives to inpatient care. However, since 1984, the rate has been stable. This corresponds to the reality that patients who are admitted are sicker and require more intensive care.

3. **Average occupancy rate.** For the 933,318 community hospital beds available in 1989, the average daily census was 618,000 individuals for an average occupancy rate of 66.2%. Occupancy rates of 73% were common during the last 25 years until recently. This is an important factor economically, as it reflects the average number of revenue-producing beds. Obviously, hospitals cannot control easily the number of admissions at all times. Sometimes a large bed capacity is needed to accommodate the ill, while, at other times, there is less demand. Low occupancy, however, is bad financially for any hospital.

4. **Labor intensity.** Hospitals are labor intensive. In 1989, an average of 415 employees was needed for every 100 patients. This essentially is unchanged from the 418 employed in 1983. However, hospital statistics reflect wide regional variations. For example, the West Coast hospitals employed 497 people per 100 daily patients, while Kentucky, Tennessee, and Alabama hired on average 361—a 38% difference. These differences are important because 54% of community hospital expenditures are payroll and benefits. The average annual salary plus benefits for an employee in a community hospital in 1989 was $29,600. Staffing is both an important patient care and financial issue.

5. **Hospital costs** constituted 39% of total health care dollars in 1988, or $211.8 billion. This was a 9% increase over the prior year and was twice the general rate of inflation of 4.1%. In 1983, the average community hospital spent $370 per inpatient day. Today, that figure is over $650.

F. Trends in hospital care. Health care has become big business in the last 2 decades. Major health care corporations have developed with national networks of institutions to earn a share of the 12.2% of the gross national product (GNP) spent on health. Between 1980 and 1983, these for-profit hospitals increased by 4% (i.e., from 730 to 757). The current number of 724 reflects the number of consolidations and closures that have occurred in the last 5 years. Voluntary general hospitals, by comparison, have declined from 3363 in 1983 to 3123 today, a 7% (i.e., from 3363 to 3123) decline.

1. **Costs.** Hospital care is expensive, and costs continue to rise. The average community hospital spent $586 per inpatient day in 1988, compared with $370 in 1983 and $20 in 1950. Three factors have contributed to this trend.
   a. As the **population ages,** there is an increased demand for medical services, the costs of which are concentrated among the elderly. Fifty percent of an individual's lifetime medical expenditures are in the last 2 years of life. Thirty percent are in the last year. As the "baby-boom" generation of individuals born between 1945 and 1969 reaches old age, there will be enormous increases in the demands for medical services.
   b. As the **technical quality of care** increases, so does cost. Computed tomography (CT) scanners, costing $2 million each, are now being replaced by magnetic resonance imagers (MRIs), which cost two to three times as much as CT scanners.
   c. The **cost of labor and supplies** always increases. Inflation in health care continues to outstrip inflation in other sectors of the economy. The consumer price index rose by 4.8% for all items in 1989. All medical care items, by contrast, increased 7.7%.

2. **Outpatient care.** Costly hospital care has led to an increased emphasis on outpatient care, thereby decreasing admissions and length of stays. More care is given at home, in nursing homes, and on an outpatient basis.

IV. LONG-TERM CARE INSTITUTIONS.

Long-term care is delivery of ongoing medical, rehabilitative, and maintenance care to chronically impaired individuals. The AHA defines long-term institutions as facilities where the average length of stay is greater than 30 days. In contrast, the Commission on Chronic Illness considers care long-term when it extends beyond 90 days. Regardless of the definition, the concept conveys the need for services for months at a time.

A. Need for long-term care

1. **Decreased length of stay at acute care hospitals** has led to an increased need for institutions where less expensive, low-intensity care can continue until the patient is ready to return home.

Between 1979 and 1983, short-stay hospital use measured in days of care per 1000 population declined by 10%. In the last 10 years, this has continued to decline. Some of this was accomplished by early discharge to nursing homes.

2. **Increased care for Americans over 65 years of age,** who comprise only 10% of the population, accounts for 75% of the use of long-term care facilities. Only 5% of individuals over 65 years of age are in nursing homes at one time. Yet, over their lifetimes, 20% of the elderly will use such institutions. However, the elderly over 85 years old (i.e., the "old, old") will number over 1.4 million more in the year 2000 than in 1980. The elderly over 65 needing institutionalization will increase from 1,541,000 in 1985 to 2,367,000 in the year 2000.

3. **Home care agencies,** such as the Visiting Nurse Association (VNA), are still growing to meet the demands of the elderly and young individuals discharged home but still needing assistance. About one-third of the elderly require support in their homes.

B. Funding long-term care

1. **Out-of-pocket costs.** In 1988, long-term care costs totaled $43.1 billion, the third greatest expense in health care after hospital and physicians' services. During this period, there was greater out-of-pocket payment for these services than in the past. The percent of costs paid by various payers includes:
   a. Medicare—2%
   b. Medicaid (state and federal)—44%
   c. Out-of-pocket by patients—49.3%

2. **Insurance.** Of the elderly, 59% have private nursing home insurance, but this covers only skilled care, which is similar to the Medicare coverage. Long-term care insurance has been available since the mid-1960s. Currently, only 1% of long-term costs are paid by private insurance.

C. Types of long-term care facilities. In 1980, over 24,000 nursing homes were licensed. Of these, 8% were government owned, 17% were not-for-profit, and 75% were proprietary. The National Nursing Home Survey (1977) listed four categories of nursing homes based on the nursing care provided. For the purpose of this survey, nursing care was defined as the provision of any of a number of different services including, for example, application of bandages, bladder catheterization, irrigation, and monitoring of vital signs.

1. **Nursing homes** must provide full-time nursing care by registered nurses (RNs) or licensed practical (vocational) nurses (LPNs). Skilled nursing facilities and intermediate care facilities belong to this category. Skilled nursing and intermediate care facilities are defined by each individual state, which, in turn, has the responsibility for licensing such nursing homes. Often, part of a facility will provide different levels of care on different floors. In the National Nursing Home Survey (1977), 24% of certified facilities provided both skilled nursing and intermediate care.
   a. **Skilled nursing facilities** provide the most intensive care. These services are covered by Medicare and Medicaid. Medicare Part A pays for care up to 100 days per episode of illness. A spell of illness begins on the day the patient is provided skilled nursing services and ends when the patient has not been a skilled nursing patient for 60 days. In the 1977 survey, 43% of nursing homes provided skilled nursing services. Medicare Part A eligibility requirements for skilled nursing care include:
      (1) Hospitalization in an acute care hospital for at least 3 days
      (2) Admission to the skilled nursing facility within 30 days of discharge
   b. **Intermediate care facilities** provide health-related services that are less sophisticated than skilled nursing but more comprehensive than simple room and board. Medicaid covers such care in appropriately certified homes. Medicare does not cover such services. In 1977, 56% of certified homes provided intermediate services.

2. **Personal care homes with nursing** employ RNs or LPNs but provide nursing services only to a limited number of clients. The nurses administer medication and provide personal services, such as assistance with daily activities like eating, bathing, dressing, and ambulation. Personal care homes without nursing typically provide only administration of medications and assistance with personal care.

3. **Domiciliary care homes** provide room and board and limited assistance with personal services. Such homes are appropriate for persons who are not entirely self-sufficient but require no nursing care.

D. Comprehensive long-term care. Approximately one-third of the elderly population requires some type of assistance though not institutionalization. For some, these needs can be met by home health care services. There has been growing interest in the concept of long-term care insurance and facilities that can meet the needs of the elderly who may need only minor assistance to live independently. These have been termed **lifecare centers**.

1. **Lifecare centers** provide a wide range of health and personal services up to, and sometimes including, skilled nursing care.
   a. **Payment** for these organizations may be out-of-pocket by the client or may be covered by private insurers. Premiums or monthly payments regularly cover the cost of room and board and nursing care when needed.
   b. The **number of lifecare centers** is growing. Not-for-profit centers are growing, as well as those developed by multihospital systems.

2. **Home health care** is an important and growing segment of long-term care. Home care provides health services to individuals at home in lieu of hospital services. These services promote, maintain, and restore health while maximizing patient independence.
   a. **Types of services provided** largely follow Medicare reimbursement guidelines.
      (1) Skilled nursing services
      (2) Physical and occupational therapy
      (3) Medical social services
      (4) Home health aid
   b. **Reimbursement** for home health services may be private or governmental. Home health care services are, however, less than 2% of total Medicare and Medicaid expenditures.
      (1) In 1982, for example, Medicare spent about $1 billion on home health care out of a budget of $51 billion, while Medicaid spent $310 million out of a budget of $31 billion.
      (2) Nursing home care consumes 40% of the Medicaid budget. Other types of health insurance, Blue Cross, and indemnity carriers cover services similar to those provided by Medicare.
   c. **Ownership** of the 3500 Medicare certified home health agencies is diverse. The original not-for-profit home nursing services were operated by VNAs. Today, over 85% of home health care services are operated by hospitals, nursing homes, public health departments, and private, for profit and not-for-profit organizations.
   d. **Emphasis on early discharge** under prospective reimbursement plans like DRGs have made home health care units important parts of all acute care hospitals.

V. AMBULATORY CARE FACILITIES.

Ambulatory care refers to health services provided for nonhospitalized patients. Physicians' offices, outpatient departments, emergency rooms, and community health centers are examples of ambulatory care. This section describes three new developments in ambulatory care.

A. Birthing centers specialize in the delivery of uncomplicated pregnancies. In the late 1960s and early 1970s, interest arose in returning childbirth from the hospital to a home-like environment. Medical and medicolegal concerns mitigated against home deliveries, however, and groups began developing out-of-hospital sites for childbirth. Some hospitals have since developed birthing rooms adjacent to the delivery suites.

1. **Operations.** Birthing centers are often operated by not-for-profit women's groups. In 1984, only three centers were run by hospital systems. Today, 65% of hospitals have birthing rooms. The deliveries are often performed by certified nurse midwives.

2. **Pros.** Since the first birthing center opened in 1975, proponents have argued that the centers provide a more intimate personal experience surrounding the delivery than the barren hospital delivery room. Costs have also been lower, approximately 50% of hospital charges.

3. **Cons.** Critics cite the limited knowledge of the nurse midwife and the lack of medical backup if the mother or infant develops complications. To counter these concerns, all patients are screened by an obstetrician for any potential risks, and, then, only low-risk pregnancies are followed by the midwives. Virtually all centers have physician and hospital backup. Birthing rooms in hospitals, of course, have none of these risks.

4. **Liability.** Although nurse midwives have a favorably low incidence of malpractice suits, several insurance carriers have refused to renew their liability insurance. Limited access to low-cost insurance constrains the availability of non–hospital-based birthing centers.

B. **Urgent care centers** are freestanding emergency care centers.

1. **History.** The first urgent care center opened in Newark, New Jersey, in 1973. There are currently 2000 such facilities. Growth in the number of centers has been rapid, averaging 70% per year.

2. The **purpose** of most of these centers is to compete with hospital emergency departments for acute, ambulatory medical visits. Estimates suggest that over 80% of emergency room visits are nonemergencies, requiring low-intensity care.

3. **Pros.** Proponents of urgent care centers see them as an efficient, cost-effective means of providing basic ambulatory care. Not only do such centers expand the service area (and potentially revenue) for the hospitals, but also they can increase access to care in underserved areas.

4. **Cons.** Critics contend that urgent care centers often are not equipped to handle serious injuries or medical problems. The issue of intensity of care offered is of critical importance to the economic viability of these centers. As the seriousness of the medical problem to be handled increases, so do the costs of operating the center.

C. **Freestanding outpatient surgery centers** are independent facilities designed to provide same-day surgery for selected problems.

1. **History.** The first surgery center was opened in Phoenix, Arizona, in 1970. This facility was unique in that it was a nonhospital outpatient surgery facility.

2. **Services.** Freestanding surgery centers offer a cost-competitive alternative to hospital surgery. While most surgeons perform some surgery in their offices, the lack of availability of anesthesia and recovery rooms limits the type of procedures that can be performed. Types of surgery commonly performed in freestanding centers include laparoscopy, arthroscopy, plastic surgery, and cystoscopy.

3. **Numbers.** In 1984, there were 330 freestanding outpatient surgery centers in the United States. In 1991, it was estimated that 1300 centers were in operation and performed 3 million procedures. It has been estimated that 40% of all surgery is appropriate for these surgery centers.

4. **Ownership** of surgery centers is independent (local entrepreneurs, 61%), by corporate chains (33%), or hospital affiliated (6%).

5. **Licensure and accreditation** of surgery centers are not uniform. In 1983, 22 states required licensure, while a growing number require accreditation. JCAHO and the Accreditation Association of Ambulatory Health Care (AAAHC) both accredit surgery centers.

VI. QUALITY AND COST OF CARE

A. **Quality of care** reflects the adequacy of the services provided. While desirability of quality is universally accepted, the realities of health policy and health care financing often have dressed cost-containment in the guise of quality assurance. For practical purposes, **cost-effectiveness** is an essential component of effective, quality care.

1. **Cost-effectiveness** attempts to relate the quantity of resources expended in the pursuit of a given outcome with the desirability of the outcome. Cost-effective medical care implies that the outcome of a medical intervention (e.g., polio immunization) is less costly than treating the complications of the disease (e.g., polio). Such decisions, of course, have ethical and economic consequences.

2. **Dimensions of quality assessment**

a. **Structure** refers to the characteristics of medical personnel, the organizational setting, and physical resources. For example, JCAHO has established requirements for the physical layout of a hospital to inhibit nosocomial (hospital acquired) infections.

b. **Process of care** is the manner in which health care professionals diagnose disease and implement treatments.

c. **Outcome assessment** is an essential and expanding area of health care research because it assesses the end result of medical care. The complex factors that affect outcome make the evaluation of outcomes difficult. Socioeconomic status, level of education, compliance, and health beliefs all have an impact on the outcome of a course of treatment.

3. **Definitions**
   a. **Medical audit,** which is synonymous with **quality assessment** or **appraisal,** is a technique of evaluating care based on review of the medical record. Charts may be audited by non-expert personnel, using explicit criteria (i.e., written guidelines) or by experts, using personal criteria that they may apply to the review.
   b. **Quality assurance** is a program that evaluates care and then institutes programs to improve care where needed.
   c. **Utilization review** assesses the necessity of medical services (i.e., the appropriateness of admission and length of stay). Specific procedures include:
      (1) **Certification**—a statement by the physician or reviewer confirming the need for admission
      (2) **Concurrent review**—the process of monitoring the duration of hospitalization while the patient is actually in the hospital
      (3) **Retrospective review**—the process of reviewing the charts after discharge. Such a review could lead to retrospective denial of an admission, placing the hospital or admitting physician at financial risk for the costs incurred.

B. **Assessing quality of care.** The goal of quality inputs is approached through the processes of accreditation, certification, and licensure.

1. **Accreditation** is a process carried out by nongovernmental organizations whereby an **institution or educational program** is recognized as voluntarily meeting a set of quality standards. These standards are established from within the profession to assure adequate programs of education or care. Medical schools are accredited and regularly reviewed by the American Association of Medical Colleges (AAMC). JCAHO accredits hospitals.

2. **Certification** is a process applied to **individuals**. Nongovernmental agencies establish standards of achievement and recognize individuals who attain these standards by certification. Certification is carried out by examination (e.g., a physician's assistant may become certified by successful completion of the examination of the National Commission on Certification of Physician's Assistants). Each recognized medical specialty has a certification board [e.g., internists are "board certified" by the American Board of Internal Medicine (ABIM)]. While certification has no legal status, virtually all specialists seek board certification to compete effectively for professional positions.

3. **Licensure** is the legal process that government agencies use to grant permission to individuals or institutions to practice or provide services. Licensure is a function of the individual states, and practitioners must be licensed by the jurisdiction in which they wish to practice. Disciplinary actions may lead to suspension or permanent revocation of a professional's license; however, it does not necessarily prevent that individual from working in another state.

C. **Cost assessment.** Medicare and Medicaid rapidly increased the percentage of the federal budget that is spent on health care and spurred congressional interest in the quality of care provided. As the Medicare budget mushroomed, however, quality control yielded to cost-containment. Two federal programs focus on the cost implications of the process of care.

1. **Professional standards review organizations (PSROs)**
   a. The **Bennett Amendment to the Social Security Act** (Public Law 92-603) established the PSRO program in 1972 to assess the quality of medical care that Medicare Title XIX recipients were receiving. It sought to curb cost escalation in these programs by utilization review.
   b. Associations of physicians, usually from within a hospital, constituted the utilization review committee. These committees were charged with approving the appropriateness of admissions of Medicare and Medicaid patients and monitoring the length of stays.
   c. By 1981, 182 federally funded PSROs existed. True quality of care, however, was not assessed. PRSOs were expensive themselves and appear to have had little impact on the cost of medical care. After 10 years of lackluster performance, PSROs were replaced by peer review organizations.

2. **Peer review organizations (PROs)**
   a. The **Tax Equity and Fiscal Responsibility Act of 1982** (Public Law 97-248) mandated the formation of PROs to accompany the implementation of **prospective payment systems,**

legislation for which was passed in 1983. Under prospective payment, a hospital is paid a fixed amount per admitting diagnosis. Intensive care and long stays may actually cost the hospital more than it receives; however, less care for shorts stays means a profit. Congress feared care could suffer from profiteering. Cost-containment is still the overriding concern. One year later, the Health Care Financing Administration (HCFA) issued a request for proposals for the first PROs.

b. **Function.** The 54 PROs are to monitor hospital use and quality of care for Medicare patients. Admissions, procedure, and quality objectives were established (Fig. 17-4). Quality of care has become a major issue because legislators fear that the financial incentives of the prospective payment systems lead to inadequate care.

c. **Organizationally,** most PROs are reformed PSROs. To receive an HCFA contract, a PRO must demonstrate either physician sponsorship or broad-based representation of at least 17 different medical specialties. They should not be associated with hospitals or insurance companies.

d. **PRO contracts** include lengthy lists of specific goals for reducing hospital use and monitoring quality. For example, a PRO might set an admission objective of eliminating all hospitalizations for cataract surgery. A quality objective might be a 60% reduction in urinary tract infections caused by Foley catheters.

e. **To maintain their contracts,** PROs have had to demonstrate effectiveness in achieving their selected goals. The PRO programs are an indicator that close government scrutiny of medical practice has become a fact of life.

f. **Quality intervention program** (QIP) was initiated in 1989.

(1) This program required PROs to take certain corrective actions when quality problems were identified.

(2) A point system is used to indicate the severity of the care problem. Level I problems are minor, level II problems are more severe, and level III problems have significant adverse effects on patients.

Admission and Procedure Objectives and Required Review Activities

One or more objectives are required in each of the following areas:

1. Reduce admissions for procedures that could be performed effectively and with adequate assurance of patient safety in an ambulatory surgical setting or on an outpatient basis
2. Reduce the number of inappropriate or unnecessary admissions or invasive procedures for specific diagnosis-related groups (DRGs)
3. Reduce the number of inappropriate or unnecessary admissions or invasive procedures by specific practitioners or in specific hospitals

Quality Objectives

At least one objective is required in each of the following five areas:

1. Reduce unnecessary hospital readmissions resulting from substandard care provided during the prior admission
2. Assure the provision of medical services which, when not performed, have significant potential for causing serious patient complications
3. Reduce avoidable deaths
4. Reduce unnecessary surgery or other invasive procedures
5. Reduce avoidable postoperative or other complications

Figure 17-4. The Health Care Financing Administration's (HCFA's) federal performance requirements for peer review organizations (PROs).

(3) Each level has assigned penalty points (level I, 1 point; level II, 5 points; level III, 25 points).
(4) Depending on the number of points, anything from "educational efforts" (10 points) to possible restriction of licensure (25 points) is possible.
(5) In 1990, 2% of reviewed cases resulted in quality problems, with 0.1% of cases meriting level III points.

g. Review of physicians' office services
(1) PROs are authorized to review physicians' office services to Medicare recipients. These reviews were authorized by the **Consolidated Omnibus Budget Reconciliation Act of 1986** (COBRA 1986).
(2) PROs are participating in demonstration projects in Wisconsin, Arizona, Connecticut, Indiana, North Carolina, and Utah. Physicians will be asked to send their records to the PRO for review.
(3) Medical professional associations are working to develop guidelines for ambulatory care.

h. Medicare quality review. COBRA 1986 also required the Institute of Medicine (IOM) to study Medicare quality review. The report was released in 1990.
(1) The report found PROs too focused on use and cost of care and not enough on quality. It felt that the impact of PROs on improving the quality of care was wholly unknown.
(2) The IOM report defined quality of care "as the degree to which health services for individuals and populations increase the likelihood of the desired health outcomes and are consistent with current professional knowledge."
(3) To achieve quality of care, the IOM recommended the elimination of PROs and their replacement with **Medicare quality review organizations (MQROs),** phased in over 10 years. MQROs will focus on assessing outcomes of care. Indeed, there is a rigorous movement nationally to implement outcome analysis broadly as the basis of quality assurance. Local MQROs will assess provider performance regarding quality of care and provide this information to physicians and other provider organizations to improve care.
(4) The Utilization and Quality Control Peer Review Organization was renamed Medicare Program to Assure Quality (MPAQ). The Quality Program Advisory Commission (Qual PAC) oversees MPAQ and advises Congress on quality of care issues.
(5) Lastly, the IOM report recognizes and encourages the continued development of internal quality assurance programs for hospitals and other health care institutions and organizations. These programs will continue to bear responsibility for evaluating structure and process of care.

D. Recent quality of care initiatives

1. Health Care Quality Improvement Act (HCQIA) of 1986

a. The bases of concern that led to this federal law are twofold:
(1) Congress perceived that medical malpractice was increasing, and, in the absence of national registration of licensure, incompetent practitioners freely relocate across state lines when privileges are revoked in one jurisdiction.
(2) Further, because of the important role of peer review in medical quality assurance, Congress wanted to establish incentives and provide legal protection for physicians engaging in peer review activities.

b. Content of the law
(1) **National Practitioner Data Bank.** This computerized data base became functional in 1991. It collects and provides information on disciplinary actions against physicians (MDs and DOs), dentists, and any licensed health care provider found liable in a medical liability suit. Professional review actions against physicians that restrict hospital privileges for greater than 30 days also must be reported. Hospitals must request information every 2 years on all licensed practitioners with clinical privileges at the institution. All new applicants to the medical staff must also be screened by the Data Bank.
(2) **Protection for peer review.** As an inducement to engage in peer review and to report actions taken against practitioners regularly, Congress legislated immunity from damages for all involved parties. To qualify for immunity, hospitals must meet all reporting requirements of the law. Further, to protect practitioners from unwarranted actions, the peer review body must meet elaborate standards of due process. Such standards

must be followed for the hospital peer review process to be protected under HCQIA 1986 immunity from having to pay damages if a law suit is initiated against the peer review committee.

(3) **Impact of the legislation.** Initially slated to begin in 1987, a variety of concerns delayed implementation of the Data Bank until 1991. One concern was how health care practitioners could review the accuracy of reports submitted to the Data Bank. This was resolved by requiring that a copy of the report be sent to the practitioner, who may then dispute the content. Also, the possibility that information in the Data Bank could be used by an attorney representing a law suit against a physician or other provider was also a concern. Regulation prevents such actions by the plaintiff's attorney unless the attorney can demonstrate that the hospital failed to make the required request of the Data Bank before practice privileges were granted. The concept of a national clearinghouse to monitor medical malpractice is an obvious and necessary step in restricting incompetent or criminal practitioners. It is feared, however, that even more law suits may result from inappropriate efforts to breach the confidentiality of the file.

2. **Continuous quality improvement (CQI)**
   a. **Definition.** CQI, also known as **total quality management,** is a form of quality assurance in medical care. It involves virtually all members of an organization in a process of assessing outcomes of care to streamline production processes, remove waste, and reduce errors by continuously reviewing the process of care.
   b. **Origins of CQI** date to the 1950s when C. Edwards Deming, Ph.D., a statistical studies consultant, taught the Japanese how to use statistical methods to improve the quality of industrial production. The success of these methods is evident in the dominance of Japanese industry in the global market. Only recently have these methods been applied to health care delivery.
   c. The **popularity of CQI** lies in its base premise that all individuals seek to do their best. It focuses on how to help an individual reach his fullest potential. This contrasts with current techniques that seek to throw "bad apples" out and terrorize providers into behaving better. Table 17-3 lists several characteristics of CQI, comparing them with current organizational attitudes.
   d. The **impact of CQI on health care** is growing. While currently only 100 institutions employ the process, supporters envision widespread adoption by the year 2000. By 1994, JCAHO expects formally to stress involvement in CQI for all health care institutions.

E. **Practice guidelines.** In the last 2 decades, studies show significant variation in the uses of medical services, with both important over- and underutilization of a variety of services. Fueled by the need to reduce health care spending, Congress targeted "unnecessary care." Practice parameters,

Table 17-3. Characteristics of Continuous Quality Improvement (CQI)

Quality by Inspection	Continuous Quality Improvement
Quality is fine	Quality can and must be improved
Poor quality and defects come from people	Poor quality and defects come from complex processes
Checking and data reporting insure quality *or* exhorting people and giving them incentives insure quality	Analysis and understanding of processes insure quality
Use intuition and the latest technology to address problems	Collect data and act with knowledge to address problems
Improvement must occur within functional areas	Improvement must occur among functional areas, as well as within
Customers are problems	Customers are partners
Suppliers are problems	Suppliers are partners
Quality costs money	Quality saves money
We do not have time to improve quality	We do not have time not to improve quality

or guidelines, are considered an important new tool in distinguishing appropriate levels of care from unnecessary care.

1. **Definition.** Pathway (or practice) guidelines are the direct application of guidelines to clinical practice. Leape (1990) defines practice guidelines in medical care as "formally developed highly specific guidelines based on the clinical research literature and the collective judgments of expert physicians." The result should refine recommendations for clinical care. When used by utilization review, guidelines become "standards, performance measures, or review criteria."

2. **Development.** The Agency for Health Care Policy and Research (AHCPR) was created within the PHS by the Consolidated Omnibus Budget Reconciliation Act of 1989 (COBRA 1989). Its purpose is to enhance quality, appropriateness, and effectiveness of health care services.
   a. To foster development of practice guidelines, the Office of the Forum for Quality and Effectiveness in Health Care was established within the AHCPR.
   b. Through the use of expert panels and contractors, the Forum initially will focus on the seven conditions listed below. Panels of experts will be selected to address each individual set of guidelines. Primary care physicians as well as subspecialists should be appointed to these groups. The seven medical conditions selected for development of practice guidelines by AHCPR are:
      (1) Visual impairment from cataracts
      (2) Management of benign prostatic hypertrophy
      (3) Management of decubitus ulcers
      (4) Urinary incontinence
      (5) Management of depression in primary care
      (6) Management of chronic pain
      (7) Management of sickle cell disease
   c. The **process of developing guidelines** is straightforward and contains three steps.
      (1) Detailed evaluation of available research is prepared. All pertinent studies, particularly randomized clinical trials of competing approaches to care, are analyzed for their ability to produce optimal outcomes in care.
      (2) A panel of experts reviews the results of the literature review and correlates these with their expert clinical experience. Recommendations are written. Leape provides a list of characteristics of useful guidelines (Table 17-4).
      (3) The results of the expert panel are then reviewed by the professional organization before written guidelines are issued.
      (4) **Example.** The RAND Corporation produced a set of guidelines for the use of coronary

Table 17-4. Characteristics of Useful Guidelines

Comprehensiveness	Useful guidelines should include all likely uses for procedures, even unusual cases
Specificity	Useful guidelines must clearly delineate the exact condition for which the procedure is recommended or not recommended
Detailed distinctions	Useful guidelines should be sufficiently detailed to separate clearly one indication from another
Clear statements of judgment	Useful guidelines should label unambiguously uses of the procedure as appropriate, inappropriate, or indeterminate
Inclusivity of relevant factors	Useful guidelines must include relevant factors to the decision-making process (e.g., comorbidity, severity of the disease, risk of the procedure)
Manageability	The guidelines should be written and presented in such a manner that they can be easily accessed and understood. If the form and presentation of guidelines are not manageable to the practitioner, they will seldom be used

Adapted from Leape LL: Practice guidelines and standards: an overview. *QRB* 16:44, 1990.

angiography (Chassin, 1986). An example, which readily demonstrates the clarity, specificity, and level of detail required by Leape, follows. Coronary angiography is indicated in a patient with chronic stable angina (without strong contraindications to coronary artery bypass graft surgery) who has received maximal medical management and has:

(a) Angina with mild exertion (class III or IV)
(b) A positive exercise electrocardiogram
(c) A negative exercise thallium scan
(d) A positive exercise scan

3. **Uses of practice guidelines** are potentially rewarding and punitive.
   a. **Pros.** Advocates see guidelines as a powerful tool assisting practicing physicians in achieving better clinical outcomes through better uses of technology. By maximizing the process and outcomes of care, costs of inappropriate or substandard care can be eliminated. Professional liability suits should decline.
   b. **Cons.** Critics fear that the guidelines will be subverted from voluntary educational tools to a means of reducing reimbursement and providing black-and-white guidelines for lawsuits.
      (1) Most recent efforts at quality control have been poorly disguised efforts to reduce the cost of care. Insurance companies use guidelines to deny payments for "inappropriate care." The current state of knowledge often does not offer the particular physician clear-cut right or wrong guidelines.
      (2) Unless there is a vigorous effort to assist practitioners in employing guidelines, the guidelines will be used more frequently in court to punish "adverse outcomes" than to improve care in the office or hospital. Whether the outcome was coincidental with the deficient care, or caused by it, will be difficult to assess.

4. Considerable momentum is propelling the development of practice guidelines. In 1990, $32 million were appropriated for research, and up to $185 million are authorized for 1994. The promise of guidelines is that they may be a common ground for patients, physicians, payers, and government to pursue affordable, quality care.

5. **Do guidelines work?** Despite the tremendous enthusiasm for guidelines in some circles, there is currently a dearth of evidence documenting their success in the literature. The published record shows mixed results.
   a. The American College of Obstetrics and Gynecology formulated guidelines to reduce the frequency of cesarean sections by 50%–80%. However, 2 years after the guidelines were promulgated, only 10% fewer women had this type of delivery.
   b. In Massachusetts, following institution of general anesthesia guidelines, no episodes of cerebral anoxia were reported in patients where the anesthetist followed the guidelines.
   c. Experts suggest that the problem is that guidelines are not universally implemented. As the quality of guidelines improves and the community of peers accepts these as meaningful and useful tools to improve care, guidelines should show greater impact on practice as they are more consistently employed.

VII. HEALTH CARE PLANNING.

The purpose of health care planning is the coordinated and comprehensive provision of medical treatment, prevention of disease, and promotion of health. Only in the last 20 years have serious attempts at national health care planning been initiated. The impact of these efforts remains unclear.

A. The **Comprehensive Health Planning and Public Services Amendment of 1966** (Public Law 89-749) was the first federal effort at planning and coordinating services. It established health planning as a priority and funded training for health planners. Tangible results of this legislation resulted from federal funding of regional comprehensive health planning agencies.

B. The **National Health Planning and Development Act of 1974** (Public Law 93-641) superseded the 1966 law by legislating 203 health service areas, each to be covered by a health systems agency (HSA).

1. The **purpose of health systems agencies** was strongly influenced by cost-containment pressures. The principal function of these organizations was to help hold the purse strings on health care spending.

2. **Certificate of need** laws required health systems agency approval for new capital expenditures such as hospital or nursing home construction or renovations. Office-based expensive equipment purchases were sometimes also subject to review. Certificate of need legislation was first implemented by several states in the 1960s, and federal legislation eventually required all states to pass certificate of need laws by 1981. By 1982, certificate of need laws in 11 states applied to equipment in physicians' offices. One of the most celebrated confrontations of the certificate of need process was the then newly developed computed tomography (CT) scanner. Each CT scanner, in theory, required health systems agency approval or risked denial of federal reimbursement for services.
3. Generally, certificate of need applies to expensive technology or buildings. Items costing over $100,000–$200,000, depending on the individual state, are subject to review. At the heart of this legislation is the awareness that new technology contributes substantially to higher health care costs. Unfortunately, it is doubtful that certificate of need laws significantly inhibited the spiral of health care costs. Federal requirements for certificate of need authorization were eliminated in 1986 legislation, and most states have abandoned certificate of need laws and health systems agencies.

BIBLIOGRAPHY

Berwick, DM: Sounding board—continuous improvement as an ideal in health care. *N Engl J Med* 320:53–56, 1989.

Chassin MR, et al: *Indications for Selected Medical and Surgical Procedures: A Literature Review and Ratings of Appropriateness: Coronary Angiography.* Pub No R-3204/1. Santa Monica, RAND Corporation, 1986.

Darr K: Hospitals and the Health Care Quality Improvement Act. *Hospital Topics* 68:4–6, 1990.

Gonzalez ML, Emmons DW: *Socioeconomic Characteristics of Medical Practice.* Chicago, American Medical Association, 1989.

Havlicek PL: *Medical Groups in the U.S. A Survey of Practice Characteristics, 1990.* Chicago, American Medical Association, 1990.

Health Insurance Association of America: *Source Book of Health Insurance Data.* Washington, DC, Health Insurance Association of America, 1990.

Leape LL: Practice guidelines and standards: an overview. *QRB* 16:42–49, 1990.

Roback G, Randolph L, Seidman B: *Physician Characteristics and Distribution in the U.S.* Chicago, American Medical Association, 1990.

STUDY QUESTIONS

Directions: Each of the numbered items or incomplete statements in this section is followed by answers or by completions of the statement. Select the **one** lettered answer or completion that is **best** in each case.

1. The phrase "services combining sciences, skills, and beliefs directed to the maintenance and improvement of the health of an entire population" best defines which of the following terms?

(A) Health services
(B) Public health
(C) Personal health care
(D) Quality of care
(E) National health care

2. A primary care practitioner is generally contacted directly by the public and has a practice that is characterized by a broad range of medical services. Primary care specialties include all of the following EXCEPT

(A) pediatrics
(B) internal medicine
(C) family medicine
(D) neurology
(E) general practice

3. An important decision for physicians entering practice is whether or not to practice alone or in a group. A solo practice is best characterized by which of the following statements?

(A) Two-thirds of physicians practice this way
(B) Approximately 10% more patients are seen by solo practitioners
(C) Physicians who work alone often work fewer hours by choice
(D) Physicians who have their own practice have higher incomes than those who are employed by a group
(E) Solo practice offers less autonomy without partners with whom to share the work load

4. Quality assessment includes all of the following dimensions EXCEPT

(A) structure
(B) certificate of need
(C) process
(D) outcome

5. Certificate of need legislation is characterized by all of the following EXCEPT

(A) the need for health systems agency approval of major health care expenditures
(B) a review of hospital or nursing home expenditures over $100,000
(C) a review of equipment purchases by hospitals and private physicians
(D) the refusal of several states to implement such laws

1-B
2-D
3-A
4-B
5-D

Directions: The item below contains four suggested answers of which **one or more** is correct. Choose the answer

A if **1, 2, and 3** are correct
B if **1 and 3** are correct
C if **2 and 4** are correct
D if **4** is correct
E if **1, 2, 3, and 4** are correct

6. Which of the following are major components of the DHHS?

(1) VA medical centers
(2) PHS
(3) HUD
(4) HCFA

Directions: Each group of items in this section consists of lettered options followed by a set of numbered items. For each item, select the **one** lettered option that is most closely associated with it. Each lettered option may be selected once, more than once, or not at all.

Questions 7–10

Match the following types of physician with the appropriate role.

(A) Gatekeeper role
(B) Keystone role
(C) Both
(D) Neither

7. A primary care physician who makes decisions about when and to whom to refer a patient for additional evaluation

8. A primary care physician who assists the patient with referrals as the patient chooses

9. A primary care physician who coordinates care provided by an increasing number of disparate specialists

10. A primary care physician who provides a broad scope of medical services

Questions 11–14

Match each act of accreditation or certification with the appropriate group.

(A) JCAHO
(B) AAMC
(C) AAAHC
(D) ABIM
(E) JCAHO or AAAHC

11. Accreditation of United States freestanding surgery centers

12. Accreditation of United States medical schools

13. Accreditation of hospitals

14. Certification of United States internists

6-C	9-C	12-B
7-A	10-C	13-A
8-B	11-E	14-D

ANSWERS AND EXPLANATIONS

1. The answer is B *[I B].*
Public health is defined as the "services combining sciences, skills, and beliefs directed to the maintenance and improvement of the health of an entire population." While public health deals with the health of an entire population, health services, personal health, and national health care focus on the care of a single person. Quality of care deals with adequacy of personal health care services.

2. The answer is D *[II A 2].*
The primary care specialties include family medicine, internal medicine, pediatrics, and general practice. The primary care physician is often the patient's first contact with the medical care system, for counseling as well as general diagnosis and treatment. Neurology, by contrast, is limited to the evaluation and management of the problems of only one organ system.

3. The answer is A *[II B 1, 2].*
Two-thirds of all practicing physicians currently practice alone. However, young physicians seem to be preferring group practice over solo practice. While offering less autonomy, group practice fosters a sharing of expertise and often an ease of referral without the fear of losing the patient to a consultant. In addition, solo practitioners see approximately 10% fewer patients, make less money, and work longer hours than group practitioners.

4. The answer is B *[VI A 2].*
The three dimensions of quality assessment are structure, process, and outcome. Because it is difficult to measure whether the desired outcome (e.g., a clinically competent physician) has been achieved, structure and process are more commonly measured. Certificate of need legislation, which is now defunct, attempted to limit capital expenditures on medical facilities and machinery.

5. The answer is D *[VII B 1–3].*
Certificate of need legislation is not characterized by the failure of several states to implement such laws. Certificate of need legislation was first implemented by several states in the 1960s. However, federal legislation eventually required all states to pass certificate of need laws by 1981. These laws required health systems agencies to review expensive equipment purchases and hospital building programs. While such review was targeted primarily at hospitals and nursing homes, 11 states extended it to physicians' offices as well.

6. The answer is C (2, 4) *[I B 1 a, b; Figure 17-1].*
The federal government involvement in health care is a function of the Department of Health and Human Services (DHHS). The Public Health Service (PHS) and the Health Care Financing Administration (HCFA) are two major divisions of DHHS. The PHS includes the Centers for Disease Control (CDC), the National Institutes of Health (NIH), and the Food and Drug Administration (FDA). HCFA is responsible for Medicare and Medicaid. The Veterans Administration (VA) hospitals are part of the VA, and the Department of Housing and Urban Development (HUD) is a department that is parallel to DHHS.

7–10. The answers are: 7-A, 8-B, 9-C, 10-C *[II A 3 a–c].*
The role of the primary care physician has been alternately described as a keystone or a gatekeeper. The difference is noteworthy.

The gatekeeper role of the primary care physician holds that the primary care provider controls access to other specialists and subspecialists. The patient sacrifices freedom of choice, to some extent, but the more efficient use of consultants provides better coordinated care at a lower cost.

The keystone role of the primary care physician holds that the primary care provider assists patients with referrals and then oversees these interactions. However, the patient freely chooses consultants and makes the decision of choosing a primary care physician or other specialist.

The primary care physician in both the keystone and gatekeeper roles coordinates the care provided by an increasing number of disparate specialists, each of whom is concerned with only a single aspect of an individual's overall medical condition.

11–14. The answers are: 11-E *[V C 5],* **12-B** *[VI B 1],* **13-A** *[III D 5 a, b],* **14-D** *[VI B 2].*
U.S. freestanding surgery centers are accredited either by the Joint Commission on Accreditation of Health Care Organizations (JCAHO) or the Accreditation Association of Ambulatory Health Care (AAAHC). Various organizations have overlapping jurisdictions (e.g., most states will inspect hospitals,

but the JCAHO will do the same process). In the case of surgery centers, either organization might be chosen by the facility for its accreditation.

American medical schools are accredited by the American Association of Medical Colleges (AAMC). They are also regularly reviewed by this organization.

Hospital licensure is a legal function carried out by each individual state. All states license hospitals and have standards for the construction and operation of hospitals. Accreditation, on the other hand, is, in theory, voluntary, although over 95% of allopathic hospitals are accredited. The accreditation process is carried out by the JCAHO.

Internists are certified by the American Board of Internal Medicine (ABIM). Certification is carried out by examination.

18
Health Care Financing

Anthony J. Buividas

I. OVERVIEW. The United States has no overall, coordinated program to provide or pay for health care services. In addition, because health care costs are rising at such an alarming rate without a corresponding increase in objective measures of health status and health outcomes (see II G), many people suggest reforming the current fragmented U.S. health care system (see VII).

II. RISING HEALTH CARE COSTS

A. Health care expenditures can be measured in several ways, including the following.

1. Approximately **$676 billion, or $2660 per capita, was spent in 1990** on health care in the United States—a 12% increase over 1989. A 12%–15% annual increase is expected in the 1991–1996 period.

2. Health care costs accounted for **12% of the gross national product (GNP) in 1990,** as compared to 5.3% in 1960. This percentage is far higher than that of any other industrialized nation (see II C).

3. The **medical component of the consumer price index (CPI) increased** 73.8% from 1980 to 1987, while the total CPI increased only 37.9% during the same period, meaning that health care cost inflation was almost double the rate of overall inflation.

4. **Employers spent 17% more on health care in 1990** than they did in 1989, resulting in an average cost of $3217 per employee per year. From 1965 to 1987, the amount of employer contributions to health care expressed as a percentage of corporate profits increased from 14% to 74%.

B. Categories of U.S. health care costs (Figure 18-1). Hospital care accounts for the largest percentage (43.7%) of personal health care expenditures in the United States. Although physicians' services have accounted for about 22% of U.S. expenditures since 1950, the percentage spent on nursing home care in the same period has risen dramatically—from 1.5% in 1950 to 9.1% in 1990.

C. Comparison to other economies (Table 18-1). The United States spends a far greater percentage of its GNP on health care than does any other industrialized country. In addition, all measures of U.S. health care costs increased in the last 10 years, while most of these measures remained stable or rose modestly in other industrialized countries.

D. National economic implications. Because the United States spends so much more than other countries on health care, **U.S. manufacturers have become less competitive** in a worldwide market. For example, in the late 1980s, employee health expenses added approximately $223 to the cost of an automobile manufactured in Canada, while adding $700 to the cost of a car made in the United States.

E. Health care cost inflation. The dramatic growth in U.S. health care expenditures has resulted from the following:

1. **Increased governmental funding** of programs such as Medicare and Medicaid

2. **Growth in private insurance coverage,** which increases demand (i.e., more people are willing to seek health care) while insulating the consumer from the direct cost of services (see III and Figure 18-3)

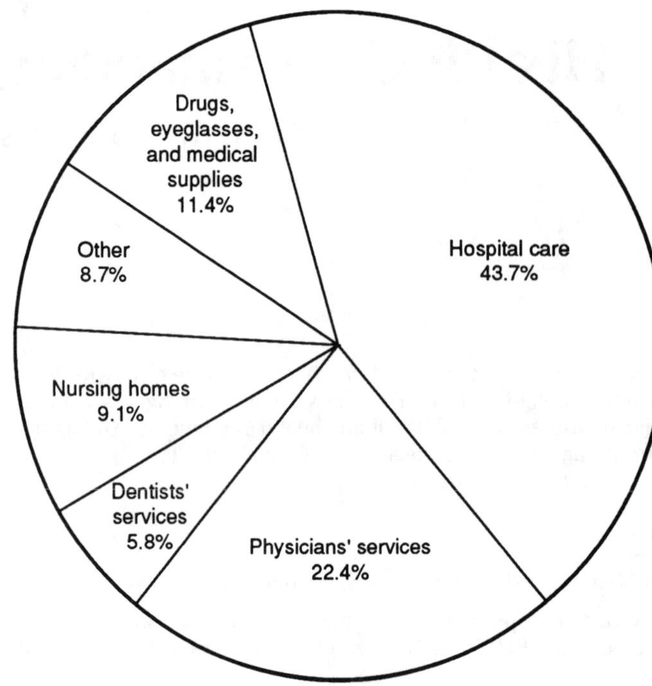

Figure 18-1. Distribution of personal health care expenditures in the United States in 1990.

3. **Expensive new technologies for diagnosis and treatment**
4. **An older U.S. population** requiring proportionately more health care
5. **Increases in labor and material costs** in the health industry disproportionate to increases in other industries
6. **An increase in the number of malpractice lawsuits,** leading to:
   a. An increase in physicians' malpractice insurance costs
   b. Physicians ordering more services (e.g., tests) in an effort to practice "defensive medicine" (i.e., medicine designed to avoid charges of malpractice)
7. **Increased governmental regulation** (e.g., fire safety codes, disposal of infectious waste material, and data reporting requirements)
8. **Costs of caring for uninsured,** including providers' bad debt (see II G 1 d)

F. Failure of the free market model. The U.S. health care industry does not respond to the usual free market mechanisms that result in strong competition and efficiency. Distortions in the competitive model include the following.

1. **Consumer insulation from the cost of health services**
   a. Payments to health care providers typically are made by **third-party purchasers,** such as governmental agencies (e.g., Medicare and Medicaid) or private insurers.
   b. With third-party payment, most health care consumers do not pay for services directly and, thus, have **little incentive to seek lower cost health care providers.**

Table 18-1. Total Health Expenditures as a Percentage of Gross National Product (GNP) by Country

Country	1970	1980	1989	% Change (1980–1989)
Canada	7.1%	7.4%	8.7%	+17.6%
France	5.8%	7.6%	8.7%	+14.5%
Japan	4.4%	6.4%	6.6%	+3.1%
United Kingdom	4.5%	5.9%	5.9%	0 %
West Germany	5.9%	8.5%	8.2%	−3.5%
United States	7.4%	9.2%	12.0%	+30.4%

2. **Failure of third-party payers to purchase health benefits wisely.** Both governmental and private third-party purchasers of health care benefits historically have exerted few restrictions on beneficiaries' choice of health care providers. Only recently have third-party payers made some effort to direct beneficiaries to cost-effective providers (see IV D 2).

3. **Poor data on providers.** Because data on providers' cost, utilization, and quality profiles (see IV D 2) historically have been sparse and unreliable, third-party payers and consumers have had to choose providers without accurate measures of cost-efficiency or quality.

4. **Fee-for-service payment structures** assess pricing for each service provided (see IV A 1). The result is a fragmented and elaborate "a la carte" billing system that **rewards physicians for providing as many of the categorized services as possible**.

5. **Inequities resulting from reimbursement structure** include **cross-subsidization,** or **cost-shifting,** whereby payers who *do not* pay a contractually set fee must compensate for the lower amounts paid by other payers (see IV B 1). This causes providers whose patients have no insurance or are covered by governmental plans with lower reimbursement levels (e.g., Medicare or Medicaid) to be at a **competitive disadvantage**.

G. Cost-benefit analysis of the U.S. health care system

1. **Poor results.** Despite leading other nations in most categories of health care spending (see II C and Table 18-1), the United States does not rank well by many objective measures of health care and health status.
   a. **The infant mortality rate** is higher in the United States than in many other industrialized countries.
   b. **Average life expectancy** is not significantly higher in the United States than in other industrialized nations.
   c. **Immunization.** A high percentage of U.S. children are not immunized thoroughly.
   d. **Uninsured population.** Approximately 15% of the population, or 35 million Americans, are not covered by health insurance. It is estimated that another 23% of the population are inadequately protected against large medical bills.
      (1) Various studies have indicated that **more than half of the uninsured are employees** (or their dependents) who are not covered by employer-sponsored health benefit plans.
      (2) A disproportionate percentage of the uninsured are **minorities and children**.
      (3) Uninsured individuals may **delay seeking care** until their condition is critical, thus jeopardizing their health and, in many cases, incurring needless suffering and expense.
      (4) Because of reimbursement structures, many **hospitals are less willing to provide non-emergency care** to those who cannot pay, thus signifying a change in hospitals' historic mission of providing care to those who need it.
      (5) Also, the **financial burden of caring for the uninsured is not shared equally**. Although uncompensated care accounts for only 5.4% of gross hospital revenues, often inner-city hospitals and poor, rural hospitals treat a disproportionate number of such cases.

2. **Call for reform.** These discouraging measures of health care performance, combined with health cost inflation and an increasingly complex and fragmented insurance system, have led many health care experts, U.S. citizens, and corporate interests to suggest restructuring the U.S. system of providing and paying for health care. Proposals for such reform are discussed in section VII.

III. SOURCES OF FUNDING.

Most health care expenses in the United States are incurred either by consumers directly or by a private insurer or a government agency (i.e., a third-party payer). Figure 18-2 illustrates the distribution of funding sources for health care in the United States in 1990. Figure 18-3 categorizes the 1988 U.S. population by health coverage type. The percentage of **total health costs paid by third-party payers has increased** dramatically, while the **percentage paid directly by consumers has declined**.

A. Third-party payers. Both public and private payers that finance health care on behalf of their beneficiaries are known as third-party payers. Typically, third-party payers provide more coverage for inpatient care and hospital diagnostic services and less for outpatient services, such as office visits, immunizations, or prescription drugs.

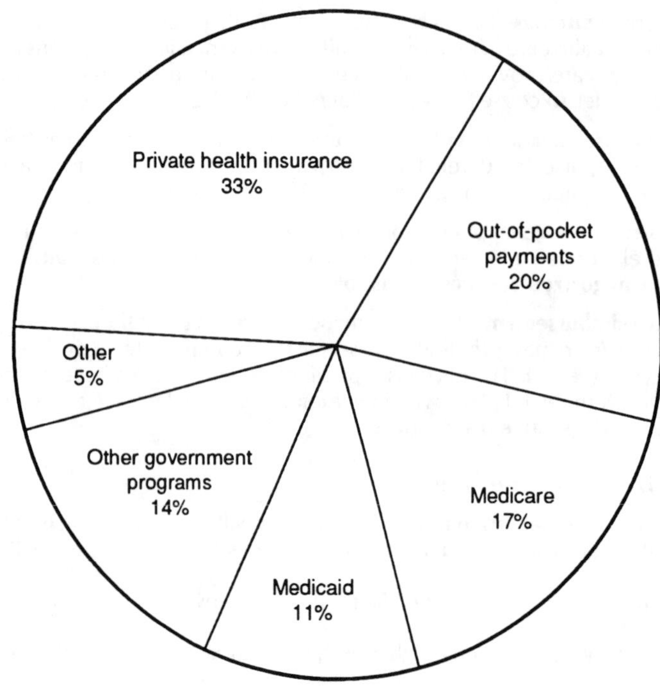

Figure 18-2. Sources of U.S. health care financing, 1990.

1. **Government** pays for approximately 42% of all personal health care expenditures in the United States (see VI). Medicare and Medicaid are the principal governmental health programs.
2. **Private health insurance** pays for 33% of all personal health care costs, with a majority of employers providing health insurance for their employees. Types of private insurance include the following.
   a. **Not-for-profit.** Blue Cross and Blue Shield insurance organizations comprise approximately 73 loosely affiliated insurers that cover nearly 71 million people, or 28% of the U.S.

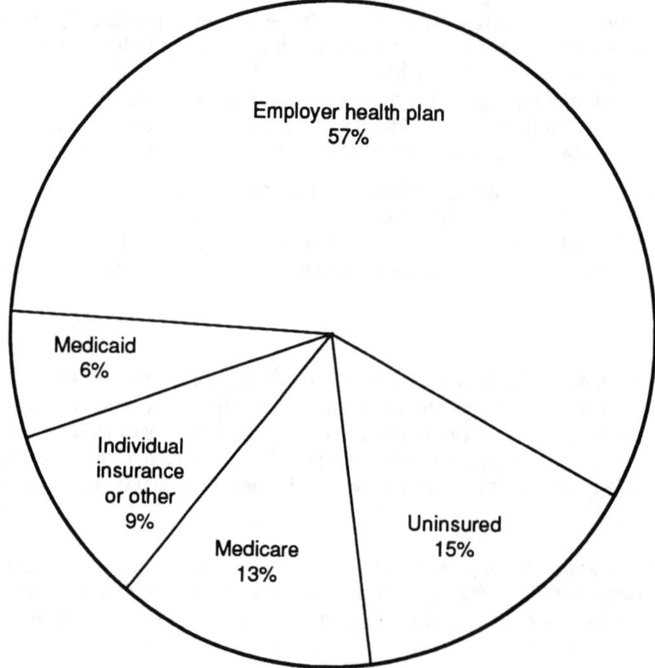

Figure 18-3. Health care coverage arrangements for the U.S. population in 1988.

health insurance market. Member plans must meet standards set by the national Blue Cross/Blue Shield association. Historically, Blue Cross plans covered hospital services while Blue Shield plans covered physicians' services. Both organizations pay health care providers directly (rather than remitting payment to the insured), according to agreed-upon fee schedules.

(1) **Blue Cross** started as a hospital-sponsored plan in the Depression, when direct payments from patients were declining and hospitals needed a steady source of income.

(2) **Blue Shield** insurance plans were developed by physicians' medical societies to provide coverage for professional services. Physicians who participate in Blue Shield accept certain fee schedules and other administrative rules.

(3) **Combined plans.** Some Blue Cross and Blue Shield plans have merged to offer the full range of health benefits. Even in locations where Blue Cross and Blue Shield organizations exist separately, the two groups often cooperate on such tasks as marketing.

b. **Commercial insurers** historically have offered indemnity coverage, whereby the insured person is reimbursed after submitting a claim form showing his or her loss. More recently, many larger commercial insurers have set up direct arrangements with providers (see V).

c. **Employer self-insurance** consists of employers assuming financial responsibility for the health care benefits offered to their employees. Sometimes expenses exceeding a defined threshold will be reinsured with an external carrier. Self-insurance has become more popular because it has cash flow advantages (benefit payments are made as incurred rather than prepaid as premiums), because self-insurance plans are not subject to extensive state regulation of benefit coverage and pricing, and because the employer has many options in benefit design and administration.

d. **Health maintenance organizations (HMOs)** and other managed health care arrangements (see V) usually pay providers (physicians and hospitals) directly, pursuant to the financial and administrative terms specified in provider participation agreements. Generally, HMOs require the insured to use designated participating health care providers in order to receive benefits.

B. Direct consumer payments. There are two broad categories of direct consumer payments.

1. **Benefits not covered** by a given insurance plan (e.g., cosmetic surgery, preexisting conditions)

2. **Out-of-pocket expenditures** required as part of the consumer's insurance policy, such as deductibles and copayments (see IV B 2, 3)

C. Uncompensated care. Those who cannot afford to pay for health care include:

1. **The uninsured** (see II G 1 d)

2. **The medically indigent**—that is, those not poor enough to qualify for Medicaid benefits but whose medical expenses when subtracted from income would lower their financial means below the poverty line

IV. METHODS OF PAYMENT

A. Four common third-party methods of reimbursing providers

1. **Fee-for-service charges** are billed on an itemized invoice. Most physicians submit itemized charge listings, categorized according to the Common Procedure Terminology (CPT) classifications published by the American Medical Association (AMA). The CPT classification contains more than 7000 discrete items, each with a unique five-digit code and description.

2. **Per diem** is an all-inclusive flat rate for each day of hospital care provided.
   a. Per diems usually include all ancillary services, supplies, and other services billed by the hospital.
   b. Per diems for different clinical services (e.g., obstetrics, surgery, intensive care, pediatrics) can be arranged to account for differences in the intensity of care provided.

3. **Per admission** is an all-inclusive flat rate for each hospital admission. The admission reimbursement can be refined further to include varying rates based on the admitting service or diagnosis, such as the diagnosis-related group (DRG) payment structure used by Medicare (see IV C 1).

4. **Capitation** is a fixed fee paid to the provider per patient per month, for each patient enrolled in the practice. In exchange for the fee, the provider renders all specified health services to enrolled patients. The reimbursement is fixed and paid regardless of the actual number or types of services provided.
   a. **Example.** An HMO might pay a particular hospital $25 monthly per insured person to provide all required inpatient services, and a general surgeon might receive $0.60 per capita per month to provide all general surgery services. Alternatively, a multispecialty group might receive a per capita amount to provide all outpatient physician and diagnostic services.
   b. **Adjustments to capitation**
      (1) Usually, the capitation amount is adjusted for the **age and gender** of the patient.
      (2) Often, **stop-loss limits** are used to protect the provider from atypical, catastrophic expenses.
      (3) Under a **risk corridor adjustment,** additional payments to or refunds from the provider would occur if the variance between actual itemized costs and the capitation amount exceeded a certain threshold percentage (e.g., 5% or 10%).

B. Other components of provider reimbursement structure (see Figure 18-3)

1. **Contractual allowance.** Although hospitals and physicians generally bill on a fee-for-service, or itemized charge, basis, they often accept less than the billed amount. The **discount given** is known as a contractual allowance and is **based on the provider's participation agreement** with the particular third-party payer. Contractual allowances have the following effects on health care costs and charges.
   a. Although providers may bill one amount for a given service, they can accept different payment amounts for the service from various third-party payers or patients.
   b. Providers often try to maximize reimbursement from patients covered by health plans with which the provider has no contractual agreement, charging such patients the full amount billed. This results in cross-subsidization, or cost-shifting, whereby payers without contractual allowances are in effect making up the difference for those able to pay lower amounts.
   c. Because of such cross-subsidization, the **itemized charge for a service may bear little relationship to the actual cost** of the service.

2. **Deductible** is a threshold amount specified in an insurance policy. It is the amount incurred directly by the patient before the third-party payer picks up coverage.

3. **Coinsurance** is a predetermined percentage of health benefit costs paid by the patient. Generally, coinsurance refers to a percentage, whereas a **copayment is a fixed dollar amount,** such as a $10 copayment per visit.

4. **Example.** In the following example, a physician participating in the Medicare program sees a Medicare patient and bills for treatment of shoulder dislocation, CPT code #90517 (see IV A 1 and Table 18-2).
   a. The physician has made an agreement with Medicare (the payer, in this case) to accept its payment level for the service [the **allowed amount;** see VI A 6 b (1)] as payment in full.
   b. The physician's usual charge for the visit is much higher than the Medicare allowance.
   c. The physician cannot recapture the difference between what is usually charged and the Medicare allowed amount. The difference is called the Medicare **contractual allowance,** or **write-off**.
   d. The physician bills the patient for any deductibles or copayments included in the Medicare program. The payment from the Medicare carrier will reflect a subtraction for applicable deductibles and copayments, so the physician must collect these payments directly from the patient.

Table 18-2. Example of Medicare Payment Format for Participating Physicians

CPT Code	Description	Qty	Billed Charge	Medicare Allowance	Deductible Applied	Patient Coinsurance	Medicare Physician Payment
23650	Treat houlder slocation	1	$250	$170	$100	$14	$56

n procedure terminology; qty = quantity.

C. Current trends in provider reimbursement methods

1. **The diagnosis-related group (DRG) payment system** was introduced in 1983 by the Health Care Financing Agency (HCFA) and is now used by both Medicare and Medicaid. Under the system, 470 treatment classifications (known as DRGs) are each assigned a fixed hospital payment rate, and hospital reimbursement is based on these rates.
   a. **DRG category ratings.** The payment for each DRG is developed by analyzing historic cost and charge data for each diagnostic category. Each category is rated in relationship to the average cost for all admissions (which is given the relative weight of 1.000) and given a relativity index. The relative weight, or **case-mix index,** of each DRG category is supposed to reflect relative hospital resource usage (Table 18-3).
   b. **Setting DRG payment rates.** Annual percentage increases in DRG payment rates are determined by Congress. The Prospective Payment Assessment Commission (ProPAC) advises Congress on the annual inflator and other price structure changes.
   c. **DRG price adjustments.** In current practice, Medicare adjusts national DRG prices according to several factors.
      (1) **Geographic variations** reflect differences in cost of living between urban and rural areas as well as other regional cost differences.
      (2) **Teaching hospitals** presently receive an adjustment to compensate them for direct and indirect costs of graduate medical education (i.e., residency programs). This hospital-specific adjustment has been lowered consistently since the DRG system began.
      (3) **Inner-city hospitals** that treat a disproportionate share of medically indigent patients also receive an adjustment.
      (4) **Capital costs.** Presently, DRG rates do not include capital costs (e.g., depreciation, interest, financing for buildings and equipment), which account for approximately 7% of total DRG expenses. Instead, capital costs, like other hospital-specific rate adjustments (known as **pass-throughs**), are calculated separately, based on each hospital's unique capital cost per admission. In the future, capital costs may be capped at a fixed percentage of the DRG payment.

2. **Prospective versus retrospective reimbursement to providers.** Prior to the DRG payment structure, a retrospective, cost-based reimbursement system was used, under which payments per admission varied dramatically by hospital.
   a. **Retrospective payment.** Under the cost-based system, each hospital's payment for inpatient care of Medicare patients was determined by complex cost-allocation formulas designed to apportion total hospital expenditures to Medicare and other third-party payers.
      (1) Although each hospital received interim payments from Medicare, adjusted for the volume of Medicare admissions, the final payment was not determined until year-end, when the cost-allocation formulas were employed to assess Medicare for its share of the hospital's total allowed costs.
      (2) Medicare used detailed definitions to differentiate allowed costs from the disallowed costs it refused to pay.
   b. **Prospective payment** refers to a predetermined pricing structure, usually based on a per admission rate, such as the DRG payment system.
      (1) **Effects due to prospective payment by Medicare.** The hospital industry has complained that setting price levels in the political budgetary arena has resulted in reduced profit margins (necessary for new capital expenditures and technologic enhancements) and diminished quality of care. Hospitals' overall profit margins under the Medicare prospective payment system have declined from 14.5% in 1984 to 1.8% in 1988 to approximately 0.2% in 1990.

Table 18-3. Example of Diagnosis-related Group (DRG) Payment Schedule in which Relative Weight of 1.000 = $5000

DRG Number	DRG Category	DRG Relative Weight	DRG Fee
2	Craniotomy for trauma	4.1379	$20,690
103	Heart transplant	13.2352	$66,176
163	Hernia procedure	0.7729	$ 3865
167	Appendectomy (without complications)	0.7922	$ 3961
373	Vaginal delivery (without complications)	0.2987	$ 1494

(2) **Prospective payment adopted by other insurers.** Blue Cross plans historically have employed the cost-based retrospective method of reimbursing hospitals. Since 1980, however, many Blue Cross plans and state Medicaid programs have switched to prospective payment methods, such as the DRG structure.

D. New developments in physicians' fee schedules. Historically, insurance plans favored coverage of inpatient care (both hospital and physician-related services), which is less frequently used but more expensive than outpatient care. Changes in medical practice patterns, technology, and consumer demand have led to more health services being rendered in the outpatient setting. Third-party payers have responded by changing their benefit coverage to extend to outpatient coverage and by changing providers' fee schedules.

1. **Resource-based relative value scale (RBRVS)**
   a. **Overview.** Third-party payers historically paid more for inpatient and procedure-based services (e.g., invasive surgical procedures, diagnostic tests requiring medical equipment) than for outpatient and cognitive services (e.g., professional time spent making differential diagnoses, developing treatment plans, counseling patients and family). As a result, compensation per minute was much higher for rendering a procedure than for thinking or listening. Extensive debate and study of the "procedure versus cognitive" fee issue led HCFA to adopt the RBRVS for paying physicians and other health professionals. HCFA began paying physicians according to the new RBRVS fee schedule in January 1992.
   b. **Previous methods of determining fees.** Historically, third-party payers based payment on **usual, customary, or reasonable (UCR) charges** rather than on a uniform fee schedule.
      (1) The **usual fee** is the amount an individual physician most frequently charges patients for a given procedure.
      (2) The **customary fee** is the 80th or 90th percentile charge among physicians in the same specialty and the same geographic area for a given procedure. Historically, Medicare used the 75th percentile value and called it the "prevailing charge," whereas private insurers typically paid at the 80th or 90th percentile value.
      (3) In most cases, the **lesser of the usual or customary fee** is paid. Because of this, physicians often set their fees close to the customary level, thus making the UCR payment method inherently inflationary.
      (4) The **reasonable fee** is paid when the conventional "usual or customary" criteria does not fully account for additional skill, time, or experience needed because of unusual circumstances.
   c. **Changes in determining fees.** The RBRVS takes the following factors into account when determining the allowed fee for a specific service:
      (1) The amount of work (e.g., time, mental effort, judgment, technical skill, physical effort) performed by the provider in rendering the service
      (2) The typical costs of the provider's practice, including malpractice premiums
      (3) The typical cost of the provider's postgraduate specialty training, if used to perform the service
      (4) The typical office overhead costs for the service
   d. **Implications of RBRVS**
      (1) Cognitive services will receive fee increases; procedural services will command lower payments.
      (2) Surgical and procedural specialties, such as ophthalmology and radiology, will receive relatively lower payment levels and a smaller allocation of Medicare's outpatient expenditures, while cognitive services and specialties, such as internal medicine and family medicine, will receive a greater share.
      (3) Fees probably will be adjusted more frequently, particularly in response to technologic or other changes that affect the time or complexity of a procedure.
      (4) Private third-party payers, such as Blue Shield and commercial carriers, likely will follow the HCFA's lead and pay physicians according to the RBRVS.

2. **Utilization review,** or **volume control,** monitors the necessity, as well as the medical and economic efficiency, of health care services. It is a typical feature of managed health care (see V) but is increasingly being employed by all third-party payers.
   a. **Utilization review procedures** include:
      (1) Prior review of the medical necessity of designated procedures or hospital admissions
      (2) Prior authorization by the payer's review organization as a prerequisite to payment
      (3) Promulgation of standard treatment protocols

b. **Difficulties.** Despite third-party payer's greater focus on fee schedules (known as unit costs in economic terms), volume control, particularly of outpatient services, has proven difficult. Providers complain that utilization control procedures interfere with professional judgment and the provider-patient relationship.

c. **Payers influence providers** to control volume and, thus, reduce overall costs in the following ways.

   (1) **Risk-sharing.** A portion of the provider's reimbursement is withheld as a contingent reserve fund to be used in case health expenditures exceed the expected level.

   (2) **Expenditure targets linked to physicians' fee schedules.** Under the new Medicare payment reforms (see IV D 1), if total Medicare physician and outpatient expenditures exceed a budgeted target, physicians' annual fee schedule increases will be reduced by the percentage of the runover.

   (3) **Capitation payment arrangements** (see IV A 4). More than 70% of HMOs use the capitation method for paying some physicians.

V. MANAGED HEALTH CARE.

To manage health benefit costs better, arrangements that relate the beneficiary's coverage to the use of selected health care providers have emerged.

A. **Managed care** refers to a wide range of techniques employed by third-party payers to control health benefit expenditures, including:

1. **Provider risk-sharing** [see IV D 2 c (1)]

2. **Restrictive selection of providers,** using criteria such as cost, quality, providers' willingness to accept specified fee schedules, payment methods, peer review procedures, and administrative procedures

3. **Financial incentives** (e.g., lower health insurance coverage price, lower coinsurance, lower deductible, benefit enhancements) to encourage insureds to use selected participating providers

4. Concurrent and retrospective **peer review** procedures to control the cost and quality of care

5. Mandatory **prior approval procedures** to review medical necessity and appropriateness of costly health services

6. Contractual **provider reimbursement structures, maximum fee schedules,** and **ground rules for payment** for each service rendered, when a course of treatment or diagnosis requires multiple services

7. **Case management** of patients needing extraordinary services

B. Health maintenance organizations (HMOs)

1. **Definition.** HMOs are medical care organizations that accept responsibility for the provision and delivery of a predetermined set of comprehensive health services to insureds who voluntarily choose the HMO for health insurance coverage. The HMO differs from a health insurance company in that it arranges a health delivery network and it conditions benefit payments on both the use of this network and the observance of certain referral and authorization procedures.

2. **Enrollment trends.** From 1970 to 1991, the number of HMOs in the United States increased from 26 to approximately 550. During this period, HMO enrollment increased rapidly from approximately 2.9 million to 35 million Americans (or approximately 17% of the insured population), due primarily to price and benefit coverage advantages over traditional group health insurance.

3. **Management of health care.** HMOs can provide more health benefits per premium dollar for a given population than traditional group health insurance by:

   a. Emphasizing low-cost alternatives to inpatient care, such as outpatient services

   b. Restricting patient referrals to participating providers who agree in advance to certain fee schedules and utilization review programs, including peer review

   c. Requiring that each HMO member select a primary care physician who coordinates the member's total health care needs

   d. Employing maximum fee schedules for participating providers to control the unit cost of health benefits

e. Implementing risk-sharing arrangements with providers
f. Negotiating volume discounts with tertiary hospitals and other suppliers, such as home health agencies, medical equipment companies, laboratories, and pharmacies

C. Preferred provider arrangements (PPAs)

1. **Definition.** PPAs are agreements between health care providers (e.g., physicians, hospitals) and a health benefit purchaser (e.g., insurance company, self-insured employer). Typically, the agreement includes:
   a. A discounted provider fee schedule
   b. Peer and utilization review programs
   c. Incentives for the insured to use the preferred providers, usually in the form of a lower deductible or copayment

2. **Characteristics of PPAs** include:
   a. **Provider panel,** with provider selection based on cost, quality, and geographic access criteria
   b. **Fee schedule** accepted by the provider panel
   c. **Utilization or claims review**
   d. **Free choice of providers,** including those outside the network of participating providers on every occasion a health service is sought

3. **Operation of PPAs**
   a. Eligible employees and dependents pay lower copayments and deductibles to participating, or preferred, providers than they would pay to nonparticipating providers. For example, an insured might pay a 20% coinsurance when selecting a nonparticipating provider versus no coinsurance if a participating provider is chosen.
   b. Typically, participating providers do not bill patients directly, except for applicable copayments. In contrast, nonparticipating providers bill directly and require patients to submit claim forms to the insurer or claims administrator.
   c. PPAs may be implemented in either of the following ways:
      (1) **Direct implementation,** whereby third-party payers (e.g., insurers or employers) contract with providers
      (2) **Indirect implementation,** whereby third-party payers contract with an independent **preferred provider organization (PPO)** to manage the PPA

4. **Differences between PPAs and HMOs** are listed in Table 18-4.

5. **Evaluating PPAs.** Historically, PPAs have focused on fee schedules (price control) to win benefit purchasers' support. However, since health benefit costs are a function of unit cost (fee schedule) and volume (utilization), it is very difficult to evaluate the effectiveness of PPAs in controlling health benefit costs.

D. Health insuring organizations (HIOs)

1. **Definition.** HIOs are risk-bearing entities that arrange and provide a health benefit program for an enrolled, defined population. HIOs are paid a fixed amount per capita for each enrollee and assume the risk that the payment is adequate to provide a specified set of benefits. The HIO arrangement is a new concept that has been employed by Medicaid programs in Kentucky and Pennsylvania. It provides the purchaser (in these cases, the state Medicaid programs) a means to cap benefit expenditures, since the risk is passed to another entity.

Table 18-4. Differences between Health Maintenance Organizations (HMOs) and Preferred Provider Arrangements (PPAs)

Characteristic	PPA	HMO
Insureds lock-in to providers under contract	No	Yes
Primary physician gatekeeper	Sometimes, but not binding	Generally, yes
Provider incentives	Possible	Generally, yes
Provider risk-sharing to offset deficits	Usually capped if present	Often unlimited
Peer review and utilization review	Usually	Yes

2. **HIOs versus HMOs.** While, in most cases, individuals or groups *choose* to enroll in an HMO, HIO coverage is always mandated by the benefit purchaser. Thus, the HIO enrollee must accept the HIO benefits plan, including restrictions on provider choice and required referral and prior authorization procedures. The mandatory enrollment feature makes the HIO system very controversial. The HIO typically employs the same features the HMO uses to manage patient care (see V B 3).

VI. GOVERNMENT PROGRAMS use a variety of payment and delivery structures to address specific populations needing health care. Government programs include: Medicare, Medicaid, Department of Defense military health benefits, the Veterans Administration, the Indian Health Service, and Maternal and Child Health Programs.

A. Medicare

1. **Origin.** Medicare began on July 1, 1966, under Title XVIII of the Social Security Act to provide health insurance coverage to patients age 65 and older. Subsequently, the program was expanded to cover disabled individuals younger than 65 and people suffering from chronic renal disease.

2. **Overview**
   a. **Part A,** which covers inpatient hospital services, limited skilled nursing facility care, and home care, is funded by the Social Security payroll tax paid by employers and employees.
   b. **Part B** helps pay for physicians' services, outpatient services, and medical supplies outside the hospital. It is funded by monthly insurance premiums paid by the beneficiary and from general tax revenues. Although enrollment in Part B is voluntary, most eligible individuals choose to participate because the federal government pays approximately 75% of total costs.
   c. **HMO options.** Since January 1985, Medicare beneficiaries have been able to enroll in HMOs that meet HCFA's requirements and that contract with HCFA. As of 1990, approximately 1 million Medicare beneficiaries, or less than 4% of those eligible, have selected HMO enrollment in lieu of traditional Medicare coverage. The "Medicare risk contract" between a qualified HMO and HCFA works as follows.
      (1) The HMO receives a fixed capitation payment equal to 95% of HCFA's estimated costs for providing Medicare benefits in the particular county.
      (2) The capitation amount is then adjusted according to the beneficiary's age, sex, and institutionalization status (whether or not the person is in a hospital or nursing home upon enrollment).
      (3) The HMO retains any profit or loss realized after fulfilling the terms of its contract with HCFA (i.e., any profit or loss that arises because the actual costs of delivering defined health benefits to Medicare recipients varied from the fixed capitation payment).
      (4) Several HMOs have terminated their Medicare benefit plans citing inadequate or uncertain reimbursement levels.

3. **Benefit limitations** of Medicare are illustrated in Table 18-5.

4. **Responses to benefit limitations**
   a. **Wraparound insurance coverage.** Many Medicare recipients buy supplemental, or wraparound, policies from private insurers to fill coverage gaps. Federal legislation passed in 1990 requires these so-called "Medigap" policies to conform to 10 standardized designs, thus simplifying comparison.
   b. **Revising Medicare coverage.** Many Medicare recipients, as well as health care experts, believe that Medicare's failure to cover long-term nursing home care is its greatest shortcoming. However, a recent attempt to expand Medicare benefits to include this and other benefits met with significant opposition.
      (1) In the late 1980s, Congress passed and subsequently repealed the **Medicare Catastrophic Coverage Act,** which expanded Medicare coverage to include: a stop-loss limit on Part A and Part B copayments; unlimited acute inpatient hospital services; expanded skilled nursing facility coverage; and prescription drugs, after satisfying an annual deductible.
      (2) Political pressure from recipients who did not want to pay additional premiums or income taxes (the funding sources for expanded benefits) resulted in the repeal of the Act.
      (3) Because of the political forces against this expansion of benefits, any future expansion to provide long-term nursing facility care seems uncertain.

Table 18-5. Limitations on Medicare Coverage, 1991

	Deductibles	Coinsurance Payments	Day or Dollar Limitations	No Coverage
Part A	$628 per inpatient admission	$157 per day of inpatient costs for days 61–90 of hospitalization $314 per day of inpatient costs for days 91–150 of hospitalization* $78.50 per day of skilled nursing facility care for days 21–100	Inpatient care not covered beyond 150 days Skilled nursing facility care not covered beyond 100 days	Long-term nursing home care Private duty nursing Custodial nursing home care
Part B	$100 per year	20% after satisfying yearly deductible	No stop-loss limit on 20% copayment	Outpatient prescription drugs Routine dental care Hearing aids Eyeglasses Routine physical exams Preventive care Physician's charges above Medicare allowance†

*These 60 days allowed only once per lifetime.

†Except in states requiring physicians to participate in Medicare or prohibiting balance billing for amounts above the Medicare allowance.

5. Administration

a. The Medicare program is administered by the HCFA, which is part of the U.S. Department of Health and Human Services (DHHS).

b. HCFA regional offices contract with private administrators or insurers known as **intermediaries** (e.g., Blue Cross) to administer benefit payments under Part A and with insurance companies, known as **Medicare carriers,** to handle payments under Part B.

c. A federal advisory council advises on policy for both Medicare and Medicaid.

6. Benefit payments

a. Part A. Inpatient hospital costs are paid using DRGs (see IV C 1).

b. Part B. Medicare usually pays 80% of the allowed amount for covered outpatient services, subject to a $100 per year deductible and the following other exceptions and limitations.

(1) Medicare allowed amount. Beginning in 1992, the allowed amount will be based on the new RBRVS, a uniform relative value scale (see IV D 1). Between 1992 and 1996, the RBRVS will be phased in, with the maximum fee derived by a complex weighting of the historical maximum payment level, also known as the "prevailing charge" (see IV D 1 b), and the new maximum payment level according to the RBRVS. By 1996, there will be a uniform fee schedule based on relative value units, with small geographic adjustments.

(2) Payment methods. Medicare Part B historically paid its share of providers' bills in two ways.

(a) Direct payment to physician (also known as the **physician assignment method**). By agreeing to this method, a physician who participates in Medicare (i.e., who accepts assignment) can charge the patient only Medicare's deductible and the 20% coinsurance. That is, the physician must accept Medicare's allowed amount as payment in full.

(b) Direct payment to the patient. After the physician submits an itemized bill to the regional Medicare carrier, Medicare pays the patient the allowable amount (less any patient deductible or coinsurance). It is the patient's responsibility to pay the physician, including any difference between the billed fee and Medicare's allowance.

(3) **Balance billing** is the practice of charging the patient the difference between Medicare's allowed amount, or maximum fee, for a particular procedure and the physician's usual charge. Since 1991, physicians who do not accept assignment can charge only a certain percentage of the Medicare allowed amount. The limit was 125% of the Medicare allowance in 1991, 120% in 1992, and 115% thereafter.

(4) **Mandatory assignment.** In an attempt to reduce or eliminate balance billing, several states have adopted some form of mandatory assignment.

B. Medicaid

1. **Overview.** Established in 1965 under Title XIX of the Social Security Act, **Medical Assistance,** commonly called Medicaid, provides medical benefits for people with low income who meet certain criteria.
   - **a.** Unlike Medicare, which is entirely federally funded and administered, Medicaid is a **combined state and federal program,** with the federal government providing 41%–79% of the funds needed and state governments paying the remainder. The **federal percentage varies according to per capita income of the state**—that is, according to the state's ability to share costs.
   - **b.** **Mandated services** include inpatient and outpatient hospital services, laboratory and radiology services, basic physician medical services, and skilled nursing facility coverage for patients over 21.

2. **Population covered**
   - **a.** **Eligibility** for Medicaid benefits is determined by **county welfare boards,** using **income and means criteria**. In 1989, Congress mandated state coverage of pregnant women and children less than 6 years old whose family income is within 133% of federal poverty guidelines.
   - **b.** **The number of individuals covered** by Medicaid doubled between 1969 and 1984, from 12.1 to 22.7 million.
   - **c.** **Medically indigent programs.** Due to the variability and timing of Medicaid's income criteria, only about half of the people whose income falls below the poverty line are covered by Medicaid. In response, 33 states have joined the federal-state medically needy program, through which states have the option of participating in federal government programs for the categorically needy [e.g., Aid to Families with Dependent Children (AFDC), Aid to the Aged (AA), Aid to the Blind (AB), Aid to the Disabled (AD)]. Such programs help defray the health costs of those who do not qualify for Medicaid based on income alone.
   - **d.** Although Medicaid was created to provide health insurance for the poor, especially women and children, nursing home care for the elderly represents the single largest Medicaid expenditure, approximately one-third of all Medicaid expenditures.

3. **State-federal administration.** Medicaid is a state-directed program, with eligibility and benefit limits set within a framework established by federal law.
   - **a.** Originally, state participation was voluntary. By 1970, states had to participate or lose aid for other federal programs targeted for the blind, disabled, and aged.
   - **b.** States complain that the federal government mandates expansion of Medicaid benefits but pays for a decreasing share of Medicaid expenditures.
   - **c.** Each state must have an advisory committee composed of provider and health professional representatives that oversees policy decisions, quality assurance, and payment methods and levels within the state-approved budget.
   - **d.** A federal advisory council advises on policy for both Medicare and Medicaid.

4. **Benefits administration**
   - **a.** Medicaid applications and claims generally come under the state's public welfare or health department.
   - **b.** Many states subcontract administrative functions to private third-party administrators.
   - **c.** Formulas and methods for provider payment vary by state. Increasingly, state Medicaid programs have moved from cost-based reimbursement to prospective payment, such as per diem or DRG rates.
   - **d.** Tremendous variation in scope of benefits exists from state to state, particularly with respect to dental services, prescription drugs, physical therapy, prosthetic devices (including

dentures), optical care, and ambulance coverage. New York and California have the most extensive benefits, while many states limit coverage to basic medical and hospital services.

5. **Financial implications of Medicaid**
   a. **Rising spending**
      (1) Medicaid spending between 1980 and 1990 grew by 180%. Medicaid, the fastest growing portion of state budgets, consumes more than 15% of state spending, up from 10% a decade ago.
      (2) Provider taxation, or voluntary hospital contribution funds ("**pooling**") is increasingly used by states as a way to increase state Medicaid spending, which, in turn, bolsters states' federal matching funds. HCFA has proposed a ban on such voluntary provider assessments because of the impact on federal spending.
   b. **Monitoring costs.** In order to control the rapid increase in Medicaid costs, states have instituted several measures, including:
      (1) Copayment or deductibles
      (2) Enrollment in HMOs and HIOs (see V B, D)
      (3) Preadmission authorization procedures
      (4) Restricted provider network
      (5) Primary care "gatekeepers" (see Ch 17, II A 3 b)
      (6) Bulk purchasing for medical supplies, eyeglasses, hearing aids, and laboratory equipment
      (7) Prospective reimbursement plans, including capitation and DRG rates
   c. **Effect on health care industry**
      (1) **Medicaid as Medicare supplement.** States use Medicaid funds to pay deductibles and coinsurance under Medicare Part A (hospital insurance) and the monthly premium for Part B (outpatient and physician services).
      (2) **Reduction of hospitals' bad debt.** By paying for patients who otherwise could not pay for care and by supplementing Medicare coverage, Medicaid has reduced bad debt levels for hospitals.
      (3) **Reduced or delayed reimbursement to health care providers** has resulted from the rise in Medicaid spending and states' inability to pay full costs. The failure by Medicaid to pay its proportionate share of patients' costs exacerbates cost-shifting from governmental to private third-party payers (see II F 5). In several lawsuits, hospitals have successfully challenged the inadequacy of Medicaid reimbursement, citing federal requirements for "reasonable and adequate" reimbursement of "efficient and economically run" hospitals.

VII. UNIVERSAL COVERAGE AND OTHER INSURANCE REFORM PROPOSALS

A. **Rationale.** At its most basic, universal health care coverage is intended to provide insurance coverage and access to medical care to the entire U.S. population. Proponents of such health care reform claim that it would remedy the following shortcomings of current U.S. health care financing.

1. **Lack of insurance.** The problems associated with the number of uninsured and underinsured people in the United States are discussed in II G 1 d.

2. **Instability of coverage.** Rapidly rising health costs and the increasingly strict enrollment criteria of insurers have made insurance coverage expensive and sometimes unobtainable for employers and employees.
   a. **Chronically or seriously ill employees or those with a bad risk potential** are difficult to insure. Insurers may refuse to cover such employees or may charge significantly higher premiums to have them covered. The impact of this added expense is felt more sharply by smaller employers, who cannot spread the cost among a large and diverse population of employees.
   b. **State regulations** regarding employers' and insurers' obligations to provide health insurance vary widely, often do not address the issue of risk selection (see VII B 3 f), and do not apply to employer-sponsored self-insurance plans (see III A 2 c).

3. **Cost.** Even private employers who have implemented aggressive programs to encourage their insureds to use selected low cost providers often have experienced steep cost increases due to provider cost-shifting (see II F 5).

4. **Administrative complexity.** The current fragmented provider payment system (see IV), in which each third-party payer has its own fee schedule, utilization review procedures, and other administrative requirements, results in much confusion and inefficiency for health care providers and consumers.

B. Health care reform strategies

1. **Lack of consensus.** Although studies report that 72% of Americans support the goal of universal coverage, there is little agreement on how this goal should be achieved. For example, many people are skeptical about expanding government's role, given the following situations:
   a. The mixed success of Medicare, a system in which government is the sole payer
   b. Medicare's current trial use of a voucher system that would permit beneficiaries to choose HMOs and PPOs
   c. The introduction of more private sector initiatives and free market principles in several formerly socialist national economies
2. **Models for universal coverage** include:
   a. **Compulsory private insurance through employers,** with government insuring nonworkers and the poor
   b. **Compulsory private insurance *or* tax equivalent** for employers ("**play or pay**" plan), with government insuring nonworkers and the poor
   c. **Tax credit for purchasers of individual private insurance,** whereby individuals purchase private insurance from competing insurers independent of employers and Medicare and Medicaid beneficiaries receive vouchers to purchase private insurance
   d. **An all-government insurance system,** which could include the following features:
      (1) **Government as the single payer** (i.e., an expanded Medicare model)
      (2) **Administration** of the system either **completely by the government or through contracts** with competing private insurers and service companies (as is currently done with Medicare)
      (3) **Various sources of funding,** including payroll taxes, individual income taxes, general government revenues, or a combination of sources
3. **Comparison of models for universal coverage.** The models can be analyzed according to several components.
   a. **Administration** of the program may be handled by the private sector or by government.
   b. **Financing.** Funding sources could include employers, employees, individuals (independent of the workplace), or tax revenues.
   c. **Changes in provider reimbursement** range from significant restructuring (such as the institution of a uniform, prospective rate structure for providers) to minimal regulation, whereby providers' rates and rate structures are determined by market forces. Most proposals attempt to reduce cost-shifting—in particular, the current de facto practice of shifting costs for Medicaid, Medicare, or uninsured patients to the privately insured.
   d. **Cost-containment features**—that is, those features designed to control health expenditures—may include: global caps (e.g., Medicare's RBRVS and volume performance standards), cost-sharing by the individual patient via deductibles and coinsurance, cost controls on provider capital and operational expenditures, and regulation of expensive new technologies.
   e. **Tax deductibility and credits.** Because unlimited employer tax deductibility of health coverage expenses often is cited as inflationary, some proposals limit or eliminate tax deductibility both for the corporation and the individual. Some proposals provide tax credits or vouchers that permit individuals who cannot afford coverage to purchase private insurance. Such a tax credit or voucher system could eliminate government-sponsored plans like Medicaid.
   f. **Risk-selection rules.** In the current market system of competing private insurance, health coverage may be exorbitantly expensive or unavailable at any price for those individuals or groups who are deemed poor underwriting risks. Conversely, those deemed favorable, or preferred, risks may select lower priced coverage plans. This differentiating process is called **adverse and preferred risk selection**. Most proposals provide for coverage of higher-risk individuals either in government-financed plans or in fallback subsidized assigned risk pools. Other proposals seek to minimize the number of "uninsurables" by regulating underwriting and policy termination rules more stringently.
   g. **Compulsory coverage.** Most proposals incorporate mandatory coverage at either the employer (e.g., "play or pay") or individual level through tax levies, exemptions, credits, or

vouchers. The models differ with respect to the scope of government-sponsored coverage for individuals who fall outside the coverage mandate.

h. **Market regulation.** In order to establish more uniformity and fairness in the market, most proposals recommend increased governmental regulation of premium rating methods, benefit coverage (minimum levels and limitations on exclusions), underwriting practices, and termination rules. Often, federal rather than the current fragmented state regulation is suggested.

i. **Role of managed care.** Many proposals envision a growing role for private managed care companies with select provider networks and stringent quality and utilization standards. Some proponents of a single-source government payer system would permit beneficiaries to "opt out" and choose a private managed care plan through a voucher program.

4. **Incremental alternatives to universal coverage.** Given the lack of consensus on the design for universal coverage, short-term incremental change is more likely to occur first, including the following methods to **expand coverage for the uninsured**.

   a. **Continuation coverage.** Currently, the **Consolidated Omnibus Budget Reconciliation Act (COBRA)**, passed in 1986, requires employers with more than 25 employees to offer health benefits for 18 months to employees (and dependents, when applicable) who no longer are eligible for the employer's group coverage (e.g., due to employment termination or retirement). The insured must pay for the continuation coverage, but the cost can be no greater than 102% of group rates. A proposed plan would extend the duration of the continuation coverage and finance the coverage by some combination of government, employer, and employee funding, rather than by the employee alone.

   b. **Proposed expansion of Medicaid** would cover those below the poverty line rather than relying on the current categorical eligibility tests. Some proposals would permit private citizens within certain income brackets to buy Medicaid coverage from the state government.

   c. **Mandatory employer-sponsored coverage of the uninsured** ("play or pay" plan) likely will be the model chosen for initial health care reform because it builds upon the current employer-sponsored private health insurance structure and could be instituted gradually. The uninsured would receive coverage through either an expansion of the Medicaid program or a voucher system that would permit purchase of a private policy or HMO coverage in lieu of Medicaid.

BIBLIOGRAPHY

Anderson HJ: Looking abroad for changes to the U.S. health care system. *Hospitals* 65(12):3, 1991.

Davis K: Expanding Medicare and employer plans to achieve universal health insurance. *JAMA* 265:2525–2528, 1991.

Francis S: Health care costs: U.S. industrial outlook 1991—health and medical services. *Medical Benefits* 8(4):1–2, 1991.

Higgins AF: Health care benefits survey 1990: Indemnity plans: costs, design and funding. *Medical Benefits* 8(4):4, 1991.

Office of the Actuary, Health Financing Administration: National health expenditures, 1990. *Medical Benefits* 8(23):2, 1991.

Pallarito K: The budget deficits threaten to shut out Medicaid benefits. *Modern Healthcare* 21(25):33, 1991.

Porter MJ, Ball PA, Kraus N: *The Interstudy Competitive Edge,* vol 1, no 2. Excelsior, MN, Interstudy, 1992, p 37.

Rockefeller JD: A call for action: the Pepper Commission's blueprint for health care reform. *JAMA* 265:2507, 1991.

STUDY QUESTIONS

Directions: Each of the numbered items or incomplete statements in this section is followed by answers or by completions of the statement. Select the **one** lettered answer or completion that is **best** in each case.

Questions 1–3

A 68-year-old woman on Medicare breaks her finger. She is seen by a Medicare-participating orthopedist who sets the fracture in an outpatient setting. Although the physician's regular charge for splinting a finger is $325, Medicare's allowed charge is $250. The patient has not incurred any other outpatient expenses during the calendar year.

1. What is the amount of the patient's portion of the payment, assuming Medicare Part B deductible of $100 per year and coinsurance of 20%?

(A) $75
(B) $50
(C) $125
(D) $0
(E) $130

2. How much would the physician be reimbursed by the Medicare carrier for this procedure?

(A) $325
(B) $250
(C) $120
(D) $215
(E) Cannot be determined from information given

3. Which of the following third-party payers most likely would have paid the orthopedist the highest amount for setting the fracture?

(A) Medicare
(B) A commercial insurer using the UCR payment methodology
(C) Medicaid
(D) An HMO that set its maximum fee schedule for the procedure at the median value for all specialists in the geographic area

4. Medicare provides coverage to which of the following patient groups?

(A) Unemployed individuals
(B) Patients receiving long-term dialysis treatment
(C) AIDS patients
(D) Low-income children
(E) None of the above

5. Characteristics of Medicare coverage include all of the following EXCEPT

(A) deductibles and coinsurance for inpatient and outpatient services
(B) inpatient hospital services and skilled nursing care
(C) physicians' services and outpatient services
(D) monthly insurance premiums for Part B coverage
(E) participation by all licensed U.S. physicians

6. Under the DRG payment method used by Medicare, for which of the following diagnostic categories would a hospital receive the highest payment rate?

(A) Vasectomy without complications
(B) Tubal ligation without complications
(C) Appendectomy without complications
(D) Coronary artery bypass without cardiac catheterization
(E) Tonsillectomy

7. After hospital services expenditures, the category that accounts for the next highest percentage of total personal health care expenditures is

(A) drugs and medical supplies
(B) nursing homes
(C) physicians' services
(D) dentists' services

1-E 4-B 7-C
2-C 5-E
3-B 6-D

Directions: Each item below contains four suggested answers of which **one or more** is correct. Choose the answer

- **A** if **1, 2, and 3** are correct
- **B** if **1 and 3** are correct
- **C** if **2 and 4** are correct
- **D** if **4** is correct
- **E** if **1, 2, 3, and 4** are correct

8. Advocates of universal health coverage cite which of the following shortcomings in the current U.S. health care financing system?

(1) More than 35 million Americans have no health insurance coverage
(2) Employer-sponsored self-insurance plans are not subject to state regulation
(3) The relatively higher cost of health care in the United States threatens U.S. manufacturers' competitive position in the global economy
(4) The current Medicare hospital payment system, based on national DRG payment rates, results in lack of competition among hospitals

9. Which of the reimbursement trends can be attributed to Medicare's adoption of the RBRVS?

(1) The average income of family medicine physicians increases by a higher percentage than that of radiologists
(2) All anesthesiologists receive a fixed salary determined by the Health Care Financing Agency (HCFA)
(3) Psychiatrists receive higher percentage increases in fees than ophthalmologists do
(4) Cognitive services receive lower fee increases than procedural services

10. Factors contributing to the dramatic growth in health care expenditures during the last 20 years include

(1) a decrease in the number of hospitals
(2) an increase in governmental funding under Medicare and Medicaid
(3) significant improvements in health status in the United States (mortality and morbidity rates)
(4) an increase in the percentage of the population over 65 years of age

---

8-A
9-B
10-C

Directions: The group of items in this section consists of lettered options followed by a set of numbered items. For each item, select the **one** lettered option that is most closely associated with it. Each lettered option may be selected once, more than once, or not at all.

Questions 11–15

The information below is taken from a typical remittance advice (explanation of benefit payments) to a physician participating in the Medicare program. Match the descriptors listed below with the correct amounts.

CPT-4 code descriptor = 90620, initial consultation, comprehensive
Billed charge for this service = $200.00
Medicare allowed amount = $125.00

(A) $100
(B) $20
(C) $5
(D) $75
(E) $25

11. The annual Part B deductible, none of which had been met by the patient when this claim was processed

12. The contractual allowance or write-off made by the physician when she recorded the Medicare payment

13. The 20% patient copayment on Medicare's allowed amount (after subtracting the patient's annual deductible)

14. Medicare's allowed amount less the annual patient deductible

15. What Medicare actually paid the participating physician

11-A
12-D
13-C
14-E
15-B

ANSWERS AND EXPLANATIONS

1–3. The answers are: 1-E *[IV B 2, 3; VI A 2 b, 6 b]*, **2-C** *[IV B 1, 4]*, **3-B** *[II F 5; IV D 1 b]*.
The total payment owed by the patient is $130. The patient is responsible for a $100 deductible under Medicare Part B because she has not incurred any other outpatient expenses during the year. After the deductible is subtracted from the total allowed charge ($250 − $100 = $150), the patient must pay 20% coinsurance on the remainder of the charges, or 20% of $150 (i.e., $30). The $100 deductible plus the $30 copayment bring the total payment to $130. If the patient had already satisfied her deductible, the payment would have been 20% of $250, or $50.

The physician will be reimbursed $120 by Medicare for the procedure, calculated by subtracting the patient's financial responsibility ($130) from the Medicare allowance ($250). The difference between the physician's usual charge ($325) and the Medicare allowance ($250) is called the contractual allowance (which equals $75 in this example), which must be written off by the physician. The participating physician's regular charges have no bearing on Medicare reimbursements.

Typically, a commercial insurer using the usual, customary, or reasonable (UCR) fee scale would set its maximum allowance (i.e., the fee paid the physician) at the 80th or 90th percentile value of the various rates charged for the procedure. The median value for a geographic area would be the middle value, or the 50th percentile, of the range of values charged for that procedure in the area. This formula is often used by health maintenance organizations (HMOs) and other groups that are attempting to contain costs. Government programs like Medicare and Medicaid usually reimburse at lower levels than private carriers, resulting in cost-shifting. In this example, cost-shifting occurs when a higher fee for the procedure is paid by commercial insurance.

4. The answer is B *[VI A 1]*.
Medicare provides health coverage to people 65 years of age and older, the disabled (after a 2-year waiting period), and end-stage renal dialysis (ESRD) patients. The unemployed, unless meeting other eligibility requirements, do not qualify. Extending Medicare coverage to include ESRD patients was a unique coverage expansion applicable to one diagnostic category only. Other diagnostic categories, including acquired immune deficiency syndrome (AIDS), are not categorically covered unless the beneficiary qualifies under other criteria. Low-income children *may* qualify for state-sponsored Medicaid benefits but not for Medicare benefits.

5. The answer is E *[VI A]*.
Physician participation in Medicare is voluntary, except in the few states where state regulation mandates participation. The Medicare system has deductible and coinsurance amounts for both inpatient and outpatient services. Part A coverage, which is funded through the Social Security payroll tax, primarily covers inpatient hospital services and skilled nursing care. Part B coverage, which is funded by monthly premiums from beneficiaries and through tax revenues, covers physicians' services and outpatient services.

6. The answer is D *[IV C; VI A]*.
The payment rate for each diagnosis-related group (DRG) category is determined by its case-mix index, or relative cost, compared to the average cost for all procedures. Clearly, the coronary artery bypass procedure is more intensive than the others listed and, thus, requires greater use of the hospital's resources. The DRG relative weight (i.e., case-mix index) for a coronary artery bypass is 4.6608, whereas for all the other procedures listed, the DRG relative weight is less than 1.0000.

7. The answer is C *[II B; Figure 18-1]*.
Hospital services account for approximately 43.7% of the total health care expenditures—the largest category by far. Physicians' services account for 22.4% of the total, followed by drugs, eyeglasses, and medical supplies, (11.4%), nursing homes (9.1%), and dentists' services (5.8%).

8. The answer is A (1, 2, 3) *[II G 1 d; VII A 1–3]*.
Both the large uninsured population and the impact of high health care costs on U.S. manufacturers' competitiveness have been cited as reasons to reform U.S. health care financing. Health care providers have developed elaborate cross-subsidies to "shift" some of the cost of the bad debt incurred from uninsured patients to third-party payers. Since employer-sponsored self-insurance plans are not subject to state regulation, they may contain exclusions for particular diseases or preexisting conditions, which can result in coverage gaps for eligible employees and dependents. Such coverage gaps exacerbate the uninsured and underinsured problem. Because the United States spends a higher percentage of its gross national product (GNP) on health services than any other industrialized nation, manufacturers (e.g., automakers) complain of product price disadvantages caused by the higher employee health coverage costs.

The inpatient hospital payment system based on fixed reimbursement rates for 470 diagnosis-related groups (DRGs) rewards those hospitals that are cost-efficient and can provide the needed care and services for less than the DRG reimbursement rate. Thus, this payment system encourages competition among hospitals, which can contribute to a hospital's cost-effectiveness.

9. The answer is B (1, 3) *[IV D 1 d].*
According to the resource-based relative value scale (RBRVS), physicians are paid more for cognitive services and less for procedure-based services. For example, office visits, consultations, and psychiatric counseling sessions all are allocated higher fees than under the pre-1992 payment structure. Therefore, specialties like family medicine, internal medicine, and psychiatry receive relatively higher reimbursement under the RBRVS Medicare program, whereas radiology and ophthalmology receive relatively lower reimbursement.

10. The answer is C (2, 4) *[II E 1, 4].*
Both the increase in governmental funding for Medicare and Medicaid and the growing number of people over 65 have contributed to rising health care costs. Although the number of hospitals has declined due to mergers and bankruptcies, this phenomenon has not been a major factor in expenditure levels. Morbidity and mortality rates have not significantly improved in the United States in the last 20 years.

11–15. The answers are: 11-A, 12-D, 13-C, 14-E, 15-B *[VI A 6].*
The Part B deductible for Medicare is $100. The deductible must be satisfied before Medicare will pay any benefits. The contractual allowance is equal to the physician's usual fee for the service (the "billed charge" on the remittance advice) less the Medicare allowed amount—in this case, $200 − $125 = $75. The 20% copayment after deductible is based on Medicare's allowed amount, or $125. Subtracting the $100 deductible from Medicare's allowed amount of $125 leaves $25 in charges to be split between Medicare and the patient. The patient's copayment is equal to 20% of this $25, or $5, and Medicare's portion is 80% of the $25, or $20. Thus, Medicare actually paid the physician $20.

Comprehensive Exam

Introduction

One of the least attractive aspects of pursuing an education is the necessity of being examined on what has been learned. Instructors do not like to prepare tests, and students do not like to take them.

However, students are required to take many examinations during their learning careers, and little if any time is spent acquainting them with the positive aspects of tests and with systematic and successful methods for approaching them. Students perceive tests as punitive and sometimes feel that they are merely opportunities for the instructor to discover what the student has forgotten or has never learned. Students need to view tests as opportunities to display their knowledge and to use them as tools for developing prescriptions for further study and learning.

A brief history and discussion of the National Board of Medical Examiners (NBME) examinations [now the United States Medical Licensing Examination (USMLE)] are presented here, along with ideas concerning psychological preparation for the examinations. Also presented are general considerations and test-taking tips, as well as ways to use practice exams as educational tools. (The literature provided by the various examination boards contains detailed information concerning the construction and scoring of specific exams.)

Before the various NBME exams were developed, each state attempted to license physicians through its own procedures. Differences in the quality and testing procedures of the various state examinations resulted in the refusal of some states to recognize the licensure of physicians licensed in other states. This made it difficult for physicians to move freely from one state to another and produced an uneven quality of medical care in the United States.

To remedy this situation, the various state medical boards decided they would be better served if an outside agency prepared standard exams to be given in all states, allowing each state to meet its own needs and have a common standard by which to judge the educational preparation of individuals applying for licensure.

One misconception concerning these outside agencies is that they are licensing authorities. This is not the case; they are examination boards only. The individual states retain the power to grant and revoke licenses. The examination boards are charged with designing and scoring valid and reliable tests. They are primarily concerned with providing the states with feedback on how examinees have performed and with making suggestions about the interpretation and usefulness of scores. The states use this information as partial fulfillment of qualifications upon which they grant licenses.

Students should remember that these exams are administered nationwide and, although the general medical information is the same, educational methodologies and faculty areas of expertise differ from institution to institution. It is unrealistic to expect that students will know all

---

The author of this introduction, Michael J. O'Donnell, holds the positions of Assistant Professor of Psychiatry and Director of Biomedical Communications at the University of New Mexico School of Medicine, Albuquerque, New Mexico.

the material presented in the exams; they may face questions on the exams in areas that were only superficially covered in their classes. The testing authorities recognize this situation, and their scoring procedures take it into account.

The Exams

The first exam was given in 1916. It was a combination of written, oral, and laboratory tests, and it was administered over a 5-day period. Admission to the exam required proof of completion of medical education and 1 year of internship.

In 1922, the examination was changed to a new format and was divided into three parts. Part I, a 3-day essay exam, was given in the basic sciences after 2 years of medical school. Part II, a 2-day exam, was administered shortly before or after graduation, and Part III was taken at the end of the first postgraduate year. To pass both Part I and Part II, a score equalling 75% of the total points available in each was required.

In 1954, after a 3-year extensive study, the NBME adopted the multiple-choice format. To pass, a statistically computed score of 75 was required, which allowed comparison of test results from year to year. In 1971, this method was changed to one that held the mean constant at a computed score of 500, with a predetermined deviation from the mean to ascertain a passing or failing score. The 1971 changes permitted more sophisticated analysis of test results and allowed schools to compare among individual students within their respective institutions as well as among students nationwide. Feedback to students regarding performance included the reporting of pass or failure along with scores in each of the areas tested.

During the 1980s, the ever-changing field of medicine made it necessary for the NBME to examine once again its evaluation strategies. It was found necessary to develop questions in multidisciplinary areas such as gerontology, health promotion, immunology, and cell and molecular biology. In addition, it was decided that questions should test higher cognitive levels and reasoning skills.

To meet the new goals, many changes have been made in both the form and content of the examination. Changes include reduction in the number of questions to approximately 800 in Step 1 and Step 2 of the USMLE to allow students more time on each question, with total testing time reduced on Step 1 from 13 to 12 hours and on Step 2 from 12.5 to 12 hours. The basic science disciplines are no longer allotted the same number of questions, which permits flexible weighing of the exam areas. Reporting of scores to schools include total scores for individuals and group mean scores for separate discipline areas. Only pass/fail designations and total scores are reported to examinees. There is no longer a provision for the reporting of individual subscores to either the examinees or medical schools. Finally, the question format used in the new exams is predominately multiple-choice, best-answer.

The New Format

New questions, designed specifically for Step 1, are constructed in an effort to test the student's grasp of the sciences basic to medicine in an integrated fashion—the questions are designed to be interdisciplinary. Many of these items are presented as vignettes, or case studies, followed by a series of multiple-choice, best-answer questions.

The scoring of this exam is altered. Whereas in the past the exams were scored on a normal curve, the new exam has a predetermined standard, which must be met in order to pass. The exam no longer concentrates on the trivial; therefore, it has been concluded that there is a common base of information that all medical students should know in order to pass. It is anticipated that a major shift in the pass/fail rate for the nation is unlikely. In the past, the average student could only expect to feel comfortable with half the test and eventually would complete approximately 67% of the questions correctly, to achieve a mean score of 500. Although with the standard setting method it is likely that the mean score will change and become higher, it is unlikely that the pass/fail rates will differ significantly from those in the past. During the first testing in 1991, there was not differential weighing of the questions. However, in the future, the NBME will be researching methods of weighing questions based on both the time it takes to answer questions vis-à-vis their difficulty and the perceived importance of the information. In addition, the NBME is attempting to design a method of delivering feedback to the student that will have considerable importance in discovering weaknesses and pinpointing areas for further study in the event that a retake is necessary.

Materials Needed for Test Preparation

In preparation for a test, many students collect far too much study material only to find that they simply do not have the time to go through all of it. They are defeated before they begin because either they leave areas unstudied, or they race through the material so quickly that they cannot benefit from the activity.

It is generally more efficient for the student to use materials already at hand; that is, class notes, one good outline to cover or strengthen areas not locally stressed and to quickly review the whole topic, and one good text as a reference for looking up complex material needing further explanation.

Also, many students attempt to memorize far too much information, rather than learning and understanding less material and then relying on that learned information to determine the answers to questions at the time of the examination. Relying too heavily on memorized material causes anxiety, and the more anxious students become during a test, the less learned knowledge they are likely to use.

Positive Attitude

A positive attitude and a realistic approach are essential to successful test taking. If concentration is placed on the negative aspects of tests or on the potential for failure, anxiety increases and performance decreases. A negative attitude generally develops if the student concentrates on "I must pass" rather than on "I can pass." "What if I fail?" becomes the major factor motivating the student to **run from failure rather than toward success**. This results from placing too much emphasis on scores rather than understanding that scores have only slight relevance to future professional performance.

The score received is only one aspect of test performance. Test performance also indicates the student's ability to use information during evaluation procedures and reveals how this ability might be used in the future. For example, when a patient enters the physician's office with a problem, the physician begins by asking questions, searching for clues, and seeking diagnostic information. Hypotheses are then developed, which will include several potential causes for the problem. Weighing the probabilities, the physician will begin to discard those hypotheses with the least likelihood of being correct. Good differential diagnosis involves the ability to deal with uncertainty, to reduce potential causes to the smallest number, and to use all learned information in arriving at a conclusion.

The same thought process can and should be used in testing situations. It might be termed **paper-and-pencil differential diagnosis**. In each question with five alternatives, of which one is correct, there are four alternatives that are incorrect. If deductive reasoning is used, as in solving a clinical problem, the choices can be viewed as having possibilities of being correct. The elimination of wrong choices increases the odds that a student will be able to recognize the correct choice. Even if the correct choice does not become evident, the probability of guessing correctly increases. Just as differential diagnosis in a clinical setting can result in a correct diagnosis, eliminating incorrect choices on a test can result in choosing the correct answer.

Answering questions based on what is incorrect is difficult for many students since they have had nearly 20 years experience taking tests with the implied assertion that knowledge can be displayed only by knowing what is correct. It must be remembered, however, that students can display knowledge by knowing something is wrong, just as they can display it by knowing something is right. **Students should begin to think in the present as they expect themselves to think in the future.**

Paper-and-Pencil Differential Diagnosis

The technique used to arrive at the answer to the following question is an example of the paper-and-pencil differential diagnosis approach.

> A recently diagnosed case of hypothyroidism in a 45-year-old man may result in which of the following conditions?
>
> **(A)** Thyrotoxicosis
> **(B)** Cretinism
> **(C)** Myxedema
> **(D)** Graves' disease
> **(E)** Hashimoto's thyroiditis

It is presumed that all of the choices presented in the question are plausible and partially correct. If the student begins by breaking the question into parts and trying to discover what the question is attempting to measure, it will be possible to answer the question correctly by using more than memorized charts concerning thyroid problems.

- The question may be testing if the student knows the difference between "hypo" and "hyper" conditions.
- The answer choices may include thyroid problems that are not "hypothyroid" problems.
- It is possible that one or more of the choices are "hypo" but are not "thyroid" problems, that they are some other endocrine problems.
- "Recently diagnosed in a 45-year-old man" indicates that the correct answer is not a congenital childhood problem.
- "May result in" as opposed to "resulting from" suggests that the choices might include a problem that **causes** hypothyroidism rather than **results from** hypothyroidism, as stated.

By applying this kind of reasoning, the student can see that choice **A,** thyroid toxicosis, which is a disorder resulting from an overactive thyroid gland ("hyper") must be eliminated. Another piece of knowledge, that is, Graves' disease is thyroid toxicosis, eliminates choice **D**. Choice **B,** cretinism, is indeed hypothyroidism, but it is a childhood disorder. Therefore, **B** is eliminated. Choice **E** is an inflammation of the thyroid gland—here the clue is the suffix "itis." The reasoning is that thyroiditis, being an inflammation, may **cause** a thyroid problem, perhaps even a hypothyroid problem, but there is no reason for the reverse to be true. Myxedema, choice **C,** is the only choice left and the obvious correct answer.

Preparing for Board Examinations

1. **Study for yourself.** Although some of the material may seem irrelevant, the more you learn now, the less you will have to learn later. Also, do not let the fear of the test rob you of an important part of your education. If you study to learn, the task is less distasteful than studying solely to pass a test.

2. **Review all areas.** You should not be selective by studying perceived weak areas and ignoring perceived strong areas. This is probably the last time you will have the time and the motivation to review **all** of the basic sciences.

3. **Attempt to understand, not just memorize, the material.** Ask yourself: To whom does the material apply? Where does it apply? When does it apply? Understanding the connections among these points allows for longer retention and aids in those situations when guessing strategies may be needed.

4. **Try to anticipate questions that might appear on the test.** Ask yourself how you might construct a question on a specific topic.

5. **Give yourself a couple days of rest before the test.** Studying up to the last moment will increase your anxiety and cause potential confusion.

Taking Board Examinations

1. In the case of the USMLE exams, be sure to **pace yourself** to use time optimally. Each booklet is designed to take 2 hours. You should use all your allotted time; if you finish too early, you probably did so by moving too quickly through the test.

2. **Read each question and all the alternatives carefully** before you begin to make decisions. Remember the questions contain clues, as do the answer choices. As a physician, you would not make a clinical decision without a complete examination of all the data; the same holds true for answering test questions.

3. **Read the directions for each question set carefully.** You would be amazed at how many students make mistakes in tests simply because they have not paid close attention to the directions.

4. It is not advisable to leave blanks with the intention of coming back to answer the questions later. Because of the way Board examinations are constructed, you probably will not pick up any new information that will help you when you come back, and the chances of getting numerically off on your answer sheet are greater than your chances of benefiting by skipping around. If you feel that you must come back to a question, mark the best choice and place a note in the margin. Generally speaking, it is best not to change answers once you have made a decision, unless you have learned new information. Your intuitive reaction and first response are correct more often than changes made out of frustration or anxiety. **Never turn in an answer sheet with blanks.** Scores are based on the number that you get correct; you are not penalized with incorrect choices.

5. **Do not try to answer the questions on a stimulus–response basis.** It generally will not work. Use all of your learned knowledge.

6. **Do not let anxiety destroy your confidence.** If you have prepared conscientiously, you know enough to pass. Use all that you have learned.

7. **Do not try to determine how well you are doing as you proceed.** You will not be able to make an objective assessment, and your anxiety will increase.

8. **Do not expect a feeling of mastery** or anything close to what you are accustomed to. Remember, this is a nationally administered exam, not a mastery test.

9. **Do not become frustrated or angry** about what appear to be bad or difficult questions. You simply do not know the answers; you cannot know everything.

Specific Test-Taking Strategies

Read the entire question carefully, regardless of format. Test questions have multiple parts. Concentrate on picking out the pertinent key words that might help you begin to problem-solve. Words such as "always," "never," "mostly," "primarily," and so forth play significant roles. In all types of questions, distractors with terms such as "always" or "never" most often are incorrect. Adjectives and adverbs can completely change the meaning of questions—pay close attention to them. Also, medical prefixes and suffixes (e.g., "hypo-," "hyper-," "-ectomy," "-itis") are sometimes at the root of the question. The knowledge and application of everyday English grammar often is the key to dissecting questions.

Multiple-Choice Questions

Read the question and the choices carefully to become familiar with the data as given. Remember, in multiple-choice questions there is one correct answer and there are four distractors, or incorrect answers. (Distractors are plausible and possibly correct or they would not be called distractors.) They are generally correct for part of the question but not for the entire question. Dissecting the question into parts aids in discerning these distractors.

If the correct answer is not immediately evident, begin eliminating the distractors. (Many students feel that they must always start at option A and make a decision before they move to B, thus forcing decisions they are not ready to make.) Your first decisions should be made on those choices you feel the most confident about.

Compare the choices to each part of the question. **To be wrong,** a choice needs to be **incorrect for only part** of the question. **To be correct,** it must be **totally** correct. If you believe a choice is partially incorrect, tentatively eliminate that choice. Make notes next to the choices regarding tentative decisions. One method is to place a minus sign next to the choices you are certain are incorrect and a plus sign next to those that potentially are correct. Finally, place a zero next to any choice you do not understand or need to come back to for further inspection. Do not feel that you must make final decisions until you have examined all choices carefully.

When you have eliminated as many choices as you can, decide which of those that are left has the highest probability of being correct. Remember to use paper-and-pencil differential diagnosis. Above all, be honest with yourself. If you do not know the answer, eliminate as many choices as possible and choose reasonably.

Vignette-Based Questions

Vignette-based questions are nothing more than normal multiple-choice questions that use the same case, or grouped information, for setting the problem. The NBME has been researching question types that would test the student's grasp of the integrated medical basic sciences in a more cognitively complex fashion than can be accomplished with traditional testing formats. These questions allow the testing of information that is more medically relevant than memorized terminology.

It is important to realize that several questions, although grouped together and referring to one situation or vignette, are independent questions; that is, they are able to stand alone. Your inability to answer one question in a group should have no bearing on your ability to answer other questions in that group.

These are multiple-choice questions, and just as with single best-answer questions, you should use the paper-and-pencil differential diagnosis, as was described earlier.

Single Best-Answer–Matching Sets

Single best-answer–matching sets consist of a list of words or statements followed by several numbered items or statements. Be sure to pay attention to whether the choices can be used more than once, only once, or not at all. Consider each choice individually and carefully. Begin with those with which you are the most familiar. It is important always to break the statements and words into parts, as with all other question formats. **If a choice is only partially correct, then it is incorrect.**

Guessing

Nothing takes the place of a firm knowledge base, but with little information to work with, even after playing paper-and-pencil differential diagnosis, you may find it necessary to guess the correct answer. A few simple rules can help increase your guessing accuracy. Always guess consistently if you have no idea what is correct; that is, after eliminating all that you can, make the choice that agrees with your intuition or choose the option closest to the top of the list that has not been eliminated as a potential answer.

When guessing at questions that have choices in numerical form, you will often find the choices listed in an ascending or descending order. It is generally not wise to guess the first or last alternative, since these are usually extreme values and are most likely incorrect.

Using the Comprehensive Exam to Learn

All too often, students do not take full advantage of practice exams. There is a tendency to complete the exam, score it, look up the correct answers to those questions missed, and then forget the entire thing.

In fact, great educational benefits can be derived if students would spend more time using practice tests as learning tools. As mentioned earlier, incorrect choices in test questions are plausible and partially correct or they would not fulfill their purpose as distractors. This means that it is just as beneficial to look up the incorrect choices as the correct choices to discover specifically why they are incorrect. In this way, it is possible to learn better test-taking skills as the subtlety of question construction is uncovered.

Additionally, it is advisable to go back and attempt to restructure each question to see if all the choices can be made correct by modifying the question. By doing this, four times as much will be learned. By all means, look up the right answer and explanation. Then, focus on each of the other choices and ask yourself under what conditions they might be correct? For example, the entire thrust of the sample question concerning hypothyroidism could be altered by changing the first few words to read:

"Hyperthyroidism recently discovered in . . ."
"Hypothyroidism prenatally occurring in . . ."
"Hypothyroidism resulting from . . ."

This question can be used to learn and understand thyroid problems in general, not only to memorize answers to specific questions.

In the comprehensive exam that follows, every effort has been made to simulate the types of questions and the degree of question difficulty in the USMLE Step 1. While taking these exams, the student should attempt to create the testing conditions that might be experienced during actual testing situations. Approximately 1 minute should be allowed for each question, and the entire test should be finished before it is scored.

Summary

Ideally, examinations are designed to determine how much information students have learned and how that information is used in the successful completion of the examination. Students will be successful if these suggestions are followed:

- Develop a positive attitude and maintain that attitude.
- Be realistic in determining the amount of material you attempt to master and in the score you hope to obtain.
- Read the directions for each type of question and the questions themselves closely and follow the directions carefully.
- Guess intelligently and consistently when guessing strategies must be used.

- Bring the paper-and-pencil differential diagnosis approach to each question in the examination.
- Use the test as an opportunity to display your knowledge and as a tool for developing prescriptions for further study and learning.

The USMLE is not easy. It may be almost impossible for those who have unrealistic expectations or for those who allow misinformation concerning the exam to produce anxiety out of proportion to the task at hand. It is manageable if it is approached with a positive attitude and with consistent use of all the information that has been learned.

Michael J. O'Donnell

STUDY QUESTIONS

Directions: Each of the numbered items or incomplete statements in this section is followed by answers or by completions of the statement. Select the **one** lettered answer or completion that is **best** in each case.

Questions 1–2

Dr. Neugierig observed a rapid recovery in one of his hepatitis C patients who sat in the hospital solarium daily. A review of the literature revealed no reported effects of the sun on the convalescence of hepatitis patients, so Dr. Neugierig published a summary of this patient's unusual recovery. One year later, he published results on six similar cases.

1. Which of the following study designs has Dr. Neugierig used?

(A) Case report
(B) Case-control study
(C) Cohort study
(D) Clinical study

2. Dr. Neugierig enlists the support of several gastroenterologists and designs a study whereby hepatitis C patients, upon hospital admission, are alternately assigned to receive either 2 hours of sun exposure daily or no sun exposure. Which of the following study designs has Dr. Neugierig and his colleagues used?

(A) Case series report
(B) Case-control study
(C) Cohort study
(D) Clinical trial

3. When performing multiple comparisons and repeated testing for statistical significance, there is an increase in the likelihood of

(A) an incorrect sample size
(B) a type I, or α, error
(C) determining causality
(D) a true null hypothesis (H_0)
(E) showing clinical importance

4. Which of the following statements concerning the epidemiology of alcohol use in the United States is true?

(A) Nearly 100 million people can be considered alcoholic
(B) Between 8% and 10% of adult men and between 3% and 5% of adult women are alcoholic
(C) Native Americans have a low rate of alcoholism
(D) Alcoholics are most likely to be 55–59 years of age and belong to high socioeconomic groups
(E) Alcoholic individuals are associated with 15,000 homicides annually

Questions 5–6

Approximately 100 people attended a buffet dinner at which they were served fried chicken, sliced ham, Swedish meatballs, green beans, potato salad, and apple pie. Thirty guests developed vomiting and diarrhea within 6 hours of the dinner. An epidemiologic investigation, interviewing 60 guests (25 ill and 35 not ill), revealed the following data:

	Consumed Food			Did Not Consume Food		
Food Served	**Ill**	**Not Ill**	**Attack Rate**	**Ill**	**Not Ill**	**Attack Rate**
Chicken	20	28	42%	5	7	42%
Ham	12	17	41%	13	18	42%
Meatballs	23	24	49%	2	11	15%
Green beans	15	24	38%	10	11	48%
Potato salad	18	26	41%	7	9	44%
Apple pie	22	34	39%	3	1	75%

5. The incriminated food item is most likely

(A) chicken
(B) ham
(C) meatballs
(D) potato salad
(E) apple pie

6. The most likely etiologic agent is

(A) *Salmonella*
(B) *Staphylococcus*
(C) *Clostridium perfringens*
(D) *Bacillus cereus*
(E) *Shigella*

7. Which of the following tests is based on the chi-square distribution?

(A) Nonparametric test
(B) McNemar test
(C) Fisher's exact test
(D) Student's t test

8. The DRG payment system is best described by which of the following payment methodologies?

(A) Per diem
(B) Capitation
(C) Per admission
(D) Fee-for-service
(E) Risk corridor

9. "Police power," a term in constitutional law, describes the inherent authority of

(A) the police to order suspects to undergo medical tests that are believed necessary to obtain evidence related to a crime
(B) the police to order licensed health care professionals to perform tests on individuals suspected of having committed crimes
(C) the state to adopt and enforce measures reasonably necessary for the protection of public health, welfare, safety, and morals
(D) a public health department to enter private homes and places of business to search for public health hazards even in the absence of a court-granted search warrant
(E) a law enforcement agency to use killing or maiming force to apprehend an escaping person who has been adjudicated a felon

10. The motor vehicle–related mortality rate is greatest among which of the following age-groups?

(A) <15 years
(B) 15–24 years
(C) 25–44 years
(D) 45–64 years
(E) >65 years

11. Which of the following statements regarding the cost and extent of mental illness is true?

(A) At least 25% of the population has some mental disorder
(B) Readmission for mental disorder is rare because patients have very long stays
(C) Mental health care costs represent about 15% of the nation's total health care costs
(D) Most of mental health costs are paid by private health insurers

12. Two medical students poll a random sample of classmates concerning their choices for residency training and find that the percentage of women who plan to train in primary care is significantly higher than the percentage of men ($p < 0.05$). The probability is less than 5% that

(A) the sampled men will enter a primary care field
(B) the difference between the men and women is real
(C) all the women in the class will enter a primary care field
(D) the difference between the sampled men and women is due to chance
(E) this sample reflects the choices of the whole class

13. Investigators are asked to study an increase in infant mortality that has occurred over the past 2 years. These changes can no longer be attributed to chance fluctuations. There are limited resources, and only the birth and death certificates are available to the investigators. The first data request they should make is for the distribution of

(A) births by birth weight for the years in question
(B) deaths by cause of death for the years in question
(C) births by birth weight for the years in question and the 2 years prior to that
(D) deaths by age at death for the years in question and the 2 years prior to that
(E) deaths by race for the years in question and the 2 years prior to that

14. Which of the following statements concerning mental hospitals is true?

(A) The number of patients in state mental hospitals has steadily increased over the years
(B) Every state has a public as well as a private mental hospital
(C) Six out of seven community hospitals have separate units for psychiatric patients
(D) For-profit psychiatric hospitals have grown 8%–10% in the past 10 years

15. Which of the following is a true statement regarding HMOs?

(A) By the mid-1990s, 75% of Americans will be receiving their health care in HMOs
(B) HMOs are not required to provide mental health care
(C) The majority of HMO mental health care visits are to psychiatrists
(D) Patients with chronic mental conditions are excluded from HMO coverage

16. Health care workers are at risk for developing which of the following diseases because of occupational exposure?

(A) Silicosis
(B) Byssinosis
(C) Bagassosis
(D) Hepatitis

17. A key characteristic distinguishing HMOs from PPAs is

(A) a utilization review program
(B) a maximum fee schedule for participating physicians
(C) a participation agreement for physicians and hospitals
(D) claims review
(E) patient choice of health providers

18. The primary difference between Niemann-Pick disease type I and type II is

(A) type I disease affects infants, whereas type II is diagnosed only in adolescents and adults
(B) whereas type I disease is associated with organomegaly, type II is characterized by a lack of organomegaly
(C) type I disease is neuronopathic but type II is not
(D) type I disease is due to an absence of sphingomyelinase and the metabolic defect for type II is unknown

19. Which of the following statements best describes allopathic physicians graduating in the United States in 1990?

(A) Upon completion of medical school, interested students completed a Fifth Pathway program permitting residency training in a foreign country
(B) Most students accumulated over $46,000 in loans and debts
(C) Graduates in 1990 were more likely to enter a primary care specialty than their osteopathic counterparts
(D) There was nearly an equal number of men and women in the graduating class of each medical school
(E) When originally applying for medical school, 1990 graduates had a 1 in 5 chance of being accepted

20. A positive dose-related response in the Ames test shows that the chemical or metabolite can cause

(A) cancer
(B) mutational events
(C) teratogenic effects
(D) behavioral effects
(E) vasodilation

21. Driving under the influence of alcohol is defined in most states in the United States as a blood alcohol concentration equal to or greater than

(A) 0.001 g/dl
(B) 0.01 g/dl
(C) 0.1 g/dl
(D) 1.0 g/dl
(E) 10.0 g/dl

22. Approximately what percentage of the adolescent population 16–17 years of age reports some alcohol use in the past month?

(A) $< 10\%$
(B) 25%
(C) 50%
(D) 75%
(E) $> 90\%$

23. Physicians may disagree about answers to ethical problems but cannot ethically avoid responsibility for issues. In which of the following public health issues is the physician, by virtue of being a physician, not qualified to present testimony?

(A) Gun control
(B) Alcohol use
(C) Distribution of condoms in secondary schools
(D) Educational policy in high schools
(E) Smoking in restaurants

24. Which of the following is characteristic of the social profile of the cocaine user?

(A) Cocaine use is more prevalent among white males with incomes over $50,000 than other income groups
(B) Individuals who use cocaine almost never use alcohol
(C) Cocaine use is highest among married rather than single men
(D) Lifetime prevalence is higher among white males than among Hispanic or black adults of either sex
(E) Marijuana use has no correlation with later use of cocaine

Questions 25–27

In preparation for a national examination, 200 medical students completed 100 questions in a practice test. Each student answered between 35 and 59 questions correctly. The arithmetic mean of the number of correct answers was 47, with a standard deviation of 4. The number of correct answers per student was distributed normally.

25. The range of questions correctly answered is

(A) 12
(B) 24
(C) 36
(D) 65
(E) 94

26. The percentage of students who correctly answered 43–51 questions is about

(A) 8%
(B) 24%
(C) 34%
(D) 68%
(E) 95%

27. The percentage of students who answered at least 55 questions correctly is about

(A) 2%
(B) 5%
(C) 8%
(D) 11%
(E) 14%

28. The most common cause of occupational injury deaths is related to

(A) manufacturing equipment
(B) agricultural equipment
(C) motor vehicles
(D) homicide
(E) falls

29. A survival curve is constructed as part of the evaluation of a new surgical procedure. The study was conducted during a 5-year period, and the 10 patients who underwent the procedure were followed for a mean of 3 years. The number of person-years of patient observation in this study is

(A) 3
(B) 5
(C) 10
(D) 30
(E) 50

30. A physician decides that all of the outside influences on medical practice from government, law suits, and so on justifies an ethic of "Me first, patients and all others second." This is an example of which ethical methodology?

(A) Act deontology
(B) Act utilitarianism
(C) Egoism
(D) Rule deontology
(E) Rule utilitarianism

31. The leading cause of death among schoolchildren is

(A) congenital anomalies
(B) injuries
(C) malignant diseases
(D) communicable diseases
(E) respiratory illnesses

32. Which of the following statements is true regarding infection with HIV-1?

(A) An infected mother has a 90% chance of transmitting the virus to her fetus
(B) The number of pediatric AIDS cases has declined over the past 2 years
(C) By the first year of life, roughly 60% of HIV-infected infants will develop AIDS
(D) In the United States, male homosexuals now constitute the fastest growing group of people with AIDS

33. Volatile organic chemicals (VOCs) tend to concentrate in

(A) surface water
(B) air
(C) sediment
(D) edible fish tissue
(E) soil

34. The figure below depicts the breakdown (by age, race, and sex) of death rates (per 100,000 population) from oral cavity and pharyngeal cancer in the United States in 1987.

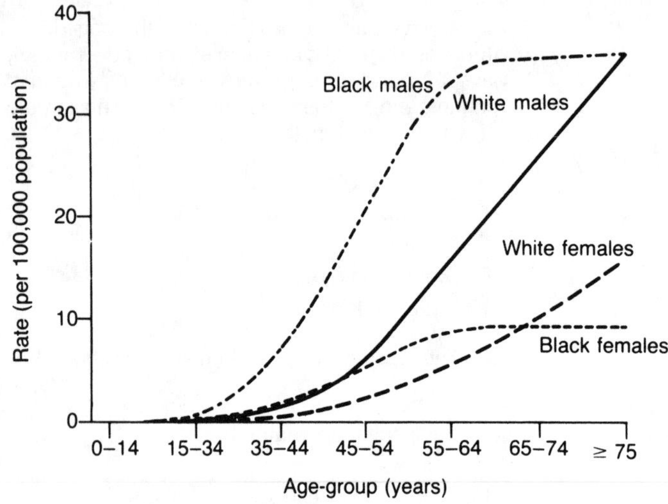

Reprinted from Centers for Disease Control: Deaths from oral cavity and pharyngeal cancer—United States, 1987. *MMWR* 39:457–460, 1990.

This figure is an example of

(A) an epidemic curve
(B) a frequency polygon
(C) a histogram
(D) a cumulative frequency graph

35. Medicaid was designed principally to serve individuals who are

(A) over 65 years of age
(B) unemployed
(C) disabled
(D) poor
(E) chronically ill

36. An Hispanic organization in a city asked a physician to support a drive for a new clinic in a location where many Hispanics live. The next week, a black group started a countermove for a clinic located in a predominantly black neighborhood. Funds for one clinic are likely to be obtained, but not for two. While the physician thinks that both groups have strong, and probably equal, claims, she chooses to build the clinic in the Hispanic community because they approached her first. The final decision was made on the basis of which form of justice?

(A) Procedural
(B) Distributive
(C) Retributory
(D) Competitive
(E) Compensatory

37. The most common STD in the United States is

(A) herpes
(B) gonorrhea
(C) syphilis
(D) genital warts
(E) chlamydial infection

38. The primary reason given for the marked increase of early syphilis is the

(A) emergence of penicillin-resistant organisms
(B) AIDS epidemic
(C) decrease in public health funds
(D) exchange of sex for drugs
(E) emergence of a virulent strain

39. Which of the following statements is true regarding drug abusers and the AIDS epidemic?

(A) The HIV-infected drug abuser population is over 50% of the total HIV-infected population
(B) Median rates for black IV drug abusers infected with AIDS exceed those of whites by 4 to 1
(C) The number of HIV-infected IV drug abusers has climbed at the same rate as the rate of HIV infection in the homosexual population
(D) The highest rate of infected drug abusers is in San Francisco
(E) IV cocaine abusers had the highest rate of HIV infection

40. The concept of managed-care systems includes which of the following?

(A) Keystone principle of primary care
(B) Financial incentives for patients to seek care outside of the plan
(C) Integration of financing and delivery of health care services
(D) Substantial patient out-of-pocket payments to help control costs

41. Health services not covered by Medicare include all of the following EXCEPT

(A) routine dental care
(B) eyeglasses
(C) outpatient prescription drugs
(D) an anesthesiologist's fees
(E) routine physical examinations

42. All of the following statements regarding occupational solvent exposure and toxicity are true EXCEPT

(A) the primary routes of exposure are by inhalation and skin absorption
(B) aliphatic hydrocarbons may cause peripheral neuropathy
(C) the primary toxicity of benzene is to the kidney
(D) CNS depression is a common effect of many solvents
(E) carbon tetrachloride typically causes liver toxicity

43. Each of the following is a true statement about the epidemiology of cancer deaths EXCEPT

(A) lung cancer is the number one cause of cancer deaths in the United States, accounting for approximately 25% of cancer mortality and 5% of all deaths
(B) lung cancer deaths among women have markedly increased but are still outnumbered by deaths from breast cancer
(C) cervical cancer deaths have increased during the past 2 decades
(D) prostate cancer kills about as many men as colon cancer does each year
(E) colorectal cancer occurs as often in men as it does in women

44. All of the following are characteristics of fatal intentional injuries EXCEPT

(A) they are caused by handguns in 60% of cases
(B) they number about 52,000 deaths per year
(C) they are associated with the acceptance of violence as an appropriate behavior
(D) they are the leading cause of death for young black males
(E) they cause fewer than 5% of fatal occupational injuries

45. All of the following are true statements regarding the cost of mental health treatment EXCEPT

(A) 40% of a general medical physician's fees come from patients' out-of-pocket payments, while only 25% of a psychiatrist's fees come from this source
(B) 70% of mental health care costs are for inpatient treatment
(C) the percentage of mental health care costs paid by private insurance is less than half the percentage of total health care costs paid by this source
(D) 25% of total mental health care costs are paid by federal funds

46. Which of the following is NOT a health care cost-containment technique included in universal health care coverage proposals?

(A) Global caps on total expenditures
(B) Cost-shifting by providers
(C) Cost-sharing by the individual patient via deductibles and coinsurance
(D) Regulation of dissemination of expensive new technologies
(E) Uniform maximum fee schedules for physicians' services

47. All of the following statements apply to both threshold and nonthreshold effects EXCEPT

(A) greater exposure increases response
(B) a chemical or metabolite causes the effect
(C) some exposure levels are safe
(D) the toxic effect is not dependent on the route of exposure

48. HIV testing of a 15-month-old infant with failure to thrive and recurrent infection should be considered in all of the following situations EXCEPT

(A) routine babysitting by a gay, HIV-positive uncle
(B) positive maternal HIV test at the birth of this infant
(C) history of maternal IV drug use
(D) routine care by a biologic father with a history of IV drug use
(E) pneumocystis pneumonia in a previously untested mother

49. All of the following are autosomal recessive disorders EXCEPT

(A) PKU
(B) Tay-Sachs disease
(C) Niemann-Pick disease type II
(D) Down syndrome
(E) homocystinuria

50. Family studies of alcoholism have shown all of the following EXCEPT

(A) there is a high prevalence of alcoholism among relatives of alcoholics
(B) children of alcoholics are vulnerable to alcoholism even if raised by nonalcoholic foster parents
(C) female relatives of alcoholics are more apt to be depressed, while male relatives are more apt to become alcoholic
(D) identical twins are more concordant for the adverse consequences of drinking than for the quantity and frequency of drinking

51. All of the following statements describe the advantages of a cohort study over a case-control study when assessing possible risk factors for disease EXCEPT

(A) a cohort study uses prospective data collection
(B) the chance for bias in data collection or subject recall is smaller for a cohort study
(C) a cohort study is more likely to explain causation
(D) true incidence rates for disease can be determined using a cohort study

52. Agents of injury include all of the following EXCEPT

(A) kinetic energy
(B) thermal energy
(C) potential energy
(D) electrical energy
(E) radiation energy

53. All of the following statements are true concerning homicide in the United States EXCEPT

(A) current homicide rates for most age-groups of both sexes are as high or higher than any previously recorded in the United States
(B) homicide is the leading cause of death for black American men between the ages of 15 and 24
(C) Hispanic men are eight to fifteen times more likely to be victims of homicide than white men
(D) use of alcohol and other drugs has been documented in about 50% of all homicides
(E) men are four times as likely to be victims of homicide than women

54. All of the following statements describing the relationship between birth weight and neonatal mortality are true EXCEPT

(A) more than one-half of very low-birth-weight infants (i.e., infants weighing $\leq$ 1500 g) die in the neonatal period
(B) low-birth-weight infants (i.e., infants weighing $\leq$ 2500 g) account for more than 65% of neonatal deaths
(C) a birth weight of 2500 g or less is believed to increase the risk of neonatal mortality, regardless of gestational age
(D) as birth weight decreases, the neonatal mortality rate (NMR) increases
(E) the major cause of neonatal mortality reflects inadequate intrauterine development

55. Blood that is used for transfusion purposes is routinely screened for serologic markers for all of the following diseases EXCEPT

(A) HBV
(B) HSV
(C) syphilis
(D) CMV
(E) AIDS

56. All of the following agents are pesticides EXCEPT

(A) insecticides
(B) herbicides
(C) vertebrate poisons
(D) cytotoxic agents
(E) fungicides

57. A physician has determined that a surgical procedure is needed to treat a condition suffered by a competent, adult patient. The physician is legally required to disclose to the patient in the course of obtaining the patient's informed consent to the procedure all of the following information EXCEPT for the

(A) nature and purpose of the proposed treatment
(B) physician's success rate in using the procedure
(C) risks and consequences of the proposed treatment
(D) reasonably feasible treatment alternatives
(E) prognosis if the proposed treatment is not implemented

58. An increase in neonatal mortality rate (NMR) in a community could be explained by any of the following factors EXCEPT

(A) an increase in the rate of lethal malformations due to a local environmental toxin
(B) an improvement in the reporting of births and deaths among infants weighing less than 500 g
(C) an increase in the rate of SIDS deaths among low-birth-weight infants
(D) a major loss in personnel in the neonatology section of the local medical center
(E) an increase in the rate of crack cocaine use in local neighborhoods

59. All of the following statements describe continuous quality improvement EXCEPT that it

(A) assumes individuals seek to do their best
(B) will soon be implemented by JCAHO
(C) must involve all members of an organization
(D) was developed by a Japanese systems engineer
(E) is also called total quality management

60. Risk factors for lung cancer include all of the following EXCEPT

(A) smoking
(B) occupational exposure
(C) air pollution
(D) radiation
(E) family history

61. All of the following are passive strategies for injury prevention and control EXCEPT

(A) vehicle anti-lock brakes
(B) carpeting
(C) a home hot water setting at 120° F
(D) seat belts
(E) air bags

62. True statements regarding allopathic medical education include all of the following EXCEPT

(A) in the last 50 years, the ratio of applicants to positions has never fallen below 1.6:1
(B) enrollment has declined in the past 5 years
(C) the number of Americans studying in foreign medical schools is increasing
(D) increased enrollment is predicted for the next decade
(E) over 29,000 students applied for first-year positions in 1990

63. All of the following physical properties are important in determining the movement of chemicals between environmental mediums EXCEPT

(A) octanol water partition coefficient
(B) water solubility
(C) viscosity
(D) bioconcentration factor
(E) vapor pressure

64. Which of the following would NOT be a factor used in developing a fee based on Medicare's RBRVS?

(A) Physician's time, mental effort, judgment, and technical skill
(B) Malpractice costs
(C) Office overhead costs
(D) Ratio of the median charge for the particular procedure to the average for all procedures in the base time period
(E) Physician's postgraduate specialty training costs

65. According to the AMA's Principles of Medical Ethics, the physician must do all of the following EXCEPT

(A) strive to expose physicians who are deficient in character or competence
(B) seek changes in requirements that are contrary to the best interests of the patient
(C) safeguard confidences within the law
(D) be free, even in emergencies, to choose when to serve
(E) continue to study, apply, and advance medical knowledge

66. The plaintiff is required to prove all of the following elements to recover damages for a defendant's alleged negligence EXCEPT

(A) duty
(B) dereliction
(C) damage
(D) proximate cause
(E) deliberate wrongdoing

67. Projections of a potential physician shortage depend on all of the following assumptions EXCEPT

(A) increased demand as baby boomers reach middle age
(B) increased demand as medical technology becomes more complex
(C) early physician retirement as Medicare reimbursement for primary care services decreases
(D) increased demand for services caused by the escalating number of AIDS cases
(E) a decreased number of medical students

68. All of the following fit the profile of a typical heroin user EXCEPT

(A) someone who lives in a big city
(B) a member of a minority group
(C) someone 18–25 years of age
(D) a male

69. Contraindications for administering a live attenuated viral vaccine include all of the following EXCEPT

(A) current febrile illness
(B) recent administration of IG
(C) immunosuppressive disorder
(D) administration of another live vaccine
(E) pregnancy

70. Residents of a rural county are tested with a screening test for a fungal disease. The probability that an individual with a positive test will have the disease depends on all of the following EXCEPT the

(A) sensitivity of the test
(B) specificity of the test
(C) false-positive rate
(D) size of the county population
(E) disease prevalence in the county

71. All of the following substances are associated with both abuse and dependence EXCEPT

(A) cocaine
(B) cannabis
(C) alcohol
(D) PCP
(E) opioids

72. All of the following diseases have a high incidence among Ashkenazi Jews EXCEPT

(A) spina bifida
(B) Tay-Sachs disease
(C) Niemann-Pick disease type I
(D) Gaucher's disease

73. All of the following organs and organ systems are significant targets of lead toxicity EXCEPT

(A) CNS
(B) liver
(C) hematopoietic system
(D) PNS
(E) kidneys

74. Documented spread of HBV has occurred in all of the following situations EXCEPT

(A) from mother to child in the prenatal period
(B) in household contacts
(C) among sexual contacts
(D) from eating food
(E) in sharing needles by IV drug abusers

75. Foundry workers may suffer all of the following diseases as a result of occupational exposure EXCEPT

(A) silicosis
(B) asbestosis
(C) stomach cancer
(D) lung cancer
(E) hearing loss

76. Factors in the system for rating severity of substance dependence in the *DSM-III-R* include all of the following EXCEPT

(A) frequency of preoccupation with seeking or taking the substance
(B) use of the substance to avoid withdrawal symptoms
(C) use of the substance in smaller doses because of lack of tolerance
(D) continuation of substance use despite a legal problem associated with the substance
(E) effort to cut down or control substance use

77. The validity of results from clinical trials can be compromised by all of the following factors EXCEPT

(A) the observer unmasked to treatment
(B) the patient unmasked to treatment
(C) a nonrandom allocation of treatments
(D) a small number of subjects
(E) the accrual of a larger study population than expected

78. All of the following are recognized foundations of morality EXCEPT

(A) social contract
(B) divine command
(C) natural law
(D) criminal law
(E) individual insight

Directions: Each group of items in this section consists of lettered options followed by a set of numbered items. For each item, select the **one** lettered option that is most closely associated with it. Each lettered option may be selected once, more than once, or not at all.

Questions 79–84

For each activity listed below, select the type or types of prevention described.

(A) Primary prevention
(B) Secondary prevention
(C) Tertiary prevention
(D) Primary and secondary prevention
(E) Primary, secondary, and tertiary prevention

79. Managing a patient with heart disease

80. Cleaning up the environment

81. Treating a case of gonorrhea

82. Health education

83. Screening programs

84. Physical therapy

Questions 85–88

Match the following definitions with the appropriate terms.

(A) PPOs
(B) IPAs
(C) Group-model HMOs
(D) Staff-model HMOs
(E) EPOs

85. A medical care plan where the physicians are employed directly by the plan

86. A medical care plan that provides financial incentives for the patient to see selected doctors but also pays for care outside of the plan, though at greater cost to the patient

87. A medical care plan in which individual physicians contract to see prepaid patients at an agreed rate or capitation but generally are occupied seeing fee-for-service patients

88. A medical care plan that contracts with a physicians' group to provide care to the prepaid patients

Questions 89–92

For each definition of fetal death, select the term that best matches it.

(A) Stillbirth
(B) Perinatal death
(C) Spontaneous abortion
(D) Neonatal death
(E) Infant mortality

89. Death of a fetus weighing less than 500 g

90. Death of a fetus before 20 weeks' gestation

91. Death of a fetus weighing less than 500 g at 21 weeks' gestation

92. Death of a fetus weighing 500 g at 28 weeks' gestation

Questions 93–95

For each definition of fetal or infant mortality, select the term that best matches it.

(A) Infant mortality
(B) Perinatal mortality
(C) Neonatal mortality
(D) Spontaneous abortion

93. Fetal or infant death between 28 weeks' gestation and 1 week postnatal, with weight > 500 g

94. Death of a liveborn infant within 28 days' postnatal

95. Death of a liveborn infant before 1 year of age

Questions 96–100

For each disease listed below, select the statement that best describes current screening strategy.

(A) Screening programs are considered cost-effective for targeted populations
(B) Screening programs are not considered cost-effective in any population
(C) Screening programs currently do not exist
(D) Screening programs for targeted populations exist, but the cost-effectiveness of the programs is controversial

96. Childhood anemia
97. Cervical cancer
98. Lung cancer
99. Peptic ulcer disease
100. Colorectal cancer

Questions 101–105

An intern sees five new patients during an afternoon clinic session. The intern counsels each patient or the patient's parent on recommended injury prevention measures. Match each patient with the most appropriate topic for age-specific injury prevention counseling.

(A) Bicycle safety helmet and the storage of matches
(B) Falls and smoking near bedding
(C) Occupational injuries and back conditioning exercises
(D) Stairway gates and window guards
(E) Violent behavior and driving while using alcohol and other drugs

101. 4-month-old infant
102. 9-year-old female grade school student
103. 17-year-old male high school student
104. 45-year-old female laborer
105. 70-year-old male retiree

Questions 106–110

Match each statement below with the health care professionals it best describes.

(A) All practicing physicians
(B) Registered nurses
(C) Diploma program registered nurses
(D) Public health nurses
(E) Osteopathic physicians

106. Although these professionals are only a small percentage of all medical personnel, they are strongly oriented to primary care

107. Although predicted by some to be in surplus by 1990, surpluses of these professionals are not evident; in fact, shortages have been predicted

108. Relatively few in number, these professionals have traditionally focused on preventive health care and health education

109. Among the most numerous of all health professionals, shortages of these professionals are still common

110. Educational programs for these professionals emphasize practical hospital-based experience, but such programs are rapidly disappearing

Questions 111–115

Match each of the following toxic effects with the metal that typically is the causative agent.

(A) Elemental mercury
(B) Nickel
(C) Zinc
(D) Arsenic
(E) Beryllium

111. Asthma
112. Metal fume fever
113. Stomatitis, gingivitis, tremor
114. Granulomatous disease
115. Peripheral neuropathy

Questions 116–120

For each of the legal principles listed below, select the case that is accredited with establishing that principle.

(A) *Helling v. Carey*
(B) *Hawkins v. McGee*
(C) *Canterbury v. Spence*
(D) *Tarasoff v. Regents of University of California*
(E) *In re Conroy*

116. When a physician makes an express promise of cure, he can be held liable on contract grounds (breach of warranty) for failure to deliver the promised result

117. A court may insist upon a higher standard of care than is currently observed in practice in the medical community

118. With proper safeguards to help assure that it would be the patient's own choice, a health care provider may legitimately discontinue the provision of nutrition and water through a nasogastric tube to a seriously ill and failing patient, even though death is certain to result

119. In obtaining a patient's consent to treatment, a physician must disclose all that a reasonably prudent patient would consider *material* to the decision of whether or not to accept treatment

120. A psychotherapist whose patient states that she intends to harm a specific third party has the duty to warn that party of the danger

Questions 121–125

For each description below, select the legislation that matches it.

(A) Health Care Quality Improvement Act of 1986
(B) Tax Equity and Fiscal Responsibility Act of 1982
(C) Consolidated Omnibus Budget Reconciliation Act of 1986
(D) Public Law 93-222
(E) National Health Planning and Development Act of 1974

121. Authorized pilot projects to review office services to Medicare patients

122. Established the 203 health service areas

123. Legislated the National Practitioner Data Bank

124. Established a network of PROs to monitor quality under prospective reimbursement

125. Was passed 10 years after the Bennett Amendment to replace PSROs

Questions 126–130

Match each phrase with the appropriate level of prevention.

(A) Primary prevention
(B) Secondary prevention
(C) Tertiary prevention

126. Early diagnosis to limit disability

127. Crisis preparation

128. Rehabilitation after disability

129. Elimination of specific diseases

130. Crisis intervention

Questions 131–134

The current severe shortage of nurses is attributed to both increased demand and decreased supply. Match each of the following factors with its impact on supply or demand.

(A) Decreases supply
(B) Increases supply
(C) Decreases demand
(D) Increases demand

131. Shift in demographics to older women

132. Increasing complexity of medical care

133. Creation of in-house nursing agencies

134. The aging of the population

Questions 135–139

The table below is a fourfold, or 2 x 2, table in which screening test results for disease Y are tabulated in relation to the true disease status of the population being tested.

	Disease Y		
Screening Test	**Yes**	**No**	**Total**
Positive	200	100	300
Negative	50	600	650
Total	250	700	950

Match each screening test parameter listed below to the appropriate numerical value.

(A) 250/950, or 26%
(B) 200/300, or 67%
(C) 200/250, or 80%
(D) 600/700, or 86%
(E) 600/650, or 92%

135. Sensitivity

136. Specificity

137. Positive predictive value

138. Negative predictive value

139. Disease prevalence

Questions 140–143

For each situation listed below, select the study design that would be most useful to solve the problem.

(A) Descriptive studies
(B) Analytical studies
(C) Both
(D) Neither

140. A drug company wants to evaluate a new vaccine before it can be marketed

141. Public health officials want to control a measles outbreak in a local school

142. Investigation of a newly identified disease, such as legionnaires' disease or AIDS, has just been initiated

143. A clinician wishes to determine the cause of an unusual cancer

Questions 144–147

Four medical students are involved in an automobile crash on a rainy Saturday night after a party that followed a national medical examination. The compact car went off the road at 70 mph and hit a tree. Two of the students died, and two were hospitalized. The driver had a blood alcohol concentration of 0.14 g/dl. None of the students was wearing seat belts. For each risk factor present in the case history, select the risk factor category that is most appropriate.

(A) Agent factor
(B) Host factor
(C) Vector factor
(D) Social environment factor
(E) Physical environment factor

144. Elevated blood alcohol concentration

145. Rainy night

146. Compact car

147. Speed of 70 mph

Questions 148–154

Match the contraceptive method listed with its typical failure rate during the first year of use.

(A) 85%
(B) 20%
(C) 18%
(D) 12%
(E) 3%
(F) 0.4%
(G) 0.15%

148. Female sterilization

149. Diaphragm with spermicide

150. Pill

151. Chance

152. Condom without spermicide

153. Male sterilization

154. Natural family planning

Questions 155–158

For each of the following illnesses resulting from a biologic hazard, choose the occupation most likely to be associated with it.

(A) Wool handlers
(B) Horticulturalists
(C) Bird fanciers
(D) Dishwashers

155. Sporotrichosis

156. Candidiasis

157. Anthrax

158. Psittacosis

Questions 159–163

Match the following statements with the appropriate STD.

(A) Gonorrhea
(B) CMV
(C) Syphilis
(D) HSV
(E) PID

159. Ranks as the number one reportable communicable disease in the United States

160. Causes sterility in approximately 150,000 women each year

161. Has been associated with carcinoma of the cervix, vulva, and penis

162. Increases the risk of ectopic pregnancy 10-fold

163. A chronic infection, which can cause blindness, psychosis, or cardiovascular disease

Questions 164–167

For each statement listed below, select the term that it best describes.

(A) Therapeutic privilege
(B) Emergency consent
(C) Abandonment
(D) Good samaritan
(E) Battery

164. To avoid liability, a physician should document carefully when a treatment relationship with a patient has terminated

165. When a health care provider undertakes, without a person's permission, to render care to that person, tort liability is possible even if no harm was intended and the patient suffered no physical injury as a result of the physician's treatment

166. Rendering care to a patient without the patient's expressed consent may not be considered a tort under certain circumstances

167. By statute, physicians who go beyond the call of their duty and act in good faith in an emergency situation will not be liable for harm caused thereby

Questions 168–171

Match each of the descriptions listed below with the type of payment to which it most likely refers.

(A) Per diem
(B) Fee-for-service
(C) Capitation
(D) Per admission
(E) DRG

168. Itemized invoice

169. A treatment classification system based on diagnostic category

170. An all-inclusive flat rate for each day of hospital care provided

171. An amount per insured per month regardless of the quantity of services rendered

Questions 172–178

For each vaccine characteristic, select the appropriate vaccine.

(A) DTP vaccine
(B) HBV vaccine
(C) OPV
(D) Pneumococcal vaccine
(E) Rubella vaccine
(F) Hib conjugate vaccine
(G) Measles vaccine
(H) Influenza vaccine

172. Developed to prevent congenital defects

173. Strain now causes more disease than the wild strain

174. Has caused persistent, inconsolable, high-pitch crying lasting 3 hours or more within 48 hours of inoculation

175. Developed to prevent one of the most common causes of preventable mental retardation

176. Protects against 23 strains of a particular organism

177. Must be updated each year by vaccine developer

178. Has not been used to protect the individuals at greatest risk of getting the disease

Questions 179–182

In tort litigation, a number of different standards are used to determine various issues involving the provision of health services. For each of the issues listed below, select the standard that is most likely to be associated with it.

(A) Objective standard of causation
(B) Subjective standard of causation
(C) Court-imposed standard of care
(D) Physician-based standard of informed consent
(E) Patient-based standard of informed consent

179. The law can require a higher standard of medical practice than is currently observed in the medical profession under certain circumstances

180. Physicians commonly tell their patients certain facts before undertaking a given medical, surgical, or diagnostic procedure

181. A patient may be entitled to damages if a physician fails to disclose information about treatment that would have caused that particular patient to refuse the treatment

182. Individuals may consider certain things material to their decision to accept a proposed treatment

Questions 183–186

Match each clinical manifestation with the most likely underlying cause of mental retardation.

(A) Syphilis
(B) Rubella
(C) Maternal iodine deficiency
(D) Fetal alcohol syndrome

183. Cretinism

184. Microcephaly, cleft palate, and cardiac atrial or ventricular defects

185. Deafness

186. Interstitial keratitis

Questions 187–190

Match the following control strategies with the appropriate communicable disease.

(A) *Shigella*
(B) Tuberculosis
(C) Rabies
(D) Measles

187. Administer a chemoprophylactic agent to kill the biologic agent inside the patient so that it cannot infect others

188. Eliminate the reservoir so that the agent has no place to live, multiply, or die in its natural state

189. Avoid contact with a potentially dangerous reservoir

190. Prevent spread of disease by good hand-washing techniques and good personal hygiene

ANSWERS AND EXPLANATIONS

1–2. The answers are: 1-A *[Ch 2 II A–B]*, **2-D** *[Ch 2 II F]*.
Dr. Neugierig first wrote a case report about his unusual observation in a hepatitis C patient. Next, he collected information from several similar patients—a case series—and reported these findings. Neither of the case reports would establish a causal relationship. While, theoretically, sunlight might aid bilirubin metabolism in the skin, it could also be true that only patients with milder disease felt well enough to walk to the solarium, thus introducing selection bias.

To determine the role of sunlight in hepatitis C treatment, Dr. Neugierig developed a nonblinded, but randomized, clinical trial. The study could not be single-blinded or double-blinded, since the physician could simply ask patients whether they had sunned that day, and, of course, the patients would know whether they had gone to the solarium. As an unblinded study, both patients and physician could easily be biased.

3. The answer is B *[Ch 3 III B 2 b, 4 a]*.
When performing multiple comparisons and repeated testing for statistical significance, there is an increased likelihood of a type I, or α, error [i.e., of rejecting a null hypothesis (H_0) that is actually true]. One method to compensate for this is to use a lower value for the type I error to determine statistical significance. The likelihood that the sample size is too small (or too large) or that the null hypothesis is true is unaffected by repeated testing. Statistical tests can evaluate a null hypothesis but do not determine causality or show clinical importance.

4. The answer is E *[Ch 11 II A 1–5]*.
Alcoholics are associated with 15,000 homicides annually. Although 100 million people in the United States drink alcohol, only 9 million Americans suffer from alcoholism. Population surveys indicate that 1%–6% of adult men and women are alcoholics. Native Americans have a particularly high rate of alcoholism. Alcoholics are most likely to be 45–49 years of age and belong to low socioeconomic groups.

5–6. The answers are: 5-C *[Ch 1 III D 2 b; V B 2 c; VII E 1–2]*, **6-B** *[Ch 1 VII C 1 e]*.
The incriminating food is most likely the meatballs. In conducting an investigation of a foodborne outbreak, the investigator must be able to demonstrate that the ill group was more often exposed to the incriminated food item than the well group. The specific attack rate must be significantly higher in the group that ate the food as compared to the group that did not eat the food. If there is no significant difference in attack rates, the food item is not responsible for the outbreak. The data given in the question show that the Swedish meatballs were responsible. Note that two ill persons did not eat Swedish meatballs. These cases could have occurred by cross-contamination of serving spoons or as a result of an unrelated diarrhea-causing agent.

The most likely etiologic agent is *Staphylococcus*. The incubation period for staphylococcal food poisoning is short because this poisoning is caused by a heat-stable enterotoxin that is produced in the food. The other bacterial causes of food poisoning require some multiplication in the gastrointestinal tract to produce symptoms; they, therefore, have a longer incubation period.

7. The answer is B *[Ch 3 III F, H 3, I, K]*.
The McNemar test is based on the chi-square distribution, as are the goodness-of-fit test and the $r \times c$ chi-square test. Student's t test is based on the t distribution. Fisher's exact test and other nonparametric tests are distribution-free.

8. The answer is C *[Ch 18 IV A 1–4]*.
Four payment methodologies are used by third-party payers to reimburse providers. Per diem is an all-inclusive flat rate for each day of hospital care provided. It usually includes all ancillary services, supplies, and other services billed by the hospital. Capitation is a fee that the provider agrees to accept per patient per month for each patient enrolled in the practice in exchange for providing all specified health services to enrollees. Risk corridor refers to a capitation adjustment whereby additional payments to or refunds from the provider would occur if the variance from the budget exceeded a certain threshold percentage. Per admission is an all inclusive flat rate for each hospital admission. The diagnosis-related group (DRG) payment system is based on a fixed hospital per admission payment rate for each of 470 treatment classifications. Fee-for-service charges are billed on an itemized invoice.

9. The answer is C *[Ch 14 VIII A 1 a, b]*.
Under the U.S. legal system, the state and federal governments, so long as they act within the bounds of their respective constitutions, have an inherent power to take reasonable steps necessary to maintain or-

der and protect the public. This power can be exercised when the state has a legitimate interest in an activity and takes action reasonably related to the protection of that interest. Police power must be balanced against the fundamental rights of the individual.

10. The answer is B *[Ch 1 V B 3 d; Ch 8 IV B 1 a, b].*
The motor vehicle–related mortality rate is greatest in individuals between 15 and 24 years of age. Approximately 49,000 people die annually as a result of motor vehicle–related injuries. The case-fatality rate (i.e., the number of deaths assigned to a specific cause divided by the total number of cases) as a result of motor vehicle–related injuries is greatest among the elderly.

11. The answer is C *[Ch 9 III A–C].*
Mental health care costs have risen from 6% of the nation's health care spending in 1955 to 15% in 1982. At least 10% of the population of the United States (about 25 million Americans) have some form of mental disorder that could benefit from professional help. Readmissions to mental hospitals are common; of the 972,000 patients admitted to mental hospitals and psychiatric services of general hospitals annually, more than a third are readmissions. Twenty-five percent of the nation's total mental health costs are paid by federal funds, 28% by state and local governments, and 12% by private health insurers.

12. The answer is D *[Ch 3 III B 2].*
The probability is less than 5% that the difference between the sampled men and women is due to chance. The study described used a null hypothesis (H_0) that there would be no difference in training choices between men and women. This null hypothesis is rejected because the likelihood that the difference found was due to chance is less than 5%. Statistical testing using probability values evaluates only the null hypothesis and not any alternate hypotheses. This is a random sample of the whole class and should be representative, as long as the number in the sample is of sufficient size.

13. The answer is D *[Ch 7 I A–E].*
The first data request that should be made is for the distribution of deaths by age at death for the years in question and the 2 years prior to that. The distinction between neonatal and postnatal deaths is especially important. Births by birth weight and deaths by cause of death for the years in question provide no comparison by which to judge the distributions. Birth weights and racial distributions may provide important information for the next rounds of investigation.

14. The answer is D *[Ch 9 IV A–D].*
In the mid-1980s, there was an 8%–10% growth in the number of for-profit psychiatric hospitals, especially those for the treatment of adolescents and substance abuse. The number of patients in state-supported mental hospitals increased steadily until 1955, after which the population has dropped continually. Although there are about 450 private psychiatric hospitals in the United States, 16 states have no private facilities. Approximately 1500 community hospitals, or one of every four, have separate units for treating psychiatric patients.

15. The answer is A *[Ch 9 V B 1–2].*
By the mid-1990s, 75% of all Americans will receive their health care from various types of managed care systems. Laws requiring health maintenance organizations (HMOs) to provide a certain level of mental health coverage have been enacted in 24 states. HMOs in states with mandated coverage cannot exclude patients with chronic mental conditions. Only 30% of HMO mental health visits are to psychiatrists; the majority are to master's level psychologists.

16. The answer is D *[Ch 12 III F 4].*
There are more than 3 million health care workers in the United States, some of whom are at risk for developing diseases, such as hepatitis B (HBV) and non-A, non-B hepatitis, tuberculosis, herpes simplex virus (HSV), and acquired immune deficiency syndrome (AIDS). HBV or non-A, non-B hepatitis can develop following needle sticks or other contact with the bodily fluids of infected patients. Byssinosis is a disease of textile workers. Silicosis is a pneumoconiosis found in foundry workers. Bagassosis is a hypersensitivity pneumonitis of sugar cane workers that results from the inhalation of the dust of bagasse, the waste of sugar cane.

17. The answer is E *[Ch 18 V B, C; Table 18-4].*
Health maintenance organizations (HMOs) are medical care organizations that accept responsibility for the provision and delivery of a predetermined set of comprehensive health services to insureds who voluntarily choose an HMO for health insurance coverage. HMOs generally restrict coverage to services

provided by physicians participating in the plan. Preferred provider arrangements (PPAs) are arrangements between a network of health providers—that is, physicians, hospitals, and other health suppliers—and a health benefit purchaser—that is, insurance companies or self-insured employers. In a PPA, the patient may choose a provider outside of the "preferred" network but usually pays a higher deductible or copayment. Both HMOs and PPAs often utilize claims review, a maximum fee schedule for participating physicians, and a participation agreement between physicians and hospitals.

18. The answer is D *[Ch 10 IV B 2 a, b].*
The Niemann-Pick group of diseases is a rare group of disorders that can be divided into two broad types on the basis of etiology. Type I includes patients who are clearly sphingomyelinase-deficient, while the underlying defect for type II disease is uncertain, although it may involve sphingomyelinase and cholesterol to varying degrees. Both type I and type II disease have three subtypes, depending on whether the disease is acute, subacute, or chronic (which usually presents in adulthood). Both type I and II appear to be autosomal recessive in their transmission, although the genetics of the type I chronic form is uncertain. Both type I and type II disease are associated with organomegaly, but the severity depends on the specific subtype of the disease. Both types are neuronopathic, although the severity of central nervous system (CNS) involvement varies according to the disease subtype.

19. The answer is B *[Ch 16 II A 1 a, b, c (4), 2 a (3), B 2, C 2].*
The rapidly rising cost of medical education as well as the perceived complexity of medical practice may contribute to the decline in medical school applicants and medical students. Projections of a sizeable surplus of physicians in 1990 led to shrinking medical school classes. Student loans are an average of $46,000 at graduation with some debt exceeding $50,000. Osteopathic physicians predominately enter primary care, while 39% of allopathic physicians currently enter pediatrics, internal medicine, or family medicine. Twice as many applicants apply for available medical school positions as there are first-year openings. Women make up approximately 37% of all medical students, and they are not evenly distributed from school to school. For example, although 39% of first-year students in 1990–1991 were women, women were a majority of the first-year enrollees in some medical schools. Fifth Pathway programs provide lectures and clinical rotations for Americans who have graduated from foreign medical schools and who wish to enter U.S. residency programs.

20. The answer is B *[Ch 13 II B 3 a (1)].*
The Ames test is a short-term genotoxic test that determines the ability of a chemical to cause point mutations. Thus, a chemical that is positive in the Ames test is a mutagen. Although cancer requires interaction with genetic material and the correlation between carcinogens and the Ames test is more than 90%, a positive Ames test is not considered sufficient to classify a chemical as a carcinogen. Teratogenic, behavioral, and vascular system effects are not measured by the Ames test either, although a chemical that is a mutagen could possibly also cause any of these other systemic effects.

21. The answer is C *[Ch 8 II A 3 d].*
In most states in the United States, a blood alcohol concentration of 0.1 g/dl is evidence of impaired driving due to alcohol. This blood alcohol concentration also is described as 0.10% (weight per volume). In several states, the legal limit has been lowered to 0.08 g/dl.

22. The answer is C *[Ch 7 III C 2 a].*
Alcohol use is decreasing among adolescents; however, close to 50% of high school students 16–17 years of age report some alcohol use within the last month. Alcohol use is a behavior that can endanger adolescent health and is often responsible for adolescent mortality. Smoking, drug use, sexual activity, and eating patterns are behaviors also associated with adolescent health problems.

23. The answer is D *[Ch 15 I C 3 a; VI D 3].*
While individual physicians may have special qualifications in education, this is not normally a part of their professional training. Issues of gun control, alcohol use, distribution of condoms in secondary schools, and smoking in restaurants directly concern matters involving public health, although a physician's support for any particular action would vary according to the personal values of the physician.

24. The answer is D *[Ch 11 II B 1 d (1)–(6)].*
The lifetime prevalence of cocaine use is higher among white males than among Hispanic or black adults of either sex. The prevalence of use in the population earning over $50,000 is low compared to other groups. Use of cocaine is highly correlated with use of both alcohol and marijuana. Cocaine use is highest among people who live together but are not married.

25–27. The answers are: 25-B *[Ch 3 II A 1, B 1]*, **26-D** *[Ch 3 III E 3 b–c; Table 3-5; Figure 3-10]*, **27-A** *[Ch 3 III E 3 b–c; Table 3-5; Figure 3-10]*.
The range of questions correctly answered is 24. The range is the spread between the highest and lowest values in a series. It is calculated by subtracting the lowest value, which in this example is 35, from the highest value, 59.

The percentage of students who correctly answered 43–51 questions is about 68%. A normal distribution curve can be characterized by the arithmetic mean and the standard deviation. In a normal distribution, about 68% of the population lies within 1 standard deviation of the mean, and 95% lies within 2 standard deviations of the mean. Conversely, 5% of the population lies outside 2 standard deviations of the mean. In this example, the mean (47) minus 1 standard deviation (4) equals 43 and the mean (47) plus 1 standard deviation (4) equals 51. Therefore, the percentage of students who correctly answered 43 to 51 questions is 68%.

The percentage of students who answered at least 55 questions correctly is about 2%. In a normal distribution, about 95% of the population lies inside and about 5% lies outside 2 standard deviations of the mean. About half of those lying outside 2 standard deviations are greater than the mean plus 2 standard deviations, and an equal number are less than the mean minus 2 standard deviations. In this example, 55 correct answers represents the mean (47) plus 2 standard deviations (each standard deviation is 4). Therefore, about 2% of the students answered at least 55 questions correctly.

28. The answer is C *[Ch 8 IV B 2 b]*.
The most common cause of fatal occupational injuries is related to motor vehicles, which account for about one-third of all occupational injury deaths. Homicide and falls, the next two most common causes of occupational injury deaths, each account for over 10%.

29. The answer is D *[Ch 3 III M 3 c]*.
The number of person-years of patient observation in this study is 30. In a clinical or demographic life table, the experience of each patient is weighted by the time the patient is under observation or followed. Although this study lasted 5 years, each patient was observed an average of 3 years, multiplied by 10 patients, for a total of 30 person-years of patient observation.

30. The answer is C *[Ch 15 II B 1 a, b]*.
When the physician decides that all actions must be judged on the basis of her needs and interests, she exemplifies the egoist theory. More than self-interest, this theory recognizes the rights of others *only* when they are beneficial to the actor. Act deontology holds that no rules can apply to specific judgments, since each situation is unique. Rule deontology holds that a rule or rules may be applied to decide ethical problems. Act utilitarianism sanctions moral conduct that results in the greatest balance of good over evil, and rule utilitarianism attempts to devise and apply rules that will result in such a balance.

31. The answer is B *[Ch 7 II A 2 b]*.
Injuries are the major cause of death among schoolchildren, accounting for 50% of all deaths. Other causes of death in this age-group include congenital anomalies, malignant diseases, infectious conditions (e.g., influenza, pneumonia), and gastroenteritis. Two approaches to prevention of injury-related childhood mortality have been identified: modification of hazards to reduce their potential to cause injury (e.g., use of products with child-proof caps) and modification of behavior to reduce exposure to hazards (e.g., use of infant car seats).

32. The answer is C *[Ch 10 V A 3 a (1)–(5)]*.
Current data indicate that, during the first year of life, the human immunodeficiency virus (HIV) infection will have progressed to acquired immune deficiency syndrome (AIDS) in about 60% of HIV-infected infants. If an HIV-infected woman becomes pregnant, there is a 30%–50% chance that the infant will become infected in utero or during delivery. Currently, there is no curative treatment for HIV, as there is for syphilis. The annual incidence of AIDS in women and children has been increasing, and these two groups now represent the fastest growing infected populations. Clinical features of HIV-infected infants include microcephaly, cerebral atrophy, and a general failure to meet developmental milestones.

33. The answer is B *[Ch 13 IV A 1 b (6)–(7), c; Table 13-13]*.
Volatile organic chemicals (VOCs) such as benzene, trichloroethylene (TCE), and vinyl chloride have high vapor pressures compared to other organic chemicals or metals and have low octanol water partition coefficients (K_{ow}) and bioconcentration factors (BCFs) compared to other organic chemicals. Thus, VOCs will concentrate in air but not in water or soil because they have high vapor pressures. Also, VOCs cannot

be transferred from water to sediment or fish tissue because of their low K_{ow} and BCF values. VOCs are found in both groundwater and soil at sites where there has been a spill. The upper layers of soil often have a lower VOC concentration than lower layers due to volatilization to air and migration down into lower soil layers.

34. The answer is B *[Ch 3 II C 1–7; Figure 3-6].*
This figure is an example of a frequency polygon. A frequency polygon is a representation of the distribution of categories of continuous and ordered data with the frequency plotted against the midpoint of each category and a line drawn through each plotted point. A histogram does not use a continuous line. An epidemic curve is a histogram that depicts the time course of an illness, disease, or abnormality in a defined population within a specified location and time period.

35. The answer is D *[Ch 18 VI B].*
Medicaid, or Medical Assistance, was established in 1965 under Title XIX of the Social Security Act. The federal government contributes 50%–83% of Medicaid costs, and each state contributes the balance for its residents. The federal share varies by state, depending on benefits covered, state income level, and other factors. Eligibility for Medicaid benefits is based on income, which must be below a certain level set by each state. Medicaid claims generally come under each state's public welfare or health department.

36. The answer is A *[Ch 15 V E 1–4].*
The decision to support a drive for a new clinic in an Hispanic neighborhood and not a black neighborhood was made on the basis of procedural justice—a means of just distribution based on the establishment of rules. The distribution of services on the basis of "first come, first served" is an example of a procedural rule. Distributive justice assesses the validity of varying claims to limited resources. Thus, one group or issue may be seen as having a more legitimate claim to the resources available. Compensatory justice compensates victims of crime or injustice (e.g., providing increased job opportunities via affirmative action, providing monetary compensation for victims of crime), while retributory justice punishes the perpetrators of a crime or injustice. "Competitive justice" is not a recogized term in the study of ethics.

37. The answer is E *[Ch 4 V A 3 a (1), E 1 a].*
Although gonorrhea is the most commonly reported disease, *Chlamydia* is believed to be the most common sexually transmitted disease (STD) in the United States, with approximately 4 million cases occurring each year. Chlamydial infection has not been a reportable disease because there is no easy way to confirm the diagnosis. However, it causes a significant proportion of the cases of nongonococcal urethritis and acute epididymitis in men and mucopurulent cervicitis and pelvic inflammatory disease (PID) in women.

38. The answer is D *[Ch 4 V B 1 d].*
Case-control studies done in different parts of the United States have shown that the exchange of sex for drugs, primarily cocaine, is a major cause of the current syphilis epidemic. Although simultaneous *Treponema pallidum* and human immunodeficiency virus (HIV) infection may alter the clinical presentation, serologic response, or response to therapy, it alone cannot explain the marked increase in early syphilis.

39. The answer is B *[Ch 11 II B 3 d (1)–(7)].*
Median rates for black intravenous (IV) drug abusers infected with acquired immune deficiency syndrome (AIDS) exceed those of whites by 4 to 1. The population of drug abusers infected with the human immunodeficiency virus (HIV) makes up only 25% of the total HIV-infected population. This rate is growing, while the rate of infection among the homosexual population is declining, perhaps because the homosexual population has heeded measures to curb HIV infection while the drug abuser population has not. San Francisco and other western U.S. cities have a low rate of HIV infection among IV drug abusers. Heroin users have the highest rate of HIV infection among infected drug abusers.

40. The answer is C *[Ch 17 II D].*
The concept of managed-care services includes integration of financing and delivery of health care services. Characteristic of managed care is the role of the financially at-risk organization [e.g., health maintenance organization (HMO) or insurance company] coordinating and monitoring the direct provision of medical care to control cost. Thus, the gatekeeper model of primary care is most common. Financial incentives exist to encourage patients to receive care within the plan, presumably at a lower cost to the insurance company or HMO. Because managed-care systems do not include a high out-of-pocket cost for the patient, patients are more willing to seek early medical care, which is a distinct advantage of this type of system.

41. The answer is D *[Ch 18 VI A 2 a, b; Table 18-3].*
Medicare pays less than one-half of the average beneficiary's total health care costs. Many Medicare recipients purchase private supplemental insurance to fill the gaps in Medicare coverage. Medicare does not pay for routine dental care, outpatient prescription drugs, hearing aids, eyeglasses, and routine physical examinations, but does pay for inpatient surgical and professional fees , such as an anesthesiologist's fee, under Part B.

42. The answer is C *[Ch 12 IV B 1–11; Table 12-4].*
Solvent use is ubiquitous in industry. Because of their relatively high vapor pressure, exposure occurs via inhalation. Skin absorption also occurs and may cause defatting of the subcutaneous tissues of the hands. Most solvents cause central nervous system (CNS) depression with acute exposure. Chronic effects include peripheral neuropathy from aliphatic hydrocarbons and liver toxicity from carbon tetrachloride. The primary site of benzene toxicity is the bone marrow, where it can cause bone marrow depression, aplastic anemia, and leukemia.

43. The answer is B *[Ch 5 II a 1, 3 b (2), 4 c; Table 5-1].*
Lung cancer deaths in women have increased so much that, by the mid-1980s, lung cancer had become the leading cause of cancer death in females. Lung cancer is also the number one cancer killer of men, although men are more likely to die from coronary heart disease (CHD) or chronic obstructive pulmonary disease (COPD) than from lung cancer. The number of people with lung cancer would be reduced by between 75% and 90% if people did not smoke.

44. The answer is E *[Ch 8 II B 2 a; IV A 1, B 2 b, D 3].*
Fatal intentional injuries, which are injuries that are purposely inflicted by one person on another or by one person on him- or herself, cause over 10% of fatal occupational injuries. There are about 52,000 fatal intentional deaths per year. Handguns, which are the leading vector for fatal intentional injuries, cause about 60% of these deaths annually. Fatal intentional injuries are associated with the acceptance of violence as an appropriate behavior. Family members and acquaintances are responsible for about 75% of the homicides. The mortality rate for homicides among blacks is more than six times greater than among whites; however, the suicide rate among whites is about double that of blacks.

45. The answer is A *[Ch 9 III C 1–6].*
In 1983, 40% of a private psychiatrist's gross income came from patients' out-of-pocket payments, while only 25% of a general medical physician's income came from that source. Approximately 25% of the nation's total mental health costs are paid by federal funds, 28% by state and local governments, and 12% by private health insurers. Approximately 70% of total mental health care costs are spent for inpatient care. The percentage of mental health care costs paid by private insurers (12%) is less than half the percentage of total health care costs paid by this source (30%).

46. The answer is B *[Ch 18 VII A 3, B 3 d].*
Global caps on total expenditures (e.g., Medicare's volume performance standards), cost-sharing by patients via deductibles and coinsurance, regulation on dissemination of expensive new technologies, and uniform maximum fee schedules for physicians' services are all proposals designed to contain health care expenditures. Universal health care coverage proposals seek to curb cost-shifting—that is, the practice of providers shifting health care costs to private third-party payers to cover shortfalls created either by governmental payers (e.g., Medicare, Medicaid), who pay at lower levels, or by the cost of providing care to the uninsured.

47. The answer is C *[Ch 13 II A 1].*
Some exposure is safe for toxic effects that show thresholds; however, for nonthreshold effects, there is some risk associated with any exposure. Increases in exposure or dose are expected to increase either the intensity of a toxic effect or the percent responding in a population, regardless of whether the effect is a threshold or nonthreshold effect. For both classes of effect, a chemical or metabolite does cause the effect, although the exact mechanism of action may not be known. Both threshold and nonthreshold effects can be independent of route of exposure because a chemical can enter the systemic circulation from inhalation or ingestion. Both nonthreshold effects that require chemical interaction with genetic material and threshold effects that require that the chemical or metabolite reach the sensitive target organ depend on absorption of the chemical.

48. The answer is A *[Ch 7 II A 2 a].*
Transmission of human immunodeficiency virus (HIV) by routine care, such as babysitting, even by an HIV-positive caretaker, has not been documented. Since most childhood HIV infection reflects maternal

transmission, situations that suggest positive maternal HIV status prior to the birth of the child would represent indications for testing. These include actual documentation of maternal infection, regular intravenous (IV) drug use or exposure to a sexual partner with such a history, or a disease indicative of HIV in a mother not previously tested.

49. The answer is D *[Ch 10 IV A 1 c, 2 c, B 1 c, 2 b (3), C 1 a–c].*
Down syndrome is not an autosomal recessive disorder; it occurs when there is excess chromosomal material relating to chromosome 21. The three types of Down syndrome are trisomy 21, translocation, and trisomy mosaic 21. Trisomy 21, the most common type, and trisomy mosaic 21, the rarest type, involve an extra chromosome 21, which is acquired due to a failure in chromosomal pairing of one of the parental germ cells. Translocation occurs when the long arm of chromosome 21 attaches to another chromosome (13, 18, or another 21). This disorder is usually inherited, and the translocation chromosome may be found in unaffected parents and siblings. Phenylketonuria (PKU), Tay-Sachs, Niemann-Pick type II, and homocystinuria are all autosomal recessive disorders. Thus, if both parents carry this gene, statistically, one in four offspring will be unaffected and not a carrier, two in four offspring will be unaffected carriers, and one in four will have the disease. Niemann-Pick type I appears to be an autosomal recessive disease, although the genetics of subtype IC (chronic) is unclear.

50. The answer is D *[Ch 11 III A 1–4].*
In one study, identical twins were more concordant for quantity and frequency of drinking but not for the adverse consequences of drinking. Most studies show a high prevalence of alcoholism among relatives of alcoholics (i.e., at least 25% of male relatives and 5% of female relatives are alcoholic). Other studies have shown that children of alcoholics are vulnerable to alcoholism whether raised by their alcoholic parents or by nonalcoholic foster parents. Family studies have shown that female relatives of alcoholics are prone to depression, while male relatives are prone to alcoholism.

51. The answer is C *[Ch 2 II D–E].*
A case-control study is an observational study in which diseased and nondiseased subjects are identified after the fact and then compared regarding specific characteristics to determine possible risk for the disease in question. A cohort study is an observational study in which exposed and nonexposed populations are identified and followed prospectively over time to determine the rate of a specific disease or event. Causality cannot be determined for either a case-control study or a cohort study. Causation is defined by various criteria in addition to risk assessment. These include biologic plausibility, appropriate temporal relationships between exposure and disease or event, consistent outcomes and observations across several studies, dose-response relationships, and finally an experimental or animal study confirmation of association. Although costly and time-consuming, a cohort study allows for determination of a population-based rate of the event under question. A case-control study, on the other hand, is relatively easy and inexpensive to conduct since prospective or long-term follow-up is not required. In a cohort study, potential bias is lessened because exposure can be determined prior to the onset of disease, while with a case-control study, there is a potential for bias in the selection of subjects since a case-control study is not population based. The incidence rate of an event or disease for exposed and nonexposed populations must be calculated for a cohort study but cannot be determined in a case-control study.

52. The answer is C *[Ch 8 II C 1–5].*
Potential energy describes the energy inherent in an object that has not yet been dissipated. Because it has yet to be transmitted, potential energy does not cause injuries. Energy is an injury-causing agent that may be transmitted quickly, resulting in injury, or over a long period of time, resulting in disease. Kinetic energy, or mechanical energy, is the most common cause of injuries (e.g., automobile collisions). Thermal energy, when excessive, is the most common cause of burns. A marked lack of thermal energy results in hypothermia and frostbite. Electrical energy causes electrocutions and burns, and radiation energy also causes burns.

53. The answer is C *[Ch 5 X A 1 b, 2, B 2–4].*
In the United States, Hispanic men are two to three times more likely than white men to be homicide victims, while black men are eight to fifteen times as likely as white men to be victims. Homicide is the leading cause of death for black American men between the ages of 15 and 24. Race, ethnicity, age, sex, and substance abuse are all risk factors for homicide. Men are four times more likely than women to be victims of homicide, and the use of alcohol and other drugs has been documented in about 50% of all homicides. In 1987, the death rate from homicide was 8.1 individuals per 100,000 population in the United States, and homicide constituted 10% of all deaths in the United States. Currently, homicide rates for most age-groups of both sexes are as high or higher than any previously recorded in the United States.

54. The answer is A *[Ch 7 I C 1 a (2) (b)].*
Between one-quarter and one-third of very low-birth-weight infants (i.e., infants weighing ≤ 1500 g) die in the neonatal period. The major cause of neonatal mortality reflects failure of intrauterine growth, which can occur as prematurity or as weight gain inappropriate to gestational age. As birth weight decreases, the neonatal mortality rate increases sharply. In general, low-birth-weight infants (i.e., infants weighing ≤ 2500 g) account for more than 65% of neonatal deaths, regardless of the gestational age of the infant.

55. The answer is B *[Ch 4 II D 2 b (2); Table 4-1].*
Blood is a common vehicle through which many diseases are transmitted; thus, blood is screened for serologic markers of biologic agents that cause disease. The American Red Cross screens blood for hepatitis B (HBV), hepatitis C (HCV), syphilis, cytomegalovirus (CMV), acquired immune deficiency syndrome (AIDS), and human T cell leukemia/lymphoma virus (HTLV-I and HTLV-II). Blood containing CMV antibodies is not given to neonates because of the severity of the disease in the perinatal period. Although blood is screened for syphilis, the chance of getting syphilis from a blood transfusion is extremely remote. Since herpes simplex (HSV) is not transmitted via blood and since most individuals have had prior herpes infections, blood is not screened for this disease.

56. The answer is D *[Ch 12 III F 5; IV D].*
Cytotoxic agents are not pesticides but chemotherapeutic agents used in the treatment of cancer and other disorders. Although the danger of exposure to these agents has not yet been documented, health care workers administering them to patients may be subject to chronic effects, including reproductive abnormalities; cancer; and irritation to mucous membranes, eyes, and skin. Pesticides are chemicals that are designed to kill, repel, or otherwise control organisms considered pests to humans. They may be grouped as insecticides, fungicides, herbicides, and vertebrate poisons. They can be further classified according to mode of entry, the pest they kill, or chemical composition.

57. The answer is B *[Ch 14 V A–C].*
While the physician's success rate for a given procedure might be important information for the patient to consider before authorizing the physician to perform the procedure, no court has yet required the physician to reveal this information. However, the physician would be bound to answer truthfully if the patient questioned the physician's success rate.

The patient is entitled to be informed about the diagnosis; the nature, purpose, and risks of the proposed treatment; feasible treatment alternatives; and the prognosis if the treatment is not carried out. In courts that apply the "new rule" on informed consent, which requires that the patient be told all that a physician would reasonably anticipate a prudent patient would consider *material* to his decision, it is conceivable that a patient could convince the court that the physician's success rate was material to that patient. However, no case has yet so held this to be true.

58. The answer is C *[Ch 7 I C 1, 2].*
Sudden infant death syndrome (SIDS) occurs in the postneonatal period, even among low-birth-weight infants; thus, it is unlikely to affect the neonatal mortality rate (NMR). However, increases in the rates of severe malformations due to whatever cause, increased documentation of births at very high risk for mortality (e.g., those born under 500 g), and changes in either the quality of perinatal and neonatal care or in addictive drug use are likely to affect the NMR. Addictive drug use operates both by decreasing use of prenatal care for fear of detection of drug use and by the specific action of crack cocaine in inducing premature delivery.

59. The answer is D *[Ch 17 VI D 2, 3].*
Continuous quality improvement (CQI), or total quality management, was developed by C. Edwards Deming, Ph.D., an American statistical studies consultant for Japanese industry. It is a form of quality assurance that emphasizes the use of statistical methods of assessing production problems and seeks to assist each employee to achieve his best. It involves virtually all members of an organization in a process of assessing outcomes of care to streamline production processes, remove waste, and reduce errors by continuously reviewing the process of care. By 1994, the Joint Commission on Accreditation of Health Care Organizations (JCAHO) expects formally to stress involvement in CQI for all health care institutions.

60. The answer is E *[Ch 5 III C 1 a–e].*
Family history has not been established as a risk factor for lung cancer. The overwhelming risk factor for lung cancer is, of course, smoking. Occupational exposure, air pollution, and radiation are all considered risk factors for lung cancer, although they account for a small percentage of cases.

61. The answer is D *[Ch 8 VI A 1, 2; Tables 8-4 and 8-5].*
Seat belts are an active, not passive, strategy for injury prevention. Passive strategies for injury prevention and control are automatic, require no individual or repetitive action to be protective, and are generally the most effective. Active strategies, on the other hand, are voluntary, require repetitive, individual action to be protective, and generally are less effective than passive strategies. Vehicle anti-lock brakes, carpeting, a safe hot water setting, and air bags require no individual or repetitive action to be protective and, thus, are considered passive strategies. Seat belts, however, must be buckled by the occupant of the automobile each time the vehicle is used in order to be effective and, thus, are considered an active strategy.

62. The answer is C *[Ch 16 II A 1 a, d].*
The number of Americans studying in foreign medical schools is unknown but appears to be declining. A total of 29,243 students applied for first-year positions in American medical schools in 1990, and 17,206 were accepted, making the ratio of applicants to position 1.7:1. In the last 50 years, the ratio of applicants to positions has never fallen below 1.6:1. Enrollment in medical schools has declined for the last 5 years but is now increasing gradually.

63. The answer is C *[Ch 13 IV A 1 b, c].*
Viscosity is a measure of how readily a liquid flows, and movement between environmental mediums cannot be predicted from viscosity information. However, all of the other properties are measures that directly predict the tendency of chemicals to concentrate in a medium. The octanol water partition coefficient (K_{ow}) predicts partitioning between water and oil-like materials such as soil or sediment. The vapor pressure (P_v) predicts partitioning between water and air. Water solubility (S_w) predicts the potential for concentration in water. Bioconcentration factor (BCF) predicts the affinity of a chemical for aquatic organisms; thus, high BCF values indicate an accumulation of the chemical in fish as compared to the water in which they swim.

64. The answer is D *[Ch 18 IV D 1].*
The resource-based relative value scale (RBRVS) is a departure from other fee schedules because it does *not* base fees on relative charges in a geographic area or over a given time period. Thus, the ratio of the median charge for the particular procedure to the average for all procedures in the base time period would not be used to determine an RBRVS fee. RBRVS was developed after extensive study and debate concerning physicians' compensation for performing a procedure versus their compensation for thinking and listening. A physician's time, mental effort, judgment, technical skill, malpractice costs, office overhead costs, and postgraduate specialty training costs are all included in determining a RBRVS fee. Medicare started implementing an RBRVS fee schedule in January 1992.

65. The answer is D *[Figure 15-2].*
According to the American Medical Association's (AMA's) Principles of Medical Ethics, in emergencies, the physician must respond to medical need. The principle of not abandoning a patient is true both for the individual and the profession. An individual physician who chooses not to serve a patient is not abandoning this patient if there is no emergency and treatment has not begun. However, in an emergency, when only one physician is available, that physician represents the profession and not providing treatment would be considered abandoning the patient.

66. The answer is E *[Ch 14 III B 1 a–d].*
Four conditions must be met if a plaintiff is to recover damages in a negligence claim. In addition to proving duty (an obligation recognized by the law and for the breach of which the law imposes sanctions), dereliction (that the defendant performed below the legally required standard of care), and damage (that the plaintiff was harmed), the plaintiff must also prove that the defendant's negligence was the proximate cause of the plaintiff's injuries. Deliberate wrongdoing, while it is an element in some tort suits, need not be proved in a negligence action, which charges that the defendant caused harm by careless or inattentive action.

67. The answer is C *[Ch 16 I B 4 c (1)].*
Reports by both the Graduate Medical Education National Advisory Committee (GMENAC) and the Council on Graduate Medical Education (COGME) have been controversial because of the difficulty in determining optimal need for medical services. Because the medical student population has steadily declined since 1984 and only recently stabilized, no growth is expected in the physician population in the 1990s. It is also felt that demand for physicians will grow significantly because of increasing numbers of acquired immune deficiency syndrome (AIDS) cases, the expanding older population, and the proliferation of complex medical technologies. While poor reimbursement for primary care deters many physicians from entering the primary care specialties, slow but steady progress has been made in correcting

the imbalances in compensation between cognitive services and surgical and invasive services. Medicare's resource-based relative value scale (RBRVS) fee schedule, for example, attempts to compensate physicians for the cognitive aspects of rendering care.

68. The answer is C *[Ch 11 II B 3 c (1)–(3)].*
The typical heroin addict is a male, 25–35 years old, an urban dweller, and a member of a minority group. Within the medical profession, the heroin addiction rate is estimated to be 1%–2%, as contrasted with the rate of 0.3% for the general population of the United States.

69. The answer is D *[Ch 4 III C 2 d (2), e (2), f (4), (5), g (1)].*
Multiple live attenuated viral vaccines may be administered on the same day, or they must be separated by at least a month. Since these vaccines require multiplication of the antigen in the body, they should not be given to immunocompromised hosts who might have trouble eliminating the infection or to pregnant women because of a theoretical harmful effect on the developing fetus. The recent administration of immune globulin (IG) can also inactivate the vaccine and prevent the vaccine from stimulating an immune response. No immunization should be given to an individual with a current febrile illness.

70. The answer is D *[Ch 3 IV F 1–4].*
The probability that an individual with a positive test will have the disease depends on the sensitivity and specificity of the test, the false-positive rate, and the disease prevalence in the county. It is not dependent on the size of the county population. Bayes' theorem is a statement of the conditional probability of a disease for an individual with a positive screening test. The false-positive rate is the probability of a positive test among those without the disease and equals 1 minus the specificity. The probability of disease given a positive test increases with increasing disease prevalence, which is also called the prior probability of disease (the probability of disease prior to knowing the test result).

71. The answer is D *[Ch 11 II].*
There are seven classes of substances that are associated with both abuse and dependence: alcohol, barbiturates, opioids, amphetamines, cannabis, cocaine, and tobacco. Phencyclidine (PCP) and hallucinogens, although illegal, are associated with abuse only; physical dependence has not been demonstrated yet.

72. The answer is A *[Ch 10 IV B 1 a, 2 a, 3 a, D 1].*
The incidence of spina bifida is highest for those of Irish ancestry. The incidence of each Tay-Sachs, Niemann-Pick type 1, and Gaucher's disease, on the other hand, is highest among Ashkenazi Jews, who are Jews of Eastern European ancestry. All of these diseases have been associated with mental retardation.

73. The answer is B *[Ch 12 IV A 5 c].*
Lead exposure is seen in the manufacture of batteries, paints, and ceramics, and in lead smelters. Exposure occurs by inhalation and ingestion. Chronic toxicity occurs in the central nervous system (CNS) [neurobehavioral disturbances], peripheral nervous system (PNS) [peripheral neuropathy], hematopoietic system (anemia due to impaired heme synthesis), and the kidneys (chronic renal failure). Reproductive effects include decreased sperm counts and fetotoxicity. Although liver involvement may be suggested by mild transaminase elevation, the liver is not a significant target of lead toxicity.

74. The answer is D *[Ch 4 VI B 2 d].*
There has never been a documented foodborne outbreak of hepatitis B virus (HBV). Carriers of the hepatitis B surface antigen (HBsAg) are allowed to work in occupations that prepare or serve food for public consumption. HBV is inactivated in its passage through the gastrointestinal tract. The mode of transmission of HBV is primarily by direct person-to-person contact via infected body fluids or by common vehicle such as a contaminated needle. Thus, transmission is likely to occur in populations with overcrowding, lack of sanitation, and poor personal hygiene; among sexual partners of infected adults; in household contacts, in intravenous drug abusers who share contaminated needles; and in infants born to infected mothers who become infected in the perinatal period.

75. The answer is C *[Ch 12 III A 1–9].*
Foundry workers who work in the metal casting industry are exposed to several hazardous substances. Silicon dioxide, which is used in the molding process, is capable of causing silicosis. Asbestos, which is used in forming gates and riser sleeves of molds as well as in the linings of furnaces and ladles, is associated with lung cancer, mesothelioma, asbestosis, and pleural disease. Noise in the foundries is associated with hearing loss and hypertension. Additional hazardous exposures include polycyclic aromatic hydrocarbons, metal dusts and fumes, formaldehyde and isocyanate compounds, carbon monoxide (CO), heat, and nonionizing radiation. Foundry workers are not known to be at increased risk for occupationally caused stomach cancer.

76. The answer is C *[Ch 11 I C 4 a–i].*
The *Diagnostic and Statistical Manual of Mental Disorders,* 3rd edition, revised (*DSM-III-R*), ranks severity of dependence on psychoactive substances according to the following factors: the degree of effort to curb the substance abuse; the frequency of intoxication or other impairment due to substance abuse; the frequency of preoccupation with seeking or taking the substance, including abandonment of important social, occupational, or recreational activity in order to seek or take the substance; regular use of the substance to avoid withdrawal symptoms; the use of the substance in larger doses or over a longer period of time than the user intended; continuation of substance use, despite mitigating physical, mental, or legal problems; evidence of withdrawal; and tolerance, which is defined as either the need for an increased amount of the substance to achieve intoxication (or a desired effect) or a diminished effect with continued use of a given amount of the substance. Thus, using smaller amounts of the substances due to a *lack* of tolerance is not one of the criteria. Other revisions made in the *DSM-III-R* regarding substance abuse include removing the distinction between drug abuse and drug dependence and using an identical set of symptoms and behaviors to determine dependence on all different classes of psychoactive substances.

77. The answer is E *[Ch 2 II F 1–5].*
A larger than expected study population will not invalidate a clinical trial, if these excess subjects are randomized equally. Study size is based on statistical determinations and cost and time constraints. Statistical accuracy usually is improved as the sample size increases. The cost of a study, however, and the time needed to recruit a larger cohort may become prohibitive. A clinical trial is an experimental design used to assess differences between two or more groups receiving different interventions or treatments. The design is such that at least one comparison group is included for the planned intervention. This comparison group, or "control group," may receive no intervention, or it may receive "standard therapy" if such exists. A population with a clinical characteristic requiring intervention must be identified. Subjects must be allocated, preferably randomly, to each of the treatment interventions. Randomization minimizes the potential adverse effect from systematic error (bias). Treatments are then administered in an identical or controlled manner to ensure uniformity of nontreatment covariants. Preferably observations should be made while observers and patients are masked to the type of interventions being made to avoid biased observations. This is called a double-blind study, as compared to a single-blind study, when only the subject or the observer is masked to the intervention. An insufficient number of subjects may lead to failure to detect true differences that may exist (β error). It should also be noted that statistically significant results can occur due to chance (α error) even in the most rigorous study design, as in a well-designed clinical trial where treatments are randomized and subjects and observers are masked.

78. The answer is D *[Ch 15 I F 1–4].*
Morality may rest on common consent of a social unit, on adherence to the will of a god, or on what is deemed consistent with normal human behavior. It may also be based on individual perception of what is right either through common sense or intuition. Criminal law is generally based on one or more of the moral sources; however, there may often be a major discrepancy between the (criminal) law and morality.

79–84. The answers are: 79-E, 80-A, 81-D, 82-A, 83-B, 84-C *[Ch 1 I B 3 a–d].*
Managing a patient with heart disease requires primary prevention (elimination of factors that cause progression of disease, such as tobacco and cholesterol), secondary prevention (treatment of underlying disease processes, such as hypertension and angina), and tertiary prevention (rehabilitation, such as graduated exercise).

Cleaning up the environment can be considered primary prevention for certain acute diseases. However, many chronic diseases cannot be prevented by environmental cleanup because most such diseases occur due to lifestyle habits. Health education is an appropriate means of primary prevention when lifestyle habits are involved.

Treating a case of gonorrhea employs both secondary prevention (the treatment of the disease) and primary prevention (preventing other people from getting the disease). The use of a condom to prevent the spread of a sexually transmitted disease (STD) also is an example of primary prevention.

Health education is a form of primary prevention. Many schools are adopting health education programs to teach children good health habits before bad health habits develop.

Screening programs are a form of secondary prevention since they are used to detect disease in the preclinical, or early, stages of the disease. Prompt treatment often can prevent further progression of the disease in the individual and possible spread of a communicable disease to others.

Physical therapy is a form of tertiary prevention. It can be used to restore mobility to an affected limb and thereby reduce disability.

85–88. The answers are: 85-D *[Ch 17 II D 3 b (3) (a)],* **86-A** *[Ch 17 II D 2 c],* **87-B** *[Ch 17 II D 2 b, 3 b (3) (c)],* **88-C** *[Ch 17 II D 3 b (3) (b)].*
Alternative delivery systems, which contrast with the traditional fee-for-service practices, have been established in an attempt to minimize costs.

Health maintenance organizations (HMOs) provide prepaid comprehensive health care, and providers are placed at financial risk for excessive use of services. Staff-model HMOs have physicians who are employed directly by the plan, while hospitals may be plan-owned or independent. Group-model HMOs have physicians' groups who contract individually with the plan, but the physicians remain employees of the group not the plan.

Preferred provider organizations (PPOs) are fee-for-service plans where insured individuals are given financial incentives to use the panel of preferred providers. Patients may choose their own physicians, though nonmember physicians require copayments or deductibles.

Independent practice associations (IPAs) are plans where physicians are in private practice but agree to accept a capitation fee for any patients referred by the plan.

Exclusive provider organizations (EPOs) are a rare form of fee-for-service plans where an employer selects hospitals and physicians with favorable charges and rates. Thus, patients are required to use the most cost-effective providers and hospitals. Providers are at no financial risk.

89–92. The answers are: 89-C, 90-C *[Ch 6 I B 1],* **91-A** *[Ch 6 I B 3],* **92-B** *[Ch 6 I C 1].*
Spontaneous abortion includes failure of embryonic development, fetal death in utero, expulsion of all or any part of the products of conception before 20 weeks' gestation, or expulsion of a fetus weighing less than 500 g. Stillbirth is fetal death after 20 weeks' gestation or spontaneous death of a fetus weighing more than 500 g. Perinatal death includes fetal as well as infant deaths between 28 weeks' gestation and 1 week postnatal, with a weight of 500 g or more.

93–95. The answers are: 93-B *[Ch 6 I C 1],* **94-C** *[Ch 6 I C 2],* **95-A** *[Ch 6 I C 3].*
Perinatal mortality refers to fetal and infant deaths occurring between 28 weeks' gestation and 1 week postnatal, in which the fetus or infant weighs 500 g or more. Neonatal mortality refers to deaths of liveborn infants within 28 days of birth. Infant mortality refers to deaths of children less than 1 year of age. Consistency in the use of definitions and collection of statistics enables comparisons to be made across space and over time.

96–100. The answers are: 96-A *[Ch 5 XII C 1],* **97-A** *[Ch 5 III D 4 a],* **98-B** *[Ch 5 III D 1],* **99-C** *[Ch 5 XI D 2],* **100-D** *[Ch 5 III D 3].*
Screening for anemia is by hematocrit. Target populations include premature infants, infants born of a multiple pregnancy or an iron-deficient woman, and individuals of low socioeconomic status. Hematocrit is considered a cost-effective method of screening for anemia for target populations.

Screening for cervical cancer is by Pap smear to detect cervical abnormalities; intervals of 1–3 years are recommended. Target populations include individuals who are between the ages of 25 and 60, are of low socioeconomic status, are prison inmates, are prostitutes, had first intercourse at an early age, have a history of sexually transmitted diseases (STDs), are unmarried mothers, have had induced abortions, or have a history of cervical squamous dysplasia. A Pap smear is considered a cost-effective method of screening for cervical cancer.

Screening for presymptomatic lung cancer is by either pulmonary cytology or chest x-ray, neither of which is considered cost-effective for target populations. In addition, although screening allows early detection of lung cancer, it has no beneficial effect on mortality from lung cancer.

Risk factors such as cigarette smoking, regular use of aspirin and acetaminophen, and prolonged use of large doses of steroids are closely associated with peptic ulcer disease. Less conclusive associations have been reported for alcohol, caffeine, diet, and psychologic stress. In spite of the awareness of these risk factors, no tests for determining a pre-ulcerous condition in asymptomatic individuals exist.

Screening for colorectal cancer is by testing the stool for occult blood in men and women over 45 years of age. Target populations include individuals with a history of colitis, familial polyposis, familial villous adenomas, or familial colon cancer. Because the tests used are not very sensitive or specific, the cost-effectiveness of this screening is debatable.

101–105. The answers are: 101-D, 102-A, 103-E, 104-C, 105-B *[Ch 8 IV D; Figure 8-3].*
The parents of a 4-month-old infant should be counseled regarding the importance of using stairway gates and window guards. In addition, the parents of infants less than 2 years old should be counseled concerning child safety seats, hot water heater temperature ($\leq$ 120 ° F), pool fences, the storage of drugs and toxic chemicals, the availabililty of syrup of ipecac, and the telephone number of the local poison control center. In high-risk settings, infants should be screened for lead exposure.

The 9-year-old female grade school student and her parents should be counseled on bicycle safety helmets and storage of matches. The storage of drugs and toxic chemicals should also be discussed.

A 17-year-old male high school student should be counseled regarding violent behavior, use of firearms, and driving while using alcohol or other drugs.

A 45-year-old female laborer should be counseled about occupational injuries and back conditioning exercises because she is likely to be at increased risk. Adults 19–64 years old also should be counseled concerning safety helmets, smoking near bedding or upholstery, and occupational injuries and illnesses. Young adults 19–39 years old, especially young males, should be counseled concerning violent behavior and firearms. Persons with children in the home should be counseled concerning childhood injuries, and persons with older adults in the home should be counseled concerning falls in the elderly.

A 70-year-old male retiree should be counseled regarding falls and smoking near bedding or upholstery. Adults 64 years old and older should also be counseled concerning hot water heater temperature (≤ 120° F).

All patients should be counseled concerning the use of safety belts in motor vehicles and the use of functioning smoke detectors in the home. Clinicians should also remain alert for signs of abuse or neglect for all patients (e.g., child abuse, domestic violence, elder abuse). Patients age 13 years old and older should be counseled concerning the use of alcohol and other drugs and clinicians should remain alert for depressive symptoms and suicide risk factors among these patients.

These recommendations are from the U.S. Preventive Services Task Force, which systematically evaluated 169 clinical interventions and made recommendations for clinicians.

106–110. The answers are: 106-E *[Ch 16 II B 2]*, **107-A** *[Ch 16 I B 4 c]*, **108-D** *[Ch 16 III A 2 b (2)]*, **109-B** *[Ch 16 I C 1]*, **110-C** *[Ch 16 III A 1 a]*.

While osteopathic physicians account for only about 5% of all practicing physicians, their numbers continue to grow (there were 31,000 practitioners in 1991). Osteopaths traditionally have been strongly oriented toward primary care, with relatively few pursuing specialties. However, the number of osteopaths who specialize is growing.

Although organizations such as the Graduate Medical Education National Advisory Committee (GMENAC) and the Council on Graduate Medical Education (COGME) had predicted physician surpluses by 1990, such surpluses are not evident in the early 1990s. In fact, shortages have been predicted due to a medical school enrollment that has been declining since 1984 and has only recently stabilized.

It is estimated that 94,500 registered nurses (RNs) were employed as public health nurses in state and local agencies in 1988. These numbers have tripled since 1966 but still reflect a small number of nurses who are available for community medicine.

From 1970 to 1990, the number of RNs in practice doubled; however, many geographic areas still felt acute shortages of RNs.

Virtually all RN diploma programs are administered by hospitals and require 3 years of training. Recent trends have shown a steady decline in the number of graduates from these programs and larger numbers of nursing students receiving associate and bachelor degrees.

111–115. The answers are: 111-B *[Ch 12 IV A 7 c (2)]*, **112-C** *[Ch 12 IV A 8 c (1)]*, **113-A** *[Ch 12 IV A 6 c (1), (2)]*, **114-E** *[Ch 12 IV A 2 c (2)]*, **115-D** *[Ch 12 IV A 1 c (4)]*.

Asthma has been linked to nickel sulfate exposure among electroplaters.

Metal fume fever is an influenza-like illness seen in welders, most typically produced by zinc oxide fumes.

The classic syndrome of elemental mercury toxicity includes stomatitis, gingivitis, tremor, and behavioral changes.

Arsenic exposure may cause a peripheral neuropathy, especially a sensory one, with high-level exposure.

Beryllium exposure causes inflammation of the mucous membranes and upper respiratory tract with acute exposure and a granulomatous disease of the lung with chronic exposure.

116–120. The answers are: 116-B *[Ch 14 IV D 2]*, **117-A** *[Ch 14 III B 2 d (1)–(3)]*, **118-E** *[Ch 14 VI B 3 b]*, **119-C** *[Ch 14 V B 2]*, **120-D** *[Ch 14 VIII D 2 d]*.

In general, courts do not like to entertain medical negligence cases under the rubric of contract suits. However, at least one court has held (*Hawkins v. McGee*) that where a very specific promise of improvement or cure is made, a health care provider may be liable if the promised result is not forthcoming. Some states insist that the promise not only be expressly stated but also that it be in writing if it is to be the basis of a breach of warranty suit.

Helling v. Carey, although not widely followed, held that customary professional practice is not absolutely determinative of reasonably prudent care. A court is normally reluctant to substitute its judgment as to what is reasonable care for that of the medical community but will do so in a clear-cut case. What made the *Helling* case clear-cut was the fact that the test involved was simple, inexpensive, painless, risk-free, and highly definitive, whereas the disease it might detect (glaucoma) was serious, degenerative, and irreversible. *Helling* stands as a limited, but significant, symbol that the medical profession cannot determine absolutely the standards by which its performance is to be judged.

The *Claire Conroy* case goes well beyond that of *Karen Quinlan* by allowing withdrawal of food and water, which some consider not to be *extraordinary* means of life support. In the *Quinlan* case, the court authorized removal of a respirator, but intravenous feeding was continued until Karen's death in 1985. Moreover, in the *Quinlan* case, the patient was comatose and was thought to have no significant chance of ever returning to consciousness. In *Conroy,* the patient was partially responsive and had some degree of interaction with her environment. The court established elaborate criteria by which to determine what the patient would have wished regarding the continuation of care had she been able to do so; thus, the doctrine of substituted judgment was followed.

Canterbury v. Spence is the landmark case that moved the physician's obligation to disclose information to the patient from a physician-based to a patient-based standard. Under this new approach, the relevant inquiry focuses on what a patient would want to know in deciding on treatment, rather than, as previously, on what physicians normally disclose to patients in such situations. It is a question of fact for the court—and for a jury when one of the parties to the suit has requested one—to determine whether a particular item of information would have been material to an individual in the patient's situation.

The *Tarasoff v. Regents of University of California* case was very controversial in the mental health community since it unsettled the traditional belief that there was an absolute privilege protecting information a patient divulged to her psychotherapist in the course of treatment. The case recognized that the mental health professional has a duty to the public that can supersede that owed to his client. The *Tarasoff* ruling, which has been adopted in a number of other jurisdictions, is limited to cases in which the therapist has sound reason to believe that the patient threatens danger to an identifiable third party. The therapist's duty is to inform the authorities or to warn the intended victim.

121–125. The answers are: 121-C *[Ch 17 VI C 2 g, h],* **122-E** *[Ch 17 VII B],* **123-A** *[Ch 17 VI D 1 b (1)],* **124-B** *[Ch 17 VI C 2 a],* **125-B** *[Ch 17 VI C 1, 2].*

The Consolidated Omnibus Budget Reconciliation Act of 1986 (COBRA 1986) contained landmark legislation authorizing pilot projects in which peer review organizations (PROs) review outpatient care. Departing from the more narrowly focused inpatient chart reviews, PROs attempt to evaluate care for Medicare patients.

The National Health Planning and Development Act of 1974 (Public Law 93-641) superceded the Comprehensive Health Planning and Public Services Amendment of 1966 (Public Law 89-749) by legislating 203 health service areas, each to be covered by a health systems agency (HSA). HSAs were empowered to restrict capital expenditures such as new buildings and new technologies [e.g., computed tomography (CT) scanners]. The elimination of excess hospital bed capacity and redundant equipment was to have reduced soaring health care costs. HSAs were ineffective and, at best, delayed rather than prevented capital expenditures.

The Health Care Quality Improvement Act of 1986 reflected the concerns of Congress that no national clearinghouse existed to monitor disciplinary actions against health care providers. As a result of this legislation, the National Practitioner Data Bank was established. This data base, which became functional in 1991, collects and provides information on disciplinary actions against physicians [doctors of medicine (MDs) and doctors of osteopathy (DOs)], dentists, and any licensed health care provider found liable in a medical liability suit. Hospitals must request information every 2 years on all licensed practitioners with clinical privileges at the institution. One function of this is to prevent practitioners who hold licenses in several states from practicing in one state when their licenses have been revoked in another.

The Tax Equity and Fiscal Responsibility Act of 1982 (Public Law 97-248) dissolved the ineffective professional standards review organizations (PSROs) and implemented peer review organizations (PROs) subject to more stringent performance guidelines. PROs are considered ineffective in monitoring quality of care, though more effective in reducing cost of care. In 1990, the Institute of Medicine recommended the elimination of PROs and the formation of quality-focused Medicare quality review organizations (MQROs).

Public Law 93-222 is the Health Maintenance Organization (HMO) Act of 1972.

126–130. The answers are: 126-B *[Ch 9 VI B],* **127-A** *[Ch 9 VI A 2 b],* **128-C** *[Ch 9 VI C],* **129-A** *[Ch 9 VI A],* **130-B** *[Ch 9 VI B 2].*

Secondary prevention encompasses early diagnosis and prompt and adequate treatment to prevent sequelae and limit disability. One of the four areas of secondary prevention is crisis intervention, which offers services immediately.

In 1964, Gerald Caplan developed a theory and techniques for preparing individuals in advance to deal with crises in the hope of avoiding the distress that usually results. This is a part of primary prevention. Primary prevention also involves the promotion of general mental health and the protection against the occurrence of specific diseases.

Tertiary prevention encompasses rehabilitation after the occurrence of defect and disability in an attempt to reduce the disability.

131–134. The answers are: 131-A, 132-D, 133-B, 134-D *[Ch 16 I C 1 a–b].*
Nurses traditionally have been single, young, white females. However, the average age of nurses has been increasing and is now 30–40 years of age. Also, many nurses are married and have children, and the demands of family life often limit the working hours of these nurses, their desire to work nights and weekends, and their availability to pursue nursing at all. Thus, these demographic factors have caused a decrease in the supply of nurses.

The more sophisticated medical care has become, the greater the demand on nursing. Although the total hospital bed count has decreased in the United States, the number of intensive care beds has increased to 10% of all beds. Intensive care requires 4–6 times as many nurses as general medical care.

In-house nursing agencies provide part-time employees, thereby saving hospitals money by decreasing the need for full-time nurses. Agency nurses usually are limited in what they can do because of their lack of familiarity with the job, but agency work is popular among nurses because of scheduling flexibility and the option of working part-time.

The elderly require more medical care than the general population does. Over 50% of an individual's lifetime health expenses will be generated in the last year of life. Over the next several decades, as the baby boomers age, there will be a steady growth in demand for health care services. By the year 2000, there will be 5 million Americans age 85 years or older as compared to only 2 million in 1980.

135–139. The answers are: 135-C, 136-D, 137-B, 138-E, 139-A *[Ch 3 IV E; Table 3-16].*
Screening test parameters are measures of the clinical usefulness of the test when compared with a definitive diagnostic test.

Sensitivity is a test's ability to identify correctly those persons who truly have the disease. In this example, the sensitivity (80%) is calculated by dividing the number of persons with the disease who screen positive (200) by the total number of persons with the disease (250).

Specificity is a test's ability to identify correctly persons who do not have disease. In this example, the specificity (86%) is the number of persons who do not have the disease and who screen negative (600) divided by the total number of persons who do not have the disease (700).

Positive predictive value is a test's ability to identify those persons who truly have the disease from among all those persons whose screening tests are positive. In this example, the positive predictive value (67%) is the number of persons with disease who screen positive (200) divided by the total number of persons who screen positive (300).

Negative predictive value is a test's ability to identify those persons who truly do not have disease from among all those persons whose screening tests are negative. Here, the negative predictive value (92%) is the number of persons who do not have disease and who screen negative (600) divided by the total number of persons who screen negative (650).

The prevalence of a disease is the proportion of people who have the disease in the population. In this example, the prevalence is equal to 250 divided by 950, or 26%. Sensitivity and specificity are independent of the prevalence of the disease, while positive and negative predictive values vary with disease prevalence.

Other screening test parameters include the false-positive rate, which is the proportion of persons without disease who screen positive among all persons without disease, and the false-negative rate, the proportion of persons with disease who screen negative among all persons with disease.

140–143. The answers are: 140-D, 141-A, 142-C, 143-B *[Ch 1 II C 1–3].*
The effectiveness of a new vaccine can only be determined by carefully designed experimental studies, which show protection in the immunized group as compared to the nonimmunized group.

In order to control a measles outbreak at a local school, descriptive studies, which describe the distribution of disease by the epidemiologic variables of person, place, and time, are used to determine who is getting the disease and why the outbreak occurred. Public health officials can then use this information to apply proper control measures to prevent further spread.

The investigation of a new disease process always begins with descriptive studies to determine which segments of the population are contracting the disease. After these segments are identified, case-control studies (analytical studies) are designed to identify risk factors that cause disease or to explain why certain individuals within these population segments develop disease.

Unusual diseases or rare diseases are usually studied with analytical studies of the case-control variety. Because of the small number of cases that occur, a case-control study must be used to identify causal relationships or factors associated with disease. Hypotheses that are generated by this technique can be tested with additional studies.

144–147. The answers are: 144-B, 145-E, 146-C, 147-A *[Ch 8 II A–D].*
Elevated blood alcohol concentration is a host factor, which indicates individual abuse of alcohol. In most states, a blood alcohol concentration of at least 0.1 g/dl defines legal intoxication. The tolerance of drunk driving, however, is a social environment factor.

A rainy night is a physical environment factor that is not controllable. However, the effects of a rainy night can be modified with road lights, improved highway surfaces, and good tires.

The compact car is a vector factor. Small cars are less safe than large cars, particularly in a collision, and are associated with an increased risk of injuries.

The speed of the car is an agent factor. The force of impact is related to the square of the speed. The force for a speed of 70 mph, for example, is four times the force for a speed of 35 mph.

148–154. The answers are: 148-F, 149-C, 150-E, 151-A, 152-D, 153-G, 154-B *[Ch 6 II A; Table 6-2].*
The first-year failure rate of leaving contraception to chance is 85%; of natural family planning, or periodic abstinence, is 20%; of diaphragm with spermicide is 18%; of condom without spermicide is 12%; of the birth control pill is 3%; of female sterilization is 0.4%; and of male sterilization is 0.15%. These are the percentages of typical couples using a particular method of contraception (not necessarily for the first time) consistently and correctly who are expected to experience an accidental pregnancy during the first year of use.

Criteria for a good contraceptive method include efficacy, safety, accessibility, acceptability, and reversibility. Risk/benefit analysis may be done for each method using these criteria and including absence of a method and the resultant unwanted pregnancy in the risk analysis.

Sterilization is the most effective method of contraception. Even though male sterilization (i.e., vasectomy) is accompanied by significantly less morbidity, mortality, time, and expense and is almost three times as effective as female sterilization, it is performed only half as often as female sterilization.

155–158. The answers are: 155-B *[Ch 12 IV I 4 e],* **156-D** *[Ch 12 IV I 4 c],* **157-A** *[Ch 12 IV I 1 d],* **158-C** *[Ch 12 IV I 1 j].*
Sporotrichosis and candidiasis are fungal diseases. Sporotrichosis is acquired from roses, sphagnum moss, and other plants and is transmitted by minor trauma, often a thorn scratch.

Candidiasis of the skin and nails is seen among workers whose hands are often wet and, therefore, prone to maceration.

Anthrax is a bacillary infection causing skin ulceration that affects handlers of hides, wool, and goat hair.

Psittacosis is a chlamydial infection transmitted by the respiratory route from infected birds and, thus, may affect bird fanciers, poultry raisers, and pet shop owners.

159–163. The answers are: 159-A *[Ch 4 V C 1 a],* **160-E** *[Ch 4 V A 5 b],* **161-D** *[Ch 4 V A 5 d],* **162-E** *[Ch 4 V A 5 c],* **163-C** *[Ch 4 V B 1 f].*
Sexually transmitted diseases (STDs) are the most common communicable diseases in this country, and gonorrhea is the most commonly reported disease. The long-term morbidity of these diseases is significant. Pelvic inflammatory disease (PID), which can be caused by a number of organisms, can cause infertility in 4% of women after a single episode and 60% after the third episode. Furthermore, 6% of pregnancies occurring in women with a previous history of PID are ectopic. Long-term sequelae of herpes simplex virus (HSV) infection cause various types of cancers, and chronic syphilis infection can lead to blindness, psychosis, and cardiovascular disease. Cytomegalovirus (CMV) is associated with Kaposi's sarcoma and teratogenicity.

164–167. The answers are: 164-C *[Ch 14 VII A 1 b],* **165-E** *[Ch 14 III C 1 a, b],* **166-B** *[Ch 14 V F 4],* **167-D** *[Ch 14 VII A 3 a, b].*
Physicians cannot unilaterally terminate a treatment relationship with a patient. They must have the patient's consent to the termination or must give the patient sufficient notice of termination to allow the patient to secure care elsewhere. A successful suit on grounds of abandonment is unlikely if the patient lives in an area where care from alternative sources is readily available.

The doctrine of battery is the root premise of the entire U.S. law on consent and informed consent. The U.S. legal system places great weight upon the individual right of bodily inviolability. Battery is regarded as a deliberate tort, even in cases where the individual doing the touching has acted in good faith and with good intentions. However, a technical violation is not likely to lead to an award of significant damages.

The doctrine of emergency consent requires that before care is rendered, steps reasonable under the circumstances are taken to locate the patient's next of kin to get authorization for treatment. In the absence of this consent, the physician is entitled to assume, unless there is a reliable indication to the contrary, that the patient would have authorized the treatment if that patient had been able to state a preference. Still, the care rendered must not extend beyond that necessary to preserve life and prevent serious harm to the patient's health.

Good samaritan statutes, which are intended to encourage physicians to render care under the difficult circumstances of emergencies, grant physicians immunity from any civil liability claims arising from the rendering of such emergency care. However, immunity usually is not provided to physicians who are grossly negligent in their emergency care or who are acting within the ordinary scope of their practice.

168–171. The answers are: 168-B *[Ch 18 IV A 1],* **169-E** *[Ch 18 IV A 3, C 1; Table 18-3],* **170-A** *[Ch 18 IV A 2],* **171-C** *[Ch 18 IV A 4].*
Providers' itemized invoices record the cost of each health care service provided; thus, they are known as fee-for-service charges.

The diagnosis-related groups (DRGs) are classifications of treatments based on diagnostic categories. Payment according to DRG is based on resources used for a given diagnosis (a relative case-mix index). Currently, Medicare uses 470 such inpatient admission diagnostic categories in the DRG payment system.

With the capitation payment method, providers agree to provide as much care as is needed in the provider's specialty to each insured person and are compensated a given amount per month per person covered. A per diem reimbursement includes all costs incurred for each day of hospital care.

172–178. The answers are: 172-E *[Ch 4 III D 3 c (2)],* **173-C** *[Ch 4 III D 2 c (3)],* **174-A** *[Ch 4 III D 1 c (4) (a)],* **175-F** *[Ch 4 VIII A 1 b (1)],* **176-D** *[III D 7],* **177-H** *[Ch 4 IV B 3 b (2)],* **178-B** *[Ch 4 VI B 3 e].*
Rubella vaccine was developed to prevent congenital defects such as blindness, deafness, cardiac defects, and mental retardation.

The problem with vaccines is that they have side effects, and they occasionally make healthy people sick. In recent years, live attenuated oral poliovirus vaccine (OPV) has caused more cases of paralysis than the wild poliovirus. Nevertheless, OPV has prevented far more disease than it has ever caused. Prevention is most important for certain diseases such as rubella, measles, and polio, since there is no therapy to treat the underlying disorder.

The pertussis component of diphtheria and tetanus toxoids and pertussis (DTP) vaccine has significant side effects such as inconsolable high-pitched crying, lasting 3 hours or more within 48 hours of inoculation; convulsions; and mental retardation. These same side effects occur with the natural disease but at a higher frequency. Therefore, although vaccines may cause significant side effects, they prevent more disease and, in the long run, do more good than harm. Unfortunately, while this overall good is for the general population, it occasionally produces significant harm to the individual.

Hemophilus influenzae type B (Hib) conjugate vaccine was developed to prevent one of the most common causes of preventable mental retardation. *H. influenzae* meningitis is treatable, but complications occur in spite of treatment.

Some vaccines have a limited effectiveness, especially the pneumococcal polysaccharide and influenza vaccines. Pneumococcal polysaccharide vaccine protects against only 23 of the most common types of the over 80 serotypes of pneumococci that cause disease.

Since the influenza virus undergoes a constant antigenic drift, the influenza vaccine must be updated each year. To be protected against the influenza virus, a person needs yearly immunization. Since the vaccine contains the influenza viruses that were circulating in the population the previous year, it may not protect against a new antigenic strain.

Even when there is an effective vaccine, it is not always used in the segment of the population most at risk of getting the disease. Hepatitis B virus (HBV) vaccine is primarily used to protect health care workers from occupational exposure because of medicolegal ramifications. However, the groups most likely to be infected with HBV are homosexual men and intravenous (IV) drug users who may not have ready access to the vaccine because of its expense.

179–182. The answers are: 179-C *[Ch 14 III B 2 d (1)–(3)],* **180-D** *[Ch 14 V B 1],* **181-B** *[Ch 14 V D 2],* **182-E** *[Ch 14 V B 2].*
Generally, the standard of care required is that of the medical community—that is, a professional community standard. However, as in *Helling v. Carey* (Washington, 1974), it is possible for a court to hold that the standard of care observed by the profession is not adequate and that "reasonable care" requires a higher standard. While the *Helling* precedent has not been widely followed, it seems clear that a court *can,* where it seems appropriate, impose its own standards of required conduct.

The older rule on informed consent, still followed in roughly half of the states, concerns the adequacy of physicians' disclosures to their patients—it is measured by what other physicians commonly would disclose under a similar circumstance. Using such a physician-based standard supports professional autonomy with regard to the provision of information to patients. Practically, it means that patients cannot sue for lack of informed consent unless they can produce expert medical testimony as to what the prevailing standard of disclosure is for the procedure in question.

Under a subjective standard of causation—that is, one focused on the "particular patient" in question—the jury attempts to decide whether that person would have chosen differently with respect to treatment if the information had been disclosed. This approach is consistent with the concept of individual self-determination, which underlies the doctrine of informed consent. The problem with this approach is that it places great weight on what patients say they would have done, since no one can really prove or disprove what a patient's response to particular information would have been.

The patient-based standard of informed consent focuses on patients' informational needs rather than on the standard practice of physicians, making it consistent with the "patient's rights" philosophy. Thus, a physician is expected to disclose all that a patient would consider material to the decision to accept or reject treatment. A factor is considered material if it is significantly likely to affect the patient's decision.

183–186. The answers are: 183-C *[Ch 10 V B 3]*, **184-D** *[Ch 10 V B 2 c]*, **185-B** *[Ch 10 V A 2 c]*, **186-A** *[Ch 10 V A 1 c (2) (c)]*.

Maternal iodine deficiency at conception or during early pregnancy can result in cretinism—a condition resulting from lack of thyroid secretion. Currently, most table salt is iodized and, thus, provides a good dietary supplement of iodine; iodine deficiency is quite rare in the United States. If a deficiency is present in a pregnant woman or an infant, supplementation should begin as soon as possible to prevent mental retardation.

Fetal alcohol syndrome has been associated with a variety of clinical features, including microcephaly, cleft palate, cardiac atrial or ventricular defects, and mental retardation. This syndrome appears to occur mostly with persistent alcohol use during pregnancy, and it has been reported in cases where the mothers consistently consumed roughly 30 ml of alcohol per day through the course of their pregnancy. Maternal abstinence from alcohol ingestion during gestation is the safest method of prevention, as even minor amounts of alcohol consumption *may* be harmful, since some proportion of the alcohol will reach the developing fetus. At the very least, strict moderation of alcohol consumption is well advised.

The most frequent clinical feature of a child affected by maternal rubella (German measles) is deafness, followed by congenital heart disease and mental retardation. Rubella generally is harmful only if contracted during the first trimester, but well-documented cases have resulted from infection several days prior to conception. The earlier in the pregnancy the infection occurs, the more likely the fetus is to be infected, and the more serious the abnormalities tend to be. Prevention of abnormalities as a result of rubella infection is best addressed via immunization.

Syphilis (infection with *Treponema pallidum*) can be transmitted in utero from mother to infant, resulting in congenital syphilis. If left untreated, this can result in numerous clinical features including interstitial keratitis, which can lead to blindness. Treating infected mothers with penicillin G (the drug of choice) before the sixteenth week of pregnancy should prevent fetal damage in utero. The fetus can be treated successfully in utero via medication given to the mother. If not treated in utero, infected infants should be treated as soon as possible in order to prevent morbidity.

187–190. The answers are: 187-B *[Ch 4 VII C 2]*, **188-D** *[Ch 4 II A 3]*, **189-C** *[Ch 4 II B 2 a]*, **190-A** *[Ch 4 II D]*.

Chemotherapeutic or chemoprophylactic agents kill biologic agents inside patients so that they cannot infect others. Isoniazid prophylaxis, for example, is administered to patients with a positive skin test for tuberculosis to prevent reactivation of a latent infection and secondary spread to other individuals.

Certain diseases, such as measles and smallpox, die out when the agent has no natural place to multiply. Thus, immunization of a susceptible population with a live attenuated measles vaccine eliminates the reservoir so that the measles virus has no place to live in its natural state.

Humans should avoid contact with potentially rabid animals and should not keep certain wild animals (e.g., skunks, raccoons) as pets. They should also make certain that their pet is properly immunized against rabies.

The transfer of organisms directly from one person to another can be blocked by simple processes such as hand washing. Hand washing is the most important procedure for preventing the spread of many enteric diseases, such as *Shigella*.

Index

Note: Page numbers in *italic* denote illustrations; those followed by t denote tables; those followed by Q denote questions; and those followed by E denote explanations.

B

C

E

F

I

N

S

U

V

W

Y

Z